QuickRef®
Orthopaedic
Procedures Atlas

Second Edition

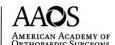

Wolters Kluwer

Philadelphia · Baltimore · New York · London
Buenos Aires · Hong Kong · Sydney · Tokyo

AAOS
AMERICAN ACADEMY OF
ORTHOPAEDIC SURGEONS

QuickRef®
Orthopaedic
Procedures Atlas

Second Edition

EDITED BY

Alexis Chiang Colvin, MD
Associate Professor
Department of Orthopaedics
Mount Sinai School of Medicine
New York, New York

Evan Flatow, MD
Lasker Professor of Orthopaedic Surgery
Leni & Peter May Department of Orthopaedic Surgery
Icahn School of Medicine at Mount Sinai
New York, New York

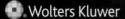. Wolters Kluwer

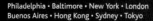
Philadelphia • Baltimore • New York • London
Buenos Aires • Hong Kong • Sydney • Tokyo

AMERICAN ACADEMY OF
ORTHOPAEDIC SURGEONS

Wolters Kluwer Health

Brian Brown, *Director, Medical Practice*

Stacey Sebring, *Senior Development Editor*

Kerry McShane, *Senior Editorial Coordinator*

Cody Adams, *Editorial Coordinator*

Erin Cantino, *Portfolio Marketing Manager*

David Saltzberg, *Production Project Manager*

Elaine Kasmer, *Design Coordinator*

Beth Welsh, *Senior Manufacturing Coordinator*

TNQ Technologies, *Prepress Vendor*

ISBN 978-1-975151-25-6

Library of Congress Control Number: Cataloging in Publication data available on request from publisher.

Printed in China

Published 2021 by the American Academy of Orthopaedic Surgeons
9400 West Higgins Road
Rosemont, Illinois 60018

Copyright 2021 by the American Academy of Orthopaedic Surgeons

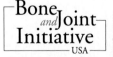

Acknowledgments

Editorial Board

QuickRef® Orthopaedic Procedures Atlas

Editors

Alexis Chiang Colvin, MD
Associate Professor
Department of Orthopaedics
Mount Sinai School of Medicine
New York, New York

Evan Flatow, MD
Lasker Professor of Orthopaedic Surgery
Leni & Peter May Department of
  Orthopaedic Surgery
Icahn School of Medicine at Mount Sinai
New York, New York

Section Reviewers

Julie E. Adams, MD, MS (Hand and Wrist)
Professor
Department of Orthopedic Surgery
Mayo Clinic and Mayo Clinic Health System
Rochester, Minnesota and Austin, Minnesota

Henry G. Chambers, MD (Pediatrics)
Professor of Clinical Orthopaedic Surgery
Department of Orthopaedic Surgery
University of California
San Diego, California

**Alexis Chiang Colvin, MD
  (Sports Medicine)**
Associate Professor
Department of Orthopaedics
Mount Sinai School of Medicine
New York, New York

**Christopher D. Harner, MD
  (Sports Medicine)**
Professor
Vice Chair of Academic Affairs
Director of the Sports Medicine Fellowship
The University of Texas Health Science
  Center at Houston
Department of Orthopaedic Surgery
Houston, Texas

Andrew C. Hecht, MD (Spine)
Chief, Spine Surgery
Mount Sinai Hospital and Mount Sinai
  Health System
Director, Mount Sinai Spine Center
Associate Professor, Orthopaedic and
  Neurosurgery
Mount Sinai Medical Center and Icahn
  School of Medicine
New York, New York

**Stephen J. Incavo, MD
  (Adult Reconstruction)**
Chief, Adult Reconstructive Surgery
Deputy Chairman, Department of
  Orthopedic Surgery
Professor of Clinical Orthopedic Surgery
Weill Cornell Medical College
Houston Methodist Hospital
Houston, Texas

Michael Pinzur, MD (Foot and Ankle)
Professor
Department of Orthopaedic Surgery
Loyola University Health System
Maywood, Illinois

**John W. Sperling, MD, MBA
  (Shoulder and Elbow)**
Consultant and Co-Vice Chair
Department of Orthopedic Surgery
Mayo Clinic
Rochester, Minnesota

Lawrence X. Webb, MD, MBA (Trauma)
Professor, Mercer University School of
  Medicine
Chairman, Orthopaedic Trauma Department
Atrium/Navicent Medical Center
Macon, Georgia

Resident Advisory Board

Robert Brochin, MD *(Shoulder and Elbow)*

Andy Chang, MD *(Hand and Wrist)*

Carl M. Cirino, MD *(Pediatrics)*

James Dowdell, MD *(Spine)*

Javier Guzman, MD *(Foot and Ankle)*

Nolan Maher, MD *(Adult Reconstruction)*

David Solomon, MD *(Sports Medicine)*

Amanda Walsh, MD *(Trauma)*

Contributors

Matthew P. Abdel, MD
Professor of Orthopedic Surgery and
  Consultant
Department of Orthopedic Surgery
Mayo Clinic
Rochester, Minnesota

Nicholas A. Abidi, MD
Attending Orthopaedic Surgeon
OrthoNorCal
Department of Orthopaedic Surgery
Dominican Dignity Hospital, Santa
  Cruz, California
El Camino Hospital
Los Gatos, California

Julie E. Adams, MD, MS
Professor
Department of Orthopedic Surgery
Mayo Clinic and Mayo Clinic Health
  System
Rochester, Minnesota and Austin,
  Minnesota

John Akins, MD
Orthopaedic Surgeon
Department of Orthopaedic Surgery
Mountain View Specialty Clinic
Mountain View, Arkansas

Craig C. Akoh, MD
Sports Medicine Fellow
Department of Orthopedics and
  Rehabilitation
Division of Sports Medicine
University of Wisconsin–Madison
Madison, Wisconsin

David W. Altchek, MD
Sports Medicine and Shoulder Service
Hospital for Special Surgery
New York, New York

Annunziato Amendola, MD
Professor in Orthopaedic Surgery
Urbaniak Sports Sciences Institute
Duke University
Durham, North Carolina

Howard S. An, MD
Professor and Director of Spine
  Surgery
Department of Orthopaedics
Rush University Medical Center
Chicago, Illinois

Steven M. Andelman, MD
Department of Orthopedic Surgery
University of Connecticut
Farmington, Connecticut

Mike B. Anderson, MSc
Research Scientist
Department of Orthopaedic Surgery
University of Utah
Salt Lake City, Utah

Robert A. Arciero, MD
Professor, Chief - Sports Medicine
  Division
Department of Orthopedic Surgery
University of Connecticut
Farmington, Connecticut

Bernard R. Bach, Jr, MD
The Claude N. Lambert, MD/Helen S.
  Thomson Professor
Director (Emeritus) - Division of Sports
  Medicine
Director (Emeritus) - Sports Medicine
  Fellowship
Department of Orthopedic Surgery
Rush University Medical Center
Chicago, Illinois

Semon Bader, MD
Muir Orthopaedic Specialists
Concord, California

Geoffrey S. Baer, MD, PhD
Associate Professor
Head Team Physician - University of
  Wisconsin–Madison
Department of Orthopedics and
  Rehabilitation
Division of Sports Medicine
Madison, Wisconsin

Contributors

Champ L. Baker, III, MD
Staff Physician
The Hughston Clinic
Columbus, Georgia

Champ L. Baker, Jr, MD
The Hughston Clinic
Columbus, Georgia

Kelley Banagan, MD
Assistant Professor, Spine Surgery
Department of Orthopaedics
University of Maryland
Baltimore, Maryland

Jarrad A. Barber, MD
Hand and Upper Extremity Fellow
Department of Orthopaedic Surgery
University of Mississippi Medical Center
Jackson, Mississippi

Jacqueline Baron, BA
Sports Medicine Research Fellow
Department of Orthopedics and
  Rehabilitation
University of Iowa
Iowa City, Iowa

Ahmad F. Bayomy, MD
Orthopaedic Sports Medicine Fellow
Cleveland Clinic Foundation
Cleveland, Ohio

Alireza Behboudi, DO
Orthopedic Surgeon
Department of Orthopedic Surgery
East Texas Medical Center
Tyler, Texas

Stephen K. Benirschke, MD
Professor
Department of Orthopaedics and
  Sports Medicine
University of Washington
Seattle, Washington

Gregory C. Berlet, MD, FRCS(C), FAOA
Orthopedic Surgeon
Orthopedic Foot and Ankle Center
Worthington, Ohio

Louis U. Bigliani, MD
Professor and Chairman
Department of Orthopaedics
Columbia University Medical Center
New York, New York

Randy Bindra, MD, FRACS
Professor of Orthopaedic Surgery
School of Medicine
Griffith University
Southport, Queensland, Australia

Scott D. Boden, MD
Director
The Emory Spine Center
Emory University School of Medicine
Atlanta, Georgia

Davide Edoardo Bonasia, MD
Orthopaedic Surgeon
Department of Orthopaedics and
  Traumatology
AO Ordine Mauriziano Hospital
University of Torino
Torino, Italy

Christopher M. Bono, MD
Associate Professor of Orthopaedic
  Surgery
Harvard Medical School
Chief, Orthopaedic Spine Service
Brigham and Women's Hospital
Boston, Massachusetts

Karl F. Bowman, Jr, MD
Orthopaedic Surgeon
EmergeOrtho, Triangle Region
Raleigh, North Carolina

Anthony D. Bratton, MD
Assistant Professor
Department of Orthopaedics
University of Nevada Las Vegas School
  of Medicine
Las Vegas, Nevada

Jaycen C. Brown, MD
Temple, Texas

Christopher L. Camp, MD
Assistant Professor
Department of Orthopedic Surgery
Mayo Clinic
Rochester, Minnesota

Eben A. Carroll, MD
Associate Professor
Director of Orthopaedic Trauma
Wake Forest Health Sciences
Winston-Salem, North Carolina

Danielle Casagrande, MD
Orthopaedic Resident
Department of Orthopaedics
University of Texas Medical Branch
Galveston, Texas

Thomas D. Cha, MD, MBA
Spine Surgeon
Department of Orthopaedic Surgery
Massachusetts General Hospital
Boston, Massachusetts

Jorge Chahla, MD, PhD
Sports Medicine Fellow
Department of Orthopaedic Surgery
Rush University Hospital
Chicago, Illinois

Peter N. Chalmers, MD
Assistant Professor
Department of Orthopaedic Surgery
University of Utah
Salt Lake City, Utah

Henry G. Chambers, MD
Professor of Clinical Orthopaedic
  Surgery
Department of Orthopaedic Surgery
University of California
San Diego, California

Loretta B. Chou, MD
Professor and Chief of Foot and Ankle
  Surgery
Department of Orthopaedic Surgery
Stanford University
Stanford, California

Michael J. Christie, MD
Founding Partner
Southern Joint Replacement Institute
Nashville, Tennessee

Michael P. Clare, MD
Nebraska Orthopaedic and Sports
  Medicine
Lincoln, Nebraska

J. Chris Coetzee, MD, FRCSC
Twin Cities Orthopedics
Edina, Minnesota

Brian J. Cole, MD, MBA
Associate Chairman & Professor
Department of Orthopedic Surgery
Rush University Medical Center
Chicago, Illinois

Alexis Chiang Colvin, MD
Associate Professor
Department of Orthopaedics
Mount Sinai School of Medicine
New York, New York

Andrew J. Cosgarea, MD
Drew Family Professor of Orthopaedic
  Surgery *in honor of* Alec J. Cosgarea
Department of Orthopaedic Surgery
Johns Hopkins University
Baltimore, Maryland

Michael J. Coughlin, MD
Director, Saint Alphonsus Foot and
  Ankle Coughlin Clinic
Boise, Idaho
Clinical Professor, Department of
  Orthopaedic Surgery
University of California, San Francisco
San Francisco, California

Timothy R. Daniels, MD, FRCSC
Head, Division of Orthopaedic Surgery
St. Michael's Hospital,
Professor, Foot & Ankle Surgery
University of Toronto
Toronto, Ontario. Canada

Roy Davidovitch, MD
Associate Professor
Adult Reconstruction Surgery
NYU Langone Orthopedic Hospital
Hospital for Joint Diseases
New York, New York

Samuel M. Davis, MD
Assistant Professor
Department of Orthopaedic Surgery
Emory University
Atlanta, Georgia

Michael R. Dayton, MD
Chief, Section of Adult Reconstruction
Department of Orthopedics
University of Colorado School of
  Medicine
Aurora, Colorado

Thomas M. DeBerardino, MD
Associate Professor
Department of Orthopaedic Surgery
University of Connecticut Health
  Center
Farmington, Connecticut

Contributors

David DeBoer, MD
Orthopaedic Surgeon
Southern Joint Replacement Institute
Nashville, Tennessee

Gregory K. Deirmengian, MD
Assistant Professor of Orthopaedic
  Surgery
Rothman Institute
Thomas Jefferson Medical School
Philadelphia, Pennsylvania

Ian J. Dempsey, MD, MBA
Fellow, Sports Medicine and Shoulder
  Surgery
Department of Orthopedic Surgery
Rush University Medical Center
Chicago, Illinois

Edward Diao, MD
Professor Emeritus
Department of Orthopaedic Surgery
  and Neurosurgery
University of California, San Francisco
Chief of Hand Surgery, California
  Pacific Medical Center
San Francisco, California

Joshua S. Dines, MD
Sports Medicine and Shoulder Service
Hospital for Special Surgery
New York, New York

Henry J. Dolch, DO
Orthopaedic Trauma
Cooper University Hospital
Camden, New Jersey

James C. Dreese, MD
Assistant Professor
Department of Orthopaedics
University of Maryland
Baltimore, Maryland

Thomas R. Duquin, MD
Associate Professor and Director of
  Medical Student Education
Department of Orthopaedic Surgery
Jacobs School of Medicine
University at Buffalo
Buffalo, New York

Mark E. Easley, MD
Associate Professor
Department of Orthopaedic Surgery
Duke University Medical Center
Durham, North Carolina

T. Bradley Edwards, MD
Attending Shoulder Surgeon
Fondren Orthopedic Group
Texas Orthopedic Hospital
Houston, Texas

John J. Elias, PhD
Senior Research Scientist
Department of Research
Cleveland Clinic Akron General
Akron, Ohio

Brandon J. Erickson, MD
Rothman Orthopaedic Institute
Assistant Professor
Department of Orthopaedic Surgery
Zucker School of Medicine
Hofstra University
New York, New York

Joseph Featherall, BS
MD Candidate
Cleveland Clinic Lerner College of
  Medicine
Cleveland, Ohio

COL James R. Ficke, MD
Chairman
Department of Orthopaedics and
  Rehabilitation
San Antonio Military Medical Center
Fort Sam Houston, Texas

Larry D. Field, MD
Director
Upper Extremity Service
Mississippi Sports Medicine and
  Orthopaedic Center
Jackson, Mississippi

Steven J. Fineberg, MD
Research Coordinator
Department of Orthopaedic Surgery
Rush University Medical Center
Chicago, Illinois

John C.P. Floyd, MD
Associate Professor
Mercer University School of Medicine
Associate Director
Georgia Orthopaedic Trauma Institute
Macon, Georgia

John M. Flynn, MD
Richard M. Armstrong, Jr. Professor of
  Orthopaedic Surgery
Perelman School of Medicine at the
  University of Pennsylvania
Chief of Orthopaedic Surgery
Children's Hospital of Philadelphia
Philadelphia, Pennsylvania

M. Patricia Fox, MD
Fellow
Philadelphia Hand to Shoulder Center
Department of Orthopaedic Surgery
Thomas Jefferson University
Philadelphia, Pennsylvania

Brett A. Freedman, MD
Chief, Spine and Neurosurgery Service
Department of Orthopaedics and
  Rehabilitation
Landstuhl Regional Medical Center
Landstuhl, Germany

Christina E. Freibott, MPH
Researcher, Trauma Training Center
Department of Orthopedic Surgery
Columbia University
New York, New York

Carol Frey, MD
Co-Director
West Coast Sports Medicine
  Foundation/UCLA Sports Medicine
  Fellowship
Assistant (volunteer) Professor,
  Orthopedic Surgery, UCLA
Manhattan Beach, California

Freddie H. Fu, MD
Professor and Chairman
Department of Orthopaedic Surgery
University of Pittsburgh
Pittsburgh, Pennsylvania

Lauren E. Geaney, MD
Assistant Professor
Department of Orthopedic Surgery
University of Connecticut
Farmington, Connecticut

William B. Geissler, MD
Professor
Director, Hand and Upper Extremity
  Fellowship
Chief, Sports Medicine and Shoulder
  Programs
Department of Orthopaedic Surgery
University of Mississippi Medical
  Center
Jackson, Mississippi

Jeffrey A. Geller, MD
Nas S. Eftekar Professor of Orthopedic
  Surgery
Chief of Orthopedic Surgery - New
  York Presbyterian - Lawrence
  Hospital Westchester
Chief, Division of Hip & Knee
  Reconstruction - Columbia
  University Irving Medical Center
Vice Chair of Finance
Director of Research, Center for Hip &
  Knee Replacement
Department of Orthopedic Surgery
Columbia University Irving Medical
  Center
New York, New York

Neil Ghodadra, MD
Department of Orthopedic Surgery
  and Sports Medicine
Southern California Orthopedic
  Institute
Van Nuys, California

Filippos S. Giannoulis, MD, PhD
Orthopaedic Surgeon
Department of Hand, Upper Extremity
  and Microsurgery
KAT Hospital
Athens, Greece

Thomas V. Giel, III, MD
Orthopaedic Surgeon
Division of Sports Medicine
OrthoMemphis
Memphis, Tennessee

Contributors

Hilton P. Gottschalk, MD
Chief, Pediatric Orthopedic Surgery,
  Central Texas Pediatric Orthopedics
Dell Children's Medical Center of
  Central Texas
Affiliate Faculty, Dell Medical School,
  University of Texas at Austin
Austin, Texas

James A. Goulet, MD
Professor, Orthopaedic Surgery
University of Michigan Health System
Ann Arbor, Michigan

Stanley C. Graves, MD
Phoenix, Arizona

Rebecca Griffith, MD
Department of Orthopaedics
University of Colorado Denver School
  of Medicine
Aurora, Colorado

Steven B. Haas, MD, MPH
Chief, Knee Service
Hospital for Special Surgery
New York, New York

Nathan B. Haile, MD
Adult Reconstruction Fellow
Department of Orthopaedic Surgery
University of Utah
Salt Lake City, Utah

Mark E. Hake, MD
Assistant Professor, Orthopaedic
  Trauma
University of Michigan Health System
Ann Arbor, Michigan

**Mansur M. Halai, MBChB, MRCA,
  MRCS, FRCS (Edin)**
Foot & Ankle Fellow
Department of Surgery
Division of Orthopaedics
St. Michael's Hospital
University of Toronto
Toronto, Ontario, Canada

Jason J. Halvorson, MD
Assistant Professor
Wake Forest Health Sciences
Winston-Salem, North Carolina

Arlen D. Hanssen, MD
Professor of Orthopedic Surgery and
  Emeritus Consultant
Department of Orthopedic Surgery
Mayo Clinic
Rochester, Minnesota

Christopher D. Harner, MD
Professor
Vice Chair of Academic Affairs
Director of the Sports Medicine
  Fellowship
The University of Texas Health Science
  Center at Houston
Department of Orthopaedic Surgery
Houston, Texas

Katharine D. Harper, MD, FRCSC
Fellow
Department of Orthopaedics and
  Sports Medicine
Houston Methodist Hospital
Houston, Texas

Robert U. Hartzler, MD, MS
Assistant Clinical Professor
Department of Orthopaedic Surgery
TSAOG Orthopaedics and Baylor
  College of Medicine
San Antonio, Texas

Andrew C. Hecht, MD
Chief, Spine Surgery
Mount Sinai Hospital and Mount Sinai
  Health System
Director, Mount Sinai Spine Center
Associate Professor, Orthopaedic and
  Neurosurgery
Mount Sinai Medical Center and Icahn
  School of Medicine
New York, New York

Kenneth Heida, MD
Department of Orthopaedic Surgery
  and Rehabilitation
William Beaumont Army Medical
  Center
El Paso, Texas

John G. Heller, MD
Baur Professor of Orthopaedic Surgery
Department of Orthopaedic Surgery
Emory University School of Medicine
Atlanta, Georgia

Christopher B. Hirose, MD
Saint Alphonsus Foot and Ankle
  Coughlin Clinic
Boise, Idaho
Clinical Instructor University of
  Washington Medical School
Seattle, Washington

Reimer Hoffmann, MD
Consultant Hand Surgeon
HPC Oldenburg
Oldenburg, Germany

Donald W. Hohman, Jr, MD
Texas Orthopaedic Associates
Dallas, Texas

Jonathan A. Hoskins, MD
Research Associate
Department of Orthopaedic Surgery
Rush University Medical Center
Chicago, Illinois

William J. Hozack, MD
Professor of Orthopaedic Surgery
Rothman Institute
Thomas Jefferson Medical School
Philadelphia, Pennsylvania

Stephanie H. Hsu, MD
Fellow
Center for Shoulder, Elbow, and Sports
  Medicine
Columbia University
New York, New York

Jeannie Huh, MD
Assistant Professor
Uniformed Services University
Chief, Department Orthopaedics &
  Rehabilitation
Womack Army Medical Center
Fort Bragg, North Carolina

Daniel Hurwit, MD
Resident
Hospital for Special Surgery
New York, New York

Kenneth D. Illingworth, MD
Assistant Professor of Orthopaedic
  Surgery
Children's Hospital Los Angeles
University of Southern California Keck
  School of Medicine
Los Angeles, California

Stephen J. Incavo, MD
Chief, Adult Reconstructive Surgery
Deputy Chairman, Department of
  Orthopedic Surgery
Professor of Clinical Orthopedic
  Surgery
Weill Cornell Medical College
Houston Methodist Hospital
Houston, Texas

Stephen K. Jacobsen, MD
Department of Orthopaedic Surgery
Rush University Medical Center
Chicago, Illinois

Evan James, MD
Resident
Hospital for Special Surgery
New York, New York

D. Marshall Jemison, MD
Associate Professor
Department of Plastic Surgery
Clinical Associate Professor
Department of Orthopaedic Surgery
University of Tennessee College of
  Medicine
Chattanooga, Tennessee

Peter Johnston, MD
Southern Maryland Orthopaedics and
  Sports Medicine
Leonardtown, Maryland

Clifford B. Jones, MD, FACS
Clinical Professor
The CORE Institute
University of Arizona
Phoenix, Arizona

Jesse B. Jupiter, MD
Hansjorg Wyss AO Professor
Department of Orthopaedic Surgery
Massachusetts General Hospital
Boston, Massachusetts

Ryland Kagan, MD
Assistant Professor
Department of Orthopaedic Surgery
Oregon Health and Science University
Portland, Oregon

Jay V. Kalawadia, MD
Orthopaedic Sports Surgeon
Department of Orthopaedic Surgery
OAA Orthopaedic Specialists
Allentown, Pennsylvania

Contributors

Daniel G. Kang, MD
Orthopaedic Surgery Resident
Department of Orthopaedic Surgery
and Rehabilitation
Walter Reed National Military Medical
Center
Bethesda, Maryland

James F. Kellam, BSc, MD, FRCSC, FACS, FRCSI
Professor
Department of Orthopaedic Surgery
McGovern Medical School
The University of Texas – Health
Science Center at Houston
Houston, Texas

Christopher A. Keen, MD
Upper Extremity Surgeon
Citrus Orthopaedic and Joint Institute
Lecanto, Florida

Stephen Kim, MD
Attending Physician
Resurgens Orthopaedics
Kennestone Hospital
Marietta, Georgia

Mininder S. Kocher, MD, MPH
Chief, Division of Sports Medicine
Boston Children's Hospital
Professor of Orthopaedic Surgery
Harvard Medical School
Boston, Massachusetts

Patricia Ann Kramer, PhD
Professor
Department of Anthropology
University of Washington
Seattle, Washington

Simon Lee, MD
Associate Professor
Department of Orthopaedic Surgery
Rush University Medical Center
Chicago, Illinois

Jonathan H. Lee, MD
Clinical Instructor
Orthopaedic Surgery
Montefiore Medical Center
Bronx, New York

Ronald A. Lehman, Jr, MD
Chief, Pediatric and Adult Spine
Associate Professor of Surgery
Walter Reed National Medical Center
Bethesda, Maryland

Thomas P. Lehman, PT, MD
Professor of Orthopedic Surgery,
University of Oklahoma
Clinical Professor, Oklahoma Hand
Surgery Fellowship Program
Medical Director of Hand Trauma
Services, OU Medical Center
OUHSC Department of Orthopedic
Surgery and Rehabilitation
Oklahoma City, Oklahoma

Lawrence G. Lenke, MD
Jerome J. Gilden Distinguished
Professor of Orthopaedic Surgery
Chief of Spine Surgery
Department of Orthopaedic Surgery
Washington University School of
Medicine
Saint Louis, Missouri

Katrina Lewis, BA, BS
Clinical Research Coordinator II
Division of Pediatric Orthopaedic
Surgery
Cincinnati Children's Hospital Medical
Center
Cincinnati, Ohio

Albert Lin, MD
Assistant Professor
Department of Orthopaedics
Division of Sports Medicine
University of Pittsburgh Medical
Center
Pittsburgh, Pennsylvania

Sheldon S. Lin, MD
Associate Professor
Department of Orthopaedic Surgery
Rutgers University New Jersey
Medical School
Newark, New Jersey

Randall T. Loder, MD
Professor of Orthopaedic Surgery
Indiana University School of Medicine
Riley Children's Hospital
Indianapolis, Indiana

John D. Lubahn, MD
Program Director, UPMC Hamot Hand
  Fellowship
Department of Orthopaedic Surgery
UPMC Hamot
Erie, Pennsylvania

Steven C. Ludwig, MD
Associate Professor and Chief of Spine
  Surgery
Department of Orthopaedics
University of Maryland
Baltimore, Maryland

William Macaulay, MD
Chief, Adult Reconstructive Surgery
William & Susan Jaffe Professor of
  Orthopedic Surgery
Medical Director, International Patient
  Services
NYU Langone Health
Brooklyn, New York

John J. Mangan, MD
Orthopaedic Chief Resident
Sidney Kimmel Medical College at
  Thomas Jefferson University
Philadelphia, Pennsylvania

Alejandro Marquez-Lara, MD
Wake Forest Health Sciences
Winston-Salem, North Carolina

Kristofer S. Matullo, MD
Associate Clinical Professor of
  Orthopedic Surgery - Temple
  University
Chief - Division of Hand Surgery
St. Luke's University Health Network
Department of Orthopedic Surgery
Bethlehem, Pennsylvania

Augustus D. Mazzocca, MS, MD
Professor, Chairman - Department of
  Orthopedic Surgery
Department of Orthopedic Surgery
University of Connecticut
Farmington, Connecticut

Maria Romano McGann, DO
Orthopedic Surgeon
Romano Orthopaedics
Oak Park, Illinois

Michael David McKee, MD, FRCSC
Professor of Surgery
Department of Surgery
Division of Orthopaedics
St. Michael's Hospital
University of Toronto
Toronto, Ontario, Canada

Richard J. McLaughlin, MD
Resident
Department of Orthopedic Surgery
Mayo Clinic
Rochester, Minnesota

Suman Medda, MD
Wake Forest Health Sciences
Winston-Salem, North Carolina

Mitchell Meghpara, MD
Sports Medicine Fellow
Department of Orthopaedic Surgery
University of Pittsburgh
Pittsburgh, Pennsylvania

Siddhant K. Mehta, MD, PhD
Research Fellow
Department of Orthopaedic Surgery
Rutgers University New Jersey
  Medical School
Newark, New Jersey

Anna N. Miller, MD
Chief, Orthopaedic Trauma
Associate Professor
Department of Orthopaedic Surgery
Washington University in St. Louis
St. Louis, Missouri

Bradley Moatz, MD
Resident Physician
Department of Orthopaedics
Union Memorial Hospital
Baltimore, Maryland

Blake K. Montgomery, MD
Resident
Department of Orthopedic Surgery
Stanford University Medical Center
Palo Alto, California

Contributors

Scott J. Mubarak, MD
Clinical Professor of Orthopedic
  Surgery
Department of Orthopedics
University of California
Surgeon in Chief and Emeritus
  Division Chief Pediatrics
  Orthopedics
Rady Children's Hospital
San Diego, California

Daniel J. Nagle, MD, FACS, FAAOS
Professor of Clinical Orthopedics
Northwestern Feinberg School of
  Medicine
Chicago, Illinois

Neal B. Naveen, BS
Research Fellow
Department of Orthopedic Surgery
Rush University Medical Center
Chicago, Illinois

Blaise Alexander Nemeth, MD, MS
Associate Professor, Clinical Health
  Science
Department of Orthopedics and
  Rehabilitation
University of Wisconsin School of
  Medicine and
  Public Health
Madison, Wisconsin

Shane J. Nho, MD, MS
Assistant Professor
Department of Orthopaedic Surgery
Rush University Hospital
Chicago, Illinois

Gregory P. Nicholson, MD
Associate Professor
Department of Orthopaedic Surgery
Rush University Medical Center
Chicago, Illinois

Scott J.B. Nimmons, MD
Orthopaedic Surgeon
Baylor University Medical Center
Dallas, Texas

Kenneth J. Noonan, MD
Associate Professor
Department of Pediatric Orthopedics
University of Wisconsin Health
Madison, Wisconsin

Thomas S. Obermeyer, MD
Fellow, Shoulder and Elbow Surgery
Department of Orthopaedic Surgery
Mount Sinai Medical Center
New York, New York

Matthew Oglesby, BA
Research Coordinator
Department of Orthopaedic Surgery
Rush University Medical Center
Chicago, Illinois

Kelechi R. Okoroha, MD
Orthopedic Surgical Fellow
Department of Orhopedic Surgery
Rush University
Chicago, Illinois

Anthony Orio, MD
Clinical Fellow, Adult Reconstructive
  Surgery
Department of Orthopedic Surgery
NYU Langone Health
New York, NY

Nirav K. Pandya, MD
Associate Professor
Department of Orthopedic Surgery
University of California San Francisco
San Francisco, California

Loukia K. Papatheodorou, MD, PhD
Clinical Assistant Professor of
  Orthopedic Surgery
University of Pittsburgh School of
  Medicine
Department of Orthopedic Surgery
Orthopaedic Specialists - UPMC
  Pittsburgh
Pittsburgh, Pennsylvania

Wayne G. Paprosky, MD, FACS
Professor
Department of Orthopaedic Surgery
Adult Joint Reconstruction
Rush University Medical Center
Chicago, Illinois

Andrew E. Park, MD
Assistant Professor of Surgery
Texas A&M Health Science Center
  College of Medicine
Dallas, Texas

Kwan J. Park, MD
Faculty
Department of Orthopedics and Sports
  Medicine
Houston Methodist Hospital
Houston, Texas

Richard D. Parker, MD
Professor of Surgery
Department of Orthopaedics
Cleveland Clinic Lerner College of
  Medicine at Case Western Reserve
  University
Cleveland Clinic Foundation
Cleveland, Ohio

Bradford O. Parsons, MD
Assistant Professor of Orthopaedic
  Surgery
Department of Orthopaedic Surgery
Mount Sinai School of Medicine
New York, New York

Chirag S. Patel, MD
Naples Orthopedic Sports Medicine
Associates
Naples, Florida

Neeraj M. Patel, MD, MPH, MBS
Assistant Professor of Orthopaedic
  Surgery
Northwestern University Feinberg
  School of Medicine
Attending Surgeon
Ann & Robert H. Lurie Children's
  Hospital of Chicago
Chicago, Illinois

Jeffrey Peck, MD
Fellow
Department of Hip Preservation
Hospital for Special Surgery
New York, New York

Gary M. Pess, MD, FACS, FAAOS
Medical Director
Central Jersey Hand Surgery
Eatontown, New Jersey

Christopher L. Peters, MD
George S. Eccles Endowed Professor of
  Orthopaedic Surgery
Chief of Adult Reconstruction and Hip
  Preservation Services
Department of Orthopaedic Surgery
University of Utah
Salt Lake City, Utah

Steven L. Peterson, MD, DVM
Staff Hand Surgeon
Operative Care Division
Portland Veterans Administration
  Health Care System
Portland, Oregon

Stephen Petis, MD, MSc, FRCSC
Orthopaedic Surgeon
Woodstock General Hospital
Woodstock, Ontario, Canada

Terrence M. Philbin, DO
Orthopedic Surgeon
Orthopedic Foot and Ankle Center
Worthington, Ohio

Mathew W. Pombo, MD
Assistant Professor
Department of Orthopaedics
Emory University School of Medicine
Atlanta, Georgia

Maya E. Pring, MD
Professor of Clinical Orthopedic
  Surgery
University of California
Orthopedic Residency Site Director
Chair, Department of Surgery
Rady Children's Hospital
San Diego, California

Sheeraz A. Qureshi, MD
Associate Professor of Orthopaedic
  Surgery
Chief of Minimally Invasive Spine
  Surgery
Hospital for Special Surgery
New York, New York

Contributors

Steven M. Raikin, MD
Professor of Orthopaedic Surgery
Chief, Foot and Ankle Service
Rothman Orthopaedic Institute
Sidney Kimmel Medical College
  at Thomas Jefferson University
  Hospital
Philadelphia, Pennsylvania

Matthew L. Ramsey, MD
Professor and Vice Chairman
Department of Orthopaedic Surgery
Rothman Institute
Thomas Jefferson University
Philadelphia, Pennsylvania

Anil Ranawat, MD
Associate Professor of Orthopaedic
  Surgery, Weill Cornell Medical
  College
Associate Attending Orthopaedic
  Surgeon, Hospital for Special Surgery
Fellowship Director of Sports Medicine
  Surgery, Hospital for Special Surgery
Medical Director of the Physician's
  Assistant Department, Hospital for
  Special Surgery
New York, New York

Ghazi M. Rayan, MD
Clinical Professor, Orthopedic Surgery,
  University of Oklahoma
Adjunct Professor of Anatomy/Cell
  Biology, University of Oklahoma
Director of Oklahoma Hand Surgery
  Fellowship Program
Chair, Department of Hand Surgery
  INTEGRIS Baptist Medical Center
Oklahoma City, Oklahoma

K. Daniel Riew, MD
Mildred B. Simon Distinguished
  Professor
Department of Orthopaedic Surgery
Washington University School of
  Medicine
St. Louis, Missouri

David Ring, MD, PhD
Associate Dean for Comprehensive
  Care
Professor of Surgery and Psychiatry
Dell Medical School - The University
  of Texas at Austin
Austin, Texas

Pascal Rippstein, MD
Medical Director/Chief, Department
  of Foot and Ankle
Schulthess Clinic
Zurich, Switzerland

Mark William Rodosky, MD
Chief, Division of Shoulder Surgery
Department of Orthopaedic Sports
  Medicine
University of Pittsburgh
Pittsburgh, Pennsylvania

Arnaldo I. Rodriguez Santiago, MD
Shoulder/Elbow Surgeon
Department of Orthopedic Surgery
HIMA San Pablo Caguas
Caguas, Puerto Rico

Anthony A. Romeo, MD
Chief of Orthopaedics
Rothman Orthopaedic Institute
Professor
Department of Orthopaedic Surgery
Zucker School of Medicine
Hofstra University
New York, New York

Melvin P. Rosenwasser, MD
Robert E. Carroll Professor of Surgery
  of the Hand
Chief, Orthopaedic Hand and Trauma
  Service
Director, Trauma Training Center
Department of Orthopedic Surgery
Columbia University
New York, New York

Roberto Rossi, MD
Associate Professor in Orthopaedic
  Surgery
Department of Orthopaedics and
  Traumatology
AO Ordine Mauriziano Hospital
University of Torino
Torino, Italy

Aaron J. Rubinstein, MD
Resident Physician
Department of Orthopaedic Surgery
Rutgers University New Jersey
  Medical School
Newark, New Jersey

Michael J. Salata, MD
Associate Professor
Department of Orthopedic Surgery
University Hospitals Cleveland
  Medical Center
Cleveland, Ohio

Paul M. Saluan, MD
Assistant Professor of Surgery
Department of Orthopaedics
Cleveland Clinic Lerner College of
  Medicine at Case Western Reserve
  University
Cleveland Clinic Foundation
Cleveland, Ohio

Joaquin Sanchez-Sotelo, MD, PhD
Consultant and Professor
Department of Orthopedic Surgery
Mayo Clinic
Rochester, Minnesota

Nana Sarpong, MD, MBA
Resident, Orthopedic Surgery
Department of Orthopedic Surgery
Columbia University Irving Medical
  Center
New York, New York

Felix H. Savoie, III, MD
Professor
Department of Orthopaedic Surgery
Tulane University
New Orleans, Louisiana

Andrew J. Schoenfeld, MD
Assistant Professor
Department of Orthopaedic Surgery
Texas Tech University Health Sciences
  Center
El Paso, Texas

William C. Schroer, MD
Research Director
St. Louis Joint Replacement Institute
SSM DePaul Health Center
St. Louis, Missouri

Alexandra K. Schwartz, MD
Clinical Professor
Department of Orthopedic Surgery
University of California, San Diego
San Diego, California

Andrew M. Schwartz, MD
Resident
Department of Orthopaedics
Emory University School of Medicine
Atlanta, Georgia

Ran Schwarzkopf, MD, MSc
Associate Professor
Associate Division Chief
Adult Reconstruction Surgery
NYU Langone Orthopedic Hospital
Hospital for Joint Diseases
New York, New York

Laura E. Scordino, MD
Orthopaedic Surgery Resident
Department of Orthopaedic Surgery
University of Connecticut
Farmington, Connecticut

Giles R. Scuderi, MD
Vice President, Orthopedic Service
  Line
Northwell Orthopedic Institute
New York, New York

Seth L. Sherman, MD
Assistant Professor
Department of Orthopaedic Surgery
University of Missouri
Columbia, Missouri

Alexander Y. Shin, MD
Professor of Orthopaedic Surgery
Professor of Neurosurgery
Department of Orthopaedic Surgery
Division of Hand and Microvascular
  Surgery
Mayo Clinic
Rochester, Minnesota

Benjamin Shore, MD, MPH, FRCSC
Co-Director, Cerebral Palsy &
  Spasticity Center
Boston Children's Hospital
Associate Professor of Orthopaedic
  Surgery
Harvard Medical School
Boston, Massachusetts

Peter Silvero, MD
Orthopaedic Surgeon
Associates in Orthopaedic Surgery
Jordan Valley Medical Center
Salt Lake City, Utah

Kern Singh, MD
Assistant Professor
Department of Orthopaedic Surgery
Rush University Medical Center
Chicago, Illinois

Ernest L. Sink, MD
Co-Director of Center for Hip
 Preservation
Associate Professor of Orthopaedic
 Surgery, Weill Cornell Medical
 College
Department of Orthopaedic Surgery
Hospital for Special Surgery
New York, New York

David L. Skaggs, MD, MMM
Children's Hospital Endowed Chair of
 Pediatric Spinal Disorders
Director of the Children's Orthopaedic
 Center
Children's Hospital Los Angeles
Professor of Orthopaedic Surgery
University of Southern California Keck
 School of Medicine
Los Angeles, California

Dean G. Sotereanos, MD
Clinical Professor of Orthopedic
 Surgery
University of Pittsburgh School of
 Medicine
Department of Orthopedic Surgery
 Orthopaedic Specialists-
 UPMC Pittsburgh
Pittsburgh, Pennsylvania

Taylor M. Southworth, BS
Research Fellow
Department of Orthopedic Surgery
Rush University Medical Center
Chicago, Illinois

Scott M. Sporer, MD, MS
Associate Professor
Department of Orthopaedic Surgery
Rush University Medical Center
Chicago, Illinois

Scott P. Steinmann, MD
Professor of Orthopedic Surgery
Mayo Clinic
Rochester, Minnesota

MAJ Daniel J. Stinner, MD
Chief Resident, Orthopaedic Surgery
Department of Orthopaedics and
 Rehabilitation
San Antonio Military Medical Center
Fort Sam Houston, Texas

Stephanie Sweet, MD
Philadelphia Hand to Shoulder Center
Assistant Professor
Department of Orthopaedic Surgery
Thomas Jefferson University
Philadelphia, Pennsylvania

John M. Tabit, DO
Orthopaedic Traumatologist
The Orthopaedic Trauma Group
Charleston Area Medical Center
Charleston, West Virginia

Miho J. Tanaka, MD
Assistant Professor
Department of Orthopaedic Surgery
Massachusetts General Hospital
Harvard Medical School
Boston, Massachusetts

Oliver O. Tannous, MD
Resident
Department of Orthopaedics
University of Maryland Medical
 Center
Baltimore, Maryland

Nikhil A. Thakur, MD
Assistant Professor
Department of Orthopaedics
State University of New York Upstate
 Medical University
Syracuse, New York

Matthew M. Tomaino, MD, MBA
Tomaino Orthopaedic Care
Rochester, New York

Michael E. Torchia, MD
Consultant
Department of Orthopedic Surgery
Mayo Clinic
Rochester, Minnesota

P. Justin Tortolani, MD
Director, Spine Education and
   Research
Department of Orthopaedic Surgery
Medstar Union Memorial Hospital
Baltimore, Maryland

Sava Turcan, BA
MD Candidate
UQ Oshner School of Medicine
Queensland, Australia

Thomas F. Varecka, MD
Orthopaedic Surgeon
Department of Orthopaedic Surgery
Hennepin County Medical Center
Minneapolis, Minnesota

Bryan Van Dyke, DO
Orthopedic Surgeon
Summit Orthopaedics
Idaho Falls, Idaho

Carola F. van Eck, MD, PhD
Assistant Professor
Department of Orthopaedic Surgery
University of Pittsburgh
Pittsburgh, Pennsylvania

Edward M. Vasarhelyi, MD, MSc, FRCSC
Associate Professor
Department of Surgery
Western University
London, Ontario, Canada

Aaron I. Venouziou, MD
Orthopaedic Hand and Upper
   Extremity Surgeon
Orthopaedic Department
St. Luke's Hospital
Thessaloniki, Greece

Armando F. Vidal, MD
Attending Surgeon
The Steadman Clinic
Vail, Colorado
Clinical Associate Professor
University of Colorado Denver School
   of Medicine
Aurora, Colorado

Dharmesh Vyas, MD, PhD
Assistant Professor
Department of Orthopaedic Surgery
University of Pittsburgh
Pittsburgh, Pennsylvania

Eric J. Wall, MD
Director Sports Medicine, Fellowship
   Program Director
Orthopaedics
Cincinnati Children's Hospital
Cincinnati, Ohio

Arthur K. Walling, MD
Fellowship Director
Foot and Ankle Surgery
Florida Orthopaedic Institute
Tampa, Florida

Stephen Warner, MD, PhD
Assistant Professor
McGovern Medical School
The University of Texas Health Science
   Center at Houston
Houston, Texas

Lawrence X. Webb, MD, MBA
Professor, Mercer University School of
   Medicine
Chairman, Orthopaedic Trauma
   Department
Atrium/Navicent Medical Center
Macon, Georgia

Lawrence E. Weiss, MD
Hand & Upper Extremity Surgeon
OAA Orthopaedic Associates
Chief, Division of Hand Surgery
Lehigh Valley Health Network
Allentown, Pennsylvania

Robin West, MD
Orthopaedic Surgeon
Associate Professor
University of Pittsburgh Medical
   Center
Pittsburgh, Pennsylvania

Matthew J. White, MD
Physicians' Clinic of Iowa
Cedar Rapids, Iowa

Kevin W. Wilson, MD
Orthopaedic Surgery Resident
Department of Orthopaedics and
   Rehabilitation
Walter Reed National Military Medical
   Center
Bethesda, Maryland

Michael A. Wirth, MD
Professor and Charles A. Rockwood, Jr,
  MD, Chair
Department of Orthopaedics
University of Texas Health Science
  Center
San Antonio, Texas

Bryan Witt, DO
Orthopedic Surgeon
Naples Orthopedics
Naples, Florida

Brian R. Wolf, MD, MS
John and Kim Callaghan Endowed
  Chair and Director of UI Sports
  Medicine
Professor and Vice-Chairman of
  Finance and Academic Affairs
Department of Orthopedics and
  Rehabilitation
University of Iowa Hospitals and
  Clinics
Head Team Physician, University of
  Iowa Athletics
Iowa City, Iowa

John W. Xerogeanes, MD
Professor Orthopaedic Surgery
Emory University School of Medicine
Atlanta, Georgia

Jeffrey Yao, MD
Associate Professor
Department of Orthopedic Surgery
Stanford University Medical Center
Palo Alto, California

Vamshi Yelavarthi, BA
Medical Student
Boston University School of Medicine
Boston, Massachusetts

Dedication

To our families, for their love and support; to our teachers, for their wisdom; and to our patients, from whom we learned the value of our craft.

Preface

This *QuickRef® Orthopaedic Procedures Atlas* is a high-yield electronic and print version of the second edition of the *Atlas of Essential Orthopaedic Procedures*. Each of the thoughtfully selected 118 surgical procedures is distilled into the key components of patient selection, the author's procedure, and surgical pearls. In addition, the images and videos included illustrate key ideas from the experts in each specialty.

The *QuickRef® Orthopaedic Procedures Atlas* would not have been possible without the support of the AAOS and the efforts of numerous individuals. First, we thank the members of the Resident Advisory Board, who wrote the summaries: Robert Brochin, MD, Andy Chang, MD, Carl Cirino, MD, James Dowdell, MD, Javier Guzman, MD, Nolan Maher, MD, David Solomon, MD, and Amanda Walsh, MD. Second, we are grateful to the section reviewers for their outstanding work in reviewing the text and video. These busy surgeons have devoted many hours to this project, in addition to the many other demands on their time. Our gratitude goes to the following, listed in alphabetical order: Julie E. Adams, MD, MS (*Hand and Wrist*); Henry G. Chambers, MD (*Pediatrics*); Christopher D. Harner, MD (*Sports Medicine*); Andrew C. Hecht, MD (*Spine*); Stephen J. Incavo, MD (*Adult Reconstruction*); Michael Pinzur, MD (*Foot and Ankle*); John W. Sperling, MD, MBA (*Shoulder and Elbow*); and Lawrence X. Webb, MD, MBA (*Trauma*).

Finally, we thank Hans Koelsch, PhD, Director, Publishing Partner Relationships; Lisa Claxton Moore, Senior Manager, Editorial; and Steven Kellert, Senior Editor at AAOS and Brian Brown, Director, Medical Practice; Stacey Sebring, Senior Development Editor, Medicine and Advanced Practice; and Kerry McShane, Editorial Coordinator at Wolters Kluwer, all of whom were instrumental in the production of the second edition of this resource.

We hope you find this updated version of the *QuickRef® Orthopaedic Procedures Atlas* to be an indispensable resource to your orthopaedic practice.

Alexis Chiang Colvin, MD
Evan Flatow, MD
Editors

Table of Contents

Section 1: Sports Medicine

Section Editors: Alexis Chiang Colvin, MD; Christopher D. Harner, MD

Section 2: Shoulder and Elbow
Section Editor: John W. Sperling, MD, MBA

Section 3: Hand and Wrist

Section Editor: Julie E. Adams, MD, MS

© 2021 American Academy of Orthopaedic Surgeons

Section 4: Adult Reconstruction

Section Editor: Stephen J. Incavo, MD

Section 7: Spine

Section Editor: Andrew C. Hecht, MD

Section 8: Pediatrics

Section Editor: Henry G. Chambers, MD

Sports Medicine

1

Section Editors
Alexis Chiang Colvin, MD
Christopher D. Harner, MD

Arthroscopic Repair of Partial-Thickness Rotator Cuff Tears

PATIENT SELECTION

Indications

- Patient with documented clinical findings in the presence of radiographically confirmed partial-thickness articular surface rotator cuff tear
- 44% of partial-thickness tears progress in size at median of 3.3 years on serial ultrasonography examination
- 46% of partial-thickness tears develop pain and dysfunction
- Persistent symptoms despite nonsurgical measures such as rest, activity modification, medication, and physical therapy
- Acute full-thickness tears should be managed surgically

Contraindications

- Patient in poor medical health
- Patient who cannot perform postoperative rehabilitation

PREOPERATIVE IMAGING

Radiography

- Shoulder series of plain radiographs
  - AP
  - Neer AP
  - Outlet
  - Axillary
- Use to assess for possible fracture, bony abnormalities, acromion types, humeral subluxation/escape

MRI or Magnetic Resonance Arthrography

- Soft-tissue evaluation for tears
- Arthrography has better specificity for partial-thickness rotator cuff tears

---

Based on Akoh CC, White MJ, Baer GS: Arthroscopic repair of partial-thickness rotator cuff tears, in Colvin AC, Flatow E, eds: Atlas of Essential Orthopaedic Procedures, *ed 2. Rosemont, IL, American Academy of Orthopaedic Surgeons, 2020, pp 1-10.*

Ultrasonography
- Less expensive alternative to MRI
- Dynamic evaluation
- Highly operator-dependent and less sensitive than MRI
- Can be done in office setting

PROCEDURE
Room Setup/Patient Positioning
- Lateral decubitus position is the preference of the authors
- Arm holder at distal position of operating room table; arm in 20° to 40° of abduction with the assistance of a 5- to 10-lb weight

Special Instruments/Equipment
- Burr or curet for footprint decortication
- Arthroscopic shaver
- Graspers
- Spinal needle
- Variously sized arthroscopic cannulas
- Knot pusher
- Arthroscopic scissors
- Suture punch for antegrade suture passing, looped tissue penetrator for retrograde suture passing, or suture lasso device for antegrade or retrograde suture passing

Surgical Technique

VIDEO 1.1 Repair of Partial-Thickness Rotator Cuff Tears. Richard Angelo, MD (15 min)

Diagnostic Arthroscopy
- Mark bony landmarks, including the acromion and coracoid
- Portals
  - Posterior—Established first, 1 cm medial and 2 cm inferior to posterolateral corner of acromion in soft spot
  - Anterior—Use outside-in technique to place through rotator interval
  - Anterolateral
  - Lateral
  - Neviaser (used occasionally)
- Visualize entire cuff via rotation of arm to see anterior to posterior
- For far anterior or far posterior tears, use a 70° arthroscope
- Gently débride frayed tissue to identify and probe edges of intact tendon

---

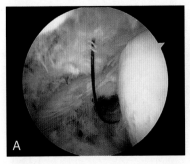 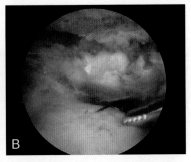

FIGURE 1 Arthroscopic views demonstrate the technique used for locating a rotator cuff tear. **A,** Monofilament suture is placed into the glenohumeral joint percutaneously to locate a partial-thickness rotator cuff tear. **B,** The monofilament suture indicates the location of the tear. A standard shaver is used to perform a bursectomy.

- Place monofilament tagging stitch through tear using spinal needle via direct visualization and pull out through anterior portal (**Figure 1**)
- Reposition arthroscope and instruments in subacromial bursa, and complete bursectomy to evaluate bursal side of tendon

Repair of Partial-Thickness Articular-Surface Tears

- Treatment is guided by Ellman classification system (**Table 1**). For A1 tears (articular surface, <3 mm deep), débridement alone is used. For A2 tears (articular surface, 3-6 mm deep), simple débridement or intra-tendon repair is used
- View through posterior portal into glenohumeral joint
- Place spinal needle lateral to edge of acromion in transtendinous fashion to locate suture anchor position (at medial margin of footprint at 45° angle)
- Use suture lasso (if extensive delamination present) from within glenohumeral joint or combination of shuttle relays in subacromial space; if delamination is not present, then tie healthy tendon edges with a tissue bridge of at least 5 mm (**Figure 2**)
- Tie with sliding knot and alternating half hitches

TABLE 1 Ellman Classification of Partial-Thickness Rotator Cuff Tears

Location	Grade (Depth of Lesion)
A (articular surface)	1 (<3 mm deep)
B (bursal surface)	2 (3-6 mm deep)
C (interstitial)	3 (>6 mm deep)

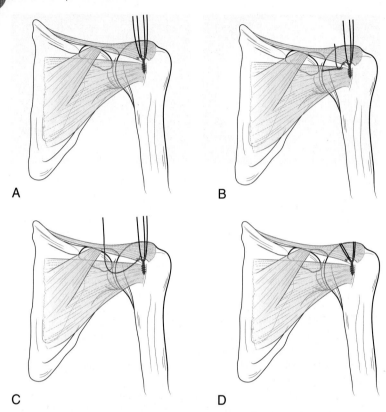

FIGURE 2 Illustrations show the arthroscopic repair of a partial-thickness articular-surface tear. **A,** A shuttle relay is passed through the spinal needle and retrieved through the anterior portal. **B,** One end of the suture also is retrieved through the anterior portal. **C,** One end of the suture is engaged in the eyelet of the shuttle relay and then pulled back out of the healthy portion of the partially torn tendon. **D,** A complete repair of a partial-thickness articular-side rotator cuff tear is shown.

Repair of Large Articular-Surface Tears
- A3 tear (articular surface, >6 mm deep)—Complete the tear from subacromial side, then perform standard rotator cuff repair
- Repair options—Single-row, double-row, or double-row transosseous equivalent

Transosseous-Equivalent Repair
- Restores anatomic footprint
- Achieves highest contact pressure between tendon and tuberosity
  - Establish anterior subacromial portal and second lateral portal in line with tear for repair

- Prepare footprint with curet or high-speed burr down to bleeding bone
- Percutaneously place one or two double-loaded anchors along medial margin at angle <45° (deadman angle)
- Can also place suture anchors through anterolateral incision by adducting arm
- Pass sutures via suture lasso/antegrade suture passer/shuttle relay in horizontal mattress configuration
- Suture management—Pass all sutures first, working anterior to posterior and pulling sutures through anterior or accessory lateral cannula
- Tie with a sliding knot and alternating half hitches
- Choose pairs of suture that lie best over lateral aspect of cuff, avoiding "dog ear" configuration
- Take one suture from each pair through medium-size knotless lateral-row anchor (**Figure 3**)

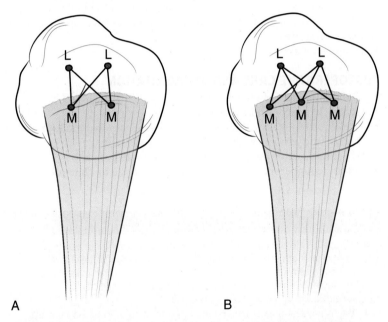

A   B

FIGURE 3 Illustrations show suture configuration possibilities for transosseous-equivalent rotator cuff repair. **A,** Two medial-row pairs of sutures are tied down with sliding/locking knots. Then, one suture from each suture stack is brought to a lateral anchor placed at the anterolateral aspect of the tear, and the second suture from each suture stack is passed to a second lateral anchor at the posterolateral aspect of the tear. **B,** In large tears requiring three pairs of medial sutures, one suture from each knot stack may be brought out to either an anterolateral or posterolateral anchor, creating the transosseous-equivalent repair with compression of the cuff tissue over the footprint. L = lateral anchor, M = medial knot stack.

- Place suture anchor in position off lateral aspect of greater tuberosity
- Place second suture from knots into second lateral-row anchor, and fix on lateral aspect of the greater tuberosity
- Number of anchors depends on size of the tear and should be adjusted appropriately
- Goal—Tension-free, well-approximated cuff repair with lateral edge compressed to greater tuberosity

COMPLICATIONS

- Continued pain—Could be secondary to failed decompression or to unaddressed pathology, including biceps tendinopathy, labral pathology, acromioclavicular joint spurs, degenerative joint disease
- Retear—Related to tissue quality as well as initial tear size; revision indicated if tissue is in reasonable condition
- Stiffness—Can occur when patient lacks commitment to rehabilitation protocol or secondary to adhesive capsulitis; treat with anti-inflammatory medications or injection, individually directed rehabilitation; if nonsurgical treatment fails, arthroscopic capsular release indicated
- Loss of strength

POSTOPERATIVE CARE AND REHABILITATION

- Abduction sling for 4 to 6 weeks
- Gentle Codman exercises for first 2 weeks
- Weeks 2 to 6—Passive range-of-motion exercises in formal physical therapy and at home with stick-and-pulley system
- At 6 weeks, active range-of-motion exercises are initiated
- Return to higher impact activity is delayed until 6 to 12 months

PEARLS

- A patient who has pain with resisted rotator cuff testing but demonstrates normal strength could have a partial-thickness rotator cuff tear. If MRI is the modality of choice in the surgeon's practice, magnetic resonance arthrography should be considered to increase the specificity for identification of the partial-thickness tear.
- We fix any tear greater than 6 mm or greater than 50% of the thickness of the tendon. The easiest way to determine the size of the tear is with a calibrated probe or shaver of known size.
- Suture management probably is the most important aspect of rotator cuff surgery. Keeping sutures "docked" or "parked" away from the set with which the surgeon is working makes visualization much easier and limits the chance of crossing the sutures, especially when using a transosseous-equivalent technique.

- To make it easier to locate the partial-thickness tear on the subacromial side, a spinal needle can be placed percutaneously through the tear. Then a monofilament suture can be passed through the needle and parked out of the anterior glenohumeral portal. The location of the partial-thickness tear is indicated by the monofilament suture position when viewed from the subacromial side.

- A thorough bursectomy enhances visualization and minimizes the possibility of getting the sutures snagged in the tissue. In addition, it affords full identification of the tear, which facilitates surgical planning.

Anterior Shoulder Stabilization Procedures: From Arthroscopic to Open to Latarjet

PATIENT SELECTION
Indications
- Overhead and contact athletes with a history of anterior-inferior glenohumeral instability
- Older and recreational athletes without engaging Hill-Sachs lesions or large (>25%) bony Bankart lesions who have recurrent instability/physical symptoms despite physical therapy
- Arthroscopic Bankart repair equivalent to open techniques
- Significant bone loss (>25%) recommended to be treated with bony reconstruction via open approach rather than soft-tissue reconstruction alone

Contraindications for Arthroscopic Bankart Repair
- At least 25% glenoid bone loss
- Engaging Hill-Sachs lesion
- Glenohumeral capsulolabral attenuation
- Connective tissue disorders
- Concomitant subscapularis tears
- Humeral avulsions of the glenohumeral ligament
- Chronic recurrent instability after surgical or nonsurgical treatment (relative contraindication)
- Contraindications for bony reconstruction
  - Concomitant irreparable rotator cuff
  - First-time dislocation in elderly population
  - Voluntary dislocators
  - Patients with epilepsy
  - Shoulder microinstability
  - Posttraumatic inferior subluxation
  - Static anterior subluxation
  - Anterior instability with soft-tissue incarceration

Based on McLaughlin RJ, Camp CL: Anterior shoulder stabilization procedures: From arthroscopic to open to latarjet, in Colvin AC, Flatow E, eds: Atlas of Essential Orthopaedic Procedures, *ed 2. Rosemont, IL, American Academy of Orthopaedic Surgeons, 2020, pp 11-20.*

PREOPERATIVE IMAGING

- Standard radiographic views—AP, axillary lateral, scapular Y
  - Assess glenohumeral relationship and rule out associated fractures.
  - Apical oblique, West Point, and Didiee are not routine but can be useful for bony glenoid defects.
  - Stryker notch can better assess for Hill-Sachs defects.
- MRI with gadolinium arthrography to assess capsule, labrum, rotator cuff, cartilage, bony anatomy (**Figure 1**)
- CT in setting of significant bony defects; subtract humeral head to get direct view of glenoid face.

PROCEDURE

Room Setup/Patient Positioning

- Authors prefer beach chair, with waist flexed to 45° and the knees to 30° while raising torso. Can be used for arthroscopic or open (**Figure 2**).
- Lateral decubitus position is alternative with beanbag and lateral arm traction
  - Axillary nerve is protected with a gel pad; pillows are placed between legs and under contralateral leg to protect peroneal nerve (**Figure 3**).

Special Instruments/Equipment/Implants

- Standard shoulder arthroscopy equipment
- Success depends more on the surgical technique than the devices used.
- Author preference—1.5-mm flat, nonabsorbable, high-strength suture mm paired with small biocomposite bone anchors
- Curved suture shuttling devices

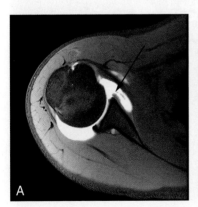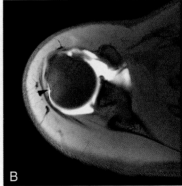

FIGURE 1 **A**, Preoperative T2-weighted magnetic resonance arthrograms of the shoulder of a patient with an anterior-inferior labral tear, or Bankart lesion (arrow). **B**, Hills-Sachs lesion (arrowhead).

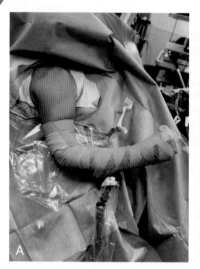 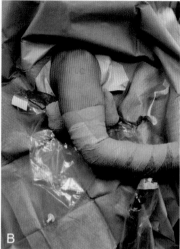

FIGURE 2 A, Photograph showing the beach chair positioning for shoulder arthroscopy. A pneumatic arm holder is used to control shoulder positioning. Cervical spine is kept in neutral positioning. This position is also used for the open Latarjet procedure. **B,** Photograph showing the surgical extremity in increased internal rotation and adduction.

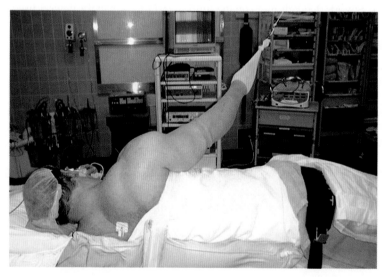

FIGURE 3 Photograph shows lateral decubitus positioning for shoulder arthroscopy. A beanbag and an axillary roll are used, and pillows are placed underneath and between the legs, padding all prominences.

- Visualization is paramount during open Bankart repair, requiring:
  - Three-pronged pitchfork glenoid retractor
  - Long, narrow right-angle retractor
  - Richardson retractors
  - Humeral head depressor
  - Latarjet equipment
    - Periosteal elevator
    - Small burr
    - Right-angle saw
    - Standard drill/screw set
    - Alternatively use specialized Latarjet set

 VIDEO 2.1 Arthroscopic Shoulder Stabilization. Richard J. McLaughlin, MD; Christopher L. Camp, MD (3 min)

Surgical Technique: Arthroscopic Repair

- Perform physical examination of both arms following anesthesia induction
- Forearm traction 5 to 10 lb in 20° forward flexion and 20° to 30° abduction
- Portals
  - Posterior portal is placed first.
  - Perform diagnostic arthroscopy.
  - Anterior portal is placed in superior subscapularis margin in lateral rotator interval (working portal, aids in anchor placement); 8.25-mm clear cannula is placed.
  - Anterosuperior portal is placed high in rotator interval (used for arthroscope); 5-mm clear cannula is placed.
- Technique
  - If engaging Hill-Sachs is present, a remplissage should be performed.
    - Accessory posterolateral portal created and 5.75 mm cannula inserted
    - Débride lesion with shaver.
    - Insert 4.5 mm double-loaded corkscrew in center of lesion.
    - Use birdbeak to pass all four suture limbs through capsule.
    - Leave sutures in cannula and tie in standard fashion to reduce the capsule into the defect after labral repair completed.
  - The labrum is prepared using an arthroscopic elevator anterior to posterior (**Figure 4, A** and **B**)
    - Care is taken to avoid creating a radial split in the labrum.
    - Anterior labral periosteal sleeve avulsion—elevate if present.
  - The glenoid is prepared for anchor placement—a 4.0-mm shaver or burr is used to roughen surface.

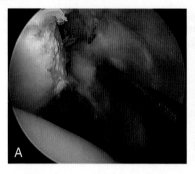 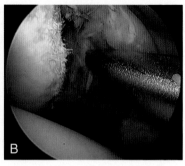

FIGURE 4 Arthroscopic views from the anterosuperior portal show labrum preparation for arthroscopic Bankart lesion repair. **A,** An arthroscopic elevator device is used to mobilize the labral tear in the interval between the glenoid rim and the anterior-inferior labrum. **B,** An arthroscopic shaver is used to prepare the glenoid rim and the labrum for repair. Note the roughened glenoid rim and bleeding tissues.

- ▹ Anchor placement
- ▹ Side-specific curved suture-passing device placed through anterior portal
  - Advance through tissue from inferior to superior at approximately 1-2 mm off glenoid near inferior 6-o'clock position. (All clockface positions described in this chapter are for a right shoulder.)
  - Loop of suture passer is brought externally through the posterior portal
  - 1.5-mm flat, nonabsorbable suture is shuttled through the joint and anterior portal
  - Suture limbs are loaded into an empty 2.9-mm biocomposite bone anchor, tagged, and set aside
  - Drill for anchor and place through anterior portal near 6-o'clock position
  - Place anchors at 45° angle to glenoid surface, 2 mm from anterior rim (**Figure 5, A** through **C**).
  - At least three anchors, 6 to 7 mm apart, marching up anterior glenoid rim
- ▹ Close portals with 2-0 nylon arthroscopic stitch.
- ▹ A sling with abduction pillow is placed; an ice pack is applied to the dressing.

Surgical Technique: Open Bankart Repair With Capsular Shift

- Position the patient beach chair as previously described.
- Deltopectoral incision beginning 1 cm lateral to tip of coracoid, extending distally to the axillary crease (**Figure 6**)

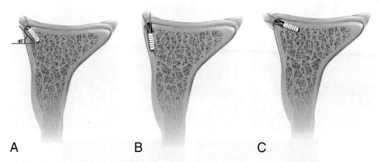

A   B   C

FIGURE 5 Illustration shows the proper angle of anchor placement: **A**, 45° from the glenoid face. The correct entry location, approximately 2 mm onto the glenoid face from the edge of the rim, is also illustrated. Illustrations show improper anchor placement, with the anchor placed too perpendicular to the glenoid and buried too far into the glenoid (**B**) and the anchor placed too parallel to the glenoid and buried too far into the glenoid (**C**).

- Subcutaneous tissues are undermined, deltopectoral interval is identified, and cephalic vein is retracted laterally. Clavipectoral fascia is incised along the lateral border. Take care to avoid acromial branch of the thoracoacromial artery lateral to coracoid; artery should be ligated.

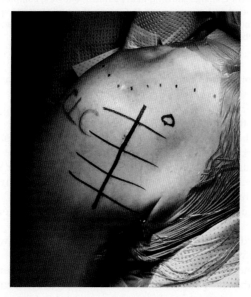

FIGURE 6 Photograph shows location of the deltopectoral shoulder incision for an open Bankart repair in a right shoulder, approximately 1 cm lateral to the coracoid.

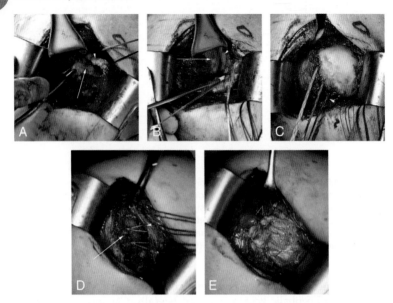

FIGURE 7 Intraoperative images of open capsular repair showing (**A**) separation of the subscapularis (arrowhead) from the anterior capsule (arrow) and (**B**) placement of the glenoid (arrowhead) suture anchors. The humeral head (arrow) is also easily seen. **C**, Image showing heavy sutures following complete glenoid and humeral head anchor placement. **D**, Closure of capsule (arrow) with sutures passing through subscapularis (arrowhead) that are yet to be tied, and (**E**) anterior view of the subscapularis after sutures are tied.

Medial retraction of the conjoined tendon is only slight, to prevent musculocutaneous nerve injury.

- The upper and lower borders of the subscapularis tendon are identified with the shoulder in 65° external rotation.
- Periosteal elevator and electrocautery used to separate subscapularis from anterior capsule
- Subscapularis tenotomy performed 1 cm medial to lesser tuberosity
- Tag both upper and lower subscapularis limbs using multiple No. 2 braided traction sutures (**Figure 7, A**).
- Release capsule off humeral head from superior to inferior and tag capsule.
- A pronged, anterior glenoid retractor may be placed between capsule and subscapularis.
- Dissect the Bankart fragment and labrum from the anterior glenoid. Prepare the rim with a small curet and burr; avoid significant bone removal.
- Self-retrieving device used to pass nonabsorbable suture in oblique mattress fashion through labrum and anterior-inferior capsule.

- Fix these sutures to glenoid using same knotless anchors and technique as for arthroscopic, beginning inferior and moving superior as needed (**Figure 7, B**).
- Four 1.6-mm all-suture anchors are placed along humeral head at previous insertion site of capsule.
- Beginning inferiorly, the sutures from these anchors are each passed through the capsule in an inferior and medialized position, advancing the capsule superiorly and laterally once tied.
- All sutures are passed before tying.
- The arm is placed in neutral adduction, flexion, and 30° of external rotation and the sutures are tied sequentially from inferior to superior, completing the capsular shift (**Figure 7, C** and **D**).
- These sutures are passed through subscapularis tendon from inferior to superior and tied to affix subscapularis to the capsule (**Figure 7, E**).
- Additional fixation of tenotomy with No. 2 suture in figure-of-8 fashion suturing free edge of tendon to stump on lesser tuberosity
- Loose reapproximation of the deltopectoral interval.
- Close the skin with running subcuticular absorbable suture.
- The arm is immobilized in a sling with an abduction pillow and ice pack.

Latarjet

- Standard deltopectoral approach as previously described
- Identify conjoined tendon and tip of acromion.
- Release pectoralis minor off the medial and interior border of coracoid.
- Release the coracoacromial (CA) ligament from the acromion, preserving length.
- Transect coracoid using right-angle saw at its base just distal to coracoclavicular ligaments to ensure maximal length.
- Two 2.5-mm drill holes placed in coracoid from inferior to superior.
- Place passing stitch through one of holes to tag coracoid.
- Place arm in maximum external rotation and identify subscapularis.
- Split subscapularis at the border between superior two-thirds and inferior one-third in line with muscle fibers.
- Internally rotate arm to relax subscapularis and place self-retaining retractor.
- Perform vertical capsulotomy just medial to glenoid.
- Use periosteal elevator to elevate capsule from anterior glenoid and place pronged anterior glenoid retractor.
- Assess size of bony defect and prepare graft bed using curettes and a burr.
- A 2.5 mm drill hole is placed in inferior glenoid and the coracoid fragment is subsequently fixed to the inferior aspect of the glenoid with a 4.0-mm partially threaded screw via the inferior-most hole previously placed in the bone block.

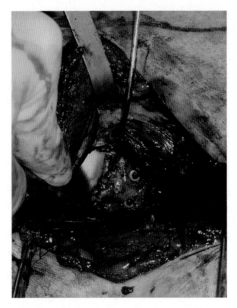

FIGURE 8 Intraoperative photograph after placement and internal fixation of bony block following coracoid transfer.

- Position graft so that inferior surface of the coracoid is adjacent to the anterior surface of the glenoid (**Figure 8**).
- Graft should be at the level of glenoid or just medial to it.
- 2.5-mm drill used to drill the superior hole in the glenoid through the superior hole that has already been created in the graft
- A 3.5-mm fully threaded screw is placed superiorly.
- If prominent, the lateral edge can be resected using a small burr.
- The capsule is closed to the remaining CA ligament.
- Subscapularis is closed in a side-to-side fashion, as is the deltopectoral interval.
- Subcutaneous tissues and skin are closed in a standard fashion.
- A postoperative radiograph is obtained showing proper placement of the graft (**Figure 9**).
- Patient is placed in a sling, with an abduction pillow, and an ice pack over the dressing.

COMPLICATIONS
Intraoperative
- Nerve injury
  - The axillary nerve lies 10 to 15 mm beneath the inferior capsule.
  - The musculocutaneous nerve lies 5 to 8 cm inferior to the coracoid.

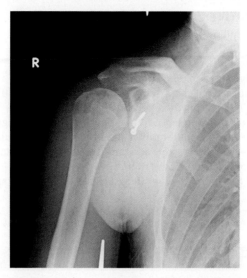

FIGURE 9 Immediate postoperative digital true AP radiograph demonstrating properly placed internal fixation along the anterior glenoid rim.

> Nerve injury to the brachial plexus is thought to result from excessive arm traction and increased cervical flexion/extension during the procedure.
- Vascular injury
- Overtensioning or undertensioning of capsulolabral complex

Postoperative
- Hardware failure
- Continued laxity
- Stiffness can result from excessive tightening of the anterior-inferior capsule leading to external rotation loss.
- Infection—up to 6% open, less than 1% arthroscopic; most common causative organism is *Cutibacterium acnes*.
- Complications higher in Latarjet than open or arthroscopic Bankart repairs
  > Infection is reported to be 1.4% to 2.5%.
  > Neurapraxia reported to range from 1% to 20%
  > Nerve injuries are typically transient.
- In a meta-analysis of 1,904 shoulders the rate of anterior dislocation following Latarjet was 2.9% and subluxation 5.8%.
  > Recurrence rates are noted in the literature between 1% and 7%.
  > Progression of the shoulder to glenohumeral arthritis in up to 20% of patients

---

POSTOPERATIVE CARE AND REHABILITATION

- Abduction pillow sling for 6 weeks
- Initial physical therapy in weeks 1 to 4
  - ▶ Elbow and wrist range-of-motion exercises
  - ▶ Passive shoulder abduction in scapular plane
  - ▶ Active internal and external rotation (weeks 1 to 2: 10°; weeks 2 to 6: 20°) with arm adducted and elbow flexed at 90°
- Weeks 6 to 12—Commence formal physical therapy program, including progressive range-of-motion and isometric periscapular exercises.
- Week 12—Goal is to restore forward flexion, internal rotation, abduction, and 50% of external rotation.
- Months 3 to 6—Progressive strengthening, plyometrics, sport-specific exercises
- Month 6—Goal is return to play for contact athletes.

PEARLS

- During arthroscopic Bankart repair, two anterior portals should be used—one in the standard position above the subscapularis tendon and one in a superior portion of the rotator interval—to prevent overcrowding.
- During arthroscopic Bankart repair, occasionally a percutaneous anchor can be placed to allow for access to the most inferior aspects of the glenoid and to prevent oblique trajectories for suture tying.
- During the approach for open Bankart repair, the subscapularis should be separated from the underlying capsule to facilitate capsuloligamentous repair and lateral/superior shifting of the capsule
- The Latarjet procedure is indicated in the presence of significant (>25%) anterior glenoid bone loss; however, it may be performed for smaller bone defects in higher risk patients or revision settings.
- Unique complications following the Latarjet include progression of osteoarthritis as well as bone block resorption.

VIDEO REFERENCE

 Video 2.1 McLaughlin RJ, Camp CL: *Arthroscopic Shoulder Stabilization* [video]. Rochester, MN, Mayo, 2020.

Arthroscopic Superior Labrum Anterior-to-Posterior Repair

INTRODUCTION

- Detachment of the superior labrum with or without biceps anchor involvement is common to all superior labrum anterior-to-posterior (SLAP) tears.
- First described in 1985

Snyder Classification

- Four original types (**Figure 1**)
  - ▸ Type I—Fraying of inner margin of superior labrum, which remains attached
  - ▸ Type II—Detachment of superior labrum and biceps tendon from superior glenoid rim; most common type that requires repair; in 1998, others subclassified type II SLAP tears into three subvariants.
    - – Anterior: Anterior detachment of superior labrum and biceps complex
    - – Posterior: Posterior detachment of superior labrum and biceps complex; most common type in throwing athletes
    - – Combined
  - ▸ Type III—Bucket-handle tear of the superior labrum with intact biceps anchor
  - ▸ Type IV—Bucket-handle tear with extension into the biceps tendon
- Three additional types described in 1995
  - ▸ Type V—A type II lesion with anterior extension to anterior-inferior labrum
  - ▸ Type VI—A type II lesion with unstable anterior or posterior flap of superior labrum
  - ▸ Type VII—A type II lesion with separation of the biceps attachment extending to the middle glenohumeral ligament (MGHL)
- Three more types described in 2004
  - ▸ Type VIII—A type II lesion with posterior labral extension
  - ▸ Type IX—A type II lesion with a circumferential labral tear
  - ▸ Type X—A type II lesion with a posteroinferior labral tear

---

Based on Dreese JC, Casagrande D: Arthroscopic superior labrum anterior-to-posterior repair, in Colvin AC, Flatow E, eds: Atlas of Essential Orthopaedic Procedures, *ed 2. Rosemont, IL, American Academy of Orthopaedic Surgeons, 2020, pp 21-30.*

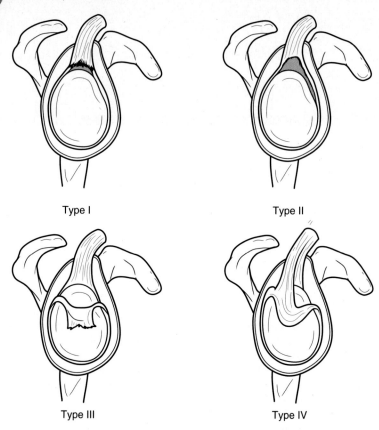

Type I

Type II

Type III

Type IV

FIGURE 1 Illustrations show the Snyder classification of superior labrum anterior-to-posterior (SLAP) tears. Type I: Local degeneration and fraying on the inner margin of the superior labrum are seen. Type II: The superior labrum and biceps tendon anchor are detached from the superior glenoid rim. Type III: A bucket-handle tear of the superior labrum is present; the biceps anchor is intact. Type IV: The bucket-handle tear extends into the biceps tendon.

Clinical Diagnosis

- Sharp or aching anterior or posterior shoulder pain is the most common presenting symptom.
- Nonsurgical treatment—Rest, NSAIDs, scapular stabilizers, posterior capsule stretching, and strengthening of the rotator cuff (RTC); intra-articular injection for temporary pain relief and confirmation of the glenohumeral joint as the source of discomfort.

PATIENT SELECTION

Indications

- Failure of 3-month trial of nonsurgical management
- Arthroscopy is the benchmark for diagnosis and management of SLAP lesions.
- Type I tears are normal and do not require treatment.
- Type III and IV tears have a stable biceps anchor and can often be treated nonsurgically with simple débridement of the torn biceps tendon.
- Types II and V through X are unstable lesions that benefit from restoration of labral and ligamentous attachment.
- Avoid repair of degenerative SLAP tears in older patients with RTC tears; better results were seen with RTC repair and biceps tenotomy than with RTC and SLAP repair.
- Tenodesis versus tenotomy—Active patients with partial-thickness tears of the biceps tendon greater than 25%, chronic atrophic changes of the tendon, tendon subluxation in the bicipital groove, and a tendon less than 75% normal width secondary to tendon atrophy benefit from biceps tenodesis; low-demand patients with extensive partial-thickness tearing and/or subluxation are candidates for biceps tenotomy.
- Types V through X are suited to anatomic restoration of the labral and ligamentous attachments.

Contraindications

- Absolute
  - Active infection
  - Medical comorbidities that outweigh the potential benefits of repair
  - Presence of a normal anatomic variant such as a sublabral foramen or Buford complex
- Relative
  - Older patients with concomitant findings such as RTC tears that explain the disability
  - Adhesive capsulitis
  - Extensive tearing of the long head of the biceps

PREOPERATIVE IMAGING

- Standard shoulder radiographs
  - Glenoid AP
  - Acromioclavicular AP
  - Scapular Y
  - Axillary views
- MRI—Study of choice to evaluate pathology.
  - Paralabral cyst within spinoglenoid notch is suggestive of SLAP tear
  - Understanding normal anatomic variants helps identify SLAP tears: 3.3% incidence of sublabral foramen; 8.6% incidence of sublabral foramen with cord-like MGHL; 1.5% incidence of Buford complex

- Magnetic resonance arthrography—Extravasation of contrast into/underneath the superior labrum/biceps complex is suggestive of SLAP pathology.

PROCEDURE

Patient Positioning

- Modified beach-chair with arm holder or lateral decubitus with 5 to 10 lb traction in 30° to 45° abduction and 10° to 20° forward elevation (**Figure 2**); with lateral decubitus, pad contralateral knee well to protect peroneal nerve.
- Mark bony landmarks (acromion, clavicle, acromioclavicular [AC] joint, coracoid process) (**Figure 3**); important to correctly localize coracoid process to avoid injuring the neurovascular structures.

Equipment

- 30° arthroscope; 70° arthroscope may be used if needed.
- One to three 7-mm clear cannulas
- Probe, elevator, rasp, shaver, burr, drill, cannulated drill sleeve, suture anchor(s), suture passer, looped suture grasper, knot pusher, suture cutter

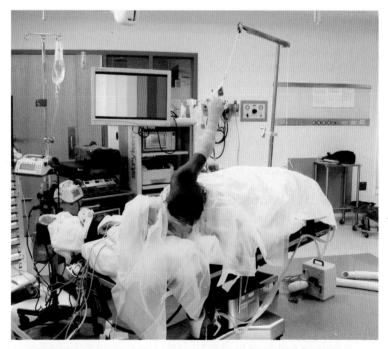

FIGURE 2 Photograph shows a patient in the lateral decubitus position.

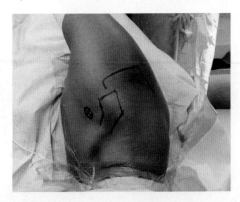

FIGURE 3 Photograph shows bony landmark demarcation on the right shoulder of a patient in the lateral decubitus position. The coracoid process is indicated with an encircled X.

Technique

Diagnostic Arthroscopy via Posterior Viewing Portal (Figure 4)

- Beach-chair position—Portal is made distal and medial to posterolateral corner of acromion.
- Lateral decubitus position—Portal is made distal and lateral to posterolateral corner of the acromion.
- Anterior portal—Place cannula using spinal needle localization high in rotator interval lateral to the coracoid.
- Inspect glenohumeral joint to rule out Bankart and Hill-Sachs; also examine the superior glenohumeral ligament (SGHL) and MGHL, anterior-inferior and posteroinferior labrum, anterior and posterior bands of the inferior glenohumeral ligament, and axillary pouch; inspect the subscapularis insertion on the lesser tuberosity and the intra-articular side of the supraspinatus and infraspinatus for tear.
- Probe superior labrum for evidence of SLAP; evaluate the long head of the biceps (both intra-articular and intertubercular segments), and rule out anatomic variants.

Cannula Placement

- Establish second cannula low in rotator interval just above subscapularis tendon to assist in suture management.
- Débride unstable superior labrum–biceps complex fragments.
- Types II and V through X—Gently mobilize superior labrum and expose bleeding surface on glenoid rim with shaver.

Suture Anchor Placement

- Port of Wilmington (**Figure 5**)
  - Localize port of Wilmington using spinal needle.
  - A 3-mm drill sleeve with sharp trocar is placed through the musculotendinous junction of the RTC.

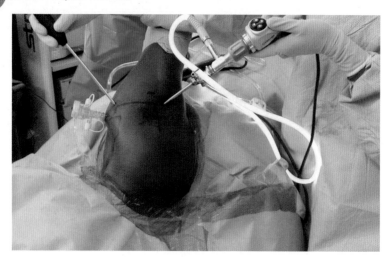

FIGURE 4 Photograph shows the placement of the drill sleeve through a rotator interval approach.

- ▶ One to two anchors are placed posterior to biceps anchor; sutures are retrieved through anterior cannula.
- Anterosuperior cannula
    - ▶ Advance cannula over superior labrum–biceps complex; pass suture passer through superior labrum at far posterior position; grasp superior-most suture in far posterior anchor; tie down with sliding locking knot with three alternating half hitches.
    - ▶ Repeat with posterosuperior anchor sutures.
    - ▶ Place anterosuperior anchor at 1-o'clock position (right shoulder) (**Figure 6**).
    - ▶ Pass the suture though the labrum so as not to overconstrain the MGHL and SGHL; tie as above.

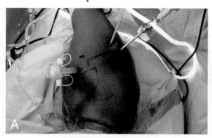
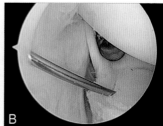

FIGURE 5 Photograph shows the placement of the drill sleeve through the port of Wilmington (**A**). Arthroscopic view shows the approach to the posterosuperior glenoid using spinal needle passage through the port of Wilmington (**B**).

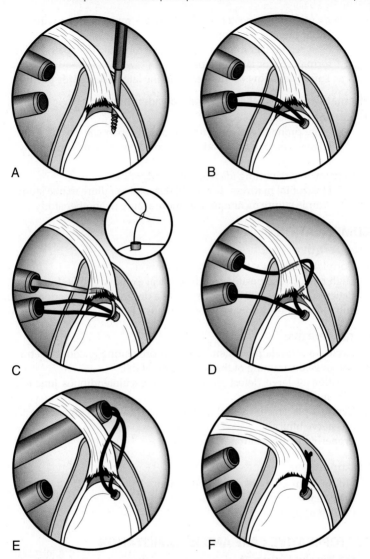

FIGURE 6 Illustrations demonstrate the arthroscopic suture anchor technique for the repair of type II SLAP tears. **A,** Suture anchor insertion is directed at a 45° angle to the glenoid rim to limit the risk of articular cartilage injury. **B,** The suture limbs are retrieved through the anterior-inferior portal. **C,** A wire suture passer then is passed under the torn superior labrum and retrieved through the anterior-inferior portal. **D,** The medial suture limb of the suture anchor is fed through the wire suture loop. The suture loop is advanced under the superior labrum and retrieved through the anterosuperior cannula. **E,** A standard arthroscopic knot-tying technique is used to secure the repair. **F,** The completed SLAP repair is shown.

- When anterior and posterior labral repairs must be done with SLAP, the author preference is to:
  - ▶ First repair the anterior labrum, perform SLAP repair, and perform posterior labrum repair.
  - ▶ This order allows better access in the lateral decubitus position.

Alternative Repair Techniques and Considerations
- Knotless anchors
  - ▶ More prone to early gap formations at repair site
  - ▶ Higher comparative load to 2-mm gapping with similar load to failure
- Controversy regarding ideal suture configuration
  - ▶ Horizontal mattress showed better load to failure in one study.
  - ▶ Simple suture technique was more secure in another study.

COMPLICATIONS
Preoperative
- Correlate pathology to clinical examination
- High rate of false-positives with physical examination findings
- Patients older than 40 years may have a degenerative superior labrum and not a tear or may have a concomitant RTC tear causing symptoms.

Intraoperative
- Accurate cannula placement is key to preventing anchor penetration and overconstraining of the MGHL and SGHL.
- Creation of large defect through the musculotendinous junction of RTC may result in pain.
- Cannula placement medial to the coracoid can cause musculocutaneous nerve injury.
- Properly identify anatomic variants.

Postoperative
- Stiffness caused by late immobilization
- Infection
- Persistent pain

POSTOPERATIVE CARE AND REHABILITATION
0 to 4 Weeks (Table 1)
- Patients younger than 25 years begin physical therapy at 1 week.
- Those older than 25 years begin physical therapy within 3 to 4 days.
- Sling is worn 3 to 4 weeks.
- Home program includes wand exercises and overhead pulley.
- Exercises include elbow range of motion; squeezing a tennis ball for grip; contraction of biceps/triceps at 0°, 30°, 60°, 90°, and 120°; pendulum exercises; passive range of motion from 0° to 120° of forward elevation in scapular plane; and external rotation to 30° with arm at the side.

TABLE 1 Range-of-Motion Goals Following SLAP (Superior Labrum Anterior-to-Posterior) Repair

Weeks Postoperative	Forward Elevation	External Rotation
0-2	90°	10°
2-4	120°	30°
4-6	140°	45°
6-8	160°	60°
8-10	Full[a]	Full[a]

[a]Preferably within 5° of the contralateral side.

4 to 12 Weeks

- Forward flexion 140° at 4 to 6 weeks, 160° at 6 to 8 weeks, and full at 8 to 10 weeks
- External rotation 45° at 4 to 6 weeks, 60° at 6 to 8 weeks, and full at 8 to 10 weeks

PEARLS

- The surgeon should look for pathologies other than SLAP lesions in patients older than 40 years, particularly in patients with no history of traumatic injury.
- Degenerative SLAP tears in patients older than 40 years are good candidates for biceps tenodesis or tenolysis rather than SLAP repair.
- Types I, III, and IV SLAP lesions have a stable biceps anchor and often can be treated nonsurgically or with simple débridement of the torn biceps tendon.
- Type II and types V through X SLAP tears are unstable lesions that benefit from restoration of the labral attachment.
- Placement of arthroscopic cannulas through the rotator cuff should be avoided. If a trans–rotator cuff portal is used, precise placement of a 3-mm drill sleeve with a sharp trocar through the musculotendinous junction can be used to limit the risk of injury to the tendinous insertion which may result in disability. Localization of the approach with a spinal needle facilitates efficient placement of the drill sleeve and limits traumatic injury to the rotator cuff musculature.

4 Biceps Tenotomy and Tenodesis

PATIENT SELECTION

Long Head of the Biceps Tendon

- The long head of the biceps tendon (LHBT) is the primary pain generator of the anterior shoulder.
- It ascends through the intertubercular groove proximally and turns 30° medially and posteriorly, where the coracohumeral ligament, superior glenohumeral ligament (SGHL), supraspinatus tendon, and subscapularis tendon form a "pulley" supporting the LHBT.
- Travels intra-articularly but extrasynovially through the glenohumeral joint and inserts on the supraglenoid tubercle and/or superior labrum
- Pathology split into three zones:
  - Inside zone—superior labrum and biceps anchor
  - Junction zone—intra-articular portion of LHBT and LHBT pulley
- Bicipital tunnel zone—extra-articular portion of LHBT from humeral head margin to subpectoral regions
- Etiology
  - Osteophytes
  - Microtrauma from repetitive overhead activities
  - Acromial morphology
  - Internal impingement
  - Subacromial impingement
  - Tendon instability
  - Trauma
  - Ischemia
  - Rotator cuff (RTC) pathology
  - Tears of the anterior capsuloligamentous complex
  - Labral tears
  - Glenohumeral instability
  - Acromioclavicular arthrosis
- History
  - Elicit patient's occupation and sports activities.
  - Pain with overhand or underhand throwing and lifting or extending of the arm

Based on Erickson BJ, Chalmers PN, Romeo AA: Biceps tenotomy and tenodesis, in Colvin AC, Flatow E, eds: Atlas of Essential Orthopaedic Procedures, *ed 2. Rosemont, IL, American Academy of Orthopaedic Surgeons, 2020, pp 31-36.*

- Pain begins in anterior shoulder and radiates distally into biceps muscle belly.
- Snapping, grinding, or popping may be described.
- Physical examination
  - Inspection, palpation, and range of motion (ROM) of shoulder
  - Neurovascular examination
  - Provocative maneuvers to test for
    - Subacromial impingement
    - RTC tear
    - Instability
    - Acromioclavicular pathology
- Physical examination maneuvers often unreliable due to crossover pathology
  - "Three pack"—excellent reliability, sensitivity, and negative predictive value
    - Biceps tunnel tenderness—most sensitive
    - Positive O'Brien test
    - Positive throwing test

Indications
- The indications for biceps tenotomy and tenodesis are similar.
- Lesions involving 25% to 50% of tendon
- Type II or IV superior labral anterior-to-posterior (SLAP) tears in older, less active patients
- LHBT instability
- Failed SLAP repair
- Failed nonsurgical treatment, including rest, ice, NSAIDs, ROM exercises, stretching, physical therapy, iontophoresis, phonophoresis, glenohumeral or subacromial steroid injections, or selective LHBT sheath injection

Contraindications
- Few exist
- Pseudoparalysis of the shoulder is a relative contraindication.

PREOPERATIVE IMAGING
Radiography
- AP, lateral, axillary, scapular Y views
- The intertubercular groove can be visualized in profile by placing the cassette at the apex of the externally rotated shoulder with the X-ray beam collinear with the humeral shaft.

MRI Findings
- Ovalization of the tendon
- Increased intrasubstance signal intensity on T2-weighted images
- Tendon dislocation of intertubercular groove

Other Modalities
- Magnetic resonance arthrography increases the sensitivity and specificity and can delineate other injuries.
- Ultrasonography is sensitive and specific, although technician dependent and limited delineation of associated intra-articular pathology
- The benchmark diagnostic test is arthroscopy.

PROCEDURE
Surgical Decision Making
- Biceps tenodeses and tenotomies are increasing in prevalence, whereas SLAP repairs are decreasing
- Perceived notion by surgeons that patients fare better with tenodesis/ tenotomy versus SLAP repair

Tenotomy
- More simple procedure than tenodesis
- Associated with several complications
  - "Popeye" deformity in up to 70% of patients
  - Weakness with elbow flexion/supination
  - Loss of anatomic length-tension relationship can lead to muscle contraction and atrophy.
  - May be preferable in patients who are older, less active, or unwilling/unable to engage in postoperative therapy or to adhere to postoperative restrictions

Tenodesis
- Preferable for active or young patients (<50 years)
- Several methods have been described.
  - Arthroscopic transfer of LHBT to conjoint tendon
  - At proximal end of intertubercular groove (arthroscopic approach)
  - Residual LHBT can produce anterior shoulder pain or may rupture because of osteophytes impinging on the tendon in the groove.
    - More technically challenging
    - Obscures re-creation of tendon length-tension relationship
    - Bulk of tenodesis at proximal end of intertubercular groove could contribute to postoperative subacromial impingement
    - High failure in proximal tenodesis secondary to tenodesis in inflamed zone
  - Soft-tissue tenodesis can be performed under the inferior edge of pectoralis major insertion (open approach).
    - May predispose to adhesions/scar tissue in subacromial and subpectoral spaces
    - Places shear stress on structures sutured to tendon, including coracohumeral ligament, SGHL, and supraspinatus and subscapularis tendons

- May increase severity of subacromial impingement by increasing superior muscular pull on humerus
- Allows recurrent subluxation within the groove
- May not reconstruct LHBT anatomy
  ▶ Osseous tenodesis can be performed using
    - Bone tunnel
    - Keyhole
    - Suture anchor
    - Interference screw (least loosening with cycling)

VIDEO 4.1 Demonstration of a subpectoral biceps tenodesis using a tenodesis screw as fixation. Brandon J. Erickson, MD; Peter N. Chalmers, MD, Anthony A. Romeo, MD (3 min)

- Author preference is osseous subpectoral tenodesis with interference screw fixation. Both subpectoral and proximal osseous tenodesis techniques are described in this chapter.

Alternate Procedure for Isolated LHBT Instability—Repair of Pulley
- Soft tissues that form the pulley include the subscapularis tendon, supraspinatus tendon, coracohumeral ligament, and SGHL.
- Poor outcome; 25% risk of rupture after repair; positive Speed test in 33% of tendons not ruptured.

Setup/Patient Positioning
- Interscalene block
- Standard preoperative intravenous antibiotics
- Beach-chair position and articulated arm holder

Surgical Technique
- Mark acromion, distal clavicle, and coracoid.
- Enter joint posteriorly with 18-gauge spinal needle 2 cm medial and inferior to the posterolateral corner of acromion, aiming toward coracoid.
- Place camera through posterior portal.
- Examine LHBT dry, so as not to obscure "lipstick" lesions.
- Insert probe through anteromedial portal to examine LHBT within intertubercular groove.
- Displace tendon medially and laterally to assess for instability and occult coracohumeral and SGHL injuries.
- Perform the peel-back test by abducting and externally rotating the humerus while observing the LHBT for SLAP tears.
- Perform the active compression test by placing the arm in 90° flexion, full elbow extension, and 15° internal rotation; test is positive for instability if LHBT moves medial and inferior and becomes entrapped.

- If surgeon elects to perform a subpectoral tenodesis (**Figure 1**):
  - ▶ Arthroscopically release LHBT from the supraglenoid tubercle.
  - ▶ Recline additional 30° from beach-chair position.
  - ▶ Tension the insertion of the pectoralis major using internal rotation and abduction.
  - ▶ Make a 3-cm longitudinal incision with the proximal edge 1 cm superior to the inferior edge of pectoralis major insertion. The incision can be placed in the axilla for cosmesis provided surgeon is intimately familiar with the anatomy.
  - ▶ Place self-retaining retractor and clear adipose tissue to identify the inferior edge of the pectoralis major, coracobrachialis, and the LHBT (at anteromedial humerus).
  - ▶ If cephalic vein is visible, dissection is too lateral and too proximal.
  - ▶ Fascia overlying coracobrachialis and LHBT should be incised from proximal to distal.
  - ▶ Retract pectoralis tendon proximally and laterally with a pointed Hohmann retractor, and gently retract the coracobrachialis and short head of the biceps medially with a blunt Chandler retractor.
  - ▶ With a right-angle clamp, pull tendon out of the groove and deliver it through the wound. Resect the tendon to leave 20 to 25 mm of it proximal to the musculotendinous junction.
  - ▶ Place a Krackow whip-stitch into the proximal 15 mm of the tendon.
  - ▶ Reflect a 2-cm × 1-cm patch of periosteum 1 cm proximal to the inferior edge of the pectoralis major. Place guidewire into this prepared bed. Guidewire should be placed in center of the groove at the intersection of the middle and distal thirds of the groove. Use an 8-mm cannulated acorn reamer to make a 15-mm-deep tunnel over the guidewire. Do not violate posterior cortex.

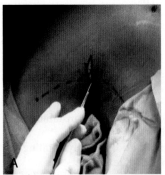
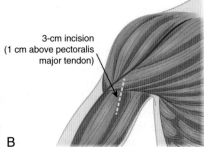

3-cm incision
(1 cm above pectoralis
major tendon)

A   B

FIGURE 1 Intraoperative photograph (**A**) and illustration (**B**) show the incision for subpectoral biceps tenodesis. A 3-cm longitudinal incision is made, with its proximal edge 1 cm superior to the inferior edge of the pectoralis major insertion.

▶ Irrigate field, and thread one limb of suture through tenodesis screwdriver loaded with an 8 × 15-mm polyetheretherketone tenodesis screw. Screw into the prepared hole and tie and cut suture after removing guidewire (**Figure 2**).

- If arthroscopic proximal tenodesis is chosen, several additional steps are performed before tendon release.

  ▶ Transfix the tendon with a spinal needle at entrance to intertubercular groove, and pass marking suture.

  ▶ Use an additional anterolateral portal made 3 cm from the anterior acromion and 3 cm lateral to the anteromedial portal to identify the groove; open groove with electrocautery, and remove tendon from groove.

  ▶ Drill guidewire into the center of the groove 1 cm distal to the superior border of the groove.

  ▶ Overdrill the guidewire with an 8-mm cannulated acorn reamer to 25 mm.

  ▶ Load marking suture through the tenodesis screwdriver loaded with an 8 × 25-mm screw, and seat into bone tunnel until screw is flush. Tie and cut or just cut suture. Assess tendon tension with a probe.

  ▶ May also use bicortical button, endocortical button, suture anchor, or bone tunnel as alternative method of fixation

Tenotomy

- Setup, positioning, and approach are the same as that for tenodesis.
- Arthroscopically identify the LHBT, and release from supraglenoid tubercle.
- Resect any tendon remaining in the joint.

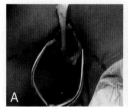 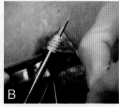 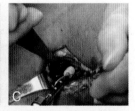

FIGURE 2 Intraoperative photographs show biceps tenodesis. **A,** The proximal cut edge of the tendon is delivered out of the wound. **B,** A tenodesis screw is loaded onto the driver. Note that one limb of the suture fixating the tendon must then be loaded onto the screwdriver. **C,** The tendon is pushed into the deepest aspect of the tunnel, and the tenodesis screw is advanced over the tendon.

COMPLICATIONS
- Loss of ROM, hematoma, seroma, infection, irritation from hardware, axillary nerve injury, musculocutaneous nerve injury, brachial artery injury, axillary artery injury, heterotopic ossification, and proximal humeral fracture
- Popeye deformity
- Complex regional pain syndrome
- Infection
- Neurapraxia
- Proximal humeral migration
- RTC arthropathy

POSTOPERATIVE CARE AND REHABILITATION
- A sling is worn for 3 to 4 weeks.
- Full passive and active ROM for first 6 weeks, with restriction on active flexion and supination of the surgical arm
- Patients can resume a lightened work schedule at 3 to 4 weeks, depending on occupation.

PEARLS

- Identification of LHBT pathology on the history and physical examination can be difficult, but careful patient selection leads to a reliable response to tenodesis.
- Patients with LHBT instability should be evaluated for other lesions. Because of the anatomic arrangement of the pulley, tendon subluxation is inevitably associated with concomitant pathology.
- LHBT tenodesis is associated with other injuries; it should be examined for in patients with subacromial impingement, RTC pathology, tears of the capsuloligamentous complex, labral tears, glenohumeral instability, and acromioclavicular arthrosis.
- Tenotomy and tenodesis outcomes may be similar, but each procedure can provide a maximum benefit to different populations. In young, active patients, tenodesis may prevent complications potentially associated with tenotomy. In older, less active, and obese patients, tenotomy may provide equivalent outcomes, with reduced surgical times, expense, and difficulty.
- Subpectoral tenodesis has several advantages over arthroscopic proximal tenodesis and should be considered in the appropriate patient.
- Interference screw fixation provides biomechanically superior fixation.

Anatomic Acromioclavicular Joint Reconstruction

PATIENT SELECTION

- Acromioclavicular (AC) joint injuries are common; they account for up to half of all athletic shoulder injuries.
- Typically due to a direct fall onto an adducted shoulder with the acromion displaced inferiorly and medially with respect to the clavicle
- Presentation—Local swelling, prominent distal clavicle, and AC joint pain with palpation and cross-body adduction or abduction
- In high-energy injuries, suspect associated injuries to the clavicle, scapula, proximal humerus, and neurovascular structures.
- AC joint separations are classified by the Rockwood classification system (**Table 1**).

Indications for Surgical Treatment

- Type IV, V, and VI separations represent high-energy mechanisms of injury and associated soft-tissue disruption.
  - Type IV—Posterior displacement of the clavicle through the trapezius
  - Type V—Detachment of the deltoid, trapezius, and fascia or the dynamic stabilizers of the AC joint from the clavicle
  - Type VI—A rare inferior displacement of the clavicle under the coracoid with associated brachial plexus and shoulder girdle fractures
- Type III—Represents injuries to both the AC joint capsule and the coracoclavicular ligaments, resulting in horizontal and vertical instability.
  - Surgical treatment is typically reserved for patients who have persistent pain after a 3-month trial of nonsurgical treatment.
  - A relative indication is a sport or job that places a high demand on the shoulder.

Contraindications

- Type I and II injuries
- Coracoid fracture

Based on Lin A, Rodosky MW: Anatomic acromioclavicular joint reconstruction, in Colvin AC, Flatow E, eds: Atlas of Essential Orthopaedic Procedures, *ed 2. Rosemont, IL, American Academy of Orthopaedic Surgeons, 2020, pp 37-42.*

TABLE 1 **Rockwood Classification of Acromioclavicular Joint Injuries**

Type	AC Ligaments	CC Ligaments	Delto-pectoral Fascia	Radio-graphic CC Distance Increase	Radio-graphic AC Appearance	AC Joint Reducible?
I	Sprained	Intact	Intact	Normal (1.1-1.3 cm)	Normal	N/A
II	Disrupted	Sprained	Intact	<25%	Widened	Yes
III	Disrupted	Disrupted	Disrupted	25%-100%	Widened	Yes
IV	Disrupted	Disrupted	Disrupted	Increased	Posterior clavicle displacement	No
V	Disrupted	Disrupted	Disrupted	100% to 300%	N/A	No
VI	Disrupted	Intact	Disrupted	Decreased	N/A	No

AC = acromioclavicular, CC = coracoclavicular, N/A = not applicable.

Adapted from Simovitch R, Sanders B, Ozbaydar M, Lavery K, Warner JJ: Acromioclavicular joint injuries: Diagnosis and management. *J Am Acad Orthop Surg* 2009;17(4):207-219.

- Clavicle fracture
- Glenohumeral arthritis
- Patients who cannot comply with postoperative rehabilitation protocols

PREOPERATIVE IMAGING

Radiography

- True AP
- Axillary lateral view (for type IV injury [**Figure 1**])
- Zanca view (10° to 15° cephalic tilt) with arm unsupported
- Contralateral views may be helpful to compare injury with uninjured shoulder.
- Stryker notch view if coracoid fracture is suspected but not visualized on other films.

Computed Tomography

- Rarely obtained in isolated AC joint injuries
- Can be helpful in the setting of suspected sternoclavicular joint disruption, physeal fracture in patients with open physes, scapular fractures, glenoid fractures, distal clavicle fractures, or proximal humerus fractures

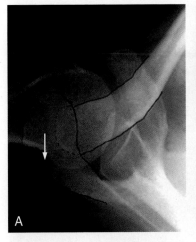 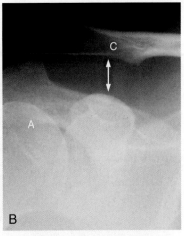

FIGURE 1 Axillary lateral (**A**) and Zanca view (**B**) radiographs demonstrate posterior displacement of the clavicle (posteriorly directed arrow in **A**) and increased coracoclavicular interspace distance (double-headed arrow in **B**), distinguishing this injury as a type IV acromioclavicular joint separation. The acromion (**A**) and clavicle (**C**) are outlined in **A**. (Reproduced from Simovitch R, Sanders B, Ozbaydar M, Lavery K, Warner JJ: Acromioclavicular joint injuries: Diagnosis and management. *J Am Acad Orthop Surg* 2009;17[4]:207-219.)

PROCEDURE

Room Setup/Patient Positioning

- Elevation of 60° on a standard operating table or in beach-chair position (**Figure 2**)
- Support head with foam and turn away from surgical site.
- Place bump under medial scapular border to elevate coracoid anteriorly.
- Preparation area is wide, extending from midline of the chest to midline of the chin and neck to expose sternoclavicular joint; this step is important in case of an unforeseen complication of the underlying subclavian vessels, brachial plexus, or lung.
- Arm draped free

Equipment

- Gelpi retractors, needle-tip Bovie electrocautery, small periosteal elevator, No. 2 nonabsorbable suture, cannulated reamer set, low-profile malleable guidewire, threaded guide pins for cannulated reamers
- Reduction clamps
- Mini C-arm
- Graft-harvesting station if hamstring autograft is obtained
- Suture-passing devices

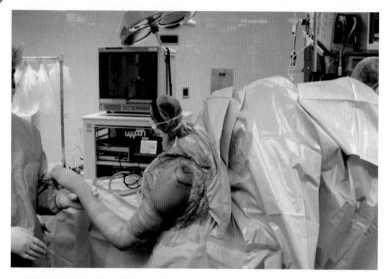

FIGURE 2 Photograph shows beach-chair positioning. The arm is draped free to allow manipulation and manual reduction. (Reproduced with permission from Mostofi A, Rios C, Tennent T, Arciero R, Mazzocca A: Acromioclavicular joint injuries. *Orthop Knowl Online J* 2008;6[4]. https://www.aaos.org/OKOJ/vol6/issue4/SHO020/. Accessed January 25, 2019.)

SURGICAL TECHNIQUE

Exposure

- Make saber-cut incision 3 to 3.5 cm medial to the AC joint in line with the Langer lines and curving medially toward the coracoid (**Figure 3**).
- Using a needle-point Bovie, make full-layer thickness skin flaps down to the deltotrapezial fascia in line with the skin incision.
- "Skeletonize" the clavicle by incising the deltotrapezial fascia off the clavicle in a medial-to-lateral direction, creating anterior and posterior flaps (**Figure 4**).

Trial Reduction

- The fully exposed AC joint is subjected to a trial reduction by pushing up on the elbow, which reduces the scapulothoracic complex toward the anatomically positioned distal clavicle.
- Interposing soft tissue on the distal clavicle may prevent reduction and must be completely cleared to allow the reduction.

Graft Technique

- Gracilis autograft or tibialis allograft can be used.
- Whipstitch the free ends and remove excess tissue to facilitate passage of bone tunnels.

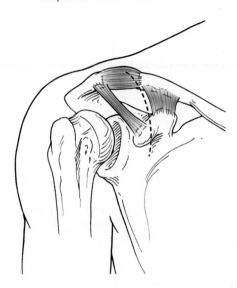

FIGURE 3 Illustration shows the saber-cut skin incision (dashed line) used for acromioclavicular (AC) joint reconstruction. The incision must be lateral enough to allow exposure of the AC joint and extend medial enough to allow access and exposure of the coracoid.

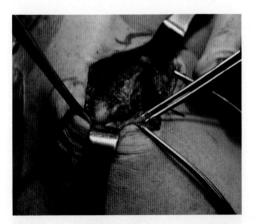

FIGURE 4 Intraoperative photograph shows the elevation of full-thickness deltotrapezial fascial flaps to skeletonize the clavicle; the flaps are preserved for later closure. (Reproduced with permission from Mostofi A, Rios C, Tennent T, Arciero R, Mazzocca A: Acromioclavicular joint injuries. *Orthop Knowl Online J* 2008;6[4]. https://www.aaos.org/OKOJ/vol6/issue4/SHO020/. Accessed January 25, 2019.)

- Expose the coracoid medially and laterally.
- Use a curved suture passer in a medial-to-lateral direction under the coracoid to avoid neurovascular injury; shuttle a looped wire across the coracoid; use the wire to pull the graft and nonabsorbable suture around and underneath the coracoid.

Ligament Reconstruction

- Place threaded cannulated guide pin posteromedially on the clavicle approximately 4.5 cm away from the AC joint for the conoid reconstruction.
- Place a second pin approximately 3 cm from the AC joint centered on the clavicle parallel to the previously placed pin for the trapezoid reconstruction (**Figure 5**).
- Pass a cannulated reamer on power over the guide pins to create bone tunnels; size tunnel according to the graft size; take particular care when reaming over the conoid so as not to breach the posterior cortex of the clavicle.
- Use a Hewson suture passer from superior to inferior to bring the graft ends through the bone tunnels.
- An assistant reduces the AC joint by pushing up on the elbow; be sure to overreduce the AC joint because some long-term displacement is common following reconstruction.

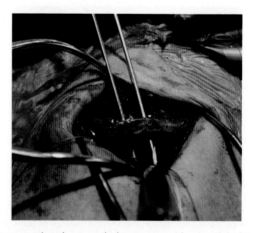

FIGURE 5 Intraoperative photograph shows two guide pins placed in parallel fashion. The conoid guide pin is placed approximately 4.5 cm from the acromioclavicular (AC) joint posteromedially on the clavicle. The trapezoid guide pin is placed about 3 cm from the AC joint lateral to the conoid guide pin and centered on the clavicle. (Reproduced with permission from Mostofi A, Rios C, Tennent T, Arciero R, Mazzocca A: Acromioclavicular joint injuries. *Orthop Knowl Online J* 2008;6[4]. https://www.aaos.org/OKOJ/vol6/issue4/SHO020/. Accessed January 25, 2019.)

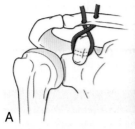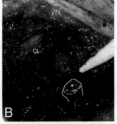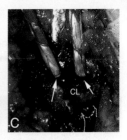

FIGURE 6 Images demonstrate the reconstruction of the coracoclavicular ligaments. **A,** Illustration shows the graft and nonabsorbable suture passed around the coracoid and crossed as the free ends are brought through the conoid and trapezoid bone tunnels. **B,** Intraoperative photograph shows a suture passer passed from medial to lateral around the coracoid tip (*) and used to retrieve the anterior tibialis allograft around the coracoid process. **C,** The graft ends are pulled through two bone tunnels (arrows) in the clavicle (CL) to approximate the pull of the conoid and trapezoid ligaments. (Panels **B** and **C** are reproduced from Simovitch R, Sanders B, Ozbaydar M, Lavery K, Warner JJ: Acromioclavicular joint injuries: Diagnosis and management. *J Am Acad Orthop Surg* 2009;17[4]:207-219.)

- Cycle the graft several times to ensure no displacement or migration is present once the graft is fixed in place.
- With the AC joint overreduced, suture is tied in place in a side-to-side fashion (**Figure 6**).

Closure
- Close deltotrapezial fascia with 0 Vicryl sutures.
- Close deep dermal layer with 2-0 or 3-0 Vicryl sutures.
- Close skin with 4-0 Monocryl suture (Ethicon).

COMPLICATIONS
- Early or late fracture of the coracoid process or clavicle
- Osteolysis of the coracoid or clavicle from nonabsorbable nonbiologic fixation
- Persistent pain
- Recurrent instability
- Loss of reduction
- Persistent deformity
- Subclavian vessel or lung injury secondary to medial and inferior overdissection
- Iatrogenic injury to the brachial plexus or axillary artery

POSTOPERATIVE CARE AND REHABILITATION
- A sling is used for 2 weeks in a normal resting position.
- Initiate pendulum exercises at 2 weeks with continued sling.
- Discontinue sling at 4 weeks; start light activities of daily living.

- At 8 weeks, begin formal physical therapy with active and passive range of motion.
- Initiate light resistance at 3 months.
- Once full strength is regained, return to labor or sports at 4 to 6 months.

PEARLS

- A bump is placed under the medial scapular border for stabilization and anteriorization of the coracoid.
- The head should be tilted maximally away from the surgical field; this will facilitate drilling of the conoid tunnel.
- Full-thickness flaps of the deltotrapezial fascia are made when exposing the clavicle. This is critical for later closure.
- When passing the graft, the medial coracoid must be adequately exposed. Passage of the graft medial to lateral is recommended to avoid injury to the brachial plexus and axillary artery.
- The size of the reamer must be accounted for when placing the guide pins to avoid breaching the posterior or anterior cortex of the clavicle.
- Frayed edges at the whipstitched ends should be adequately débrided to facilitate easy graft passage through the bony tunnels.
- Using heavy, ultra-high-strength nonabsorbable sutures for nonbiologic fixation should be avoided because this increases the risk of late osteolysis of either the coracoid or the clavicle.
- If doubt exists about the size of the bone tunnel, the surgeon should start with a smaller reamer and incrementally increase the reamer size.
- When fixing the graft in place, the joint should be overreduced, because some loss of reduction often occurs over time.
- The graft is cycled several times back and forth through the tunnels to ensure no displacement or migration of the graft is present after it is fixed in place.

Open Reduction and Internal Fixation of Clavicle Fractures

INTRODUCTION
- Clavicle fractures account for 2.6% to 5% of adult fractures
- Historically, nonsurgical management was standard, but with improved surgical techniques, growing evidence shows that surgical management may be beneficial in select patients

CLASSIFICATION
- Clavicle fractures are classified based on their location and the degree of comminution and angulation
- Allman classification system
  - Proximal (2% to 3%)
  - Midshaft (70% to 80%, high-energy, younger patient population)
  - Distal (21%)

PATIENT SELECTION
Indications
- Open fracture
- Floating shoulder
- Impending skin necrosis
- Associated neurovascular injuries
- Multiply injured trauma patients
- Improved outcomes associated with shortening greater than 15 to 20 mm, with 100% displacement, or with comminution

Contraindications
- Nondisplaced or minimally displaced fractures in older, sicker patients
- Low-demand patient or unfit to undergo surgery
- If nonsurgical management pursued, use a sling and course of non–weight bearing

---

Based on Scordino LE, DeBerardino TM: Open reduction and internal fixation of clavicle fractures, in Colvin AC, Flatow E, eds: Atlas of Essential Orthopaedic Procedures, *ed 2. Rosemont, IL, American Academy of Orthopaedic Surgeons, 2020, pp 43-47.*

PREOPERATIVE IMAGING

- Orthogonal views of the clavicle
- AP chest views (**Figure 1**) to rule out chest injury (eg, rib fractures, hemothorax, pneumothorax)
- Apical oblique view—Shoulder tilted 45° anterior, and radiograph beam 20° cephalad
- Abduction lordotic view—X-ray directed 25° cephalad with shoulder abducted above 135°; useful to assess healing postoperatively
- Preoperative CT can help to evaluate nonunion and medial fractures extending to the sternoclavicular joint

PROCEDURE FOR MIDSHAFT CLAVICLE FRACTURE
Room Setup/Patient Positioning

- Supine or modified beach-chair position on radiolucent table with intraoperative fluoroscopy available
- Bump placed at medial portion of scapula
- Arm in pneumatic arm positioner (**Figure 2**)

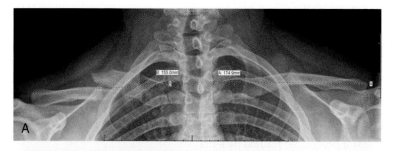

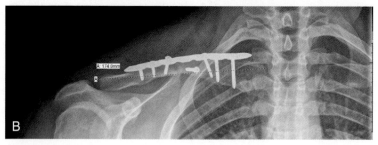

FIGURE 1 AP radiographs of a patient with a right midshaft clavicle fracture. **A**, Preoperative radiograph demonstrates 2 cm of shortening. **B**, Postoperative radiograph shows that clavicle length symmetric to the uninjured left side is restored with plate fixation. An interfragmentary screw and a contoured clavicle fracture plate were used.

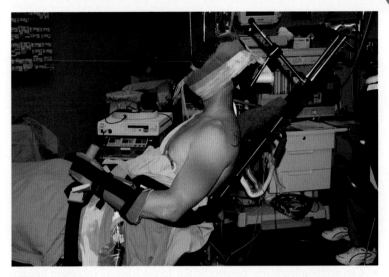

FIGURE 2 Photograph shows a patient with a pneumatically controlled arm positioner in place for left shoulder surgery.

- Palpate and mark the acromion borders, coracoid, triangular soft spot in acromion; acromioclavicular (AC) joint is anterior to soft spot and lateral to coracoid; palpate S-shaped clavicle
- Location of incision depends on fixation technique used

Surgical Technique

Plate Fixation

- Position plate superiorly or anteroinferiorly; if placed anteroinferiorly, extraperiosteally elevate the deltoid and pectoralis major. An anteriorly placed plate has less hardware prominence and avoids neurovascular structures with posteriorly directed screws
- Assigned laterality contoured clavicle plates for superior plating. Using contralateral plate or flipping the plates can help with contouring
- A standard 3.5-mm limited-contact dynamic compression plate can be bent to fit the clavicle
- Make a longitudinal incision inferior to and in line with the clavicle (**Figure 3**)
- Preserve the supraclavicular nerves as they cross perpendicular to the clavicle deep to the platysma (**Figure 4**)
- Apply the plate to the clavicle with a minimum of three bicortical screws on either side of fracture

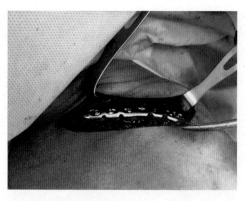

FIGURE 3 Intraoperative photograph shows the typical incision for a left midshaft clavicle fracture. A contoured clavicle plate and screws are used to maintain reduction.

- Can apply a lag screw perpendicular to the fracture fragment to compress fracture fragments in simple fracture patterns
- In comminuted fractures, a bridge plating technique can be used extraperiosteally without fracture exposure

Intramedullary Nailing
- Used for simple fractures of the middle third of the shaft with good cortical contact after fixation
- Drawback—Does not resist torsional forces as well as plating

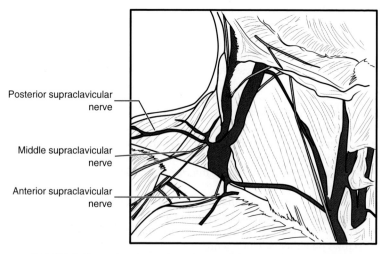

FIGURE 4 Illustration shows the anatomy of the supraclavicular nerves.

- Advantages—Smaller incisions, less soft-tissue stripping, easier removal of hardware
- Technique:
  - Make a 2- to 3-cm incision over fracture fragment; dissect off platysma while protecting middle branches of supraclavicular nerve
  - Elevate medial fragment with bone-reducing clamp, prepare canal, and avoid disruption of the medial cortex
  - Elevate lateral fragment (externally rotate the arm), and pass drill through the posterolateral cortex of the lateral fragment; avoid placing the opening too superior to prevent pin prominence
  - Pass pin into the lateral fragment out the posterolateral opening; make a small incision over the palpable tip; reduce fracture, and drive the pin medially into the medial segment and toward the anterior cortex
  - Place two nuts on lateral portion of the pin to provide compression against the lateral cortex of the clavicle and to provide means to advance and remove the clavicle pin throughout fixation and prevent medial pin migration
  - Clavicle pin can be removed under general or local anesthesia at 10 to 12 weeks

Additional Considerations for Lateral Clavicle Fractures

- Lateral fractures are often nondisplaced and occur most commonly in low-demand, elderly patients
- Higher risk of nonunion with nonsurgical treatment but with little effect on quality of life
- Fixation options include coracoclavicular screws, plate or hook-plate fixation, or the suture and sling technique; late intervention for AC joint arthritis may include arthroscopic or open distal clavicle resection

Additional Considerations for Medial Clavicle Fractures

- Largely nonsurgical management
- Usually extra-articular and minimally displaced
- Posterior fracture displacement and compression on superior mediastinal structures mandate treatment
- Closed reduction attempted first
- Fixation with either suture or nonabsorbable wide fiber suture obviates need to return to the operating room for hardware removal

COMPLICATIONS

- Infection (0% to 18%)
- Nonunion, which is often symptomatic in younger patients; incidence of 2.2% with plate fixation, 2.0% with intramedullary nail fixation, 15.1% after nonsurgical treatment
- Malunion, which is symptomatic, especially with greater than 15 to 20 mm initial displacement; need for hardware removal

- Neurologic complications usually result from the initial injury, with fracture compression of nerves, or as a late complication such as from hypertrophic callus, that is, thoracic outlet syndrome, which is associated with ulnar symptoms (0.3% to 20% [**Figure 4**])
- Refracture can result from a too-early return to sports, alcohol abuse, or epilepsy, as well as after removal of hardware (0% to 8%)
- Osteoarthritis of AC joint, which is treated with distal clavicle excision
- Subclavian artery or vein injury (rare), which typically occurs secondary to drill penetration or during fracture mobilization; repair by a vascular or cardiothoracic surgeons may be indicated

POSTOPERATIVE CARE AND REHABILITATION

- Sling used for 4 weeks
- Range of motion at wrist and elbow and active-assisted motion of shoulder to 90° of forward flexion to be performed at least five times a day can be performed immediately postoperatively
- Once radiographic and clinical healing occurs at 6 weeks, begin resisted activity
- Return to sport no earlier than 3 months after injury

PEARLS

- Landmarks should be drawn out, including the superior/inferior clavicle margins, the sternoclavicular joint, the AC joint, and the planned incision.
- The patient should be in a modified beach-chair position.
- A bump placed under the medial portion of the scapula to be operated on helps with reduction.
- A pneumatically controlled arm positioner allows precise positioning of the arm, negates the weight of the arm, facilitates the surgery, and frees fellows and residents to assist with the operation rather than hold the limb during the case.
- Placing the incision inferior to the clavicle avoids hardware that lies directly under the skin.
- Fracture reduction is aided by reduction clamps.
- The authors of the chapter prefer anterior-inferior plating, because it avoids hardware prominence, for patients who will carry heavy loads over their shoulders, such as firefighters.
- In addition to standard radiographs, an apical oblique view is helpful to evaluate fracture reduction.
- Nonabsorbable suture can be looped around small segmental fragments to bring them into apposition with the main fracture lines.

Open Treatment of Medial and Lateral Epicondylitis

PATIENT SELECTION
- Symptoms include pain, local tenderness, and limitations of activity.
- Typically managed nonsurgically with rest and restriction
- Surgical intervention is reserved for patients with persistent symptoms after 6 months of nonsurgical treatment
- For lateral epicondylitis, must rule out:
  - Cervical radiculopathy
  - Radial tunnel syndrome
  - Posterolateral impingement
  - Posterolateral rotatory instability
  - Radiocapitellar arthrosis
- For medial epicondylitis, must rule out:
  - Ulnar neuritis
  - Attenuation of the ulnar collateral ligament with instability
  - Flexor/pronator muscle ruptures

PREOPERATIVE IMAGING
- Lateral and medial epicondylitis are clinical diagnoses; use imaging to rule out other conditions
- Plain radiographs can identify calcifications in 20% of patients
- MRI can evaluate for intra-articular pathology, assess the collateral ligaments, or aid in determining the extent of tears in the extensor flexor or pronator origin; increased signal intensity on T2-weighted images may be seen in extensor carpi radialis brevis (ECRB) tendon origin or common flexor origin

PROCEDURE
Room Setup/Patient Positioning
- General anesthesia preferred provided patient comorbidities permit; regional anesthesia used if needed, but may not allow for postoperative neurologic examination

---

Based on Baker CL III, Akins J, Baker CL Jr: Open treatment of medial and lateral epicondylitis, in Colvin AC, Flatow E, eds: Atlas of Essential Orthopaedic Procedures, *ed 2. Rosemont, IL, American Academy of Orthopaedic Surgeons, 2020, pp 48-51.*

- Supine position with surgical arm on arm board with tourniquet; hand and lower arm in stockinette

Special Instruments/Equipment/Implants

- No special equipment required for open treatment of either condition
- If a surgeon prefers to drill the epicondyle to stimulate a healing response, a 0.062-in Kirschner wire or a 5/64-in drill bit is needed

Surgical Technique

Lateral Epicondylitis

- Make incision 4 cm anteromedial to the epicondyle (**Figure 1**); divide subcutaneous tissues to level of deep fascia over extensor tendons
- Identify and split (to a 2- to 3-mm depth) the interval between the extensor carpi radialis longus (ECRL) and the extensor digitorum communis

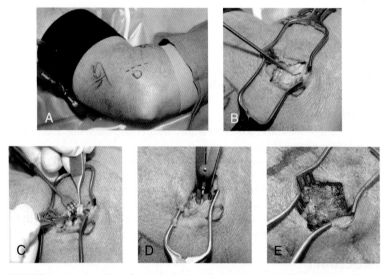

FIGURE 1 Intraoperative photographs demonstrate open treatment of lateral epicondylitis. **A**, The planned incision is marked anteromedial to the palpable and outlined lateral epicondyle. **B**, The interface between the anterior extensor carpi radialis longus (ECRL) and the more posterior extensor digitorum communis (EDC) is identified and superficially split. **C**, The pathologic extensor carpi radialis brevis tendinosis tissue is resected en bloc with a scalpel. **D**, A rongeur is used to roughen the lateral condyle to create a healing response. **E**, The ECRL/EDC aponeurosis is repaired with a running No. 1 absorbable suture (not visible in this photograph). Débridement and closure of the extensor split is complete.

- Separate the ECRL from deep ECRB by scalpel dissection and retract anteriorly; the ECRB tendon is visible
- Pathologic angiofibroblastic tendinosis is typically dull, gray, and friable in appearance
- Excise abnormal tissue en bloc with scalpel
- Perform Nirschl scratch test, using a scalpel to scrape away remaining abnormal edematous tendinosis tissue, which should peel away, exposing healthy tissue
- Use a drill or rongeur on the lateral condyle to enhance vascular supply, and reapproximate the ECRL and extensor digitorum communis aponeurosis with running No. 1 absorbable suture
- Place in well-padded posterior splint at 90° after closure

Medial Epicondylitis

- Identify medial epicondyle, olecranon, and position of ulnar nerve.
- Make a 4- to 5-cm incision starting at the medial epicondyle and directed distally (**Figure 2**); divide subcutaneous tissues to level of flexor pronator deep fascia; avoid damaging the medial antebrachial cutaneous nerve
- Sharply detach and reflect the pronator teres and flexor carpi radialis from the medial epicondyle; identify abnormal dull, gray, edematous tissue, and complete resection with scalpel scratch test
- Manage the ulnar nerve depending on preoperative clinical examination; if preoperative symptoms were present, decompress; if moderate/severe ulnar neuropathy or a subluxating or dislocating nerve was present, transpose the ulnar nerve into the anterior subcutaneous tissue

COMPLICATIONS

- Persistent pain
- Surgical dissection can cause iatrogenic injury to the lateral ulnar collateral ligament, leading to posterolateral rotatory instability
- Injury to the medial antebrachial cutaneous nerve with neuroma formation
- Inadequate flexor pronator mass repair can lead to flexor pronator weakness and pain
- Valgus instability due to ulnar collateral ligament injury
- If ulnar neuropathy is not identified preoperatively, progression of symptoms and poor outcome can result

POSTOPERATIVE CARE AND REHABILITATION

- Brace for therapy and vigorous activities of daily living
- At 1 week, remove splint and begin range-of-motion exercises for wrist and elbow

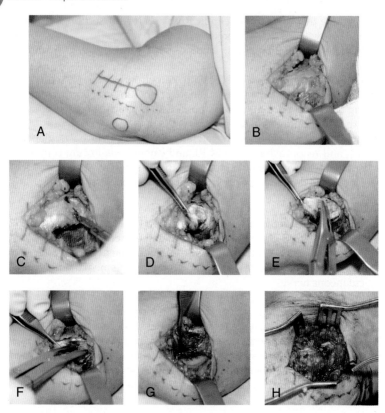

FIGURE 2 Intraoperative photographs demonstrate open treatment of medial epicondylitis. **A,** The planned incision is marked, progressing distally from the medial epicondyle. The medial epicondyle, the olecranon, and the position of the ulnar nerve are outlined on the skin. **B,** Dissection progresses through the subcutaneous tissues to the deep fascia of the flexor pronator mass. **C,** The planned area of detachment of the flexor pronator origin is outlined and scored with a scalpel. **D,** A portion of the flexor pronator origin is detached from the medial epicondyle and reflected distally. A good cuff of tissue remains proximally for later repair. **E,** The tendinosis tissue is removed from the undersurface of the flexor pronator tendons. **F,** A rongeur is used to roughen the medial epicondyle to create a healing response. **G,** The ulnar nerve is identified and either simply decompressed or transposed, based on the presence and severity of preoperative ulnar nerve symptoms. **H,** The flexor pronator mass is securely repaired back to the medial epicondyle with No. 1 absorbable sutures.

- At 4 to 6 weeks, begin gentle strengthening exercises once full painless motion obtained
- At 3 to 4 months, when painless full motion and strength are achieved, full sports may be resumed

PEARLS

- When detaching the flexor pronator origin, the surgeon must leave a healthy cuff of tissue to the medial epicondyle to permit a secure repair that will allow early rehabilitation.
- The Nirschl scratch test is an effective method to separate and remove the pathologic tissue from the healthy tendon.
- Appropriate postoperative rehabilitation greatly aids the return of painless full elbow motion and strength.

8 Distal Biceps Repair

PATIENT SELECTION
- Single traumatic "pop" at time of rupture
- Aching pain persisting weeks to months
- Grossly palpable and visible signs of proximal retraction of the distal biceps
- Weakness with elbow flexion and forearm supination
- The O'Driscoll hook test can identify absence of the distal insertion; elbow is at 90° flexion with forearm supinated; if distal tendon is intact, examiner can hook finger underneath the tendon

Indications
- Acute, complete rupture of distal biceps tendon
- Typically seen in middle-aged active men
- Failure of 3 to 4 weeks of physical therapy (PT), if patient does not initially want surgery

Contraindications
- Partial ruptures
- If pain continues despite physical therapy and weakness is unacceptable, then surgical repair is performed

PREOPERATIVE IMAGING
- AP and lateral radiographs
- MRI (**Figure 1**)
  - ▶ May help confirm diagnosis or be of use in the case of partial ruptures
  - ▶ Can identify amount of tendon retraction for preoperative planning

 VIDEO 8.1 Cadaveric Demonstration: Distal Biceps Tendon Fixation. Anthony A. Romeo, MD, Augustus D. Mazzocca, MS, MD (32 min)

Based on Andelman SM, Geaney LE, Arciero RA, Romeo AA, Mazzocca AD: Distal biceps repair, in Colvin AC, Flatow E, eds: Atlas of Essential Orthopaedic Procedures, ed 2. Rosemont, IL, American Academy of Orthopaedic Surgeons, 2020, pp 52-58.

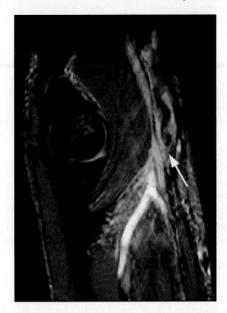

FIGURE 1 Sagittal MRI shows a torn biceps tendon (arrow) retracted 6 cm.

PROCEDURE

Special Instruments/Equipment/Implants

- Author preference: Cortical button with interference screw fixation using an 8 mm × 12 mm interference screw
- Other options include bone tunnels, suture anchors, a cortical button, or interference screw alone

Surgical Technique

- Anatomic technique—Reinsert the tendon to the radial tuberosity
- Nonanatomic technique—Suture biceps tendon to brachialis

 VIDEO 8.2 Distal Biceps Repair. Steven M. Andelman, MD, Anthony A. Romeo, MD, Augustus D. Mazzocca, MS, MD, Robert A. Arciero, MD (6 min)

Two-Incision Approach

- Historical approach is an anterior S-shaped incision, through which the tendon is identified, and a posterolateral incision, through which the lateral epicondylar extensor muscle group is detached from the radial tuberosity

- Current incisions include the S incision, horizontal incision, and vertical incision
- Make a transverse incision 2 to 4 cm long over anterior elbow
- Incise deep fascia; identify and tag biceps tendon (can be retracted up to 7 cm)
- Protect lateral antebrachial cutaneous nerve where it exits between the biceps and brachioradialis
- Dissect down to radial tuberosity; with forearm supinated, advance Kelly clamp along medial border of the radial tuberosity to dorsolateral aspect of proximal forearm (**Figure 2**)
- Flex elbow and make second posterolateral incision over palpated clamp
- Incise fascia over muscle mass
- Develop interval between anconeus and extensor carpi ulnaris; take care not to go too posterior and disrupt the periosteum
- Incise the supinator to expose the radial tuberosity with the arm in maximal pronation to protect the posterior interosseous nerve (PIN)

Single-Incision Approach

- Make a transverse incision 2 to 4 cm long over anterior elbow, three fingerbreadths distal to elbow crease
- Dissect subcutaneous tissue carefully to identify lateral antebrachial cutaneous nerve
- Identify biceps tendon; usually found in the interval between the flexor and extensor muscle groups; if the tendon cannot be localized secondary to chronicity and retraction, a second incision may be made proximally over the palpated stump; identify the nerve in the antecubital fossa, where it exits between the biceps and brachioradialis; hemostasis is imperative at this point

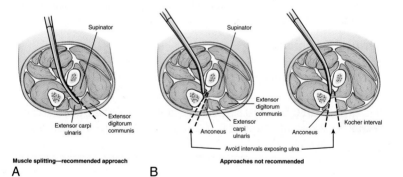

FIGURE 2 Illustrations demonstrate the two-incision approach for distal biceps repair. **A,** With the arm supinated, a clamp is advanced along the medial border of the radial tuberosity to the dorsolateral aspect of the proximal forearm. **B,** Exposure of the ulna should be avoided to reduce the risk of heterotopic ossification.

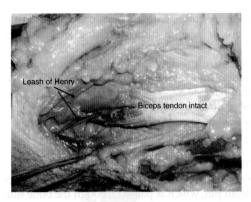

Leash of Henry

Biceps tendon intact

FIGURE 3 Intraoperative photograph shows the leash of Henry, an arcade of veins that is identified during the dissection.

- Identify the leash of Henry (**Figure 3**); dissect down to radial tuberosity; hypersupinate to expose radial tuberosity; place a blunt, small Hohmann retractor on the ulnar side to avoid injury to the PIN

Tendon Preparation

Two-Stitch Preparation

- Starting 12 mm proximal to stump, place Krackow locking stitch traveling distally through the prepared tendon; pass through the inner two holes of the cortical button 2 to 3 mm from the end, and travel up the tendon in Krackow stitch
- Second suture is passed through the distal tendon and cortical button, then travels proximally to the level of the first suture and again distally to meet the starting point

FiberLoop (Arthrex) Preparation

- Use a Keith needle attached to a loop of No. 2 FiberWire (Arthrex) starting 3 cm from the end of the tendon
- Thread distally in Krackow-type fashion
- Débride distal end into a bullet shape
- Supplement with No. 2 FiberWire traveling proximally then distally— two or three stitches if an interference screw is to be used; cut the FiberLoop and load through the center holes of the cortical button

Bone Preparation

- Identify tuberosity and ream the proximal cortex
- Place cannulated reamer guide pin in the central area of the tuberosity with at least 2 mm of good bone on either side
- Hypersupinate arm to ensure perpendicular drilling and place 7- or 8-mm cannulated reamer down the pin to make sure no cortical blowout will occur

POSTOPERATIVE CARE AND REHABILITATION

- Arm in soft dressing, immediate active-assisted flexion, active extension with gravity
- Sutures are removed at 7 to 10 days
- Full active range of motion at 3 to 4 weeks
- Strength training at 10 weeks
- Return to work between 3 and 6 months

PEARLS

- The lateral antebrachial nerve usually travels with superficial veins, which will help with identification.
- The position of the bicipital tuberosity coincides with the position of the thenar eminence.
- Hypersupination allows maximal exposure of the tuberosity.
- Permanent retraction on the radial side should be avoided to minimize PIN injuries.
- The tunnel should be angled ulnarly to avoid damaging the PIN.
- The insertion of the distal biceps tendon is 2 mm × 14 mm. It twists 90° from the musculotendinous junction to the insertion of the ulnar side of the tuberosity.
- Every attempt should be made to recreate the anatomy after rupture with the tendon on the ulnar side.
- Polyetheretherketone screws are recommended because they are stronger and will not strip as easily as bioabsorbable screws.
- A tap should be used on the tuberosity.

Ulnar Collateral Ligament Reconstruction

INTRODUCTION

Ulnar Collateral Ligament Anatomy

- The ulnar collateral ligament (UCL) is composed of multiple bundles
  - Anterior bundle is the primary restraint to the valgus forces of up to 290 N and angular velocities exceeding 3,100°/s that occur during throwing of a baseball
  - Posterior bundle
  - Transverse bundle
- The UCL originates at the inferior surface of the medial epicondyle of the humerus and inserts onto the sublime tubercle of ulna

History of UCL Reconstruction (Figure 1)

- The Jobe technique returned athletes to their previous level of play; as originally described, it involved the submuscular transposition of the ulnar nerve, elevation of the flexor-pronator mass to expose the tunnel sites, and figure-of-8 graft configuration through a tunnel on the ulnar side and three large holes in the medial epicondyle
- Author preference is the docking technique, a muscle-splitting approach using a single bony tunnel with two small converging holes, which simplifies graft tensioning and reduces the risk of medial epicondyle fractures

 VIDEO 9.1 Ulnar Collateral Ligament Reconstruction Using the Docking Technique. Joshua S. Dines, MD; David W. Altcheck, MD (5 min)

- An alternate hybrid technique is called the DANE TJ technique

PATIENT SELECTION

Indications

- Medial-side elbow pain with UCL insufficiency that prevents patient from competing at the normal level

Based on Dines JS, Altchek DW: Ulnar collateral ligament reconstruction, in Colvin AC, Flatow E, eds: Atlas of Essential Orthopaedic Procedures, ed 2. Rosemont, IL, American Academy of Orthopaedic Surgeons, 2020, pp 59-64.

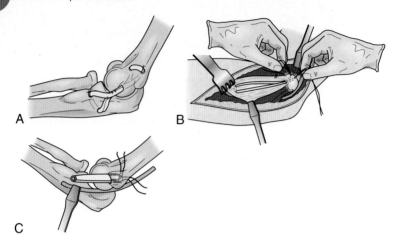

FIGURE 1 Illustrations show elbow ulnar collateral ligament reconstruction techniques. **A,** The figure-of-8 graft configuration as described by Jobe et al. **B,** Graft configuration using the docking technique. **C,** A hybrid technique of interference screw fixation on the ulna and the docking technique in the humerus, also referred to as the DANE TJ technique.

- During history, examiner must ask about the location of pain and presence of ulnar nerve symptoms
- Radiographs may show calcification in ligament, bone spurs, or avulsion fractures
- MRI can confirm UCL insufficiency and identify associated injuries, including flexor-pronator tears, loose bodies, and cartilage injury

Contraindications
- The use of biologics to augment conservative treatment has improved outcomes, particularly in partial tears
- Athlete with no plans or options to continue playing the same sport
- Patient who is unwilling or unable to complete a lengthy rehabilitation

PROCEDURE
Preoperative Planning
- Determine type of graft
  - ▶ Most common are the gracilis and palmaris longus tendons
  - ▶ Less common are the split flexor carpi radialis, toe extensor, and plantaris tendon
- Arthroscopy should be used in patients with preoperative physical and imaging findings consistent with valgus extension overload
- Ulnar nerve transposition is not indicated unless persistent preoperative paresthesias, motor symptoms, or nerve subluxation are present

Patient Positioning/Special Equipment

- Supine position with arm draped free on arm board
- Equipment includes a nonsterile tourniquet, No. 1 nonabsorbable suture, suture shuttle, and 1.5-mm, 3.5-mm, 4-mm, and 4.5-mm burrs; if a fracture of the sublime tubercle is present or in revision cases, a Bio-Tenodesis screw (Arthrex) or EndoButton (Smith & Nephew) may be required for graft fixation

Surgical Technique

- Authors' preferred harvest graft is palmaris longus tendon
  - Make a transverse incision proximal to the wrist flexor crease
  - Use No. 1 braided nonabsorbable suture on an OS-2 needle to place a Krackow locking stitch in the tendon
  - Harvest tendon using a tendon stripper
  - Multiple-incision harvesting technique—After initial incision is made, make two additional transverse incisions about 7 and 15 cm proximal to wrist to expose entire length of tendon
  - Amputate graft proximally at musculotendinous junction
- Place graft in moist sponge on back table, then exsanguinate the arm
- Use a medial approach to the elbow (**Figure 2**)
  - Begin just proximal to the medial epicondyle, extending distally over the UCL to a point 2 cm past sublime tubercle. Protect the medial antebrachial cutaneous nerve (**Figure 3**)
  - Split the common flexor mass through the posterior third within the anterior fibers of the flexor carpi ulnaris
  - Use a periosteal elevator to bluntly expose anterior bundle of the ligament
  - Incise ligament in line with its fibers to expose the joint; recommend tagging each side of the ligament with 2-0 Vicryl suture (Ethicon) to aid in closure; be mindful of the ulnar nerve when placing suture in posterior half of the ligament
- Prepare ulnar tunnel
  - Expose the sublime tubercle while protecting the ulnar nerve posteriorly
  - Use a 3.5-mm burr to make holes anterior and posterior to the tubercle; maintain a minimum of a 1-cm bone bridge between the holes
  - Connect the holes with a curved curet
  - Use looped surgical steel on a curved needle to place a looped suture through the tunnel, which will be used later to pass the graft
- Prepare humeral tunnel
  - Use a 4- or 4.5-mm burr, adjusted to graft size, to drill longitudinally along the axis of the medial epicondyle to a depth of 15 mm to make a humeral socket on the anterior-distal aspect of the medial epicondyle

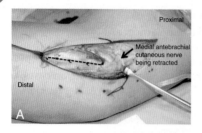
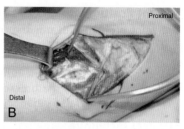
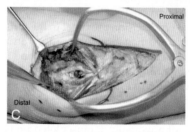

FIGURE 2 Intraoperative photographs show the initial steps in the docking technique for elbow ulnar collateral ligament reconstruction. **A,** The dashed line shows the planned muscle-splitting approach through the posterior third of the common flexor mass within the anterior fibers of the flexor carpi ulnaris. **B,** The native ligament is exposed and then incised in line with its fibers. **C,** The ulnar tunnel has been created, taking care to preserve at least a 1-cm bone bridge between the holes.

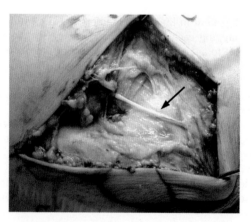

FIGURE 3 Intraoperative photograph shows the medial antebrachial cutaneous nerve (arrow), which frequently crosses the incision site. It should be protected throughout the case.

- ⟩ Place a straight curet in the socket, and use a 1.5-mm burr to make two puncture holes with at least a 1-cm bony bridge connecting to the socket anterior to the intermuscular septum
- ⟩ Bring two separate shuttling sutures through the exit punctures with looped surgical steel, and clamp the sutures
- Prepare graft (**Figure 4**)
  - ⟩ Pass graft through the ulnar tunnel using the previously placed shuttling suture
  - ⟩ Repair the native ligament with the previously placed sutures with the arm in 30° elbow flexion and forearm supination while applying varus stress
  - ⟩ Using shuttling suture from the posterior humeral puncture hole, the posterior limb of the graft is shuttled, "docking" it into the medial epicondylar socket
  - ⟩ Applying tension through the grasping suture maintains docking; by applying varus force with the elbow flexed and forearm supinated, the elbow is reduced while the graft is cycled and tensioned

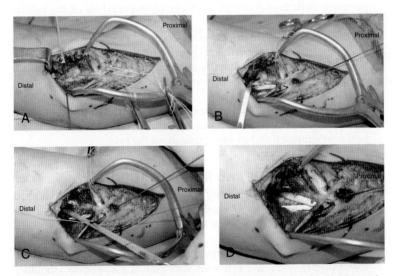

FIGURE 4 Intraoperative photographs show graft placement for the docking technique in elbow ulnar collateral ligament reconstruction. **A,** The graft is brought into the ulnar tunnel using the previously placed shuttling suture. **B,** The posterior limb of the graft is docked into the humeral socket, after which the anterior limb is marked where it will enter the socket. **C,** A running Krackow stitch is placed from the mark to a point 1 cm proximal. **D,** The final graft configuration is shown.

▸ Position the second (anterior) graft limb next to the humeral tunnel to approximate the length of graft that will fit in the humeral socket

▸ Pass No. 1 braided nonabsorbable suture in Krackow fashion for the estimated length to be positioned in the tunnel, typically between 10 and 15 mm

▸ Maintain tension on the posterior limb and reduce the elbow with varus stress and supination; using the previously placed suture shuttle, bring the Krackow suture through the humeral socket and out the anterior exit hole

▸ Tension the Krackow stitch to dock the anterior limb adjacent to the posterior limb within the humeral socket; tie down grasping sutures over the bone bridge

▸ Deflate the tourniquet, repair fascia with 0 Vicryl suture, close wound in layers, and immobilize the arm in a posterior splint with the elbow flexed 45° and the forearm supinated

COMPLICATIONS

- Ulnar nerve injury—The nerve is susceptible during drilling of the posterior ulnar tunnel and the posterior connection hole on the medial epicondyle
- Fracture of ulnar bone bridge—Can occur intraoperatively or late in postoperative period; minimize risk by preserving at least 1 cm of bony bridge between the anterior and posterior drill holes on the ulna; potential fracture salvage intraoperatively is a Bio-Tenodesis screw and/or an EndoButton
- Medial antebrachial cutaneous nerve injury—Can lead to painful neuroma; minimize through meticulous subcutaneous dissection; identify nerve on approach and protect throughout the case

POSTOPERATIVE CARE AND REHABILITATION

- At 7 to 10 days postoperatively, switch from plaster splint to hinged elbow brace with 40° to 90° motion
- Advance range of motion until 15° to 105° by week 4
- Discontinue brace at 6 weeks
- During first 3 to 4 months, physical therapy focuses on rotator cuff, forearm, core, and lower extremity strengthening and elbow/shoulder range of motion
- Interval throwing program begins at 4 months
- Throwing off mound begins at 8 months
- Discourage competitive pitching until 9 to 12 months after surgery

PEARLS

- Meticulous dissection during the surgical approach will help prevent medial antebrachial cutaneous nerve injury.

- Maintaining at least 1 cm of bone between the holes of the ulnar tunnel is important to prevent fracture.

- The surgeon must take care to not be too shallow in the medial epicondyle when drilling the humeral socket.

- After both limbs of the graft have been docked into the humerus, the arm is held in about 30° of flexion, with the forearm supinated and a varus stress applied when tying the sutures.

- A structured postoperative protocol focusing on strengthening and motion of the elbow and shoulder, as well as throwing mechanics, is critical to achieving a successful outcome.

Arthroscopic Management of Femoroacetabular Impingement

PATIENT SELECTION

- Femoroacetabular impingement syndrome (FAIS) is a bony incongruity that results in a cascade of pathological hip issues
  - Femoral side—Cam lesion
  - Acetabular side—Pincer lesion
  - Both sides—Combined cam and pincer lesion

Symptoms

- Groin pain or pain lateral and posterior to the hip with walking, running, sports
- Difficulty sitting for prolonged periods or putting on socks or shoes
- Clicking or catching sensation in hip joint

Evaluation

- History, including queries about childhood hip abnormalities
- Physical examination
  - Range of motion (ROM)
  - Strength of hip muscle groups
  - Stinchfield test (examiner resists active hip flexion)
  - Posterior impingement test
  - Flexion, abduction, and external rotation (FABER) test
  - Flexion, adduction, and internal rotation (FADIR) test
- Rule out hernia and other extra-articular pathology
- Intra-articular anesthetic injection response correlates with intra-articular abnormality

Indications

- Failed nonsurgical management, including NSAIDs, physical therapy
- Try nonsurgical management for at least 6 to 12 weeks

Contraindications

- Advanced arthrofibrosis or ankylosis of hip joint

Based on Colvin AC, Chahla J, Nho SJ: Arthroscopic management of femoroacetabular impingement, in Colvin AC, Flatow E, eds: Atlas of Essential Orthopaedic Procedures, *ed 2. Rosemont, IL, American Academy of Orthopaedic Surgeons, 2020, pp 65-70.*

- Severe obesity
- Arthritis
- Advanced osteonecrosis

PREOPERATIVE IMAGING

- Standard AP pelvis radiographs
  - ▹ Distance between sacrococcygeal junction and pubic symphysis should be 32 mm in males and 47 mm in females
  - ▹ Lateral center-edge angle (LCEA)—Borderline normal is 20° to 24°; dysplastic is less than 20°
  - ▹ Pincer impingement—LCEA greater than 39°
  - ▹ Tönnis angle—Represents acetabular volume and femoral head coverage
    - − Horizontal line drawn from teardrop to teardrop, and a line tangential to sourcil
    - − Normal is −10° to 10°
    - − >10° indicative of acetabular dysplasia
    - − <−10° indicative of pincer deformity
- Dunn view—Obtained at 45° or 90° used to evaluate femoral head sphericity and contour of head-neck junction
  - ▹ Alpha angle characterizes anterior deformity of cam type (>50° for cam)
- AP and frog-lateral or cross-table lateral hip radiographs to assess
  - ▹ Acetabular version
  - ▹ Presence/absence of cam lesion (**Figure 1**)
  - ▹ Herniation pits in femoral neck
  - ▹ Joint space narrowing
  - ▹ Os acetabuli
- False-profile view—To measure anterior CEA
- CT—Three-dimensional reconstructions help determine bony abnormalities

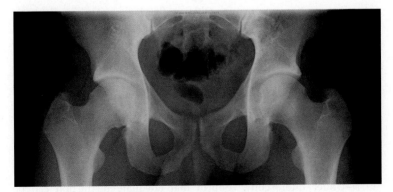

FIGURE 1 AP pelvis radiograph demonstrates bilateral cam lesions.

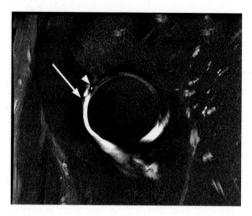

FIGURE 2 Sagittal T2-weighted magnetic resonance arthrogram demonstrates a paralabral cyst (arrow) and a perforation in the anterosuperior labrum (arrowhead).

- Magnetic resonance arthrography—Better than MRI at assessing intra-articular soft-tissue pathology (labral tears)
- MRI/MRA findings
  - Paralabral cysts (**Figure 2**)
  - Herniation pits at head-neck junction
  - Os acetabuli

VIDEO 10.1 Arthroscopic Management of Pincer- and Cam-Type Femoroacetabular Impingement. Christopher M. Larson, MD; Rebecca M. Stone, ATC (8 min)

PROCEDURE
Room Setup/Patient Positioning
- Supine position on fracture table or flat table with hip distractor (**Figure 3**)
  - General anesthesia, followed by examination under anesthesia to assess for side-to-side differences in ROMWell-padded feet and peroneal post
  - Position pelvis at level of peroneal post and slide toward nonsurgical side
  - Hip in neutral flexion, 0° of abduction, and 20° of internal rotation of the foot pad and position ipsilateral arm over chest, away from surgical field
  - Slight traction on contralateral leg before distracting surgical side to stabilize torso
  - Under fluoroscopy, confirm that adequate distraction can be obtained, then release traction for preparation and draping

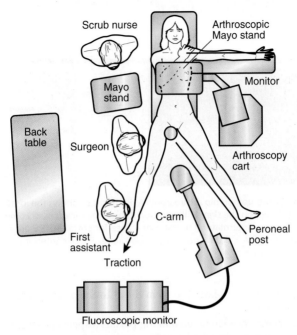

FIGURE 3 Illustration depicts the room setup for hip arthroscopy.

Special Instruments/Equipment/Implants

- C-arm fluoroscopy
- Fracture table or hip distractor
- 30° and 70° arthroscopes
- Slotted cannula
- Concave extended-length 4.2-mm shaver
- Arthroscopic 5.5-mm burr
- Flexible electrothermal probe
- Suture-passing device
- Small biocomposite bone anchors

Surgical Technique

- Portals (**Figure 4**)
  - ▷ Anterolateral—Mark at anterior border of superior aspect of greater trochanter
  - ▷ Posterolateral (used only for posterior pathology)—Mark at posterior border of superior aspect of greater trochanter
  - ▷ Anterior—Make at the intersection of a vertical line drawn distally from the anterior superior iliac spine and a horizontal line drawn medially from top of greater trochanter

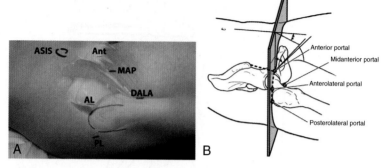

FIGURE 4 Portals used in hip arthroscopy. **A,** Photograph shows the locations of the portals drawn on the skin. **B,** Illustration depicts the locations of commonly used portals. AL = anterolateral portal, Ant = anterior portal, ASIS = anterior superior iliac spine, DALA = distal anterolateral portal, MAP = midanterior portal, PL = posterolateral portal

> ▶ Midanterior—Mark 4 to 6 cm distal to the anterolateral portal at a 60° angle
> ▶ Cut only the skin when making portals (especially anterior portal) to avoid injuring the lateral femoral cutaneous nerve
> ▶ Distal anterolateral portal (DALA) important for most anterior anchors

- To identify anterolateral portal, use a 17-gauge spinal needle placed under fluoroscopy; confirm placement in joint with air arthrogram (**Figure 5**)
- Insufflate joint with 40 mL normal saline mixed with 1% lidocaine with epinephrine
- Avoid penetration into the labrum with spinal needle
- Turn bevel of needle to avoid damaging cartilage; pass nitinol guidewire through the spinal needle, and confirm with fluoroscopy that guidewire does not go past the medial wall of the acetabulum
- Dilate portal 5 to 6 mm to allow insertion of the arthroscopy sheath
- Introduce 70° arthroscope and visualize outside-in placement of midanterior portal
- Identify triangle formed by the labrum, femoral head, and joint capsule
- With arthroscope in anterolateral portal, use a beaver blade to make capsulotomy, then switch arthroscope to the anterior portal, and use banana blade in anterolateral portal to make lateral capsulotomy; connect to previous capsulotomy
- Débride capsule with shaver
- Capsular suspension sutures can be placed to improve visualization

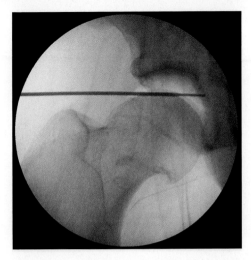

FIGURE 5 Air arthrogram visualized on fluoroscopy confirms intracapsular placement of the spinal needle.

- Perform diagnostic arthroscopy, first through the anterolateral portal then through the anterior portal
  - The 70° arthroscope is best for visualizing the periphery of the hip joint, labrum, and inferior acetabular fossa
  - The 30° arthroscope is best for visualizing the central acetabulum, femoral head, and superior acetabular fossa
  - Assess quality of cartilage
    - Wave sign (bubbling of cartilage) at chondrolabral junction indicates unstable cartilage
    - Microfracture is done on any focal Outerbridge grade IV chondral lesions
  - Assess quality of labrum
    - Once a pincer-type impingement is identified, with the arthroscope in anterolateral corner and banana knife in anterior portal, separate labrum from edge of acetabulum; use shaver or burr to prepare acetabulum edge
    - Under fluoroscopy, address pincer lesions and anterior wall overcoverage
    - Use a punch or biter to trim unstable cartilage from the acetabular rim
    - Place an 8.5-mm cannula in the working portal to pass instrumentation for repair
    - With arthroscope in midanterior portal, place 3-mm or smaller anchors through the anterolateral portal beginning superiorly on the acetabular rim; suture anchor or knotless repair can be performed using device of surgeon's choice

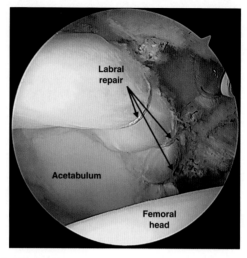

FIGURE 6 Arthroscopic view demonstrating a labral repair in a right hip.

- Place arthroscope in anterolateral portal, and place remaining anchors through DALA portal along anterior rim as needed
- Degenerative labral tissue cannot be repaired and should be débrided to a stable transition zone (**Figure 6**)
- Examine femoral head-neck junction for a cam deformity
  - Release traction, and flex hip 45° to allow inspection
  - Can perform T-capsulotomy to improve visualization
  - Intraoperative fluoroscopy helps locate lesion
  - Internal rotation allows visualization of the lateral aspect of cam lesion, and external rotation allows visualization of its medial aspect
  - Identify lateral retinacular vessels and medial synovial fold; do not resect farther than these landmarks of resection
  - Use a 5.5-mm arthroscopic burr for resection
  - At completion of cam resection, take hip through full ROM to identify persistent impingement
  - Close T-capsulotomy longitudinal portion using three simple interrupted No. 2 high–tensile strength sutures passed with a suture-shuttling device. Close the interportal capsulotomy in similar fashion

COMPLICATIONS

- Incomplete resection of cam, pincer, or both lesions
- Neurapraxia of sciatic, pudendal, femoral, and/or lateral femoral cutaneous nerves
- Instrument breakage

- Iatrogenic cartilage injury
- Femoral neck fracture
- Postoperative dislocation
- Fluid extravasation leading to abdominal compartment syndrome

POSTOPERATIVE CARE AND REHABILITATION

- Continuous passive motion machine immediately after surgery
- Physical therapy, beginning with passive ROM, starts on postoperative day 2
- Stationary bike without resistance immediately after surgery
- For surgery without osteoplasty, 20-lb foot-flat weight bearing for 2 weeks
- With osteoplasty, restricted weight bearing for 4 weeks
- With microfracture, restricted weight bearing for 6 to 8 weeks
- Progressive strengthening begins 6 weeks after full weight bearing is allowed
- Between 3 and 6 months, running and sport-specific training may begin
- Return to sport once strength and power are optimal, usually at 6 months postop

PEARLS

- Confirmation that adequate distraction can be obtained on the hip should be obtained under fluoroscopy before preparation and draping.
- A distal accessory anterolateral portal often is helpful when both intra-articular pathology and a cam lesion need to be addressed.
- An adequate capsulotomy facilitates the use of instruments.
- A DALA portal can help avoid fixation failure for the most anteriorly placed anchors (use of curved instruments can also help with the attack angle of the cannula).
- If the hip has been under traction for 2 consecutive hours, the traction should be released. It can be reapplied later if the intra-articular work has not been completed.

VIDEO REFERENCE

 Video 10.1 Larson CM, Stone RM: *Instructional course lectures*, in *Arthroscopic Management of Pincer- and Cam-Type Femoroacetabular Impingement* [video]. Edina, MN, AAOS, 2009, vol 58, chap 39, pp 423-436.

11 Meniscectomy

INTRODUCTION

- Most symptomatic meniscal tears are irreparable
- Subtypes of meniscal tears
  - Simple patterns
    - Radial
    - Vertical/longitudinal
    - Horizontal
  - Complex patterns
    - Displaced bucket-handle
    - Parrot-beak
    - Multiplanar
    - Degenerative
  - Meniscal root tear
- Location of tear directly affects the capacity for repair (**Figure 1**)
  - Peripheral third of meniscus—Red-red zone
  - Middle third—Red-white zone
  - Central third—White-white zone

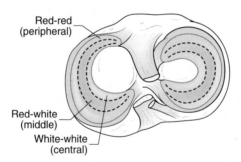

FIGURE 1 Illustration of the vascular zones of the meniscus. The medial meniscus is on the left, and the lateral meniscus is on the right.

Based on Bayomy AF, Bader S, Parker RD, Saluan PM: Meniscectomy, in Colvin AC, Flatow E, eds: Atlas of Essential Orthopaedic Procedures, ed 2. Rosemont, IL, American Academy of Orthopaedic Surgeons, 2020, pp 71-79.

- The menisci occupy 60% of the contact area between the tibia and femur
- They transmit 50% of compression forces across the joint
- The medial meniscus is a secondary stabilizer against anterior translation in the anterior cruciate ligament–deficient knee
- The lateral meniscus plays a much greater role in force transmission than the medial meniscus; the convexity of the lateral plateau leads to point loading after meniscal débridement, increasing peak contact pressures in the lateral compartment (235% to 335% in total meniscectomy)
- Relative medial joint congruity buffers the effect of the meniscectomy on peak pressures
- Circumferential meniscal collagen fibers distribute hoop stresses; disruption may lead to degeneration

PATIENT SELECTION

Indications for Repair

- Repair should be attempted for young patient with red-red and red-white zone tears
- For radial tears, repair red-red and red-white zones and débride white-white zone
- Stable partial-thickness vertical tears less than 10 mm in the red-red zone may be treated with abrasion or trephination or left alone if showing healing

Indications for Meniscectomy

- Irreparable tears due to
    - Degeneration
    - Fragmentation
    - Tearing of avascular tissue
- Goals of meniscectomy
    - Resect irreparable and/or unstable meniscal tissue
    - Leave a contoured and smooth tissue remnant
    - Preserve over 50% of meniscal rim
- Controversial in patients with underlying degenerative arthritis.
    - FIDELITY study group published in 2017 had 2-year follow-up of arthroscopic partial meniscectomy (APM) versus sham surgery. No statistical difference in outcomes. Multiple recent systematic reviews show that APM has equal or worse outcomes to nonsurgical management

DIAGNOSIS

- History—Symptoms include
    - Knee pain
    - Mechanical locking

- Pain or swelling with activities of daily living, work, or sports
- Knee effusion
- Physical examination
  - McMurray test
  - Apley grind test
  - Thessaly test has an accuracy greater than 94% in anterior cruciate ligament–intact knees
- Discoid meniscal tears
  - Typically present in a child younger than 10 years
  - Intermittent painful episodes of dramatic popping or snapping of the knee
  - Unable to fully extend knee
  - Clunk is elicited on examination with flexion, extension, and circumduction

PREOPERATIVE IMAGING

- Radiographs include 30° flexion lateral, Merchant, AP weight-bearing in extension, and 45° PA flexion weight-bearing views
- Best MRI sequences (**Figure 2**)
  - 3-T MRI
  - Proton-density weighted
  - High-resolution
  - Fast spin-echo sequences
  - Can identify and delineate tear morphology and location
  - Used to rule out other intra-articular pathology
- Discoid meniscus
  - Radiographic indicators
    - Tibial spine hypoplasia
    - Widening of lateral joint line
    - Flattening of lateral femoral condyle on PA view
  - MRI indicators diagnostic of discoid meniscus
    - Thickened bow tie on coronal view
    - Greater than three cuts with continuity of the anterior and posterior horn on a 5-mm-thick sagittal cut view

PROCEDURE
Setup/Equipment

- Supine position
- Spinal, regional, or general anesthesia
- With or without antibiotic prophylaxis
- The authors do not use a tourniquet
- Sequential compression device on contralateral leg
- Positioning
  - Leg holder placed 5 to 8 cm proximal to superior pole of the patella; a post can suffice
  - Drop foot of the table

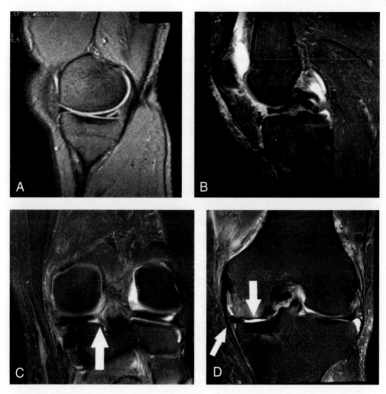

FIGURE 2 Magnetic resonance images (3-T) show meniscal tears. **A**, Horizontal tear of the posterior horn extending to the inferior surface. **B**, Double posterior cruciate ligament sign, indicative of a displaced bucket-handle tear. **C**, Meniscal root tear (arrow) on coronal view. **D**, A tear at the root (large arrow) and extrusion of the meniscus (small arrow).

- Equipment includes
  - Standard arthroscopy pump
  - Meniscal shaver (4.5-mm or 5.0-mm), straight and curved
  - Meniscal punches—Straight and curved, backbiter, and 90° punch
  - Toothed grasper
- Preoperative examination under anesthesia
- Intra-articular injection—10 to 50 mL of 1% lidocaine or 0.25% bupivacaine, both with at least 1:400,000 epinephrine

Surgical Technique

Arthroscopy

- Portal placement
  - Landmarks—Inferior pole of patella and edges of patellar tendon

- Lateral portal is placed 0.5 to 1 cm off lateral edge of patellar tendon at level of inferior pole of patella; used for joint insufflation
- Medial portal is placed 1 to 2 cm off medial edge of patellar tendon in soft spot
- Outflow portal, if physician prefers, can be placed superolateral or superomedial
- Additional portals
  - Posteromedial portal is useful for loose bodies in back of knee; create under direct visualization to avoid injury to neurovascular structures
  - Transpatellar portal (rare) can be used to do work in the center of the knee
  - Anteromedial portal created under direct visualization
- Begin with routine diagnostic arthroscopy; visualize all three compartments through full range of motion (ROM) and medial and lateral gutters as well as suprapatellar pouch
  - Medial compartment
    - Application of valgus stress with foot externally rotated at 10° to 20° of knee flexion improves visualization of posterior horn
    - Avoid iatrogenic injury by slowly stressing ligaments, avoiding sharp movements
  - Lateral compartment
    - Apply varus stress in figure-of-4 position through distal fibula to avoid ankle injury
    - Option of resting lower leg on well-padded Mayo stand with knee at 45° to 90° of flexion

Evaluation and Tear Morphology

- Flounce sign reassures for an intact medial meniscus
- Identify tear and evaluate for stability, size, extent, location, configuration, and vascularity (position on meniscus) (**Figure 3**)

Radial Tears

- Hybrid repair/débridement technique should be considered for tears extending into red-red zone or red-white zone, especially in young patients
- Use curved biter to remove the meniscus en bloc to minimize free body generation
- Portal size must accommodate fragment removal
- Use shaver to remove any additional debris
- For lateral meniscal tear in right knee
  - Use right-curved or straight biter from medial portal
  - Resect anterior to the tear; create a gentle contour to minimize unstable/acute edges
  - Hybrid repair/débridement can also be performed with repair of the peripheral segment of the tear

Posterior

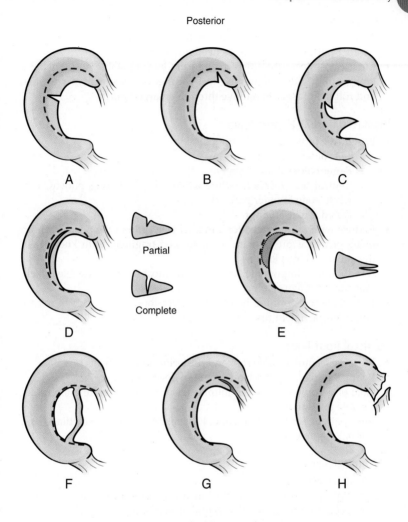

Anterior

FIGURE 3 Illustrations show meniscal resections. **A** and **B**, Radial tears (**B** is radial root tear). **C**, Parrot-beak tear. **D**, Vertical/longitudinal tears. **E**, Horizontal tear. **F**, Bucket-handle tear. **G**, Root tear. **H**, Root avulsion. The resection line is shown by red dashes.

Horizontal Cleavage Tears

- Preserve larger leaf of tear (either superior or inferior)
- Use biter for most of resection with smoothing by shaver; alternatively, a shaver can be used for the entire resection

Vertical Tears

- Tears less than 10 mm in length can be trephinated or abraded
- Smaller partial-thickness tears need no treatment
- Must excise tears that displace into the joint to stable tissue using a grasper and "gator" technique; lock the meniscal segment in a grasper, and roll the grasper to remove through enlarged portal

Displaced Bucket-Handle Tears

- Prognostic indicators against repair
  - Tear older than 6 months
  - Patient older than 30 years
  - Central tear location (white-white zone in young patient, red-white zone in older patient)
  - Failed repair attempt
- Reduce with blunt trocar; for a medial tear, offload the posterior horn using posterior pressure on the displaced fragment with knee at 20° flexion and valgus loading
- If reduction is impossible, amputate the most easily accessible attachment and remove en bloc
- Posteromedial portal is helpful to access the posterior horn; release anterior attachment first

Meniscal Root Tears

- Preserve as much stable root and posterior horn tissue as possible
- Poor prognosis, rapid advancement of degeneration
- Goal of débridement is to minimize tissue removal while establishing a stable transition zone
- Ideal patient has healthy meniscal tissue, intact articular cartilage, and normal alignment

Discoid Meniscus

- Watanabe classification
  - Type 1—Normal tibial attachment, covers plateau
  - Type 2—Normal tibial attachment, semilunar
  - Type 3—Wrisberg ligament variant; no discoid shape; only femoral attachment; more mobile than normal meniscus
- Assess anterior meniscus for instability
- Perform saucerization if symptomatic; preserve as much peripheral rim as possible; start at free edge of tear and resect back to front using standard biters and shavers
- Outcomes of symptomatic discoid meniscus débridement are favorable when saucerization is performed over subtotal or total meniscectomy

COMPLICATIONS

- Infection
  - Typically presents 7 to 10 days postoperatively; best treated with immediate aspiration for organism identification and urgent arthroscopic lavage
  - Intravenous antibiotics for 2 to 4 weeks
  - Maintain ROM to avoid arthrofibrosis
- Deep vein thrombosis (DVT) and pulmonary embolism (PE) in high-risk patients

POSTOPERATIVE CARE AND REHABILITATION

- Early mobilization is key
- May bear weight as tolerated with crutches
- Thigh-high compression stocking on surgical limb helps reduce venous stasis
- Chemical prophylaxis for DVT prevention as deemed necessary
- Physical therapy is prescribed to regain mobility, ROM, and quadriceps function and strength as needed
- Postoperative patient expectations and risks for progression of arthritis should be discussed at length
- DVT/PE prevention measures
  - Sequential compression device placement
  - Consider chemical prophylaxis if history of DVT/PE, hypercoagulable state such as factor V deficiency, or use of oral contraceptive

PEARLS

- Current evidence does not support a benefit of arthroscopic partial meniscectomy (APM) in patients with degenerative meniscal tears.
- Placing the leg holder just proximal to the superior pole of the patella maximizes control of the limb.
- A well-padded Mayo stand placed under the lateral malleolus helps facilitate control of the limb for exposure of the lateral compartment.
- Consider tear morphology with respect to the zones of the meniscus, particularly with radial tears, because hybrid resection/repair techniques may help preserve the peripheral third if the tear extends to the capsule.
- Preserve as much stable posterior horn and root attachment as possible when treating nonrepairable posterior horn and root tears.
- Take patient status and tissue health into account when deciding when to perform meniscal resection and how much is necessary.

PATIENT SELECTION

- A strong correlation exists between meniscectomy and the increased risk of developing radiographic signs of knee osteoarthritis.
- Goal of meniscal preservation surgery is to protect the articular cartilage from changes in joint contact pressures seen with meniscal deficiency.

Indications

- Based on patient age, chronicity, and concomitant injuries
- Classification of tears
  - ▹ Tear location—Meniscal zones classify tears based on the vascular supply.
    - – Red-red zone—Richly vascular
    - – Red-white zone—Transitional
    - – White-white zone—Avascular
  - ▹ Tear pattern (**Figure 1**)
    - – Longitudinal—Ideal for repair
    - – Radial split—Amenable to repair
    - – Horizontal flap
    - – Parrot beak—Amenable to repair
- Ideal candidate is young patient with longitudinal tear involving red-red zone.
- Other factors
  - ▹ Healing improved if concomitant cruciate ligament is reconstructed at time of surgery likely due to the increased marrow elements in the knee from drilling the tibial and femoral tunnels.
  - ▹ Isolated repairs can be enhanced with fibrin clot, capsular rasping, or microfracture of intercondylar notch.

Relative Contraindications

- Significant intrasubstance degeneration
- Isolated tearing in avascular white-white zone
- Presence of tricompartmental arthritis
- Unstable displaced meniscal fragments

Based on Bowman KF Jr, Harner CD: Meniscal repair, in Colvin AC, Flatow E, eds: Atlas of Essential Orthopaedic Procedures, ed 2. Rosemont, IL, American Academy of Orthopaedic Surgeons, 2020, pp 67-72.

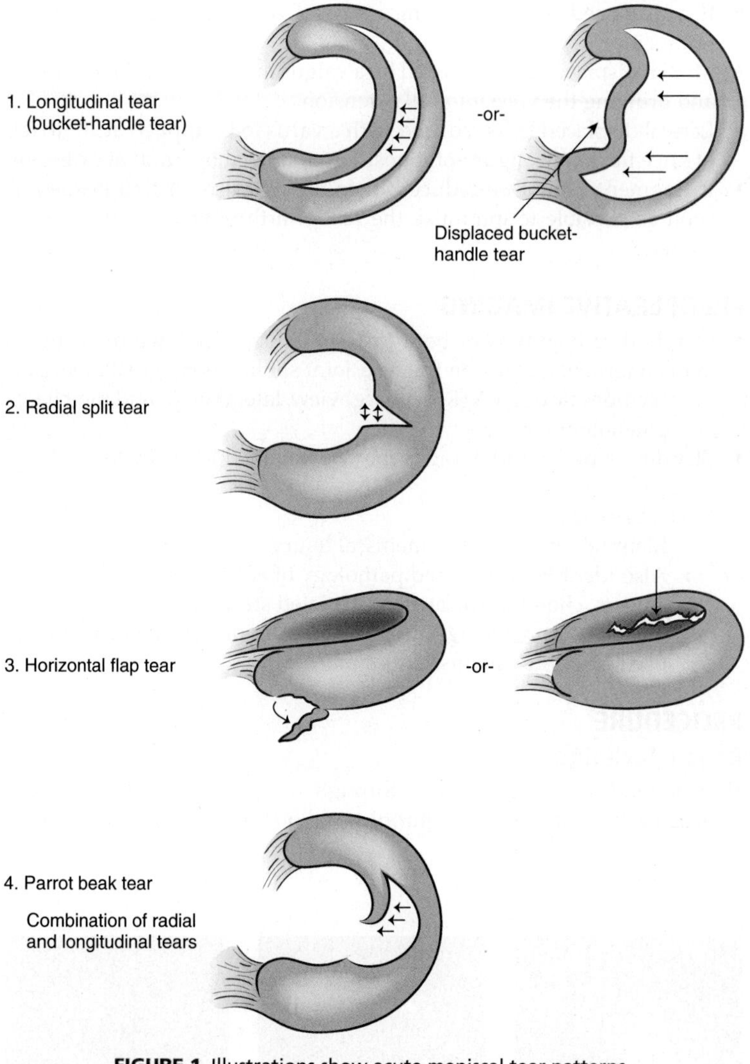

1. Longitudinal tear (bucket-handle tear)

-or-

Displaced bucket-handle tear

2. Radial split tear

3. Horizontal flap tear

-or-

4. Parrot beak tear

Combination of radial and longitudinal tears

FIGURE 1 Illustrations show acute meniscal tear patterns.

Clinical Evaluation

- Knee is evaluated for:
  - Signs of joint line tenderness
  - Effusion
  - Limitation of range of motion
  - Ligamentous laxity
  - Apley's and McMurray's test

- If a displaced tear is blocking range of motion, attempt to reduce fragment.
- Medial displaced tears reduced by a valgus force at 10° to 30° of flexion and bringing the knee into full extension
- Lateral displaced tears reduced with a varus force applied at 20° to 60° of knee flexion (ie, figure-of-4 position) followed by gradual extension
- If fragment cannot be reduced, then a surgical reduction needed as soon as possible to minimize the risk of arthrofibrosis and chondral damage.

PREOPERATIVE IMAGING

- Standard radiographs of both knees; evaluate for fracture, arthritis, joint congruency, avulsion fracture, joint subluxation, patellar height.
  - Includes flexion PA (Rosenberg) view, lateral view, and merchants patellofemoral view
- Standing long leg radiographs may be obtained to evaluate mechanical alignment.
- MRI (**Figure 2**)
  - Identifies and classifies meniscal injury
  - Also identifies associated pathology of cruciate and collateral ligaments, chondral surfaces, and related structures
  - Oblique coronal images in plane of anterior cruciate ligament are used to identify meniscal root pathology.

PROCEDURE

Repair Technique

- Inside-out: passing sutures through cannulas introduced intra-articularly and retrieved through a counter incision in the skin (author's preference)

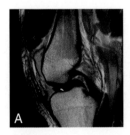 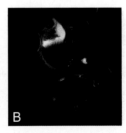 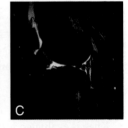

FIGURE 2 Sagittal magnetic resonance images demonstrate various meniscal tear patterns. **A**, T1-weighted MRI shows a displaced longitudinal (bucket-handle) tear of the medial meniscus. The displacement into the notch creates the classic "double posterior cruciate ligament" sign. **B**, A radial split tear of the lateral meniscus presents as a gap on the T2-weighted MRI. **C**, T2-weighted MRI shows a nondisplaced longitudinal tear of the lateral meniscus in the red-red zone.

- Outside-in: passing a cannula, usually an 18-gauge spinal needle, from an extra-articular location and passing a suture that is retrieved within the joint
- All-inside: placing sutures arthroscopically without using a counter incision

Room Setup/Patient Positioning
- Supine position
- Bump under ipsilateral sacroiliac joint, lateral post at level of greater trochanter
- 10-lb sandbag secured to operating table to let limb rest at 90° knee flexion
- No tourniquet
- Well-padded contralateral extremity
- IV antibiotics within 60 minutes of incision

Special Instruments/Equipment/Implants
- Standard meniscal repair surgical set consists of various rasps.
- Henning retractor for suture passage
- Pre-bent metallic cannulas for zone-specific targeting of meniscal pathology
- Multiple suture options—Authors prefer a 2-0 nonabsorbable suture with a non-Kevlar core (prevents further injury to meniscal tissue during suture passage).

Surgical Technique
- Landmarks—Inferior patellar pole, tibial tubercle, Gerdy's tubercle, fibular head, and medial and lateral joint lines; the soft spot at fibular neck is palpated and marked (corresponds to location of peroneal nerve).
- Anterolateral portal placed 2 to 3 mm lateral to edge of patellar tendon at level of inferior pole of patella
- Anteromedial portal placed 1 cm medial to patellar tendon at same level
- Superolateral outflow portal placed 1 cm proximal to superior pole of patella
- Posteromedial portal (if needed) determined under direct visualization with spinal needle
- Inject incisions with 0.25% bupivacaine and 1:100,000 epinephrine for hemostasis
- Diagnostic arthroscopy includes evaluation of presence and pattern of meniscal injury.
- Method of repair chosen based on location and pattern
- Most tears can be addressed with an inside-out technique, but far anterior tears may require the use of outside-in sutures.
- Lateral meniscal repair

- ▶ Incision (**Figure 3**)—3- to 4-cm longitudinal incision immediately posterior to the lateral collateral ligament; two-thirds of incision inferior to joint line, one-third superior.
- ▶ Approach
  - – Skin sharply incised
  - – Dissection down to level of biceps femoris
  - – Plane between long and short heads of the biceps femoris developed
  - – Underlying tendon of lateral head of gastrocnemius identified
  - – The space between the lateral head of the gastrocnemius muscle and lateral joint capsule is developed.
- Medial meniscal repair
  - ▶ Incision (**Figure 4**)—3- to 4-cm incision centered over junction of middle and posterior thirds of medial femoral condyle, with two-thirds of incision distal to the joint line
  - ▶ Approach
    - – Skin sharply incised
    - – Dissection carried down to first medial retinacular layer
    - – Saphenous nerve and branches are protected.
    - – Open first retinacular layer in line with skin incision.
    - – Blunt dissection to identify joint line and medial joint capsule
  - ▶ The interval formed by the posteromedial capsule, medial head of the gastrocnemius, and semimembranosus tendon is used.
- Fibrin clot
  - ▶ Can be used to aid healing when isolated meniscal tear is present
  - ▶ Prepared on surgical field and placed into meniscal tear after suture placement (**Figures 5** and **6**) but before the sutures are tied down to the capsule

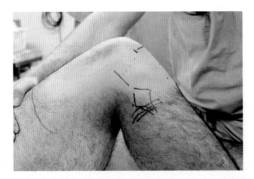

FIGURE 3 Photograph shows lateral meniscal procedures being performed through a 3- to 4-cm longitudinal incision placed posterior to the lateral collateral ligament at the junction of the middle and posterior thirds of the lateral femoral condyle. The incision is placed 1 cm proximal to the joint line and extended 2 to 3 cm distal to the joint line.

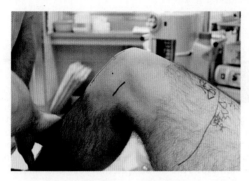

FIGURE 4 Photograph shows medial meniscal injuries being addressed through a 3- to 4-cm incision that is centered over the junction of the middle and posterior third of the medial femoral condyle.

- Following the surgical approach, the edges of the meniscal tear and adjacent synovium are rasped to promote healing.
- Arthroscope is placed in portal adjacent to site of repair, and arthroscopic cannulas are placed in contralateral portal; this improves suture angle and protects posterior neurovascular structures.

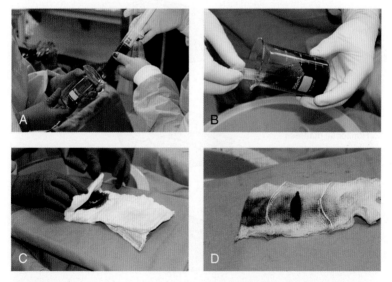

FIGURE 5 Photographs show preparation of an autologous fibrin clot, which is frequently used to augment healing in the setting of isolated meniscal repair. **A,** After harvesting from the patient, 60 mL of sterile venous blood is transferred to a beaker. **B,** The blood is gently rolled/stirred with a frosted glass stir rod to create the clot. The clot is gently compressed with gauze (**C**) into a fibrinous matrix (**D**).

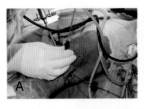 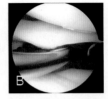 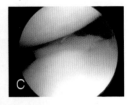

FIGURE 6 Images show the placement of the fibrin clot during meniscal repair.
A, Photograph shows the introduction of the clot into the knee through a 5-mm cannula. The arthroscopic inflow is turned off to facilitate clot placement.
B, Arthroscopic view shows the clot being manipulated into the meniscal repair.
C, Arthroscopic view shows the clot secured with additional sutures.

- Configurations for meniscal repair (**Figure 7**)
  - Performed from anterior to posterior, ideally using vertical mattress sutures
  - Horizontal mattress sutures are also acceptable for additional reinforcement.

1. Vertical mattress 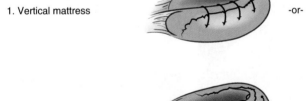 -or-

2. Horizontal mattress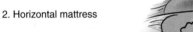

3. Combination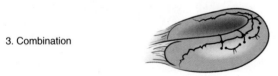

FIGURE 7 Illustration shows the suture configurations for meniscal repair. Meniscal sutures are ideally placed in a vertical mattress fashion to maximize the biomechanical strength of the repair. Horizontal mattress sutures also can be used if the tibiofemoral compartment is tight or to augment the vertical mattress sutures for complete reapproximation of the tear edges.

- Sutures are passed through the meniscus and capsular tissue and retrieved through the surgical incision.
- The knee is brought into 20° of extension, and the sutures are tied onto the joint capsule.

COMPLICATIONS

- Rare, but could have significant consequences, so must be identified and treated promptly
- Immediate postoperative complications include surgical-site infection, deep vein thrombosis, and stiffness.
  - Neurovascular injuries from posterior placement of needle-type all inside meniscus repair devices have also been reported.
  - Patients are routinely seen within 5 to 7 days.
  - Antibiotics are not routinely prescribed.
  - Deep vein thrombosis prophylaxis only for those with elevated risk
  - If flexion or extension deficits are seen, physical therapy and postoperative clinical visits are increased; if no improvement in 3 to 4 months, manipulation under anesthesia, arthroscopic lysis of adhesions, and application of an extension drop-out cast are performed.

POSTOPERATIVE CARE AND REHABILITATION

- Hinged knee brace for 6 weeks
  - Placed at the end of the case
  - Isolated meniscal tear—Locked in 20° of flexion
  - With anterior cruciate ligament reconstruction—Locked in full extension
- Toe-touch weight bearing, with crutches, for 6 weeks, followed by transition to full weight bearing under guidance of physical therapist over the next 6 to 8 weeks
- Knee flexion restricted to 0° to 90° for 6 weeks, then progressive unrestricted flexion
- Home exercises—Isometric quadriceps sets, straight-leg raises, and ankle/calf pumps twice daily for the first week
- Progressive strength training initiated; light jogging allowed at 12 to 16 weeks

PEARLS

- Approach all meniscal tears as potentially repairable.
- The maximum amount of meniscal tissue should be preserved in young patients.
- Success of repair can be enhanced by using autologous fibrin clot, meniscal rasping, or microfracture of the intercondylar notch.

13 Meniscal Root Repair

INTRODUCTION

- Medial meniscal root tears (MMRTs) are a subset of meniscal injuries.
- They are radial tears located within 1 cm of tibial meniscal attachment.
- MMRTs can lead to meniscal extrusion, loss of normal meniscus function, altered knee kinematics, and increased peak contact pressures leading to arthritis.
- Posterior MMRTs more common in middle-aged women. Lateral meniscal root tears (LMRTs) are more common in those with anterior cruciate ligament (ACL) tear

PATIENT SELECTION

Indications

- Isolated symptomatic MMRTs with minimal arthritis
- Failure of nonsurgical management with continued activity-limiting pain
- LMRTs with a concomitant anterior cruciate ligament (ACL) tear

Contraindications

- Medial joint space narrowing with Fairbank changes on flexion weight-bearing PA radiographs
- Asymmetric varus alignment (>3°) and medial joint space narrowing on long-cassette radiographs
- Diffuse International Cartilage Repair Society grade 3 or 4 chondral changes

PREOPERATIVE IMAGING

- Radiography
  - 45° flexion weight-bearing PA views of both knees, lateral views, and Merchant patella views
  - Assess for arthritis, patellar height (lateral), patellar tilt/subluxation (Merchant).
  - Long-cassette AP view to determine overall limb alignment

---

Based on Meghpara M, Harner CD, Vyas D: Meniscal root repair, in Colvin AC, Flatow E, eds: Atlas of Essential Orthopaedic Procedures, *ed 2. Rosemont, IL, American Academy of Orthopaedic Surgeons, 2020, pp 88-94.*

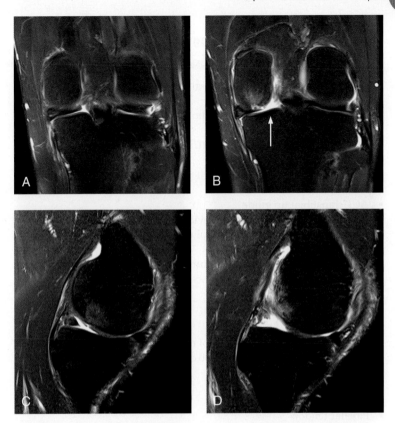

FIGURE 1 Coronal (**A** and **B**) and sagittal (**C** and **D**) T2-weighted MRIs demonstrate a medial meniscal root tear (MMRT) (arrow), which is identified by increased signal intensity within the meniscal root that extends to the articular surface. Extrusion of the medial meniscus also is noted. As a result of a complete radial tear, the two fragments are separated and take on the appearance of an empty meniscal space (**C** and **D**). An associated medial femoral condyle articular cartilage lesion also can be seen.

- MRI
  - Identify tear on contiguous coronal images and sagittal images (**Figure 1**).
  - A varying degree of injury is seen, from mild fraying to a full-thickness tear.
  - A tear is identified by increased signal intensity in the meniscal root that extends to the articular surface on T2-weighted images.
  - Extrusion of the meniscus more than 3 mm beyond the margin of tibial plateau and an empty meniscus sign also may be present in root tear.

PROCEDURE

Room Setup/Patient Positioning

- Supine position
- Ipsilateral hip bump
- 10-lb sandbag to support flexed knee at 90°
- Lateral post at level of midthigh
- We do not use tourniquet or leg holder.

Special Instruments/Equipment/Implants

- 30° arthroscope
- 4.5-mm full-radius resectors (straight and curved)
- Arthroscopic curet
- ACL transtibial tip guide
- Self-retrieving suture passing device
- Suture shuttle with looped nitinol wire
- Meniscal rasp
- No. 2 nonabsorbable braided sutures with a closed loop on one end
- 4.5-mm cancellous screw with washer or cortical fixation device

Surgical Technique

Examination Under Anesthesia

- Performed to assess knee range of motion, effusion, ligamentous laxity
- Inject 1% lidocaine with 1:100,000 epinephrine for hemostasis

Key Landmarks

- Patella
- Patellar tendon
- Medial joint line
- Tibial tubercle

Portals and Incisions

- Portals
    - Anterolateral—viewing portal
    - Anteromedial
- A 2 cm longitudinal incision is made on the anteromedial aspect of the tibia to drill the tibial tunnel.

Diagnostic Arthroscopy

- Perform diagnostic arthroscopy with the arthroscope in anterolateral portal and probe in anteromedial portal.
- Can perform reverse notchplasty by using a 4.5 mm full-radius resector (shaver) to remove bone from the posterior aspect of the notch to improve visualization for medial meniscus root repairs
- Figure-of-4 position is used to visualize the lateral root.

- Under direct visualization and tactile probing, the root should be confirmed to be repairable.

 VIDEO 13.1 Arthroscopic posterior medial meniscus root repair using a single transtibial tunnel. Video by Dharmesh Vyas, MD, PhD; Mitchell Meghpara MD (3 min)

Preparation of the Insertion Site
- Use the curved shaver, a meniscal rasp, and/or an arthroscopic curet to prepare a broad tibial insertion site down to bleeding bone
- Débride edges of meniscal root to aid in healing

Suture Passage
- Arthroscope is in anterolateral portal
- Self-retrieving suture passing device is passed through the anteromedial portal loaded with a No. 2 nonabsorbable suture in the lower jaw. A medial meniscus root repair is illustrated in **Figure 2**.
- Open lower jaw under the root of the meniscus near its normal bony attachment
- Deploy trigger and the upper jaw captures the suture, and then remove from joint, forming a cinch stitch.
- Repeat so that two cinch stitches are placed side by side for added security.

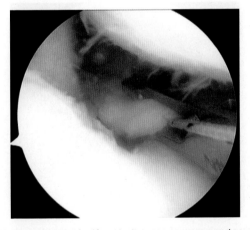

FIGURE 2 Arthroscopic view of self-retrieving suture passer used to pass a No. 2 nonabsorbable suture.

Tunnel Preparation

- Place arthroscope in anterolateral portal.
- Insert ACL transtibial tip guide through the anteromedial portal and position it at the native root insertion site (**Figure 3**).
- Make a 2 cm incision over anteromedial skin with dissection down to the periosteum.
- Elevate 2 to 3 cm of soft-tissue off tibia.
- Reposition the ACL tip guide on the root insertion and place drill sleeve onto the tibia.
- Drill a 3/32-in (2.4-mm) guide pin up to (but not through) the posterior cortex of the tibia on power; tap guide pin with gentle mallet blows to pierce cortex.
  - For LMRT repair at the same time as ACL reconstruction, can either pull sutures through ACL tibial tunnel or create separate tunnel posterior to the ACL tibial tunnel.

Tear Fixation

- Withdraw guide pin, and a shuttle with a looped nitinol wire is introduced in its place.
- Through anteromedial portal, retrieve the loop of nitinol wire and both sutures (**Figure 4**).
- Pull out of joint and avoid soft-tissue bridge.
- Place sutures through nitinol wire loop, and the free end is pulled from tibial tunnel.

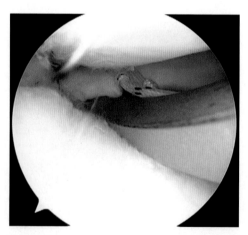

FIGURE 3 Arthroscopic view of a transtibial drill guide positioned at the native root insertion site on the tibia.

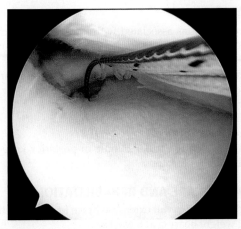

FIGURE 4 Arthroscopic view of a looped nitinol wire inserted through the tibial tunnel and both strands of the suture being grasped with a suture retriever.

- Verify reduction of the root arthroscopically by pulling tension on the sutures (**Figure 5**).
- Tie sutures over a post on the anteromedial aspect of the tibia using a 4.5-mm cancellous screw with a washer.
- If a backup post screw is used for an ACL reconstruction, the sutures from the meniscal root repair can be tied over the same ACL post.
- Sutures can also be placed through a cortical fixation device and tied to the tibia.
- Keep knee in 30° flexion during suture tying.

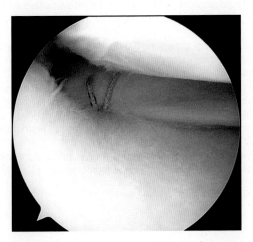

FIGURE 5 Arthroscopic view of completed repair with the meniscal root reduced back to its insertion with two cinch stitches.

COMPLICATIONS

- General complications associated with knee surgery, including infection, arthrofibrosis, deep vein thrombosis, and failure of meniscal root healing.
- Complications specific to meniscal root repair surgery are most commonly associated with inadequate exposure of the repair bed (insufficient reverse notchplasty), resulting in:
  - Insufficient root tissue captured with repair stitch
  - Iatrogenic damage to ACL
  - Damage to neurovascular bundle in posterior knee with poorly visualized pin passage

POSTOPERATIVE CARE AND REHABILITATION

- Non–weight bearing in full extension brace for 4 weeks, then progression to full weight bearing at 8 weeks
- Postoperative range of motion from 0° to 90° is encouraged.
- Physical therapy
  - First month—Straight-leg raises, quadriceps sets, heel slides, calf pumps.
  - Second and third months—Formal supervised physical therapy
  - Return to full activity usually is achieved by 4 months.

PEARLS

- The majority of the procedure can be done without the use of a tourniquet or leg holder.
- A reverse notchplasty or fenestration of the medial collateral ligament can be performed to help visualize the posteromedial compartment for MMRT repairs.
- A cinch stitch is easy to perform if a braided suture has a closed loop on one end and the self-retrieving suture passer is placed through the loop before inserting the device into the joint.
- Multiple passes of the suture shuttle device through the meniscal root should be avoided because this will result in irreparable fraying of already injured tissue.
- Check for an aberrant popliteal artery on MRI before performing a lateral meniscus root repair.
- If performing MMRT and LMRT repairs concomitantly, the MMRT repair should be performed first as this is the more posterior structure of the two.

INTRODUCTION
- Articular cartilage has limited intrinsic healing capacity; microfracture is one of various different cartilage repair strategies.
- Marrow-stimulating techniques such as microfracture rely on perforation of the subchondral plate, allowing pluripotential mesenchymal cells to fill the defect and create a hybrid fibrocartilage repair.
- Augmentation of microfracture using biologic acellular scaffolds may retain the mesenchymal cells and growth factors at site of defect.

PATIENT SELECTION
- Microfracture is often the first-line treatment of full-thickness cartilage lesions (Outerbridge grade IV) because of its success, relative ease, and cost-effectiveness.
- When unsuccessful, it does not preclude use of other techniques.
- Selection criteria are very specific for a successful outcome.

Indications
- Lesion size less than 2 cm^2 is ideal, not exceeding an area of 4 cm^2
- Location of lesion
  - Femoral condylar lesion is favorable.
  - Patellofemoral compartment lesions are less favorable.
- Unipolar lesion, well contained
- Intact meniscus
- Body mass index less than 30 kg/m^2 and age younger than 40 years associated with better outcomes
- Symptomatic lesion

Contraindications
- Bipolar lesions
- Diffuse degenerative joint disease
- Uncorrected malalignment
- Patients unable to comply with or fulfill postoperative protocol

---

Based on Vidal AF, Griffith R: Microfracture, in Colvin AC, Flatow E, eds: Atlas of Essential Orthopaedic Procedures, *ed 2. Rosemont, IL, American Academy of Orthopaedic Surgeons, 2020, pp 95-100.*

- Subchondral bone loss or uncontained lesions such as an osteochondral defect
- Body mass index over 30 kg/m² and older age
- Longer duration of preoperative symptoms is associated with poorer outcomes.
- Significant loss of meniscal tissue

PREOPERATIVE IMAGING

- Radiography
  ▹ Weight-bearing AP, weight-bearing 45° PA, lateral, and Merchant views to assess for loose bodies, arthritis
  ▹ Long leg alignment radiographs
    – Assess for angular deformity
    – Focal lesion with varus malalignment can be treated with microfracture and high tibial osteotomy.
- MRI
  ▹ Cartilage-specific MRI sequences
    – Proton density–weighted fast spin-echo imaging with or without fat saturation
    – T2-weighted fast spin-echo imaging with or without fat saturation
    – T1-weighted gradient-echo imaging with fat suppression
- Assess for concomitant meniscal or ligamentous pathology.

VIDEO 14.1 Microfracture: Technique and Pearls. Armando F. Vidal, MD (10 min)

PROCEDURE

Setup/Patient Positioning

- General, spinal, or regional anesthesia
- Supine position
- Preparation for standard knee arthroscopy is based on surgeon's preference.
- No tourniquet necessary
- Examination under anesthesia
- Diagnostic arthroscopy through anterolateral and anteromedial portals

Surgical Technique

- Address meniscal, loose body pathology before microfracture and ligamentous reconstruction after.
- Identify the cartilage lesion (**Figure 1**).
- Débride unstable cartilage flaps.
- Determine if lesion is amenable to microfracture treatment.

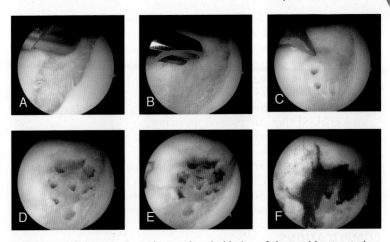

FIGURE 1 Arthroscopic views show a chondral lesion of the trochlea treated with the microfracture technique. **A,** Initial débridement of the lesion. **B,** A shaver is used to remove the calcified cartilage layer. **C,** Beginning at the periphery of the lesion, a microfracture awl is used to create holes perpendicular to the subchondral bone. **D,** The completed holes are shown. **E** and **F,** Inflow has been clamped off, allowing visualization of blood emanating from the holes.

- Assess the arc of motion in which lesion bears weight.
- Use shaver and curet to débride and prepare the lesion; create perpendicular edges at the transition between the lesion and stable healthy cartilage; author preference is to use a ring curet (**Figure 2**).
- Débride the central calcified cartilage layer; this enhances the ability of the repair tissue to bond to the underlying subchondral plate.

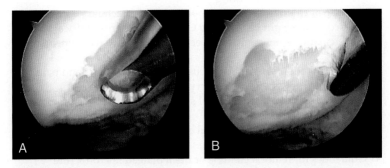

FIGURE 2 Arthroscopic views demonstrate débridement and preparation of a chondral lesion before microfracture. **A,** A ring curet removes the calcified cartilage layer. **B,** The ring curet creates shoulders.

- Use awls of various angles to create holes within the base of the lesion that are perpendicular to the subchondral plate.
  - ⏵ Start at periphery and work toward center of lesion
  - ⏵ May use a drills as opposed to awls
  - ⏵ Leave 3 to 4 mm of space between holes.
  - ⏵ Make holes 2 to 4 mm deep.
- Assess adequate marrow access by visualizing fat droplets or the presence of blood after clamping off the inflow.
- Clear bony debris created during microfracture process with a shaver.
- Postoperative drains are not necessary.
- Apply compressive wrap and cryotherapy to help with postoperative swelling and pain.
- For patellofemoral lesions, immobilize knee in hinged knee brace locked in full extension; no brace necessary for other lesions.

COMPLICATIONS

- Relatively few complications
- Joint effusion is typical for several postoperative weeks and again with return of weight bearing.
- Consider aspiration if effusion is present for greater than 1 month.
- Anterior knee pain generally is due to quadriceps weakness; resolves with return of strength.
- Osseous overgrowth has been seen on subsequent MRI studies in 25% to 62% of patients; this may contribute to failure of the technique.
- Intralesional bone formation and elevation of the subchondral bone plate are characteristic problems.

POSTOPERATIVE CARE AND REHABILITATION

- Critical to success of the procedure
- Rehabilitation principles
  - ⏵ Protected weight bearing
  - ⏵ Use of continuous passive motion (CPM) machine
- Protocols for weight bearing and CPM machine are empirical because a systematic review has not been done; author recommendations include:
  - ⏵ During first 7 to 10 days, focus on control of edema and pain.
  - ⏵ Compressive bandage and cryotherapy
  - ⏵ CPM machine started day of surgery, protected weight bearing
  - ⏵ Avoid rigorous activity.
- The goal is to provide the optimal environment for a super clot to form and adhere.
- Guidelines for femoral condyle or tibial plateau microfracture
  - ⏵ Start on CPM machine within first 24 hours, at either 0° to 60° or 30° to 70° at a rate of one cycle per minute.
  - ⏵ Use CPM machine for 6 to 8 hours per day for 6 weeks.

- Advance range of motion in 10° increments as tolerated until full range of motion is achieved.
- Protected weight bearing is maintained for 6 to 8 weeks; no weight bearing or touchdown weight bearing, based on surgeon preference; the patient may then progress slowly to full weight bearing.
- Strength training
  - Isometric quadriceps and hamstring strengthening begin immediately.
  - At 2 weeks, initiate stationary bike with low resistance
  - Progressive active strengthening begins at 8 weeks.
  - Running is allowed at 3 to 4 months.
  - Activities involving cutting or pivoting are restricted until 4 to 6 months after surgery.
- Guidelines for patellofemoral microfracture
  - Hinged knee brace locked in full extension
  - Full weight bearing permitted with brace
  - CPM machine started within the first 24 hours without brace
  - Early isometric strengthening is allowed, but progressive strength training is limited to the arc of motion (noted at the time of surgery) that does not subject the lesion to compressive forces in the patellofemoral compartment.

PEARLS

- Lesion should be defined with well-shouldered borders.
- The calcified cartilage layer that remains must be débrided.
- Lesion should be measured after débridement.
- Use awls or drills from peripheral to central part of lesion.
- Use sharp awls or drills to avoid coalescence of the holes.
- Perforate the subchondral bone 2 to 4 mm apart and 2 to 6 mm deep.
- All holes should be checked for bleeding at the conclusion of the case (if you are using a tourniquet, consider deflating). It is common for some of the microfracture holes to become impacted with bone, and preventing the marrow elements from emanating. Holes that do not actively bleed should be revised. Try not to have microfracture holes coalesce to avoid larger break out of bone.

Surgical Treatment of Osteochondritis Dissecans Lesions

INTRODUCTION

- Osteochondritis dissecans (OCD) is a pathologic joint disorder that affects the subchondral bone and the overlying articular cartilage.
- Results in subchondral bone loss and destabilization of articular cartilage
- End result is fragmentation of cartilage and bone that can progress to early degenerative changes and loss of function in the affected compartment.
- Site of lesions
  - 80% affect the medial femoral condyle (MFC), usually the lateral aspect of the MFC intersecting the intercondylar notch near the femoral footprint of the posterior cruciate ligament.
  - 15% in lateral femoral condyle
  - 5% in patellofemoral region
- Course of treatment dependent on stability, which is most accurately determined arthroscopically. MRI only has 53% accuracy in determining stability.
- Nonsurgical options
  - Can be successful in the case of a stable lesion and short duration of symptoms
  - Consists of hiatus from sports and high-impact activities for 6 to 8 weeks; normal weight bearing is allowed in the compliant patient.
  - "Relative rest program" can maintain joint health without compromising healing potential of a symptomatic OCD lesion; length of rest is highly variable and is a factor to consider when deciding whether to intervene surgically.
- Surgical options
  - Fragment removal
  - Drilling (antegrade or retrograde)
  - Internal fixation
  - Marrow stimulation
  - Autologous chondrocyte implantation (ACI)
  - Osteochondral autograft/allograft transplantation
  - Joint arthroplasty—last resort in advanced cases.

Based on Salata MJ, Naveen NB, Southworth TM, Dempsey IJ, Cole BJ: Surgical treatment of osteochondritis dissecans lesions, in Colvin AC, Flatow E, eds: Atlas of Essential Orthopaedic Procedures, ed 2. Rosemont, IL, American Academy of Orthopaedic Surgeons, 2020, pp 101-114.

- Decision-making debate—Treat lesions early with cartilage restoration versus initial fragment excision, which leaves many patients clinically normal.

PATIENT SELECTION

- Thorough history mandatory
  - Inciting events
  - Underlying metabolic or systemic conditions
  - Duration of symptoms
  - Previous treatments
- Risk factors for OCD include:
  - Male sex
  - African-American race
  - Presence of discoid lateral meniscus
  - Family history of OCD
  - Active sports participation
- Typical presentation
  - Pain and swelling related to activity
  - Mechanical symptoms such as catching or locking if fragment has destabilized or completely detached
  - Physical examination findings
  - Localized tenderness, antalgic gait, leg externally rotated while walking (Wilson sign)
  - Joint effusion, loose-body symptoms, reduced range of motion (ROM), and quadriceps atrophy are variably present

Indications

- Failed nonsurgical management
- Unstable fragment in an active, symptomatic patient
- Can comply with postoperative weight bearing and activity restrictions
- Classic location in MFC; this site has a resolution rate of less than 30%, but nonclassic lesions more likely to heal in adolescent population, with 88% to 100% healing rates with nonsurgical management.

Contraindications to Surgical Management

- Physeal status stratifies OCD into juvenile OCD (JOCD) or adult OCD (AOCD).
- Nonsurgical management recommended for stable lesion in JOCD
- Activity modification has good outcomes in juveniles because of increased regenerative capacity from chondrocytes and mesenchymal cells.
- Primary surgical fixation not recommended if lesion is free-floating loose body and underlying subchondral bone is compromised

---

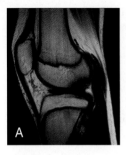 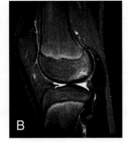 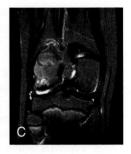

FIGURE 1 Magnetic resonance images show the appearance of an osteochondritis dissecans (OCD) lesion. **A,** T1-weighted sagittal view. **B,** T2-weighted sagittal view. **C,** T2-weighted coronal view of an OCD lesion presenting concomitantly with compromised subchondral bone. An area of high signal intensity between the OCD lesion and the subchondral bone suggests instability.

PREOPERATIVE IMAGING

- Crucial to diagnosis
- Radiography
  - AP weight-bearing knee, weight-bearing 45° flexion PA, lateral, Merchant views
  - Open physes are a positive predictor for healing of an OCD lesion.
- MRI (**Figure 1**)
  - Evaluate for bone edema, subchondral separation, cartilage breakdown, lesion size, lesion location.
  - Meeting one of the following four criteria offers up to 97% sensitivity and 100% specificity in predicting lesion stability.
    - A thin, ill-defined, or well-demarcated line of high signal intensity, measuring 5 mm or more in length at the interface between the lesion and underlying subchondral bone
    - A discrete, rounded area of homogeneous high signal intensity
    - A focal defect with a width of 5 mm or more in the articular surface of the lesion
    - A high signal intensity line traversing the articular cartilage and subchondral bone plate into the lesion

PROCEDURE

- Goal—To enhance the healing potential of the subchondral bone, fix the unstable fragment, or replace the abnormal cartilage and bone with implantable tissue.
- Surgical treatment algorithm determines the type and extent of surgery needed (**Figure 2**).

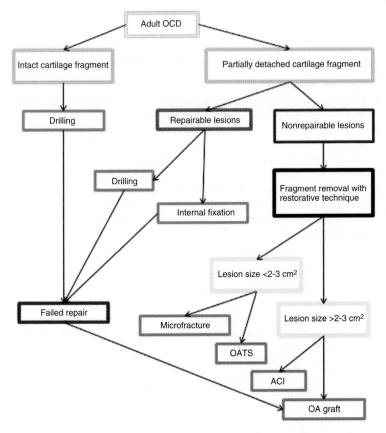

FIGURE 2 Diagram depicts the surgical treatment algorithm for osteochondritis dissecans (OCD). The surgical goals should always incorporate an attempt to reestablish the joint surface using the least invasive procedure first. ACI = autologous chondrocyte implantation, OA graft = osteochondral allograft, OATS = osteochondral autograft transfer system

Room Setup/Patient Positioning
- Supine position, ACL leg holder with foot of bed dropped, permits full extension, flexion including hyperflexion, valgus loading, and figure-of-4 position
- Examination under anesthesia to assess ROM and ligamentous stability
- Patellofemoral and tibial lesions may be more difficult to access arthroscopically and thus may require mini-open technique to treat.

Surgical Technique

- Diagnostic arthroscopy
- Assess stability and boundaries of the lesion; in lesions with intact articular cartilage, surgeon can feel defect with the probe.

Reparative Procedures

- Goal is to restore integrity of subchondral bone, improve blood supply, and restore and preserve overlying articular cartilage.
- Typically, primary reduction and fixation of fragment; often accompanied by removal of fibrocartilaginous scar at interface between lesion and underlying subchondral bone, coupled with restoration of blood flow to lesion by microfracture or drilling of host tissue bed.
- In presence of cystic changes or attritional bone loss, local bone graft procedures that harvest cancellous bone from Gerdy tubercle or distal femur using small-diameter osteochondral autograft harvesting tube are effective.

Drilling

- Stable lesion with intact articular cartilage that remains symptomatic despite nonsurgical management
- Favorable in younger patients
- Antegrade drilling—Done through articular surface of lesion; violates articular surface, resulting in reparative tissue similar to that created by microfracture.
- Retrograde drilling (authors' preference) is extra-articular; done to avoid fibrocartilage formation at the fragment site; drill enters proximal to lesion and penetrates sclerotic proximal border without violating the overlying articular cartilage; fluoroscopic guidance is recommended.
- When possible, drill via intercondylar notch or along the lateral nonarticulating border of the distal femur using a 4.5-mm Kirschner wire.
- Can augment larger lesions with one or two bioabsorbable compression screws that are buried deep to the level of the subchondral plate

Internal Fixation

- Attempt reduction and fixation for detached lesions with loose bodies or articular cartilage flaps that have sufficient subchondral bone to provide biologic and mechanical support for fixation.
- Prepare the bed of the defect with a curet, a shaver, and a microfracture awl.
- Trim the edges of the fragment to aid in anatomic reduction.
- Can fill cystic subchondral defects with bone graft
- Achieve internal fixation with cannulated screws, metal pins/Kirschner wires, or bioabsorbable pins and screws.

- The authors prefer cannulated variable-pitched metal screws placed deep to the level of the articular cartilage; a second procedure is performed 8 weeks later for hardware removal.
- Bioabsorbable screws may remain intact for at least 12 months.
- Use two fixation points to ensure compression and rotational stability.
- Recess prominent screw heads beneath the chondral surface.
- Heel-touch weight bearing postoperatively; maintain knee ROM with continuous passive motion (CPM) machine for up to 6 weeks.

Restorative Procedures

- Attempt to replace damaged articular cartilage with hyaline or hyaline-like tissue.
- Consider if reparative options have failed and patient presents with recurrent joint effusion, pain, and reduced ROM or if fragment at time of index procedure is determined to be unsuitable for primary reduction and fixation.
- Treatment should begin with least invasive and progress to most invasive options.
- Decision to repair OCD lesion or perform microfracture is rarely associated with decision to simultaneously address concomitant pathology (eg, meniscal deficiency, malalignment).
- Higher level procedures (eg, ACI, osteochondral autograft/allograft transplantation for OCD lesion) often undertaken simultaneously with meniscal allograft transplantation and osteotomy when appropriate

Marrow Stimulation (Microfracture)

- Involves perforation of the subchondral bone (**Figure 3**), formation of a super clot, subsequent cell differentiation, and formation of "cartilage-like" fibrocartilage
- This new fibrocartilage is mechanically inferior to native cartilage and less tolerant to shear forces.
- Pluripotent stem cells and growth factors are released from marrow.

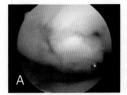 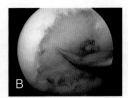 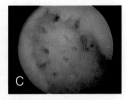

FIGURE 3 Arthroscopic views demonstrate microfracture of an osteochondritis dissecans (OCD) lesion. **A,** An unstable OCD lesion. **B,** Defect site is prepared with vertical wall formation. A surgical awl is used to penetrate the subchondral bone. **C,** Completed microfracture; the holes are about 3 to 4 mm apart. Microfracture holes are started at the periphery, adjacent to the stable cartilage rim.

- Considered as first-line treatment, especially in the setting of fragment removal in small, shallow defects ranging between 2-3 cm^2
- Not pursued in treatment of bipolar defects, damage more than 4 cm^2, or suspicion of subchondral bone damage on MRI
- Postoperatively, 6 weeks of protected weight bearing and CPM machine use for 6 hours a day
- Given activity restriction and postoperative rehabilitation protocol, authors recommend removal of fragment without microfracture in cases of deep, sclerotic, uncontained defects.
- Overall, the decision to perform microfracture may have no bearing on the future progression of the defect.

Osteochondral Autograft Transfer System

- For small lesions where underlying subchondral bone integrity has been significantly compromised
- Addresses both the underlying structural support of the subchondral plate and the articular surface
- Involves transplantation of osteochondral autograft tissue from a non–weight-bearing region of the joint such as the area proximal and far medial or far lateral of the trochlea or the lateral intercondylar notch to the defect site (**Figure 4**)
- Use single autograft plug for lesions less than 1 cm^2; use mosaicplasty with multiple smaller plugs for larger defects.
- Harvesting tool positioned perpendicular to surface and the impacted donor cartilage plug is procured by impacting tool to depth of 12 to 15 mm.
- Limited to small lesions because of low supply of donor tissue and donor-site morbidity
- Ideal for lesions smaller than 2 cm^2, however, may be used for lesions up to 8 cm^2
- Postoperative rehabilitation—Immediate CPM and protected weight bearing for 4 to 6 weeks; return to sport considered at 8 to 12 months.
- Good clinical outcomes have been reported.

Autologous Chondrocyte Implantation

- For full-thickness, isolated osteochondral defects larger than 4 cm^2; no previous cartilage procedures and no subchondral involvement
- Two-step procedure (**Figure 5**)
    - Initial healthy chondrocyte biopsy performed arthroscopically; extract tissue from non–weight-bearing intercondylar notch region or from OCD loose body if grossly healthy.
    - Extracted cells are dedifferentiated in vitro over 4 to 6 weeks and reimplanted at the lesion site, which can be as large as 10 cm^2.
- Defect preparation for reimplantation
    - Preserve the calcified cartilage layer.

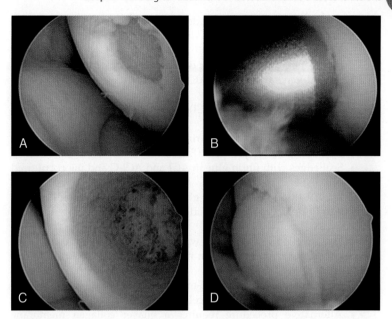

FIGURE 4 Arthroscopic views demonstrate osteochondral autograft for an osteochondritis dissecans (OCD) lesion. **A,** An unstable OCD lesion. **B,** Using the osteochondral autograft transfer system (OATS) transfer tool, the defect site is prepared to an appropriate depth. **C,** View of the recipient site. **D,** Implantation of a donor osteochondral plug into the recipient site.

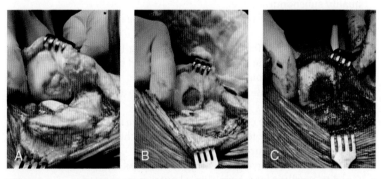

FIGURE 5 Intraoperative photographs demonstrate autologous chondrocyte implantation (ACI) for an osteochondritis dissecans lesion. **A,** Patellar defect. **B,** The defect site after vertical wall formation, ready for suturing of the type I/III collagen patch. The patch is sutured with 6-0 Vicryl. **C,** The lesion following injection of the dedifferentiated cultured chondrocytes and suturing and gluing of the collagen patch. The patch is sutured and then glued over the defect using a fibrin glue.

- ▶ Create a vertically walled defect to act as a reservoir for the implanted cells and better distribute force at the edges of the lesion.
- ▶ First-generation ACI—cover defect with periosteal flap
- ▶ Second-generation ACI (ACI-C)—cover defect with collagen based membrane
- ▶ Third-generation ACI (MACI)—cover defect with chondroinductive matrix
- ▶ Attach membrane to the perimeter of the healthy articular cartilage using 6-0 Vicryl suture (Ethicon).
- ▶ Seal edges with fibrin glue in ACI and ACI-C and inject cultured cells beneath the patch.
- In MACI, a thin layer of fibrin glue is placed in defect, and matrix is cut to fit defect, placed cell side up. Edges are sealed with fibrin glue.
- Postoperatively, 6 weeks of non–weight bearing and CPM use
- Defects deeper than 8 to 10 mm need a concomitant or staged bone grafting.
  - ▶ Staged procedure requires 6-month wait for bone graft incorporation before implantation of cells.
  - ▶ Alternative procedure requires a bilayer collagen membrane (periosteal "sandwich" technique).

Osteochondral Allograft

- For large lesions; salvage procedure; ideal for patients whose initial treatment has failed and who have deeper, cavitating lesions with poor quality subchondral bone.
- Convert host defect to cylindrical socket using commercially available systems.
- Shape a prolonged fresh allograft into a plug that matches the diameter and depth of the resultant socket; should be implanted before 28 days of donor asystole to maximize viability.
- At time of implantation, use minimal force to avoid damage to donor chondrocytes.
- Use a bioabsorbable compression screw in the center of the graft with the head advanced to the level of the subchondral bone to ensure proper fixation (**Figure 6**).
- Postoperatively, no weight bearing for 6 weeks and CPM
- Good to excellent long-term clinical outcomes reported

VIDEO 15.1 Fresh Osteochondral Allografting to the Knee for Osteochondritis Dissecans. Joseph Yu, MD; William Bugbee, MD (8 min)

© 2021 American Academy of Orthopaedic Surgeons

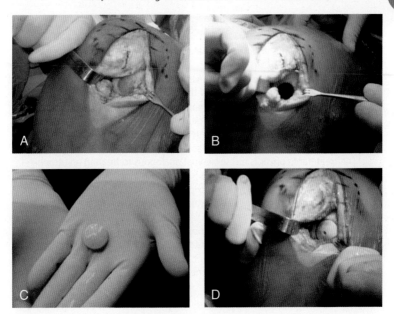

FIGURE 6 Intraoperative photographs show osteochondral allografting for an osteochondritis dissecans lesion. **A,** Arthrotomy reveals the chondral defect. **B,** The defect site is prepared to receive a donor cartilage plug. A counterbore is used to drill to a depth of 6 to 8 mm or until a bleeding bone is established. **C,** A donor cartilage plug is procured from a donor condyle that has been sized and contour matched to the recipient site. **D,** The donor plug is press-fit into place, and a bioabsorbable compression screw is used to ensure fixation.

COMORBIDITIES

- Combined pathologies such as meniscal injury or deficiency, malalignment, and ligamentous instability are commonly encountered when treating articular defects; these pathologies contribute to development of articular lesions.
- Surgical management of combined pathologies ensures integrity of primary cartilage repair without affecting patient's ability to return to activities of daily living.
- To avoid prolonged rehabilitation, address combined pathologies at time of primary cartilage repair.

PEARLS

- Early recognition is important; initiate treatment once the diagnosis is made.
- Advanced imaging, including MRI, is helpful in making the diagnosis and determining the relative stability of the lesion.
- In skeletally immature patients, initial nonsurgical therapy can be employed with some success, but persistently painful lesions may still require surgical fixation despite skeletal immaturity.
- For an unstable lesion that is favorable to repair, preserve the fragment. The treatment concepts are somewhat analogous to treating an atrophic fracture nonunion.
- If the fragment is irreparable, remove it with or without concomitant microfracture; consider a trial of return to activities; can perform an ACI biopsy at fragment removal.
- The condition of the subchondral bone and the size of the lesion should be used to select the appropriate cartilage augmentation or restoration procedure.
- Address comorbidities with the same decision making as that for any cartilage repair procedure.

16 Anterior Cruciate Ligament Reconstruction: Single-Bundle Transtibial Technique

INTRODUCTION

- Surgical reconstruction of the anterior cruciate ligament (ACL) is recommended for active patients.
  - ▶ Restores instability and normal knee kinematics
  - ▶ Improves function and return to active lifestyle
- Benefits of bone–patellar tendon–bone (BPTB) autograft
  - ▶ Biomechanical strength
  - ▶ Accessibility and ease of graft harvest
  - ▶ Bone-to-bone healing
  - ▶ Rigid initial interference screw fixation
  - ▶ Track record of clinical success

PATIENT SELECTION

Indications

- Younger than 40 years with an active, athletic lifestyle
- Other considerations—Type of sports involvement, hours per week played, concomitant meniscal pathology, failure of nonsurgical care, ability to participate in postoperative physical therapy
- Delay surgery until postinjury effusion has fully resolved and patient has attained full range of motion.

Contraindications

- Open physes
- Symptomatic preoperative patellar tendon disease or patellar malalignment
- Relative contraindications—Degenerative joint disease, sedentary lifestyle, inability to comply with postoperative rehabilitation protocol

---

Based on Okoroha KR, Bach BR Jr: Anterior cruciate ligament reconstruction: Single-bundle transtibial technique, in Colvin AC, Flatow E, eds: Atlas of Essential Orthopaedic Procedures, *ed 2. Rosemont, IL, American Academy of Orthopaedic Surgeons, 2020, pp 115-125.*

PREOPERATIVE IMAGING

- Radiography
  - Weight-bearing AP in full extension
  - Weight-bearing PA 45° flexion
  - Non–weight-bearing 45° flexion lateral
  - Merchant view
  - Plain radiographs may identify Segond fracture (<1%), tibial spine fracture, "lateral notch" sign, or loose bodies if present.
- KT-1000 arthrometer (MEDmetric) used by authors to assist in physical examination diagnosis; anterior translations greater than 10 mm or side-to-side differences exceeding 3 mm are highly suggestive of ACL tear.
- MRI
  - Use as an adjunct to history and physical examination to support diagnosis.
  - Sensitive and specific for ACL tears
  - Provides information about status of other intra-articular structures, such as the menisci, posterior cruciate ligament, medial collateral ligament, lateral collateral ligament, and chondral surfaces, as well as bone bruises

VIDEO 16.1 Anterior Cruciate Ligament Reconstruction: Single-Bundle Transtibial Technique. Eric J. Strauss, MD; Adam Yanke, MD; Bernard R. Bach, Jr, MD (19 min)

PROCEDURE

Room Setup/Patient Positioning

- Supine position; waist of operating table is reflexed to reduce lumbar extension.
- Examination under anesthesia
  - Lachman test
  - Varus/valgus knee stability
  - Pivot shift test; if positive, BPTB graft harvest can proceed before diagnostic arthroscopy.
  - Assessment of posterolateral corner
- Tourniquet applied (rarely inflated)
- Contralateral leg in gynecological leg holder
- Surgical leg in arthroscopic leg holder with foot of table flexed completely to allow the surgical knee to flex to at least 110°

Special Instruments/Equipment/Implants

- Standard arthroscopy instruments, including arthroscopic scissors and a basket

- Graft harvest—No. 10 scalpel, forceps with teeth, two Senn retractors, an Army-Navy retractor, a metal ruler, 3/8- and 1/4-in curved osteotomes, mallet, Metzenbaum scissors
- Bone plug creation—Oscillating saw with 10-mm-wide blade
- Graft preparation
  - Rongeur
  - 10- and 11-mm sizing tubes
  - Kirschner wire (K-wire) driver with 0.062-in smooth K-wires
  - Two No. 5 sutures
- Tibial tunnel
  - Tibial aiming device
  - 11-mm acorn reamer
  - Chamfer reamer
  - Hand rasp
- Femoral tunnel
  - 7-mm offset aimer
  - 10- and 11-mm acorn reamers
- Notch preparation
  - Large shaver
  - Curved 7-mm osteotome
  - Large spherical burr
- Graft passage—Satellite pusher
- Graft fixation
  - 14-in hyperflex nitinol wire
  - 7- × 25-mm metal interference screw for femoral tunnel
  - 9- × 20-mm metal interference screw for tibial tunnel

Surgical Technique

Graft Harvest

- Mark anatomic landmarks—Distal aspect of patella, tibial tubercle, borders of patellar tendon
- Make 8-cm incision from distal patellar pole to tibial tubercle at medial edge of patellar tendon.
- Take incision down through paratenon, then elevate paratenon from the patellar tendon medially and laterally.
- Measure patellar tendon width.
- Ideal graft is 10 mm wide with 10- × 25-mm bone plugs
- Cut the central third of the patellar tendon from the center of the distal patellar tendon to the center of the tibial tubercle at a width of 10 mm; extend the incision 2.5 cm past the tendo-osseous junction on the tibial tubercle (**Figure 1**).
- Repeat process on the other side, creating a 10-mm-wide graft.
- Bone cuts using oscillating saw (**Figure 2**)
  - Create tibial bone plug in equilateral triangle shape; make the transverse bony cut with the saw angled at 45°.

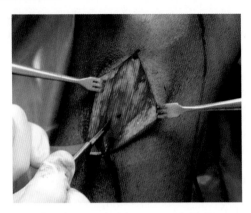

FIGURE 1 Intraoperative photograph shows a central-third bone–patellar tendon–bone autograft harvest using a No. 10 scalpel blade starting on the patella and continuing into the patellar tendon.

▸ Create patellar bone plug in trapezoidal shape no deeper than 6 to 7 mm to avoid injuring patellar articular surface; make transverse bony cut angled at 45°.

▸ Free bone plugs from osseous beds with osteotome (**Figure 3**).

Graft Preparation

- Measure graft length, length of tendinous portion, and length of each bone plug.
- Fine-tune bone plugs with rongeur to 10- × 25-mm dimensions.
- Save removed bone for bone graft of harvest sites.

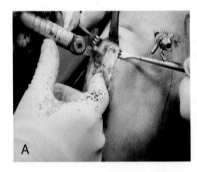
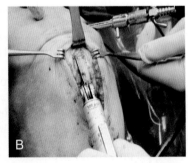

FIGURE 2 Intraoperative photographs depict bone cuts made using an oscillating saw with a 10-mm (No. 238) blade. Cuts on the right side are made with the saw in the surgeon's right hand (**A**) and those on the left are made with the saw in the surgeon's left hand (**B**).

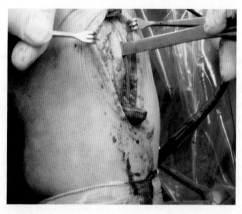

FIGURE 3 Intraoperative photograph shows the patellar bone plug being freed from its osseous bed with an osteotome.

- Drill two holes in tibial bone plug with smooth 0.062-in K-wire, parallel to cortex; place No. 5 suture through each hole.
- Mark tendo-osseous junction of femoral side of graft to aid in fully seating the graft in the femoral tunnel.

Diagnostic Arthroscopy and Notch Preparation

- Create superomedial outflow portal proximally.
- Create standard inferolateral and inferomedial portals within the graft harvest site.
- Perform diagnostic arthroscopy and assess ACL and associated pathology; address any associated pathology that needs management.
- Clear the lateral wall of the intercondylar notch of soft tissue and any fat pad or ligamentum mucosum that is impeding visualization.
- Notchplasty limits the possibility of graft impingement.
  - Insert 1/4-in curved osteotome through medial portal; this is used to begin the notchplasty at the level of the articular surface of the lateral wall.
  - Remove fragments with arthroscopic grasper; save fragments for later use as graft for distal patellar and tibial tubercle defects.
  - Use 5.5-mm spherical burr to widen the notch in an anterior-to-posterior direction, working toward the over-the-top positions.
  - Alternatively, a bone cutting shaver can be used to perform notchplasty.
  - Use arthroscopic probe to check adequacy of notchplasty; should be possible to hook the probe around the sharp edge of posterior wall of the notch.
  - Authors aim to have 10 mm width from lateral portion of the PCL to the lateral intercondylar wall

Tibial Tunnel Placement

- Use a variable-angle tibial aimer (**Figure 4**) to create the tibial tunnel.
  - ▶ Angle depends on length of soft-tissue component of graft.
  - ▶ Use "N + 10" rule to set angle to no less than 55° (45 mm of tendon equates to a setting of 55°).
- Authors' approach—Place an accessory incision through the patellar tendon rent, 1 cm distal and 1 cm lateral to the standard inferomedial portal; this creates an obliquely oriented tunnel that will enable creation of a more anatomic femoral tunnel.
- Insert the tip of the tibial aimer through this accessory midpatellar portal; ideal guide-pin placement is just lateral to the medial tibial spine at the level of the posterior aspect of the anterior horn of the lateral meniscus and/or 7 mm anterior to the posterior cruciate ligament.
- Rotate the cannulated portion of the aimer into position using the upper border of the pes anserine and the anterior edge of the superficial medial collateral ligament as landmarks.
- Perform provisional guide-pin placement using a 3/32-in smooth Steinmann pin; ensure that no impingement occurs on the superior notch with knee extension, then advance guide pin with mallet to lateral wall of intercondylar notch.
- Use appropriately sized (usually 11-mm reamer in tibial tunnel) cannulated acorn reamer to ream over guide pin.

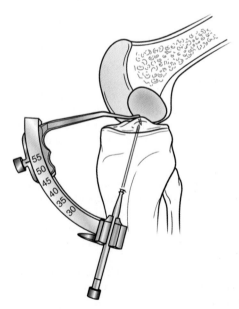

FIGURE 4 Illustration shows a variable-angle tibial aimer used to create the tibial tunnel.

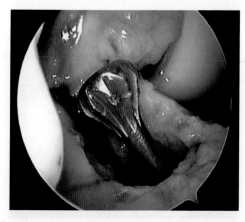

FIGURE 5 Arthroscopic view showing that after the tibial tunnel is reamed using an 11-mm acorn reamer, a chamfer reamer is used to smooth the posterolateral edge of the tunnel.

- Tibial tunnel sizes smaller than 9 mm may result in a nonanatomic femoral tunnel placement.
- Smooth posterior edge of tunnel with chamfer reamer, shaver, or arthroscopic hand rasp (**Figure 5**).
- Remove excess soft tissue at the aperture of tibial tunnel with a rongeur to avoid impingement of the bone block during passage.

Femoral Tunnel Placement

- Insert a 7-mm offset aimer through tibial tunnel into intercondylar notch with the knee flexed to 80° to 90°; tip of aimer is hooked over posterior wall and rotated laterally to permit guide-pin placement lower on lateral wall of the intercondylar notch (**Figure 6**).
- Drill 3/32-in Steinmann pin into lateral wall to depth of 3 cm.
- Overream guide pin with a 10-mm reamer advanced 1 cm; 1 to 2 mm of posterior cortex should remain; confirm integrity of the posterior cortex before continuing to ream.
- Complete reaming to a depth of 30 to 35 mm.
- Confirm lateral wall placement from both an inferolateral and inferomedial viewing portal.

Graft Passage and Interference Screw Fixation

- Advance BPTB autograft into joint using push-in technique.
- Place two-pronged pusher at base of femoral bone plug as the graft is inserted into the tibial tunnel.
- Insert hemostat to guide plug into femoral tunnel with cortical surface facing posteriorly.
- With femoral bone plug seated 75%, place nitinol wire at 1-o'clock (left knee) or 11-o'clock (right knee) position.

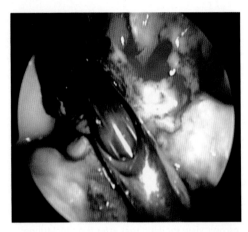

FIGURE 6 Arthroscopic view shows a 7-mm offset aimer inserted through the tibial tunnel into the intercondylar notch, with its tip hooked around the back wall and rotated laterally, to allow guide-pin placement low on the lateral wall at the anatomic femoral footprint of the anterior cruciate ligament.

- Fully seat the femoral bone plug with the knee flexed.
- Hyperflex knee to 100° to 115° and place a 7- × 25-mm metal interference screw over wire; remove wire once screw is seated halfway.
- Cycle the graft with tension on the tibial bone plug sutures.
- With the knee in full extension/hyperextension and axial load applied, use a hemostat to externally rotate the tibial bone plug 180° so that the cortical surface is facing anteriorly.
- Place the nitinol wire anterior to the plug.
- Insert the 9- × 20-mm metal interference screw over the wire while tension is held on the sutures; seat the screw until just below the cortical surface of the tibia.
- Do not bury screw within tibial tunnel as subsequent removal can be difficult.
- Remove the wire.
- Test for graft tension and knee stability.

Closure
- Reapproximate the patellar tendon with the knee in flexion to avoid excessive shortening.
- Place bone graft collected from reaming into the patellar and tibial bony defects.
- Close the paratenon with running 2-0 Vicryl (Ethicon) suture.
- Perform skin closure with subcutaneous 2-0 Vicryl sutures followed by running 3-0 Prolene pullout stitch (Ethicon).

- Close superomedial outflow arthroscopic portal with simple 3-0 Prolene suture.
- Inject surgical incision with 0.5% bupivacaine and cover with adhesive skin closure strips and sterile dressings.
- Place cryotherapy device over gauze bandage and overwrap with compressive elastic wrap.
- Place leg in hinged knee brace locked in extension for walking but allowing full range of motion as tolerated in the unlocked resting position.

COMPLICATIONS
- Arthrofibrosis
- Infection
- Patellar fracture
- Anterior knee pain
- Deep vein thrombosis
- Complex regional pain syndrome
- Compartment syndrome

POSTOPERATIVE CARE AND REHABILITATION
- Full weight bearing postoperatively in hinged knee brace locked in extension
- Brace is removed for motion activities.
- Physical therapy starts 1 week postoperatively.
- Authors emphasize regaining full extension by 10 days, with 80° to 90° of knee flexion.
- Weeks 2 to 4—Closed-chain exercises, hamstring curls, stationary bike
- Weeks 4 to 6—Flexion goal of 120° usually obtained
- Weeks 8 to 10—Patients advanced to light jogging and outdoor biking
- Return to play at 4 to 6 months postoperatively

NATURAL HISTORY
- Systematic review of ACLR versus no reconstruction (at least 10-year follow-up):
  - ACLR had fewer subsequent meniscal injuries, less need for further surgery, and significantly greater improvement in activity levels.
  - No significant differences in development of radiographic osteoarthritis (OA), Lysholm scores, or IKDC scores
- Whether or not ACLR alters course of OA has yet to be determined

PEARLS

- Position patient to allow the knee to be flexed to at least 110° intraoperatively.
- Place the tibial aiming guide in an accessory midpatellar portal to improve the surgeon's effort to gain proper obliquity of the tibial tunnel, which will allow a more anatomic placement of the femoral tunnel.
- Ream the tibial tunnel with an 11-mm reamer to permit easy passage of the 10-mm bone plug.
- With the femoral plug seated in the femoral tunnel, the tibial bone plug should be checked for evidence of graft-tunnel mismatch; if present, perform recession of the femoral bone plug to improve tibial plug position.

VIDEO REFERENCE

 Video 16.1 Strauss EJ, Yanke A, Bach BR Jr: Anterior cruciate ligament recon-struction: Single-bundle transtibial technique, in Fu FH, Howell SM, eds: *Arthroscopic Surgical Techniques: Anterior Cruciate Ligament Reconstruction* [video]. Rosemont, IL, American Academy of Orthopaedic Surgeons, 2010.

Anterior Cruciate Ligament Reconstruction: Two-Tunnel Technique

INTRODUCTION

- An untreated anterior cruciate ligament (ACL)–deficient knee can develop recurrent instability, meniscal instability, meniscal pathology, and articular cartilage damage
- Authors' preferred ACL reconstruction—Single-bundle reconstruction primarily using a bone–patellar tendon–bone (BPTB) autograft
  - Using medial portal technique rather than transtibial for femoral tunnel placement
  - Versatile technique—Appropriate for all autograft and allograft types and fixation methods

PATIENT SELECTION

- Physical examination demonstrates ACL insufficiency
- Surgical indications depend on
  - Degree of perceived instability
  - Associated knee injuries
  - Chronicity of ligament insufficiency
- Prior to surgical intervention
  - Physical therapy to achieve full range of motion (ROM), symmetric quadriceps strength, and reduced effusion
  - Most patients meet these criteria in 3 to 4 weeks
- Contraindications
  - Partial tears with minimal reported instability and no joint laxity on examination
  - Elderly, low-demand patients with minimal instability
  - Comorbidities that make surgery unsafe for the patient

GRAFT CHOICE

- Individualized for patient's age and activity level, partial versus complete tear, associated injuries, and return-to-play timeline (**Figure 1**)
- Autograft indications—Patients younger than 35 years (generally more active lifestyle)

Based on Bratton AD, Vyas D, Harner CD: Anterior cruciate ligament reconstruction: Two-tunnel technique, in Colvin AC, Flatow E, eds: Atlas of Essential Orthopaedic Procedures, *ed 2. Rosemont, IL, American Academy of Orthopaedic Surgeons, 2020, pp 126-133.*

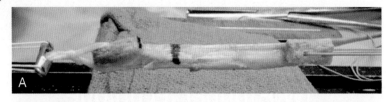

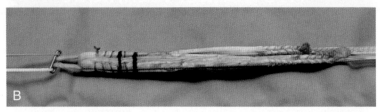

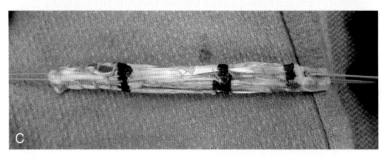

FIGURE 1 Photographs depict autograft options. **A**, Bone–patellar tendon–bone: femoral side with EndoButton CL BTB (Smith & Nephew Endoscopy) and tibial side with Ethibond (Ethicon) lead sutures. The first blue mark is at the bone-tendon junction, and the second marks the amount of graft needed in the femoral tunnel for the EndoButton to engage the lateral femoral cortex. **B**, Quadrupled hamstring: semitendinosus and gracilis. **C**, Quadriceps with patellar bone block.

- Allograft indications—Reserved for older patients
- Authors' preferences
  - BPTB autograft—For younger, active athletes, especially those involved in cutting sports, and in larger patients
  - Hamstring autograft—For those who require single-bundle augmentation, those with contraindications to BPTB graft, and female patients with donor site cosmesis concerns
  - Quadriceps autograft—Authors prefer to harvest without bone block, useful in revision cases when other autografts have been used

PREOPERATIVE IMAGING

- Radiography
  - ▶ 45° flexion weight-bearing PA of bilateral knees, lateral view, Merchant patella view
  - ▶ Used to identify/assess
    - – Associated fractures (avulsion, plateau, or subchondral impaction)
    - – Joint space narrowing, if present
    - – Patellar height (alta/baja), tilt, and subluxation
    - – Presence of physis in younger patients
- MRI (noncontrast)
  - ▶ Discontinuity of ACL on T1 or T2 image sequences indicates a tear
  - ▶ Helps identify associated injuries, such as meniscal tears, chondral damage, bone bruises, and associated ligamentous injuries

PROCEDURE

Room Setup/Patient Positioning

- Femoral and sciatic nerve blocks are not routinely used, as authors have found that femoral blocks increase risk for quadriceps weakness and loss of extension
- Adductor canal block or local anesthetic may be used if necessary
- Supine position, no tourniquet or leg holder, prophylactic antibiotics
- Lower extremity in neutral rotation, gel bump under ipsilateral hip
- 10-lb sandbag to support knee at 90° flexion (**Figure 2**)
- Alternative setup is to use a pneumatic leg holder

Special Instruments/Equipment/Implants

- 30° arthroscope
- 30° Steadman awl
- ACL drill guide with 3/32-in Kirschner wire (K-wire) guide pin
- EndoButton CL BTB
- 3.2-mm EndoButton cannulated drill
- Cannulated compaction reamer
- Tunnel dilators (round, 0.5-mm increments)
- Beath pin
- 4.5-mm cortical screw with washer
- 0.25% bupivacaine with 1:200,000 epinephrine; inject before arthroscopy for hemostasis

Surgical Technique

Examination Under Anesthesia

- Assess range of motion
- Look for presence of effusion or ligamentous laxity
- Perform Lachman, pivot-shift, and anterior drawer tests

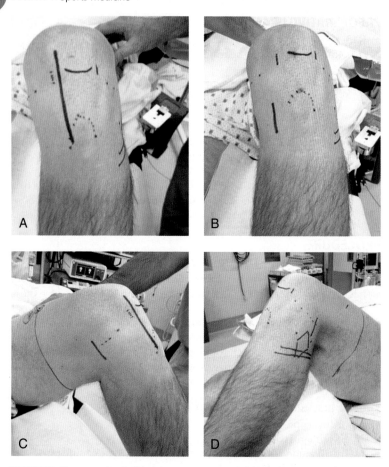

FIGURE 2 Photographs show surface anatomy and skin incisions marked on the skin for anterior cruciate ligament reconstruction procedures. **A,** Bone–patellar tendon–bone (BPTB) autograft. Marked are the inferior pole of the patella, the tibial tubercle, the graft harvest incision, the medial and lateral joint lines, the lateral portal, and the provisional position of the medial portal. This portal is made through the BPTB incision and only after identification of the appropriate location with a spinal needle. **B,** Hamstring autograft. **C,** Medial meniscus inside-out repair (as needed). **D,** Lateral meniscus inside-out repair (as needed). Markings include the lateral joint line, the fibular head and neck, and the position of the peroneal nerve.

Landmarks

- Inferior pole of patella
- Medial and lateral joint lines
- Tibial tubercle
- Medial parapatellar skin incision for BPTB autograft harvest

- Anteromedial (AM) tibial skin incision
- Meniscal repair landmarks—medial, medial joint line, posterior border of superficial MCL; lateral, lateral joint line, and fibular head

Portals and Incisions

- Authors use three portals—anterolateral (AL; viewing), AM (working), and superolateral (outflow) (**Figure 3**)

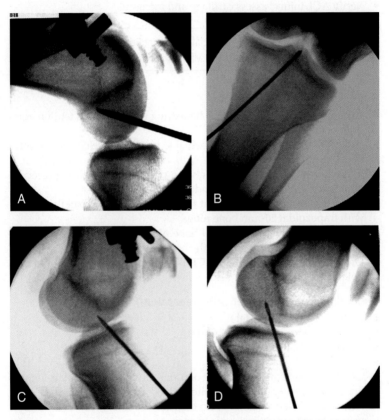

FIGURE 3 Intraoperative fluoroscopic views show confirmation of tunnel positions before drilling. **A,** Position of the femoral tunnel as marked using the Steadman awl through the medial portal. The awl is used to mark the center of the anterior cruciate ligament footprint, with the goal of anatomic positioning of the tunnel. **B,** AP view of the knee shows correct guidewire placement in the coronal plane. This corresponds to the midpoint between the tibial spines. **C,** Lateral image of the knee shows correct position of the tibial guidewire for bone–patellar tendon–bone grafts. The proper placement is parallel and in line with the Blumensaat line. **D,** Lateral view of the knee shows the correct position of the tibial guidewire for soft-tissue grafts. Proper placement is parallel and 2 to 4 mm posterior to the Blumensaat line.

- Make medial portal under direct visualization
  - Provides adequate clearance from medial femoral condyle to avoid cartilage damage
  - Allows proper trajectory for the reamer into the anatomic location on the wall of the lateral femoral condyle

Diagnostic Arthroscopy
- Place arthroscope in AL portal
- Verify ACL injury; assess cartilage and meniscus

VIDEO 17.1 Anterior Cruciate Ligament Reconstruction: Medial Portal Technique. Dharmesh Vyas, MD, PhD; Christopher D. Harner, MD (16 min)

Graft Harvest and Preparation
- Authors prefer BPTB graft, but hamstring or quadriceps tendon autograft used in select cases
- Make a 5- to 6-cm incision just medial to midline; develop full-thickness flaps
- Make a vertical incision through the paratenon, which is preserved and meticulously lifted from underlying tendon
- Harvest a 10-mm wide segment from middle third of patellar tendon with trapezoidal 20-mm bone plugs
- Drill two 1.5-mm holes in tibial bone plug, and thread No. 5 braided nonabsorbable suture through the holes
- On femoral plug, EndoButton CL BTB is attached via a 1.5-mm drill hole in the plug

Femoral and Tibial Insertion Site Preparation
- Arthroscope in AL portal
- Working instruments in AM portal
- Evaluate ACL tear pattern
- Leave fat pad intact
- On femoral side, using remnant of torn ACL as guide for placement of graft, mark center of insertion site with 30° Steadman awl
- Remove ACL remnant and expose wall of lateral femoral condyle using shaver and arthroscopic burner
- Authors do not routinely do notchplasty unless better visualization is needed or graft impingement is present

Femoral and Tibial Tunnel Placement
- Confirm tunnel placement via intraoperative fluoroscopy before drilling
- Femoral tunnel placement
  - Perform placement via medial portal, independent of tibial tunnel
  - Native ACL footprint is generally 4 to 6 mm anterior to posterior femoral cortex with knee at 90° flexion

- Maximally flex the knee (>120°) and, through the medial portal, mallet the guide pin into the position marked by the awl
- By hand, make a shallow provisional footprint using the 0.5- to 1-cm undersized cannulated acorn reamer over the guide pin
- Evaluate placement with reference to posterior cortex, and if acceptable, power ream to predetermined depth for the fixation technique of choice
- Sequentially dilate the tunnel to a size 1 mm larger than bone block diameter
- Use 3.2-mm EndoButton drill to breach the lateral femoral cortex
- Tibial tunnel placement
    - ACL tip-guide set at 50° to 55° is positioned at the intersection between the free edge of the anterior horn of the lateral meniscus and the midline between the tibial spines
    - Usual tunnel length is 30 to 45 mm
    - Insert guidewire approximately 3 cm below the medial joint line and 1.5 to 2 cm medial to the tibial tubercle
    - Advance K-wire until the tip is visible under direct arthroscopic visualization
    - Verify placement of K-wire via fluoroscopy and arthroscopically
    - On the AP view, the wire should be directly between the two tibial spines
    - On the lateral view, pin should be parallel to Blumensaat line and within the anterior 20% to 40% of the tibial plateau
- Check for guide pin impingement on the notch with full knee extension
- Use cannulated compaction reamer (0.5-1 cm smaller than final graft size) to drill the tunnel
- Dilate the tunnel in increments of 0.5 mm to a final size 0.5 mm larger than bone block
- Pass Beath pin with attached suture loop from medial portal into femoral tunnel and out the skin on the lateral thigh; pull the suture loop through the tibial tunnel

Graft Passage and Fixation

- Pull sutures from the femoral side of the graft out through the lateral side of the thigh
- Advance graft up the tibial tunnel, and maintain the tendinous portion of the BPTB graft in the posterior aspect of both tunnels
- After clearing the lateral femoral cortex with the EndoButton, the device is engaged and seated on the cortex; view on fluoroscopy
- Apply tension to the tibial sutures, and cycle the knee
- Tibial fixation
    - Tie sutures over a post
    - Use 4.5-mm AO fully threaded cortical screw with bicortical purchase over a washer; place screw 1 to 2 cm below the tunnel

---

> Tie sutures individually around the post with the knee in full extension
- Examine the knee to ensure stability

COMPLICATIONS
- Incorrect placement of medial portal can lead to iatrogenic injury
  > Cartilage damage of medial femoral condyle
  > Meniscal injury
  > Tibial spine injury
- Infection, arthrofibrosis, deep vein thrombosis, failure of graft healing

POSTOPERATIVE CARE AND REHABILITATION
- First week—Weight bearing as tolerated with crutches in hinged brace locked in extension; basic home exercises in brace
- After first week—Formal physical therapy with unlocked brace
- Early emphasis to regain full extension and reset the quadriceps muscle to pull patella superiorly. This will avoid patellar entrapment, which can be a problem with BTB and quadriceps autografts
- Wean off crutches at 1 month
- Begin running at 6-9months
- Return to full activity at 9 to 12 months

PEARLS

- The medial portal technique is universal to all autograft and allograft choices. An accessory medial portal is not necessary.
- The majority of the procedure can be done with the knee at 90° of flexion; final fixation on the tibia is accomplished with the knee in full extension.
- We do not use a tourniquet or leg holder.
- Positioning of the BTB vertical incision just medial to the midline minimizes scar-induced anterior knee pain during kneeling.
- Closure of the paratenon over the patellar tendon helps restore normal anatomic fascial planes.
- The medial portal is made under direct arthroscopic visualization with a spinal needle. This provides three benefits: avoidance of iatrogenic damage to the medial meniscus; adequate clearance of the medial femoral condyle articular cartilage and prevention of damage during the passage of reamers; and facilitation of the proper angle for direct access to the anatomic positioning of the graft on the lateral femoral condyle.
- Use of half acorn reamers also helps to minimize the chances of iatrogenic damage to the medial femoral condyle during passage of the drill bits.
- Use of intraoperative fluoroscopy ensures precise and reproducible positioning of the femoral and tibial tunnels.

- Minor adjustments to the tibial guidewire positioning can be made quickly and easily using a 3- or 5-mm offset drill guide.
- Intraoperative fluoroscopy is critical to verify that the EndoButton has seated and engaged the lateral femoral cortex.
- The tibial and femoral tunnels are dilated 0.5 mm larger than the BTB bone block size to facilitate easy passage of the graft.
- Meniscal repair sutures are passed before the ACLR is undertaken but are not tied until after the graft is passed and secured. This avoids tearing of the repair sutures during hyperflexion of the knee for the femoral tunnel drilling.
- Postoperative rehabilitation focuses on quadriceps strength and function as soon as possible to avoid loss of extension, the most common complication after surgery.

CHAPTER 18

Individualized Anatomic Anterior Cruciate Ligament Reconstruction

INTRODUCTION

- The anterior cruciate ligament (ACL) is a dynamic, neurovascularly rich structure
- Distinct bundles function synergistically and in concert with other ligaments, meniscus, and capsular attachments to facilitate normal kinematics
- Traditionally, only one of the two native ACL bundles has been reconstructed; this "single-bundle" reconstruction places the ACL in a nonanatomic position
- Anatomic double-bundle reconstruction better re-creates the native knee kinematics and function

Patient Selection

- ACL ruptures are secondary to noncontact trauma to the knee during cutting or pivoting sports
- Audible pop, immediate effusion
- Lachman and pivot-shift tests
- Isolated ACL injuries typically involve both bundles, but in rare cases only one bundle may be torn
  - ▶ Isolated posterolateral (PL) bundle injury—Positive pivot shift test and negative Lachman test
  - ▶ Isolated anteromedial (AM) bundle injury—Positive Lachman test and negative pivot shift test
- KT-1000 and KT-2000 arthrometer testing (MEDmetric) can assist with diagnosis.

Indications

- Indications for anatomic ACL reconstruction are well known and not discussed in this chapter
- Use reconstruction algorithm for decision making on treatment (**Figure 1**)

Based on van Eck CF, Fu FH: Individualized anatomic anterior cruciate ligament reconstruction, in Colvin AC, Flatow E, eds: Atlas of Essential Orthopaedic Procedures, *ed 2. Rosemont, IL, American Academy of Orthopaedic Surgeons, 2020, pp 134-143.*

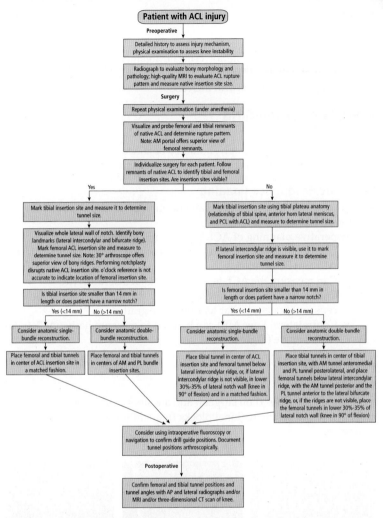

FIGURE 1 Diagram depicts the algorithm used for anatomic single- and double-bundle ACL reconstruction. ACL = anterior cruciate ligament, AM = anteromedial, PCL = posterior cruciate ligament, PL = posterolateral. (Adapted with permission from van Eck C, Lesniak B, Schreiber V, Fu F: Anatomic single- and double-bundle anterior cruciate ligament flowchart. *Arthroscopy* 2010;26[2]:258-268.)

Contraindications

- Relative (as per senior author)
    - ◗ Small femoral or tibial insertion site; tibial site smaller than 14 mm will not support the necessary bone tunnels
    - ◗ Notch size less than 12 mm in medial-to-lateral dimension

- Absolute
  - Active infection
  - Malalignment
  - If incompetent posterior cruciate ligament, posterior corner, or medial collateral ligament not addressed, the rate of failure of ACL reconstruction will increase

PREOPERATIVE IMAGING

Radiography

- Weight-bearing radiograph should be obtained
- Evaluate for bony avulsions such as spine fractures or Segond fractures

Magnetic Resonance Imaging

- Evaluate for concomitant ligament injury, meniscal pathology, or chondral injury
- Preoperative planning of ACL bundles and insertion sites
  - Use oblique sagittal and oblique coronal planes to evaluate the AM and PL bundles
  - Can measure the ACL femoral and tibial insertion sites
  - Can determine autograft length and the diameter of the quadriceps and bone–patellar tendon–bone graft
  - Contralateral knee MRI can be used to measure native ACL inclination angle (**Figure 2**)

PROCEDURE

Anesthesia

- Regional used based on surgeon and anesthesia experience
- Femoral and sciatic regional blocks frequently used, as well as spinal anesthesia

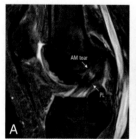 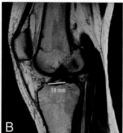 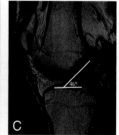

FIGURE 2 Sagittal MRIs of the knee show a cut through the anterior cruciate ligament (ACL). **A,** The two-bundle anatomy of the ACL can be observed, as well as the presence of an isolated anteromedial (AM) bundle tear; the posterolateral (PL) bundle remains intact. **B,** The ACL insertion site is measured on MRI; it measures 18 mm in this patient. **C,** The inclination angle of the ACL is measured on MRI; it measures 46° in this patient.

Examination Under Anesthesia

- Passive range of motion (ROM) assessed; Lachman (translation and end point) and pivot-shift tests (compare with contralateral side)
- Varus/valgus stability, dial test, posterior drawer test to evaluate other ligaments

Room Setup/Patient Positioning

- Place tourniquet high on surgical extremity
- Supine position with leg holder
- Foot of operating table dropped to allow greater than 125° of knee flexion

Surgical Technique

Portals and Diagnostic Arthroscopy

- Three portals—Anterolateral, central, and accessory medial (**Figure 3**)
- Make anterolateral portal first—Located high, above joint line and 2 cm lateral to patella
- Perform diagnostic arthroscopy (**Figure 4**)
- Under direct visualization, make central and accessory medial portals

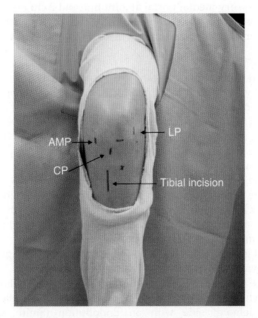

FIGURE 3 Photograph shows markings on the knee for the three-portal technique for anterior cruciate ligament reconstruction. The locations of the anterolateral portal (LP), the central portal (CP), and the accessory medial portal (AMP) are shown, as well as the location of the tibial incision for drilling the tibial tunnels and possible hamstring tendon harvest.

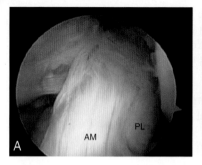 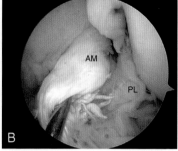

FIGURE 4 Arthroscopic views show the anterolateral portal view of the left knee in 90° of flexion. **A,** Intact native anterior cruciate ligament (ACL) displays the two-bundle anatomy. **B,** Torn ACL; the anteromedial (AM) and posterolateral (PL) bundles are ruptured and separated from each other.

- Place central portal just above the meniscus, on medial border of the patellar tendon or through the medial half of the tendon; provides visualization of the notch
- Place accessory medial portal at joint line and 2 cm medial to patellar tendon; a spinal needle should be able to pass into the notch with 2 mm of clearance from the medial femoral condyle

Graft Preparation

- Autograft or allograft can be used, including quadriceps tendon (with or without bone block), hamstring, or bone–patellar tendon–bone
- Benefit of quadriceps autograft—It can be assessed preoperatively, and large size provides enough graft for both bundles (**Figure 5**)
  - ▶ Make standard midline incision 1 cm proximal to superior pole of the patellar tendon and extending 5 cm proximal
  - ▶ Make 1-cm transverse incision through the tendon 8 cm proximal to the superior pole of the patella; make lateral incision
  - ▶ Mark a rectangle 20 mm in length by 10 mm in width on the anterior surface of the patella; harvest a bone block sized to appropriate tunnel size; place drill hole for passing sutures
  - ▶ Split graft longitudinally up to the bone block through its natural cleavage plane
  - ▶ Place modified Bunnell locking stitch within both tails of the graft, which will become PL and AM grafts; mark PL bundle
  - ▶ Fix femoral side with an EndoButton (Smith & Nephew Endoscopy)
  - ▶ Only one femoral tunnel is drilled at the center of the AM and PL femoral tunnels; two tibial tunnels receive the tails of the graft

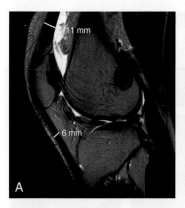
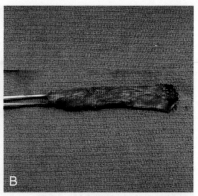

FIGURE 5 Images show graft selection for anterior cruciate ligament (ACL) reconstruction. **A,** Sagittal MRI shows the quadriceps tendon and the patellar tendon. The size of these tendons for use as autograft material for ACL reconstruction can be measured. In most patients, the quadriceps tendon (11 mm in this patient) is larger than the patellar tendon (6 mm in this patient). **B,** Photograph shows freshly harvested soft-tissue–only quadriceps tendon.

Soft-Tissue Débridement

- Evaluate the ACL tear pattern; entire ACL should be affected for double-bundle reconstruction versus isolated PL or AM bundles
- Use remnants of the native ACL to determine the location for the AM and PL tibial and femoral tunnels (**Figure 6**)
- Remove residual ACL, and identify the anatomy of the lateral femoral condyle
- Preserve the local bony anatomy; identify the lateral bifurcate ridge separating the AM and PL bundles and the lateral intercondylar ridge (resident's ridge); the steps of the double-bundle procedure are illustrated in **Figure 7**

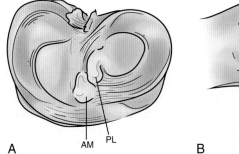
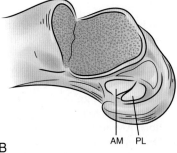

FIGURE 6 Illustrations show the two-bundle anatomy of the anterior cruciate ligament. **A,** Tibial anteromedial (AM) and posterolateral (PL) bundle insertion site locations. **B,** Femoral AM and PL bundle insertion site locations.

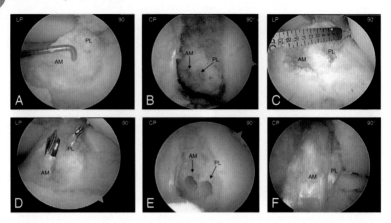

FIGURE 7 Arthroscopic views show anatomic double-bundle anterior cruciate ligament (ACL) reconstruction in a left knee in 90° of knee flexion. The tibial (**A**) and femoral (**B**) ACL insertion sites are marked. **C**, The tibial insertion site is measured; in this patient, it is 20 mm. Two tibial (**D**) and two femoral (**E**) tunnels are created. **F**, The AM and PL grafts are passed, and the two-bundle anatomy is restored. AM = anteromedial, CP = central portal view, LP = anterolateral portal view, PL = posterolateral

Femoral Tunnel: Posterolateral

- Mark the center of the footprint with a Steadman awl
- Place a guidewire in the awl punch site via accessory medial portal
- Place arthroscope in central portal; knee is hyperflexed (>125°)
- Use a mallet to impact the guidewire
- Drill the femoral PL tunnel with a size 6 reamer to a depth of 20 to 25 mm
- Use EndoButton reamer to break the lateral cortex
- Perform dilation of the tunnel to desired size by hand

Tibial Tunnels

- With arthroscope in anterolateral portal, introduce ACL guide in accessory medial portal; set guide to 45° for the PL bundle and 55° for the AM bundle
- Make a 3- to 4-cm incision over AM tibia midway between the tibial tubercle and posterior border of the tibia
- Advance two guide pins per ACL guide, and view them through the arthroscope to ensure they are in the center of the previously marked tibial AM and PL insertion sites
- Drill guide pins with size 6 reamer; use hand dilators until desired diameter is reached
- Use rasp to smooth posterior aspect of each tunnel, and remove with a shaver any soft tissue that could prevent graft passage

Femoral Tunnel: Anteromedial
- AM tunnel can be drilled anatomically from one of the three entries
  - PL tibial tunnel (possible in 60% of cases)
  - AM tibial tunnel (possible in 5%)
  - Accessory medial portal (possible in 99%)
- Drill tunnel to size 6, and dilate by hand to final diameter

Routing the Grafts
- Route PL graft first, and then AM graft
- Pass Beath pins with No. 5 Ethibond sutures (Ethicon) from the accessory medial portal and out the PL and AM tunnels
- Retrieve the suture from the respective tibial tunnel, and pass the graft

Femoral Fixation
- EndoButton is routinely used for fixation
- After EndoButton is delivered though the lateral cortex, it is toggled and viewed fluoroscopically to verify its flipped position

Cycling the Graft
- Cycle 25 times with tension on the grafts as they exit the tibial tunnel
- View grafts through lateral and central portals to ensure that they do not impinge along the roof in full extension or along the posterior cruciate ligament

Tibial Fixation
- Use bioabsorbable interference screws of equal diameter to tunnel
- Secure AM bundle first with the knee in 30° of flexion
- Then the PL bundle with the knee in 0 to 10° of flexion

Single-Bundle Anatomic Reconstruction
- Prepare tunnels in manner similar to that for double-bundle reconstruction
- Use oval dilators to better approximate local anatomy of femoral ACL footprint

Closure
- Layered wound closure
- Periosteum and deep fascia over the tibial incision are closed with 0 Vicryl (Ethicon)
- Subcutaneous tissue closed with 2-0 Vicryl
- Skin closed with absorbable monofilament
- Portals closed with 3-0 nylon suture
- Apply sterile dressings, as well as elastic bandage starting at the foot
- Ice pack over knee and hinged knee brace locked in full extension are placed before transfer to recovery room

COMPLICATIONS

- Graft failure
  - ◗ Main cause is malposition of the tunnel
  - ◗ Other causes—trauma, poor biologic incorporation of graft, early return to sport
- Rare complications—Infection, deep vein thrombosis, pulmonary embolism; early mobilization can prevent last two

POSTOPERATIVE CARE AND REHABILITATION

- First week—Hinged knee brace locked in extension, toe-touch weight bearing
- After first week—Full ROM allowed in brace, weight bearing as tolerated
- Brace is discontinued at 6 weeks postoperatively
- Physical therapy is initiated during the second week for ROM and quadriceps strength
- Continuous passive motion machine is started after the first week; begun at 0° to 45° and advanced 10° per day to goal of 0° to 100°; 2 hours twice a day is desired
- No running until 3 months postoperatively
- No return to sports until 9 to 12 months after surgery
- Recommend using a functional ACL brace for sports until 2 years after the reconstruction

PEARLS

- When looking at the tibial insertion site, place the arthroscope in the anterolateral portal, withdrawn as far as possible and aim the optics inferior to provide a panoramic view of the tibial insertion site.
- The femoral insertion site is best viewed through the central portal, with the optics aimed slightly superior and lateral to visualize the bony ridges.
- The femoral notch width should be 12 mm for a double-bundle reconstruction.
- The tibial footprint should be 14 mm for a double-bundle reconstruction.
- Measure the width of the quadriceps and patellar tendon preoperatively on MRI to ensure it is wider than 8 mm before harvest.
- The PL graft should be routed first.
- After fixation of both the femoral and tibial sides, the knee should be rescoped to evaluate graft tension. If the ACL graft is loose, the graft should be retensioned.
- If concern about femoral or tibial fixation is present, a post and washer construct can be used as secondary fixation.

Quadriceps Tendon Anterior Cruciate Ligament Reconstruction

PATIENT SELECTION

Indications

- Ideal option for majority of patients indicated for autograft anterior cruciate ligament (ACL) reconstruction
- Quadriceps tendon (QT) graft is the author's preferred graft choice
- Strong candidates include those who frequently kneel for work or activity or those with coexisting medial collateral ligament injury

Contraindications

- Prior QT injury or surgery
- Moderate or severe preexisting quadriceps tendinopathy
- Large cavitary bony defects

PROCEDURE

Room Setup/Patient Positioning

- Perform examination after induction of general anesthesia
- Tourniquet to surgical leg; nonsurgical leg in lithotomy holder
- Surgical leg placed in padded circumferential leg holder positioned at level of tourniquet (**Figure 1**)
- Leg holder is elevated 4 inches off table and tilted 30° cephalad, allowing knee to hang at 90°
- Remove OR table's leg platform, and the knee should rest at 90° flexion
- Alternatively, a lateral post and a foot stop can be used to maintain the knee in 90° of flexion and neutral hip rotation
- Prep surgical leg up to the midthigh for QT harvest

Special Instruments/Equipment/Implants

The components of the QT harvest system are as follows (All Arthrex, Naples, FL):

- Double-blade QT harvest knife
- QT stripper/cutter with on-instrument ruler

Based on Schwartz AM, Pombo MW, Xerogeanes JW: Quadriceps tendon anterior cruciate ligament reconstruction, in Colvin AC, Flatow E, eds: Atlas of Essential Orthopaedic Procedures, *ed 2. Rosemont, IL, American Academy of Orthopaedic Surgeons, 2020, pp 144-153.*

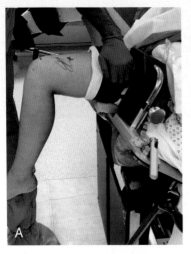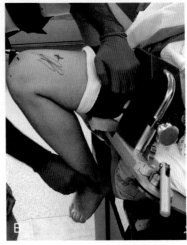

FIGURE 1 A, Photograph of leg freely hanging in leg holder. **B**, Photograph of leg passively hyperflexed in leg holder.

- FiberLoop whipstitch
- Self-retrieving suture passer (Scorpion)
- Graft sizer/compressor

Components of tunnel drilling and graft fixation are as follows:

- TightRope RT (Arthrex, Naples, FL)
- Single-fluted drill (to avoid chondral damage during far medial portal femoral drilling) (Linvatec, Utica, NY)
- FlipCutter for tibial tunnel (Arthrex, Naples, FL)

SURGICAL TECHNIQUE

General Considerations

- Exsanguinate leg and inflate tourniquet
- Anterolateral portal at junction of the lateral and inferior patellar borders made in extension
- The anteromedial portal is positioned medial of the medial border of the patellar tendon. Both the anteromedial portal and far medial accessory portal are made in 90° of flexion
- Graft harvest site is 1.5 to 2 cm in length, marked just proximal to superior pole of patella, favoring laterally to avoid the vastus medialis obliquus (VMO)

Minimally Invasive Graft Harvest

- Ideal graft length is 6 to 7 cm in length
- With knee at 90° flexion, make 1.5 to 2 cm transverse incision previously marked

© 2021 American Academy of Orthopaedic Surgeons

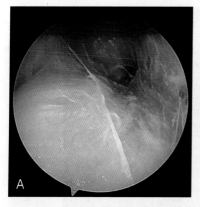 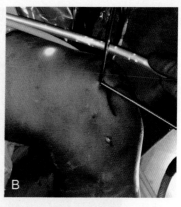

FIGURE 2 A, Arthroscopic view of proximal extent of graft harvest site. **B**, Photograph showing that the arthroscope is turned 180° to create an external landmark for proximal graft targeting.

- Widely excise subcutaneous, pretendinous fat for adequate exposure
- Excise paratenon
- Use sponge with forceps to debride soft tissue from tendon
- A key elevator is passed proximally and distally to remove residual soft tissue
- Insert dry arthroscope directed down the tendon
- Visualize triangular junction of VMO, vastus lateralis, and distal rectus femoris (**Figure 2**)
- Use arthroscope to transilluminate skin over the junction and mark spot
- Measure distance from proximal pole of patella to this spot, which is maximum achievable length of all soft-tissue graft, usually at least 7 cm
- Use double-blade harvest knife while knee held in 90° flexion
- Cut retrograde from proximal pole of patella to the mark of junction site
- Use 15-blade to extend tendon incision to superior patella and connect transverse incisions
- Alternatively, a small bone plug can be harvested if preferred
- Dissect proximally with scissors, maintaining tension on QT graft with Allis clamp
- If QT thickness is ≤7 mm on the preoperative sagittal MRI, then a full-thickness tendon is used obtain a graft diameter of at least 8 mm (**Figure 3**)
- If pre-op measurement is ≥8 mm, a partial-thickness graft is taken
- Use elevator to free graft proximally and taper distal end using scissors

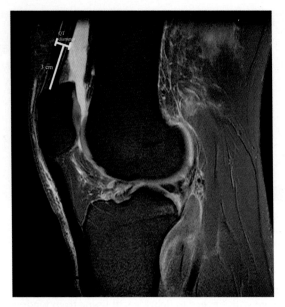

FIGURE 3 Measure quadriceps tendon thickness 3 cm above the superior pole of the patella on midsagittal MRI.

- Use #2 suture to whipstitch three to four throws in tendon starting 1.5 cm proximal to end and moving distally, exiting central portion of graft
- A stripper/cutter is used to amputate tendon from proximal attachment
- Reinsert dry arthroscope into the incision toward proximal harvest site
- Use Scorpion suture passer to close longitudinal QT defect

 VIDEO 19.1 This video shows the harvest of the quadriceps tendon graft and its preparation using an Arthrex (Naples, FL) TightRope RT fixation device for femoral fixation and an Arthrex (Naples, FL) TightRope CL fixation device for tibial fixation over an Arthrex (Naples, FL) button with backup suture fixation. Andrew M. Schwartz, MD; Matthew Pombo, MD; John W. Xerogeanes, MD (7 min)

Graft Preparation
- Smaller end of graft is used for femoral side of reconstruction
- Use #2 suture to whipstitch the musculotendinous junction end of graft
- The femoral end of the graft is then attached to the aperture fixation device

- Place needle through the loop of TightRope RT, and three whipstitches are placed back in the tendon, starting 5 mm from the end, and proceeding toward the middle of the graft
- The needle is then removed, and suture limbs are wrapped and tied about the graft
- Determine size and compress graft in Arthrex graft compressor

Tunnel Drilling

- Establish far medial portal after localization with spinal needle
- Arthroscope in AM portal with instrumentation in far medial portal
- Place femoral anatomic footprint guide loaded with spade-tipped pin centered over femoral ACL footprint
- Flex knee to or past 120° and drill pin transosseously
- Measure intraosseous condylar width, typically 30 to 40 mm
- Advance pin through lateral skin
- The drill size should correlate with the diameter of the graft, and be passed over the pin (authors drill 25 to 28 mm to leave residual lateral wall)
- Position a looped passing suture in femoral tunnel for later graft passage
- Place arthroscope in anterolateral portal to visualize and mark tibial footprint
- Authors prefer to drill tibial tunnel using FlipCutter (Arthrex), alternatively can drill tunnel conventionally
- Pass second looped suture into tibial tunnel from outside in
- Grasp tibial and femoral looped sutures and remove from joint via AM portal

Graft Passage and Fixation

- Pass the graft through the far medial portal, femoral side first
- Shorten the TightRope RT to 5 mm greater than the potential femoral length so that the button will be successfully deployed when the graft reaches the tunnel aperture
- Pull the graft sutures out the femoral side via passing suture
- Pull the graft into the tunnel and deploy button on lateral cortex
- Alternately pull white limbs of TightRope RT to advance graft in femoral tunnel until no more sutures remain visible in joint
- Place tibial sutures in passing looped suture and pull the sutures through the tibial tunnel
- The graft is then pushed into knee and pulled into tibial tunnel
- Cycle knee with tension on sutures and ensure no graft impingement
- Tibial fixation can be performed as per surgeon preference; authors prefer low-profile tie-over-post screw
- Perform final tightening of TightRope RT with knee in extension
- Close arthroscopic portals in standard fashion

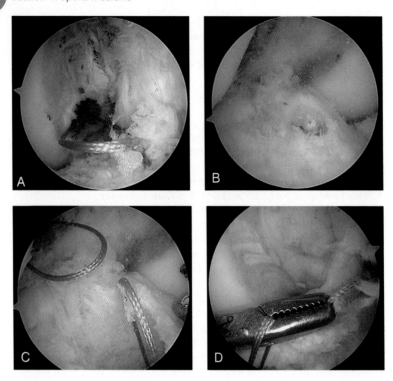

FIGURE 4 A through **D,** Arthroscopic views. **A,** Femoral tunnel with passing suture protruding. **B,** Tibial tunnel. **C,** Femoral and tibial tunnels with passing sutures to be grabbed simultaneously. **D,** Grabbing passing sutures for simultaneous removal.

- QT harvest site is closed with interrupted 3-0 polyglactin 910 for subcutaneous tissue, and running 3-0 subcuticular poliglecaprone 25 (**Figure 4**)

COMPLICATIONS AND MORBIDITY
- Residual quadriceps deficit is similar to hamstring and less than patellar tendon graft
- Rate of frontal knee pain and kneeling pain is minimal
- Very rare cases of acute thigh compartment syndrome, usually associated with graft harvest greater than 8 cm proximally
- Authors report two cases of rectus femoris retraction
- Authors report 2% postoperative wound hematoma
- Loss of extension occurs in 8.3% historically
- Authors' postoperative protocol is to begin aggressive extension exercises 3 to 4 days postoperatively. They recommend lysis of adhesions if loss of extension continues past 8 weeks

POSTOPERATIVE PAIN CONTROL

- Authors use adductor canal nerve block prior to surgery
- Patients are given instructions on pain medicine usage and prescribed oral anti-inflammatory medication and oxycodone

POSTOPERATIVE CARE AND REHABILITATION

- Emphasize early full range of motion
- No brace
- Protected weight bearing once the quadriceps musculature is recruited
- Transition off crutches as early as safe and after physical therapy initiation
- Cryotherapy used in early postoperative period
- Principles of rehabilitation are similar between QT and patellar tendon ACL reconstruction

PEARLS

- Remove all arthroscopic fluid prior to graft harvest if arthroscopy is performed prior to harvest.
- Widely excise subcutaneous fat and areolar tissue which allows for adequate visualization through the small incision.
- Coagulate any crossing vessels to minimize the risk of harvest site hematoma.
- Taper the distal end of the graft slightly as the addition of suture will add girth to the end of the graft, if free tendon graft is used.
- If fat is encountered during partial-thickness harvest, avoid deeper dissection or risk full-thickness violation.
- Trim bulky areas of graft that prevent passage of the stripper/cutter.
- Reinsert arthroscope following graft harvest to reapproximate harvest site.
- The skin incision is left open until case completion to avoid fluid collection in the pretendinous space.
- View from the anteromedial during femoral tunnel marking and drilling portal for adequate visualization and anatomic tunnel placement.
- Measure intraosseous distance also known as the "potential femoral tunnel length."
- Do not drill a femoral tunnel greater than 28 mm in length. With a graft 6 to 7 cm in length, pulling a greater amount of graft into the femoral tunnel may leave inadequate graft for the tibial tunnel.
- After placement of the tibial drill, extend the knee to see that it is not impinging on the superior notch.
- Retrieve the passing sutures through the far AM portal at the same time to ensure no tissue bridges will remain when passing the ends of the grafts.

- Shorten TightRope construct to 5 mm longer than the potential femoral tunnel length, so the button will deploy when graft end is at the tunnel aperture. Failure to shorten this length may lead to deploying the button outside the iliotibial (IT) band
- TightRope bounce test" can be used to ensure button deployment.
- Retain 5 mm of room in the femoral tunnel for final tightening following tibial fixation.
- Fix graft with the knee in full extension.

INTRODUCTION

- Treatment of anterior cruciate ligament (ACL) tears in patients with open physes remains controversial
- Pediatric ACL injuries have increased 2.3% annually from 1994 to 2013
- Surgical timing—Early versus delayed reconstruction
  - ‣ Benefits of early treatment—May improve knee function, avoid strict activity modification in competitive athletes, and reduce progressive chondral and meniscal injury
  - ‣ Benefit of delayed treatment—May avoid potential growth disturbances
- Surgical technique (**Figure 1**)
  - ‣ Physeal-sparing technique
    - – Intra-articular, extra-articular, and combined
    - – Extra-articular and combined are nonanatomic; associated with poor outcomes

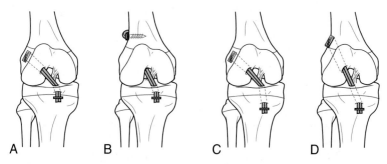

FIGURE 1 Illustrations show the most commonly used techniques for pediatric anterior cruciate ligament reconstruction. **A**, Intra-articular physeal-sparing technique. **B**, Partial transphyseal technique, with proximal over-the-top positioning of the graft (authors' preference). **C**, Partial transphyseal technique, with all-epiphyseal proximal tunnel drilling. **D**, Complete transphyseal technique.

Based on Bonasia DE, Rossi R, Wolf BR, Amendola A: Pediatric anterior cruciate ligament reconstruction, in Colvin AC, Flatow E, eds: Atlas of Essential Orthopaedic Procedures, *ed 2. Rosemont, IL, American Academy of Orthopaedic Surgeons, 2020, pp 154-162.*

- ▸ Partial transphyseal techniques
    - – Hybrid of physeal-sparing and adult-type reconstructive procedures
    - – Most commonly, the femoral physis is left intact via epiphyseal tunnel drilling or over-the-top positioning of the graft
- ▸ Complete transphyseal technique is comparable to adult-type reconstruction
- ▸ Direct repair has had inferior outcomes compared with reconstruction
- ▸ Rigid fixation for tibial spine avulsions; reconstruction of ACL is contraindicated in these cases

---

 VIDEO 20.1 Pediatric Anterior Cruciate Ligament Reconstruction. Davide Edoardo Bonasia, MD; Roberto Rossi, MD; Brian R. Wolf, MD; Annunziato Amendola, MD (18 min)

PATIENT SELECTION

- Clinical examination
    - ▸ History—Audible pop, rapid-onset hemarthrosis
    - ▸ Mechanism—Flexion-valgus-external rotation is most common
    - ▸ Evaluate joint effusion, point tenderness, range of motion (ROM), and instability
    - ▸ Perform Lachman, drawer, pivot-shift, and varus/valgus stress tests
- Conservative treatment
    - ▸ Includes ROM exercises, strengthening, functional braces, and activity modification
    - ▸ Conservative management should be discussed in all cases, especially for inactive patients
- Surgical indications
    - ▸ Failure of conservative treatment with persistent effusion, pain, instability
    - ▸ Patient is unwilling or unable to modify activity levels
    - ▸ Meniscal tear is associated with ACL tear.
- Patient age
    - ▸ In older adolescents (females older than 14 years; males older than 16 years), a complete transphyseal technique can be used
    - ▸ In younger patients (females younger than 14 years; males younger than 16 years), technique selected based on surgeon preference
    - ▸ Authors' preference—Partial transphyseal technique with proximal over-the-top positioning of semitendinosus tendon autograft

PREOPERATIVE IMAGING

Radiography

- AP, lateral, Merchant, and tunnel views of bilateral knees
- To evaluate the physis for remaining growth
- To rule out
  - Tibial and/or femoral epiphyseal fractures
  - Tibial spine avulsions
  - Malformation of tibial spine and/or femoral notch

Magnetic Resonance Imaging

- To visualize ACL tear and location of injury
- To assess associated pathology (eg, meniscal tear)
- To evaluate status of maturity of epiphyses when needed
- Evaluate the length of ACL stump for possible direct repair

PROCEDURE

Room Setup/Patient Positioning

- General or spinal anesthesia
- Supine position
- Tourniquet
- Arthroscopic leg holder or lateral post
- Table is slightly reflexed to achieve 10° of hip flexion

Surgical Technique

- Examination under anesthesia
- Harvesting of semitendinosus tendon (**Figure 2**); be sure to release all vincula to harvest full length of tendon

Graft Preparation

- Double the graft after passing it through a closed loop device
- Arm together the distal ends with No. 2 nonabsorbable braided suture
- Size and pretension graft at approximately 15 N

Arthroscopic Knee Evaluation

- Perform diagnostic arthroscopy through standard anteromedial and anterolateral portals
- Evaluate length of stump of ACL; when possible, perform ACL repair with semitendinosus autograft augmentation
- Identify and treat any associated pathology
- Remove remaining ACL stump with shaver until tibial footprint and intercondylar notch are well visualized

Lateral Approach

- Make a 3- to 4-cm incision to lateral femur at level of posterior femoral cortex proximal to the lateral femoral condyle (**Figure 3, A**)
- Incise iliotibial band longitudinally

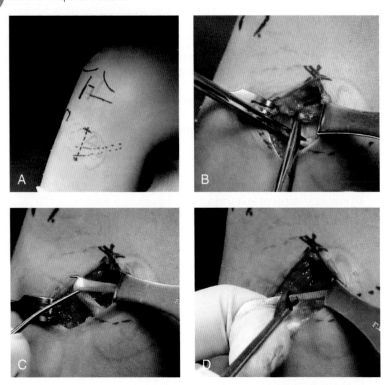

FIGURE 2 Intraoperative photographs demonstrate semitendinosus graft harvesting. **A,** The incision is placed 2 cm medial to the tibial tubercle, started 3 cm below the joint line, and prolonged 3-4 cm distally. **B,** The sartorial fascia is incised proximally and parallel to the tendons with a No. 15 blade first and then with Metzenbaum scissors. **C,** The semitendinosus tendon is then pulled out with a blunt hook, and all the vincula are released proximally, distally, medially, and laterally. **D,** An open tendon stripper is used to harvest the semitendinosus.

- Bluntly separate the vastus lateralis from intermuscular septum and retract anteriorly
- Bluntly create hole in the septum with Metzenbaum scissors, and keep them in contact with posterior femoral cortex; avoid injuring neurovascular bundle
- Use a finger to enlarge septum opening until posterior aspect of condyles and posterior capsule can be palpated (**Figure 3, B**)

Proximal Over-the-Top Preparation

- Pass a gaff hook or curved Kelly clamp from the anterolateral portal into the notch (**Figure 3, C**)
- Important to palpate the passage of the hook along the posterior cortex as it comes out laterally to prevent popliteus vessel injury

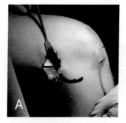 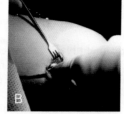 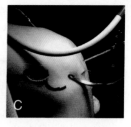

FIGURE 3 Intraoperative photographs demonstrate the lateral femoral approach for anterior cruciate ligament reconstruction. **A,** A 3-4 cm skin incision is performed at the level of the posterior femoral cortex, proximal to the lateral femoral condyle, and the iliotibial band is incised longitudinally. **B,** Metzenbaum scissors and a finger are used to create an opening in the intermuscular septum, posterior to the vastus lateralis. **C,** A gaff hook (or a curved Kelly clamp) is passed from the anterolateral portal into the notch.

- Push hook through posterior capsule and guide it with the finger outside the lateral incision
- Place a suture loop into the tip of the hook and retrieve it anteriorly through the anterolateral portal (**Figure 4**)

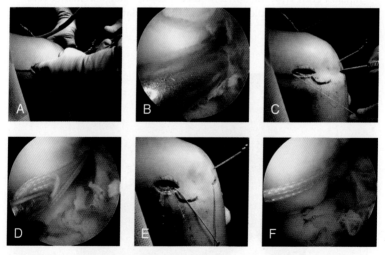

FIGURE 4 Intraoperative photographs and corresponding arthroscopic views demonstrate proximal over-the-top preparation. **A** and **B,** Once the tip of the hook is placed in contact with the posterior femoral cortex and against the posterior capsule, it can be palpated from the lateral approach with a finger. **C** and **D,** The hook is then pushed through the posterior capsule and guided with the finger outside the lateral incision. **E** and **F,** A suture loop is placed into the tip of the hook and retrieved anteriorly through the anterolateral portal.

Tibial Tunnel Preparation

- Insert ACL guide into joint through anteromedial portal and position on native ACL footprint
- Drill guide pin into proximal tibia in more vertical position than that for conventional adult ACL reconstruction to reduce injury to physis
- Drill tibial tunnel of the same size as the graft (usually 6 mm) over the guide pin
- Insert an arthroscopic grasper through the tibial tunnel to retrieve the suture loop from the anterolateral portal and bring it out of the antero-medial tibia
- Use shuttle suture to pull the proximal graft, leading suture out of the lateral incision
- Pull graft into the joint

Proximal Fixation

- Drill a hole at the center of the shaft; insert a screw with a soft-tissue washer into the femur but do not tighten until loop is placed around the screw
- Apply some tension to the graft to allow the loop to sit in a correct position; tighten (**Figure 5**)

Distal Fixation

- Tension graft with traction and knee flexion/extension maneuvers
- Place soft-tissue staple distal to epiphyseal plate to fix the graft to the tibia

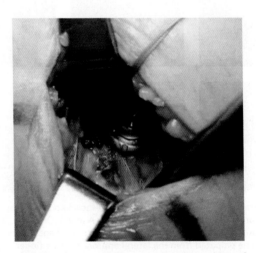

FIGURE 5 Intraoperative photograph demonstrates the position of a 6.5-mm cancellous screw with a soft-tissue washer that was used to fix the loop device that was previously placed in the proximal part of the graft.

COMPLICATIONS

- Growth disturbance
  - Limb-length discrepancy
  - Axial deformity
- Infection
- Residual instability
- Incorrect tunnel placement
- Stiffness

POSTOPERATIVE CARE AND REHABILITATION

- Immediate weight bearing as tolerated and full ROM are allowed post-operatively (**Figure 6**)
- Brace usually not necessary
- First 6 weeks
  - Achieve full ROM
  - Commence strengthening
- At 12 weeks, may begin noncutting and nontwisting sports
- Return to full activity not earlier than 8 to 9 months.

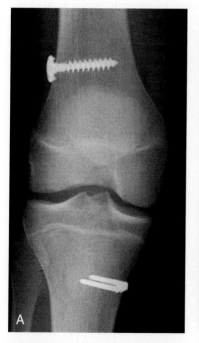 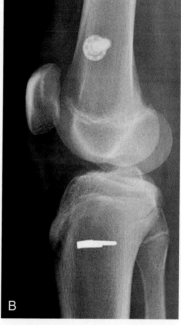

FIGURE 6 Postoperative AP (**A**) and lateral (**B**) radiographs following anterior cruciate ligament (ACL) reconstruction in a pediatric patient show hardware placement that avoids the level of the physes.

- Exceptions to protocol dictated by combined chondral or meniscal procedures and patient age and compliance
- Evidence indicates that a later return to sport may be beneficial in pediatric population

PEARLS

- Care should be taken to not place the lateral femoral incision too proximally.
- Make a small vertical tunnel (6 to 8 mm) in the tibia to minimize damage to the epiphyseal plate and reduce the risk of growth disturbance.
- During fixation of the graft, it is essential to avoid the physes (**Figure 6**). Hardware position can be viewed fluoroscopically.
- Avoid excessive tensioning of the graft to reduce risk of axial deformities.

VIDEO REFERENCE

Video 20.1 Bonasia DE, Rossi R, Wolf B, Amendola A: *ACL: Pediatric Anterior Cruciate Ligament Reconstruction* [video]. Rosemont, IL, American Academy of Orthopaedic Surgeons, 2011.

Medial Patellofemoral Ligament Reconstruction for Recurrent Patellar Instability

INTRODUCTION

- The medial patellofemoral ligament (MPFL) is the primary passive soft-tissue restraint to lateral patellar instability
  - ▶ Can tear when patella dislocates
  - ▶ Other patellar stabilizing components include
    - Bony restraints, especially lateral trochlear ridge
    - Dynamic soft-tissue restraints, especially vastus medialis
- Recent emphasis on additional soft-tissue restraints including medial quadriceps tendon femoral ligament (MQTFL), medial patellotibial ligament (MPTL), and medial patellomeniscal ligament (MPML)
- MPFL reconstruction is performed to restore patellar stability

PATIENT SELECTION

Indications

- Symptomatic recurrent patellar instability with medial soft-tissue insufficiency
- Indicated as a concomitant procedure when bony procedures alone do not restore functional stability
- Patient apprehension with lateral translation on physical examination; best candidates are those who report recurrent painful episodes of lateral subluxation or dislocation associated with twisting mechanism

Contraindications

- Medial patellar instability due to
  - ▶ Iatrogenic overaggressive lateral retinacular release
  - ▶ Hyperlaxity syndromes
- Skeletal immaturity requires modification of procedure
- Active infection

Based on Cosgarea AJ, Tanaka MJ, Elias JJ: Medial patellofemoral ligament reconstruction for recurrent patellar instability, in Colvin AC, Flatow E, eds: Atlas of Essential Orthopaedic Procedures, *ed 2. Rosemont, IL, American Academy of Orthopaedic Surgeons, 2020, pp 163-170.*

PREOPERATIVE IMAGING

Radiography

- Standard AP, notch view, PA in 45° (the latter only in suspected tibiofemoral osteoarthritis)
- Lateral at 30° flexion
  - Used to quantify patellar height using Caton-Deschamps index (**Figure 1**); surgeon can perform distalizing tibial tuberosity osteotomy to correct extreme patella alta
  - Can identify trochlear dysplasia as "crossing sign" (**Figure 2**)
- Sunrise view at 45°—May suggest need for an anteromedializing osteotomy to reduce reactive joint forces in those with arthritic patellofemoral joint

Magnetic Resonance Imaging

- Can assess integrity of articular surfaces
- May lead to additional procedures if necessary, including
  - Cartilage débridement, marrow stimulation, osteochondral replacement procedures

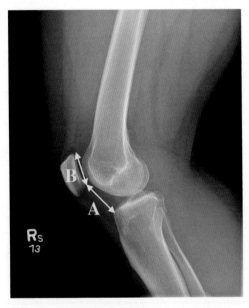

FIGURE 1 The lateral radiograph is used to determine relative patellar height. The Caton-Deschamps index is a measurement of patellar height, calculated by dividing the distance from the inferior articular pole of the patella to the anterior margin of the tibia (**A**), by the articular length of the patella (**B**).

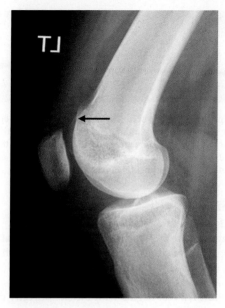

FIGURE 2 Lateral radiograph of a knee shows the "crossing sign" (arrow), indicative of trochlear dysplasia.

- For lateral patellofemoral lesions—Medialization osteotomy (eg, Elmslie-Trillat) to unload lateral patellofemoral joint
- For inferior pole patella lesions—Unload inferior pole with osteotomy (eg, Fulkerson anteromedialization osteotomy)

Computed Tomography
- Determine trochlear morphology, measure malalignment
- Measure tibial tuberosity–trochlear groove distance on superimposed axial CT cuts at Roman arch and proximal tibia at level where tuberosity is most prominent
- Dynamic CT can quantify amount of maltracking and determine flexion angle where lateral translation of the patella is greatest

PROCEDURE
Patient Positioning/Examination Under Anesthesia
- Supine position
- Examination under anesthesia
    - Assess limb alignment, hip rotation; perform knee ligament evaluation
    - Glide test assesses amount of lateral translation of patella; quantified in quadrants; compare with contralateral knee
    - Tilt test determines tightness of lateral retinaculum

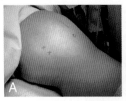 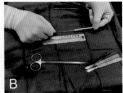 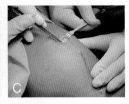

FIGURE 3 Intraoperative photographs of medial patellofemoral ligament (MPFL) reconstruction. **A,** Bony landmarks are marked on the surface of the skin. The proximal X is over the adductor tubercle, and the distal X is over the medial femoral epicondyle. **B,** A locking stitch is woven through the patellar end of the graft. **C,** An incision is made along the medial border of the patella.

Surgical Technique

- Tourniquet is optional
- Perform diagnostic arthroscopy; evaluate for chondral abnormalities to determine whether concomitant osteotomies are indicated; perform osteotomies before MPFL reconstruction
- Mark bony landmarks (**Figure 3**)
- Hamstring graft harvest begins with incision directly over pes anserine bursa
- Perform blunt dissection, electrocauterize small vessels, and expose superior edge of sartorial fascia
- Place tips of scissors under sartorial fascia and sharply release it off its insertion on proximal medial tibia
- Evert sartorial fascia to expose underlying gracilis tendon
- Gracilis hamstring autograft harvest—Use semitendinosus if gracilis is too small; a 4- to 5-mm diameter graft is adequate
- Indications for hamstring allograft are revision surgery, connective tissue disorder
- Prep graft at rear table
  - Using curved scissors, scrape muscle off the hamstring tendon at musculotendinous junction
  - Sharply débride additional tissue to create smooth graft of appropriate size (4 to 5 mm)
  - Weave No. 2 nonabsorbable suture through distal end of graft using locking technique
- Make incision over the medial patella
- Identify superomedial border of the patella and expose just distal and deep to the vastus medialis obliquus muscle

Patellar Fixation

- Interference or tenodesis screw technique—Pass a 2.5-mm drill bit medial to lateral just proximal to equator of patella (**Figure 4**); exchange drill for eyelet Kirschner wire (K-wire) and overdrill with cannulated drill bit 0.5 mm larger than diameter of graft

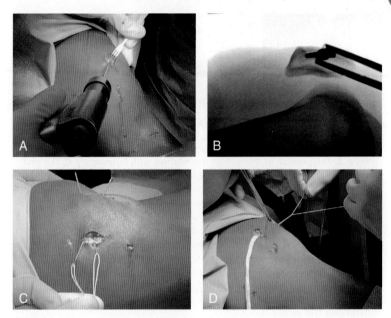

FIGURE 4 Intraoperative photographs (**A**, **C**, and **D**) and a fluoroscopic view (**B**) demonstrate the placement of the patellar tunnel. **A**, A 2.5-mm drill bit is drilled from the medial border of the patella near the junction of the proximal and middle thirds. **B**, Appropriate positioning of the drill bit in the patella is confirmed with lateral fluoroscopy (mini C-arm). **C**, Two diverging eyelet needles are then drilled laterally through the end of the socket, exiting the lateral cortex of the patella. **D**, The knot is tied over a lateral patellar bony bridge.

- Docking technique—Advantage is that femoral tunnel tends to be smaller, and no implants are necessary
  - Drill blind tunnel approximately 10 to 15 mm deep into patella
  - Drill two diverging eyelet needles laterally through end of socket, exiting lateral cortex of patella
  - Pass one end of suture through each K-wire and tie knot over bony bridge

Femoral Fixation
- Palpate to identify locations of adductor tubercle and medial epicondyle, then expose both with sharp and blunt dissection
- Electrocauterize small vessels
- Avoid injury to saphenous nerve
- Place 2.5-mm drill bit just posterior to medial epicondyle
- View position on mini C-arm (**Figure 5**)
- Evaluate graft tension as knee is taken through range of motion (ROM), and confirm that position is isometrically appropriate for the femoral tunnel before fixation of graft; may alter position of drill bit if necessary

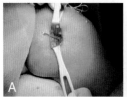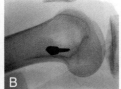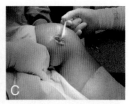

FIGURE 5 Intraoperative photographs (**A** and **C**) and a fluoroscopic view (**B**) demonstrate femoral tunnel position. **A**, Preliminary femoral tunnel position is determined by placing a drill bit just posterior to the palpable medial femoral epicondyle. **B**, The position of the drill bit is confirmed with fluoroscopy. **C**, The graft is wrapped around the drill bit, and knee range of motion is assessed to confirm appropriate isometry.

- Pass graft deep to residual MPFL and superficial to joint capsule; dock in blind femoral tunnel after using a cannulated drill to enlarge the tunnel 0.5 mm larger than diameter of graft (**Figure 6**)
- Place interference screw 1 to 2 mm larger than diameter of femoral tunnel over guidewire and advance

Tensioning the Graft
- 2 N of graft tension restores normal patellar translation
- Avoid overtightening the graft; determine appropriate tension by ranging the knee before fixation of the graft in the femoral tunnel

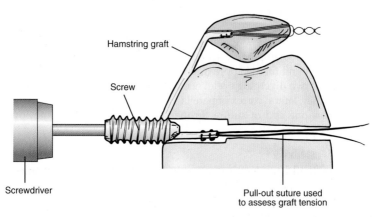

FIGURE 6 Illustration shows fixation in the femoral tunnel. The graft is first fixed to the patella using the docking technique, then into the blind femoral tunnel. With manual traction placed on the pull-out suture, the surgeon assesses knee range of motion to confirm appropriate graft tension and isometry before fixation with the femoral screw.

- MPFL should become looser with flexion beyond 70°
- Repeat glide test; compare with contralateral knee

Wound Closure

- Close wounds in layers in outpatient setting with judicious use of local anesthetic and cryotherapy devices
- Drain used if desired
- Apply adhesive skin closure strips, followed by cryotherapy unit and loosely applied compression dressing and thromboembolic stocking
- Apply hinged brace to facilitate progression to full weight bearing as soon as possible
- Physical therapy recommended for quadriceps strengthening and knee ROM exercises

COMPLICATIONS

- Meta-analysis reported complication rate of 26.1%
- Reduced ROM is the most common complication
- Femoral tunnel malpositioning
  - Especially the femoral tunnel because graft tensioning relationships are more sensitive to femoral tunnel position than to patellar tunnel position
  - If too proximal, can cause excessive graft tension with greater flexion angles, loss of flexion, articular cartilage overload, or graft failure
- Overtensioning of the graft
  - Decreased lateral patellar excursion
  - Increased pressure on patellofemoral cartilage
  - Iatrogenic medial patellar subluxation
- Injury to physis in pediatric cases—Must alter fixation method for femoral tunnel
- Patellar fracture
  - Uncommmon yet devastating complication
  - Can occur after transverse or long tunnels that extend the entire width of the patella
  - Can occur from large diameter or multiple tunnels
- Soft-tissue complications
  - Wound dehiscence
  - Hematoma
  - Implant pain

POSTOPERATIVE CARE AND REHABILITATION

- Immediately postoperatively
  - Quadriceps contractions, straight-leg raises
  - Partial weight bearing
  - Hinged brace locked in extension

- At 1 week, unlock brace; discontinue brace at 6 weeks
- Formal physical therapy three times per week; goals are full extension immediately postoperatively, 120° flexion by 4 weeks, full flexion by 8 weeks
- Jogging by 12 weeks
- Return to sports by 4 to 5 months
- Modify postoperative care if osteotomy has been performed—Crutches for 6 weeks, jogging by 16 weeks, return to sports by 6 to 8 months

PEARLS

- Tibial tuberosity osteotomy may be a preferred surgical approach in patients with excessive tuberosity lateralization, patella alta, or high-grade inferior or lateral chondral lesions. After completing the osteotomy, a concomitant MPFL reconstruction can be performed if the patella is still unstable.

- Surgical stabilization can reliably prevent recurrent instability in most cases but is less reliable in treating concomitant anterior knee pain unrelated to instability episodes.

- If the patient's symptoms, preoperative radiographs, and physical examination are consistent with excessive lateral pressure, then a concomitant arthroscopic lateral retinacular release or lengthening should be considered.

- A common technical error is to place the femoral tunnel too proximally. Malpositioning of the femoral tunnel by as little as 5 mm can result in substantially increased graft force pressure applied to the medial patellofemoral cartilage.

- After fixing the patellar end of the graft in place, the femoral end is wrapped around a drill bit placed just posterior to the medial femoral epicondyle. If graft isometry is not optimal (tension should decrease with flexion beyond 70°), the position of the drill bit should be modified before drilling the femoral tunnel.

- The glide test is used to determine the normal amount of lateral patellar translation in the asymptomatic contralateral knee. This amount of excursion is reproduced in the graft on the symptomatic knee before final graft fixation.

Realignment for Patellofemoral Arthritis

PATIENT SELECTION
- Multiple causes of patellofemoral arthritis
  - Limb alignment
  - Bony architecture of trochlea and patella
  - Integrity of surrounding soft tissues
- Surgical treatment indicated in patients for whom nonsurgical measures—activity modification, bracing treatment, physical therapy, medications, and injections—have failed
- Patellar realignment consists of anteromedialization of the tibial tubercle with osteotomy
  - First described by Fulkerson for patellar instability
  - Excellent option for patients with isolated lateral facet arthritis
- Other procedures for patellofemoral arthritis include lateral release, cartilage restoration, patellofemoral arthroplasty, total knee arthroplasty, and patellar realignment

Indications
- Isolated distal/lateral patella facet or lateral trochlear chondrosis with no chondrosis of the proximal/medial patellofemoral joint
- Central patellar wear in patients with patellar subluxation seen on radiographs

Contraindications
- Severe medial and/or proximal patellar chondrosis
- Standard osteotomy contraindications—Nicotine use, osteoporosis, nonspecific pain, complex regional pain syndrome, infection, inflammatory arthropathies, patella baja, or arthrofibrosis
- Relative contraindications
  - Varus knee, medial compartment arthritis, post–medial meniscectomy knee
  - Severe medial and/or lateral compartment arthritis of the knee—requires a more global procedure

---

Based on Lin A, West R: Realignment for patellofemoral arthritis, in Colvin AC, Flatow E, eds: Atlas of Essential Orthopaedic Procedures, *ed 2. Rosemont, IL, American Academy of Orthopaedic Surgeons, 2020, pp 171-176.*

 169

PREOPERATIVE IMAGING

Radiography

- 45° flexion weight-bearing PA shows degree of tibiofemoral joint space narrowing
- Merchant view assesses patellar tilt, subluxation, and trochlear dysplasia
- Lateral view evaluates patellar height and trochlear dysplasia

Magnetic Resonance Imaging

- Assess for medial patellofemoral ligament injury or other ligamentous or meniscal pathologies
- Find degree and location of articular cartilage loss
- Determine tibial tuberosity–trochlear groove distance—Lateral offset of tibial tuberosity from the deepest point in the trochlear groove; greater than 20 mm nearly always is associated with patellar instability

CT

- Rarely ordered in treatment of patellofemoral arthritis
- Occasionally ordered in treatment of patellofemoral instability in patients with correlating femoral anteversion, increased tibial torsion, and patellar maltracking
- Can determine tibial tuberosity–trochlear groove distance, femoral anteversion, and patellar tracking at different knee flexion angles

PROCEDURE

Room Setup/Patient Positioning

- Supine position
- Tourniquet (for osteotomy portion of case only)

VIDEO 22.1 Anterior Medialization via Tibial Tubercle Osteotomy. Albert Lin, MD; Robin West, MD (21 min)

Special Instrumentation/Equipment/Implants

- 30° and 70° arthroscopes
- Microsagittal saw
- Standard Steinmann pins and Kirschner wires
- 4.5- and 3.2-mm drill bits
- 4.5-mm threaded standard AO cortical screws

Surgical Technique

Examination Under Anesthesia

- Compare with contralateral knee

© 2021 American Academy of Orthopaedic Surgeons

- Document range of motion, presence of effusion, ligamentous laxity, and patellar tracking/tilt/crepitus/glide
- Examine the patella in full extension and at 20° to 30° flexion (when patella is engaged in trochlea)

Landmarks, Portals, Incisions

- Mark landmarks (patella, patellar tendon, tibial tubercle, Gerdy tubercle, tibial crest), arthroscopic portal sites, and skin incisions (**Figure 1**)
- Superolateral portal with a 70° arthroscope is best viewing portal to evaluate the patellofemoral joint

Diagnostic Arthroscopy

- To assess the articular cartilage and confirm no contraindication to the realignment exists
- Involves two portals
- View the patellofemoral joint while flexing/extending the knee
- Anterolateral portal with a 30° arthroscope is standard for diagnostic knee arthroscopy
- Open lateral release is performed only if retinaculum is taut (negative patellar tilt) and tilt cannot be passively restored to neutral (**Figure 2**)
  - Make a 2- to 3-cm longitudinal incision from midportion of patella to just proximal to superior pole of patella
  - Release only from inferior pole to superior pole

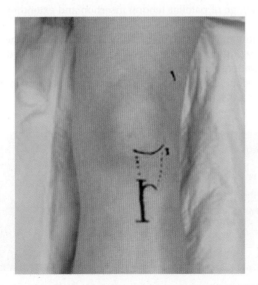

FIGURE 1 Preoperative photograph shows the standard incisions used for patellofemoral realignment, including a superolateral and an inferolateral portal site marked on the skin.

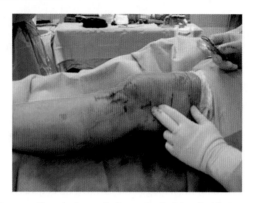

FIGURE 2 Intraoperative photograph shows the incision for the open lateral release.

Realignment

- Make a 5- to 7-cm incision just medial to the tibial tubercle, extending from 1 cm proximal to patellar tendon insertion distally
- Dissect and elevate fascia from lateral tibia to expose anterolateral tibial crest and Gerdy tubercle
- Protect patellar tendon
- Mark osteotomy site with Bovie on anteromedial tibial crest, starting at medial edge of patellar tendon insertion and extending distally for 5 cm
- Place Steinmann pin from medial tibial crest to indicate the slope of the osteotomy (**Figure 3**); slope can be adjusted for more medialization or anteriorization (**Figure 4**)
- Once the slope is determined, use a microsagittal saw to perform the osteotomy freehand (**Figure 5**)

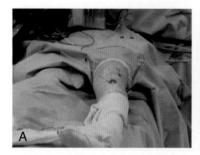
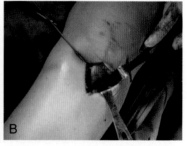

FIGURE 3 Intraoperative photographs show use of a Steinmann pin to mark the osteotomy angle for patellofemoral realignment. **A,** View from the end of the table with the Steinmann pin in place. **B,** Close-up view with the Steinmann pin exiting the lateral tibial cortex.

© 2021 American Academy of Orthopaedic Surgeons

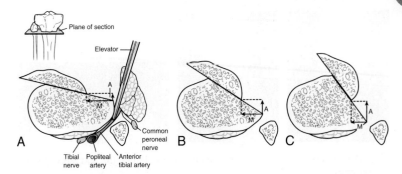

FIGURE 4 Drawing demonstrates the determination of osteotomy slope for tibial tubercle realignment. **A,** A flat (no-angle) osteotomy allows medialization of the tibial tubercle. The elevator protects the neurovascular bundle. **B,** A steeper cut provides equal anteriorization and medialization of the tibial tubercle. **C,** A very steep cut provides maximum anteriorization of the tibial tubercle with less medialization. A = distance of anteriorization, M = distance of medialization

- Complete the osteotomy with a 1/4-in curved osteotome proximally in a transverse fashion; hinged distally and completed only if patella alta present
- Tibial tubercle shifted anteromedially up to 1 cm with at least 50% contact with underlying tibia to ensure good healing potential
- Fix with two fully threaded 4.5-mm screws with compression technique
- Countersink to prevent painful prominent hardware
- Confirm with mini C-arm before wound closure

COMPLICATIONS

- Detachment of vastus lateralis obliquus from overzealous lateral release
- Injury to patella tendon
- Iatrogenic tibial metaphyseal fracture

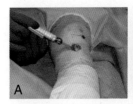
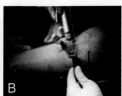
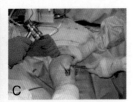

FIGURE 5 Intraoperative photographs show the tibial tubercle osteotomy. The sagittal saw angle is shown from the end of the table (**A**) and from the side (**B**). **C,** The proximal transverse cut is completed under the patella with the 1/4-in curved osteotome.

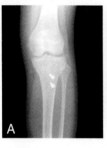 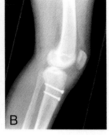 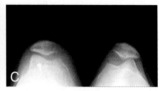

FIGURE 6 Postoperative non–weight-bearing AP (**A**), lateral (**B**), and Merchant (**C**) radiographs.

- Complications related to any bony surgery near knee—Infection, non-union, malunion, compartment syndrome, arthrofibrosis, patella baja, worsening or no improvement in symptoms

POSTOPERATIVE CARE AND REHABILITATION

- Full weight bearing with crutches
- Brace locked in full extension—Unlocked at 6 weeks with radiographic confirmation of osteotomy healing
- Radiographs at first postoperative visit—Assess screw lengths, position of the osteotomy, and patellar tilt and subluxation (**Figure 6**)
- Continuous passive motion started within a few days of surgery; heel slides allowed to 90° of knee flexion until osteotomy healed
- Physical therapy to help regain quadriceps control and patellar mobility
- Return to sports without restrictions at 4 to 5 months postoperatively

---

PEARLS

- Lateral release done in conjunction with the tibial tubercle transfer to help "balance" the soft tissues. Overzealous lateral release can lead to poor outcomes.
- Fracture at osteotomy site can occur in patients with osteoporosis or who use nicotine.
- Complete osteotomy with 1/4-in curved osteotome to avoid fracture extension into lateral plateau.
- Countersink screws to prevent painful prominent hardware.
- To aid in healing, 50% contact between tibia and tubercle is maintained.
- Brace locked in extension postoperatively to prevent excessive forces at the osteotomy site. Full weight bearing is allowed.

Surgical Treatment of Traumatic Quadriceps and Patellar Tendon Injuries of the Knee

INTRODUCTION

Background

- Ruptures of the extensor mechanism are debilitating injuries that typically require surgery and prolonged physical therapy
- Knee extension plays a central role in activities of daily living

Epidemiology

- Quad tendon ruptures typically occur in patients older than 40 years; patella tendon ruptures typically occur in patients younger than 40 years
- Patella fractures are the most common cause of extensor mechanism failure
- Indirect injury accounts for twice as many quad tendon injuries and three times as many patella tendon injuries as direct injury
- Males are more likely to have quad or patella tendon rupture

Biomechanics and Pathology

- The relatively low frequency of tendinous rupture is partly due to the relative strength of tendons
  - Biomechanical studies have shown that a force 17.5 times body weight is required for rupture of extensor mechanism
  - Nondirect traumatic tendinous rupture is likely to occur through a region of pathologic change
    - End-stage renal disease, diabetes mellitus, rheumatoid arthritis, gout, obesity, hyperparathyroidism, systemic lupus erythematosus, systemic steroid use, infection, and repetitive microtrauma predispose to rupture
    - Incidence of systemic conditions is 70% in bilateral quadriceps ruptures and 20% in unilateral ruptures
  - One study showed poor blood supply in the quadriceps tendon in a zone 1 to 2 cm from insertion site of the quadriceps tendon into the patella; this finding coincides with the observation that most tears occur within 2 cm of the superior pole of the patella

---

Based on Featherall J, Hurwit D, James E, Turcan S, Ranawat, AS: Surgical treatment of traumatic quadriceps and patellar tendon injuries of the knee, in Colvin AC, Flatow E, eds: Atlas of Essential Orthopaedic Procedures, *ed 2. Rosemont, IL, American Academy of Orthopaedic Surgeons, 2020, pp 177-189.*

PATIENT SELECTION

- Symptoms—Pain, inability to perform a straight-leg raise due to lack of active knee extension, a palpable suprapatellar or infrapatellar tendinous defect, large knee effusion, ecchymosis
- Timing—Surgical repair done more than 2 weeks post injury is associated with increased surgical complexity and more unsatisfactory results
  - ❱ Chronic tears are more likely to need graft augmentation
- Relative contraindications
  - ❱ Nonambulatory patients
  - ❱ Significant medical comorbidities
  - ❱ Compromised soft tissues around the knee from infection, trauma, radiation
  - ❱ Known noncompliance with rehabilitation
  - ❱ Chronic irreparable tears
- Incomplete tear of the extensor mechanism can be treated nonsurgically
  - ❱ Incomplete tears—Evident when patients retain active knee extension against gravity while supine but have compromised extension against resistance while seated
  - ❱ Such patients lack a large palpable tendinous defect and radiographic findings of patella baja or alta

PREOPERATIVE IMAGING
Radiography
- AP and lateral views
- Quadriceps tendon tear—Characteristic findings are patella baja, interruption of quadriceps tendon soft-tissue shadow, and suprapatellar soft-tissue mass
- Patellar tendon tear—Characteristic finding is patella alta

Ultrasonography
- Operator dependent
- Expeditious and inexpensive way to determine location and completeness of the tear (**Figure 1**)

Magnetic Resonance Imaging
- Can accurately diagnose difficult cases (**Figure 2**)
- Can identify concomitant injuries; 30% of patellar tendon tears and 10% of quadriceps tendon tears are associated with concomitant injuries, usually anterior cruciate ligament and medial meniscus tears

PROCEDURE
Positioning and Preparation
- Regional anesthesia
- Supine position with bump under ipsilateral hip

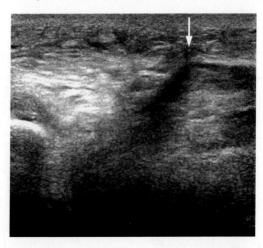

FIGURE 1 Sagittal ultrasonographic image shows a ruptured quadriceps tendon. The anechoic shadow within the substance of the tendon (arrow) represents the rupture.

- Tourniquet
- Examination under anesthesia to evaluate for soft-tissue injuries or confirm presence and extent of injuries identified on preoperative imaging

Quadriceps Tendon Repair

- For osteotendinous junction tear repair (**Figure 3**)
  - Most common repair is transosseous tunnel technique, which involves interlocking sutures through proximal tendon

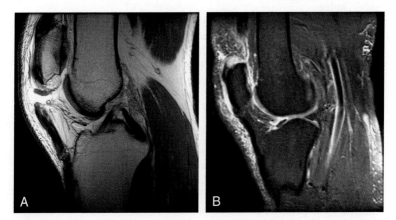

FIGURE 2 Extensor mechanism injuries of the knee. **A,** Sagittal T1-weighted MRI demonstrates an acute patellar tendon rupture. **B,** Sagittal fluid-sensitive, fat-suppressed MRI demonstrates an acute quadriceps tendon tear.

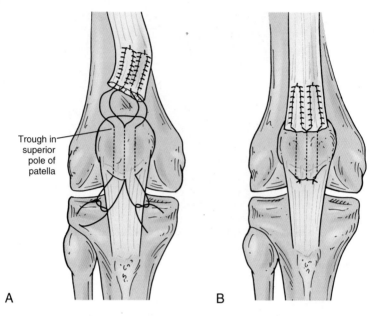

Trough in superior pole of patella

FIGURE 3 Illustrations show acute quadriceps tendon repair. **A,** The four suture limbs of the Krackow stitch are passed through the three transosseous drill holes. **B,** The suture limbs are tied together over the patellar bone bridge.

    ▸ Pass sutures through longitudinal transosseous patellar drill holes

    ▸ Tie sutures over patellar bony bridge

- On rare occasions you can do a quadriceps turndown technique or augmented with an Achilles allograft
- Use of suture anchors—recent biomechanical studies have demonstrated that suture anchors are equally as strong or superior to transosseous tunnels
- Authors' preferred technique for repair is using transosseous tunnels

Surgical Technique

- Make midline longitudinal incision 5 cm proximal to superior border of patella extending to inferior pole of patella distally
- Create full-thickness flaps down to extensor mechanism
- Débride and irrigate scar tissue/hematoma
- Deflate tourniquet to allow full mobilization of the tendon; hemostasis is achieved using electrocautery

Quadriceps Tendon Repair Using Transosseous Tunnels

- Débride degenerative tendon of proximal segment, then place two No. 5 nonabsorbable sutures using a Krackow stitch through the full-thickness medial and lateral aspects of the tendon; it is critical to maximize the number of sutures across the tendon
- Débride the superior pole of the patella of remaining tendon, and create a bleeding cancellous bone bed
- Use 2.5-mm drill to create medial, middle, and lateral longitudinal holes through the patella (**Figure 4**); avoid iatrogenic damage to patella cartilage
- Use a suture passer to pull the four suture limbs through the three bone tunnels with two sutures passed through the middle tunnel
- With the knee in full extension and the patella maximally elevated superiorly with a bone clamp, tie the sutures over the patellar bone bridges

VIDEO 23.1 Repair of Injuries to the Extensor Mechanism: Quadriceps and Patellar Tendons. Spero G. Karas, MD; Richard J. Hawkins, MD, FRCSC; J. Richard Steadman, MD (10 min)

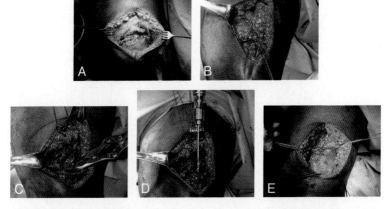

FIGURE 4 Intraoperative photographs demonstrate the surgical repair of an acute quadriceps tendon rupture. **A**, Exposure of the tear. **B**, The quadriceps tendon is mobilized after two sutures are placed in the tendon using a Krackow stitch. **C**, Débridement of the superior patellar pole. **D**, Creation of the transosseous patellar tunnels using a 2.5-mm drill. Careful attention is paid to drill orientation to avoid iatrogenically violating the articular cartilage. **E**, Medial and lateral retinaculum repair.

- Repair the medial and lateral retinaculum with No. 2 nonabsorbable suture using a figure-of-8 suture technique
- Gently take knee through range of motion (ROM) from 0° to 90° to assess integrity of repair
- Place drain subfascially
- Irrigate and close wound superficially, using interrupted 0 and 2-0 absorbable sutures to close the deep fascia and superficial subcutaneous tissue; close skin with interrupted 3-0 nylon sutures and cover with sterile dressing
- Fit hinged knee brace locked in extension

Acute Patellar Tendon Repair

- Most commonly occurs at the patella–patellar tendon junction; repair with locking stitch through tendinous component, passed through longitudinal transosseous patellar drill holes, and tied over a patellar bone bridge proximally (**Figure 5**)
- Suture anchors have superior biomechanical properties to transosseous sutures

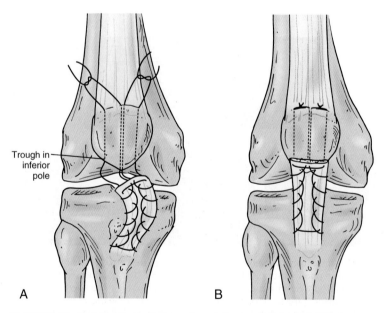

FIGURE 5 Illustrations demonstrate acute patellar tendon repair. **A,** The four suture limbs are passed through the three transosseous drill holes. **B,** The sutures are tied over the patellar bone bridge, reapproximating the torn superior portion of the patellar tendon with the patella.

- Cortical button repair has biomechanical superiority over both suture anchors and transosseous sutures
- Distal disruption in proximity to tibial tubercle
  - Infrequent
  - Repaired with locking sutures inserted through the proximal portion of the tendon, passed through tibial drill holes, and tied
- Midsubstance tears
  - Repaired primarily
  - If augmentation required, semitendinosus autograft or allograft can be used; pass graft through horizontal tibial and patellar drill holes, and suture the graft to itself and native tendon
- Avulsion fracture of nonarticulating inferior pole of patella
  - Typically comminuted and treated with resection of distal fragments and reattachment of tendon
  - Or perform open reduction and internal fixation with basket plate and screws if nonosteoporotic bone or in minimal comminution
- Authors' preferred method is proximal osteotendinous repair

Surgical Technique

- Inflate tourniquet and then deflate after approach or before tying sutures
- Make midline longitudinal skin incision starting 2 cm proximal to the superior border of the patella, extending distally to the tibial tubercle
- Preserve paratenon if possible.

Patellar Tendon Repair Using Transosseous Tunnels

- Débride any remaining tendon from inferior pole of patella until a bed of bleeding cancellous bone is obtained
- Sew two No. 5 nonabsorbable sutures using a Krackow stitch through the full-thickness medial and lateral aspects of the tendon
- Use 2.5-mm drill to create medial, middle, and lateral longitudinal tunnels through the patella
- Bring suture through the tunnels proximally with suture passer; tie sutures over bony bridges with knee in full extension

Retinacular Repair

- Repair retinaculum with No. 2 suture in figure-of-8 fashion if necessary
- If concern for patient compliance exists, pass No. 5 nonabsorbable suture through distal quadriceps muscle and tendon immediately proximal to the superior pole of patella, and tie in a figure-of-8 pattern through a tibial drill hole made with a 2.5-mm drill bit, with knee in 45° flexion (**Figure 6**)
- Perform gentle ROM to assess integrity of repair
- Place drain subfascially
- Fit hinged knee brace locked in extension

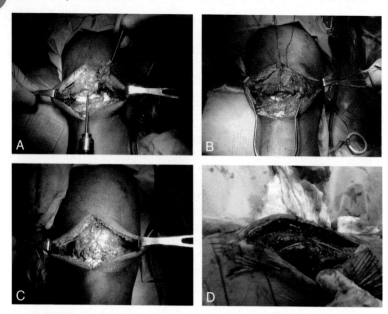

FIGURE 6 Intraoperative photographs demonstrate surgical repair of an acute patellar tendon rupture. **A**, Creation of the longitudinal patellar tunnels. **B**, Passage of the patellar tendon sutures. It is important to ensure that the tourniquet is deflated before tightening the repair, to facilitate adequate mobilization of the proximal portion of the knee extensor mechanism. **C**, Completed repair of the patellar tendon and retinaculum. **D**, Figure-of-8 augmentation suture. The suture is passed around the superior patellar pole and through a tibial drill hole before tightening to take tension off the patellar tendon repair.

Chronic Quadriceps and Patellar Tendon Repairs
- Rare but disabling injuries
- Unique challenge surgically because of
  - Retraction of the patella
  - Adhesions of the extensor mechanism
  - Quadriceps atrophy
  - Relative paucity of native tendon to use for repair
- Surgical techniques that can be used for repair/reconstruction
  - Augmentation with wire or additional nonabsorbable suture
  - V-Y quadricepsplasty when muscular contraction present

Graft Augmentation
- Autograft or allograft for reconstruction
  - Autograft options—Contralateral bone–patellar tendon–bone or autologous ipsilateral semitendinosus and/or gracilis tendon transfers
  - Allograft used is generally Achilles tendon–bone allograft

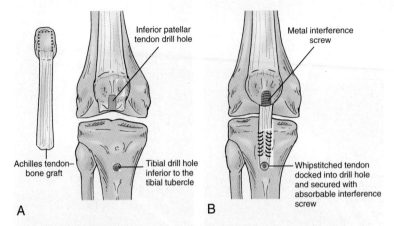

FIGURE 7 Illustrations demonstrate patellar tendon allograft reconstruction. **A,** The inferior patellar and tibial drill holes are made, and an Achilles tendon–bone allograft is prepared. **B,** The bone plug is fitted into the inferior patellar drill hole and secured with an interference screw. The distal tendinous portion of the graft is whipstitched and seated in the tibial drill hole using a docking technique.

- Authors' preferred method of repair for chronic patellar tendon rupture is patellar tendon allograft reconstruction

Approach
- Exposure is the same as that for acute patellar tendon rupture repair
- Débride extensive scar and adhesions
- Attempt repair if adequate tendon remains

Graft Preparation and Placement
- If native tendon is deficient, use Achilles allograft (**Figure 7**)
- Débride inferior pole of patella until bleeding bone bed is obtained
- Use anterior cruciate ligament tunnel guide system to drill 10-mm hole centrally in the inferior pole of patella to a depth of 30 mm
- Make a similar 10- × 30-mm hole on anterior tibia just inferior to tibial tubercle
- Prepare Achilles tendon–bone allograft with oscillating saw to create a 10- × 25-mm calcaneal bone plug
- Place allograft bone plug in inferior drill hole of the patella; secure with a 7- × 25-mm metal interference screw
- Measure allograft tendon, and whipstitch it distally with a No. 2 nonabsorbable suture
- Dock tendon into tibial drill hole; secure it with 9- × 30-mm absorbable interference screw

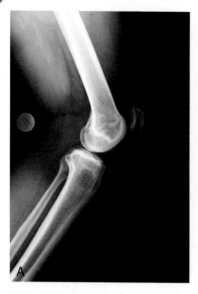 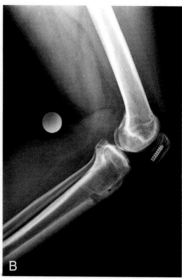

FIGURE 8 Radiographs show the knee of a healthy 39-year-old man with an extensor lag after a failed patellar tendon repair. **A,** Lateral view of the right knee demonstrates patella alta. **B,** Postoperative lateral radiograph shows the right knee after a revision patellar tendon repair using an Achilles allograft. The patient regained all extension and a normal patellar height.

Adjustment of Patellar Position

- Use fluoroscopy to determine that correct patellar height has been obtained using the Insall-Salvati ratio (**Figure 8**)
- Compare with preoperative imaging of contralateral knee
- If quadriceps contracture prevents restoration of patellar height, Z-plasty or V-Y lengthening can be performed
- For V-Y lengthening, make full-thickness inverted V-shaped incision in the quadriceps; once adequate tendon length is gained (determined via fluoroscopy), incision is repaired with nonabsorbable sutures, resulting in Y-shaped repair

Repair Augmentation

- Augment repair with No. 5 nonabsorbable suture around superior pole of patella tied in figure-of-8 pattern through a tibial drill hole with the knee flexed at 45°
- Place hinged brace locked in extension

Patellar Tendon Repair With Suture Anchor Augmentation

- After primary patella tendon repair is complete, two suture anchors loaded with tape sutures are placed medially and laterally in the inferior pole of the patella

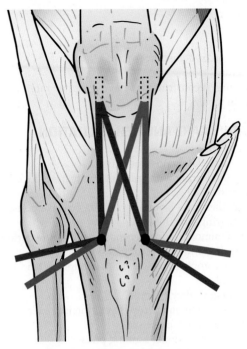

FIGURE 9 Illustration of patellar tendon repair augmentation using suture anchors and tape sutures in box-and-X configuration.

- Free needle is used to pass the sutures through the patellar tendon to its anterior aspect
- Arrange sutures in the box-and-X pattern and fix distally using suture anchors medial and lateral to the tibial tubercle (**Figure 9**)

Extensor Mechanism Disruptions After Total Knee Arthroplasty
- Uncommon complication
  - 0.1% to 1.1% incidence for quadriceps tendon rupture
  - 0.17% to 1.4% incidence for patella tendon rupture
- Surgical options
  - Direct repair
  - Transosseous bone tunnels
  - Autograft or allograft augmentation
  - Autograft or allograft reconstruction
  - Synthetic mesh

COMPLICATIONS
- Quadriceps atrophy and weakness
- Quadriceps lag

- Anterior knee pain
- Stiffness
- Rerupture
- Wound infection or dehiscence
- Patellar fracture
- Chronic repairs/reconstructions have a higher rate of complications than do acute repairs

POSTOPERATIVE CARE AND REHABILITATION

- Immobilization phase
  - ▶ Begins immediately postoperatively
  - ▶ Full weight bearing with crutches and in brace locked in extension for 1 month
  - ▶ Physical therapy—Isometric quadriceps exercises, calf pumps, and hamstring stretching
  - ▶ Length of immobilization depends on procedure performed; motion is begun sooner following inferior pole patellar fracture fixation and later in noncompliant patients with quadriceps tendon ruptures
- Passive ROM phase
  - ▶ Usually begins after 1 month
  - ▶ Passive ROM and quadriceps strengthening exercises; low-weight and high-repetition exercises
- Active ROM with functional training phase
  - ▶ Gait training with brace unlocked
  - ▶ After 1 month of active ROM and gait training, wean the patient from the crutches and brace
  - ▶ Advance from closed-chain quadriceps exercises to jogging, running, and jumping/cutting/pivoting maneuvers by the fifth postoperative month
  - ▶ Return to sport when quadriceps strength and one-leg vertical jump is greater than 90% that of contralateral leg with no visible quadriceps atrophy and ability to run and do drills without a limp

PEARLS

- Quadriceps tendon tears are more degenerative in nature than are patellar tendon ruptures and typically occur in patients who are older than 40 years.
- Fractures of inferior pole of the patella with significant comminution are patellar tendon rupture variants and can be fixed in a similar manner; however, the surgeon must avoid creating patella baja.
- The strength of a repair depends on the number of sutures that cross the repair site. In some cases, three sutures can be used but should not be used if the vascular and structural integrity of the tendon are compromised.
- Chronic repairs or reruptures are best treated with allograft augmentation.

Shoulder and Elbow

2

Section Editor

John W. Sperling, MD, MBA

24 Arthroscopic Subacromial Decompression and Distal Clavicle Resection

PATIENT SELECTION
- Subacromial impingement and degenerative changes of the acromioclavicular joint are common causes of shoulder pain; they often result from repetitive overhead use that leads to inflammation of the bursa and supraspinatus tendon as they pass under the acromion
- Pain reported with overhead activities, lateral shoulder pain, night pain, and pain with abduction and internal rotation
- Surgical intervention is indicated following failure of a 3- to 6-month course of nonsurgical management that includes anti-inflammatory medications, physical therapy with rotator cuff strengthening, and activity modification

PREOPERATIVE IMAGING
Radiography
- True AP view of the glenohumeral joint
- Outlet view to evaluate the acromion
- Axillary lateral view to rule out os acromiale
- Zanca view to evaluate acromioclavicular joint

Magnetic Resonance Imaging
- Helpful in assessing condition of rotator cuff
- Increased signal intensity at acromioclavicular joint can aid in confirming the diagnosis

 VIDEO 24.1 Subacromial Decompression and Distal Clavicle Resection. Mark Rodosky, MD; Albert Lin, MD (6 min)

Based on Lin A, Rodosky MW: Arthroscopic subacromial decompression and distal clavicle resection, in Colvin AC, Flatow E, eds: Atlas of Essential Orthopaedic Procedures, *ed 2. Rosemont, IL, American Academy of Orthopaedic Surgeons, 2020, pp 191-197.*

PROCEDURE

Room Setup/Patient Positioning

- Upright in beach-chair position (**Figure 1**)
- Acromion parallel to the floor
- Bony prominences well padded

Special Instruments/Equipment/Implants

- 30° arthroscope
- 4.5- and 5.5-mm arthroscopic shavers
- 5.5-mm arthroscopic burr
- Standard and hooked arthroscopic electrocautery devices

Surgical Technique

Examination Under Anesthesia

- Should be performed to evaluate range of motion (ROM) and ligamentous laxity
- Side-to-side comparison with nonsurgical limb can be done

Landmarks/Portals

- Mark arthroscopic portal sites and other bony landmarks (**Figure 2**)
- Use three portals: anterior working, posterior viewing, and lateral working

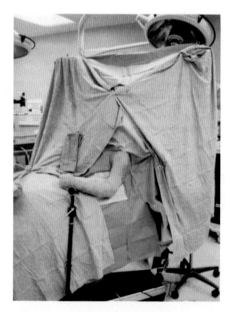

FIGURE 1 Photograph demonstrates upright beach-chair positioning of a patient for arthroscopic subacromial decompression and distal clavicle resection.

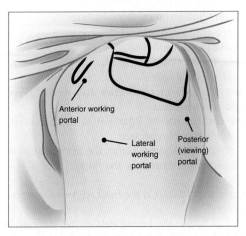

FIGURE 2 Illustration of a left shoulder shows the location of the anterior working portal, lateral working portal, and posterior (viewing) portal in relationship to the coracoid, clavicle, acromion, and scapular spine, which are marked on the skin.

- Arthroscopic subacromial decompression is best performed with arthroscope in posterior portal and instruments in lateral portal
- Distal clavicle resection is best performed with arthroscope in lateral portal and instruments in anterior portal

Diagnostic Arthroscopy

- Performed through posterior portal; make skin incision 2 to 3 cm inferior and in line with the posterolateral corner of the acromion
- Premark anterior portal: this site will be collinear with glenohumeral joint
- Always make anterior portal under direct arthroscopic visualization
- Portal position can vary depending on the pathology to be addressed
- Perform a full diagnostic arthroscopy to include assessment of the cartilage, labrum, capsuloligamentous structures, biceps, and rotator cuff
- Place arthroscope into the subacromial space
- Arthroscope should hug undersurface of acromion
- The trocar can be used to bluntly release subacromial adhesions via a sweeping motion
- Visualize the anterolateral corner of the acromion
- Establish the lateral portal under direct visualization using a spinal needle
- An anterior and low position is preferred; a high portal makes it difficult to assess the medial acromion and limits acromioclavicular joint visualization

Acromioplasty and Subacromial Decompression

- Use a 5.5-mm arthroscopic shaver to perform bursectomy and expose undersurface of the acromion
- Expose lateral aspect first to help identify the position of the shaver within the subacromial space
- Débridement proceeds in a posterior and medial direction until the scapular spine is visualized
- Preserve the coracoacromial ligament in the presence of a deficient rotator cuff or irreparable cuff tear
- Otherwise, release the ligament from the front edge of the acromion
- Place a 5.5-mm burr through the lateral portal to perform the acromioplasty
- Acromioplasty should start at the front edge of the anterolateral aspect of the acromion
- Use the burr to flatten the lateral half of the anterior third until it is collinear with the middle third of the acromion
- The depth of the acromioplasty will be equal to the width of the burr
- Resect the medial half in the same fashion, using the lateral half as a template

Distal Clavicle Resection

- Expose the acromioclavicular joint after completing the subacromial decompression
- Establish an anterior working portal in the subacromial space
- Switch the arthroscope to the lateral working portal
- Place a 5.5-mm arthroscopic shaver through the anterior portal
- Resect the inferior and anterior capsule and the intra-articular fibro-cartilage disk
- Expose and remove the distal clavicle arthritic cartilage with a shaver
- Use electrocautery to elevate the capsule from the clavicle edge; take care to preserve the posterior and superior capsule
- Place a 5.5-mm burr in the anterior portal and resect 1 cm of the distal clavicle (**Figure 3**)
- Resect the front half first and use it as a template for the posterior half

Conclusion of Procedure

- Suction fluid from the subacromial space
- Close the portal sites with buried monofilament absorbable sutures
- Apply standard dressings, a sling, and a compressive cooling device

COMPLICATIONS

- Incomplete resection of acromion or distal clavicle
- Regrowth of distal clavicle or acromion
- Continued pain
- Acromioclavicular joint instability

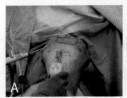 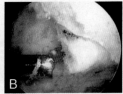 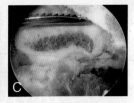

FIGURE 3 Images show distal clavicle resection. **A,** Photograph shows the arthroscope in the lateral working portal and the 5.5-mm arthroscopic burr in the anterior working portal. **B,** Arthroscopic view demonstrates the position of the burr at the distal clavicle. The anterior half has been resected from superior to inferior. **C,** Arthroscopic view demonstrates use of a rasp of known dimension to verify the width and angle of resection at the completion of the distal clavicle resection.

- Infection
- Adhesive capsulitis
- Neurovascular injury

POSTOPERATIVE CARE AND REHABILITATION
- Sling and cold device are used for 48 hours
- Pendulum exercises start immediately
- Physical therapy is started within 24 to 48 hours, with progressive passive and active ROM exercises in all planes
- Strengthening is started within a few weeks once full ROM is achieved
- Return to strenuous activities can take 3 to 6 months

PEARLS

- Avoid improper portal placement by using a spinal needle under direct visualization to localize the lateral working portal and by paying strict attention to the bony landmarks.
- An arthroscopic pump helps the surgeon to change the pressure needed for visualization and adjust for variability in the patient's blood pressure.
- Complete exposure of the anterior two-thirds of the scapula and the scapular spine before acromioplasty helps avoid leaving behind ridges.
- When performing subacromial decompression in patients with a deficient rotator cuff or an irreparable rotator cuff tear, preserve the coracoacromial ligament.
- In arthroscopic distal clavicle resections, placing the anterior working portal parallel to the acromioclavicular joint makes resection easier.
- Fully release the capsule before performing a distal clavicle resection, and resect from superior to inferior.
- Take care to avoid resecting more than 1 cm of the distal clavicle; doing so will destabilize the acromioclavicular joint.

25 Arthroscopic Management of Frozen Shoulder

PATIENT SELECTION

- Frozen shoulder is defined by a loss of range of motion (ROM), which impairs the performance of daily activities or desired recreational activities
- Etiology, pathology, natural history, diagnosis, and treatment are debated
  - ▸ Cytokines, myofibroblasts, growth factors, and matrix metalloproteinases have all been implicated
  - ▸ Similarities to Dupuytren disease and Peyronie disease have been described
- Generally affects patients aged 40 to 60 years
  - ▸ Occurs in 2% of overall population
  - ▸ Seen in up to 18% of those with diabetes
- Progresses through three stages
  - ▸ Inflammation (freezing)
  - ▸ Fibrosis with disorganization and contracture (frozen)
  - ▸ Resolution (thawing)
- Most cases resolve within 2 to 3 years, although residual loss of ROM is common
- Frozen shoulder or adhesive capsulitis is the clinical diagnosis; the terms are used interchangeably
- Primary means of diagnosis is assessment of ROM before and after local injection of anesthetic into the glenohumeral joint
  - ▸ If ROM does not resolve, diagnosis of frozen shoulder is more likely
  - ▸ If ROM improves, other conditions are considered, including impingement, rotator cuff tears, subacromial impingement, acromioclavicular joint pathology, and cervical spine pathology
- Multiple treatment options exist
  - ▸ Benign neglect
  - ▸ NSAIDs

Based on Chalmers PN, Sherman SL, Ghodadra N, Nicholson GP: Arthroscopic management of frozen shoulder, in Colvin AC, Flatow E, eds: Atlas of Essential Orthopaedic Procedures, *ed 2. Rosemont, IL, American Academy of Orthopaedic Surgeons, 2020, pp 198-204.*

 ▶ Oral steroids
 ▶ Steroid injections
 ▶ Home stretching regimens
 ▶ Supervised physical therapy
 ▶ Manipulation under anesthesia (shown to be effective in a recent meta-analysis)
 ▶ Arthroscopic synovectomy, arthroscopic subacromial decompression, arthroscopic capsular release, and open capsular release

- Nonsurgical measures should be pursued for at least 6 weeks to 3 months before considering surgery
- Arthroscopic capsular release has been shown to reduce pain, improve ROM, and possibly shorten the natural history of the disease
 ▶ Contraindications include an indwelling prosthesis or a history of instability
 ▶ Advantages over manipulation under anesthesia include additional diagnostic information, more controlled capsular release, ability to perform simultaneous brisement, ability to perform synovial débridement, and ability to perform subacromial decompression

PREOPERATIVE IMAGING

- Frozen shoulder is a diagnosis of exclusion; imaging helps exclude other pathology
- AP, lateral, outlet, and Zanca views can evaluate for glenohumeral arthritis, fracture, locked dislocations, chondrolysis, calcific tendinitis, acromioclavicular arthrosis, abnormal acromial morphology, or other disorders
- Shoulder MRI can evaluate the rotator cuff, biceps tendon, and glenohumeral coracohumeral ligaments
- Shoulder arthrography was used to document decreased joint volume but is now of historical interest only

PROCEDURE

Patient/Positioning/Equipment

- Contracted capsule can limit the visualization and mobility of the instruments within the joint
- General arthroscopy equipment and an insufflation pump, articulated arm holder, and 90° bipolar electrocautery
- Scalene block with catheter allows postoperative pain control, and general anesthesia promotes intraoperative muscle relaxation
- Beach-chair or lateral decubitus position
- Rolled towel beneath the medial border of the scapula
- Acromion, distal clavicle, and coracoid are marked
- Preoperative ROM is documented

Surgical Technique

- Enter with 18-gauge spinal needle 2 cm medial and inferior to postero-lateral corner of acromion
- Insufflation to 20 mm Hg with dilute epinephrine improves visualization
- Resistance upon trocar insertion is often found due to the thickened capsule
- Arthroscopic triangle anteriorly is identified
- Red, filmy, gelatinous proliferative hypertrophic synovial tissue is often encountered in the rotator interval
- Anterior portal is established with an outside-in technique (**Figure 1**)
- Release is performed anteriorly from superior to inferior, then posterior, using 90° bipolar electrocautery (**Figure 2**)
  - Release is performed in an extralabral fashion just below the long head of the biceps and proceeding inferiorly to the superior aspect of the subscapularis
  - Upper region of the middle glenohumeral ligament also can be released if needed
- During rotator interval release, visualization is improved by placing the joint in 30° to 40° of abduction and alternating between 30° of internal and external rotation
- Release of the subscapularis tendon is controversial
- Inferior to the subscapularis, the lower region of the middle glenohumeral ligament and the anterior band of the inferior glenohumeral ligaments are released.
- Once release is complete to the 6-o'clock position, the arthroscope is switched to the anterior portal

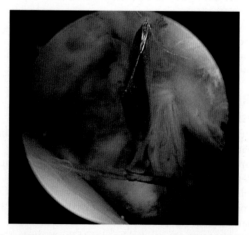

FIGURE 1 Arthroscopic view shows proliferative hypertrophic synovial tissue in the rotator interval. A spinal needle is seen entering the joint for the placement of the anterior portal.

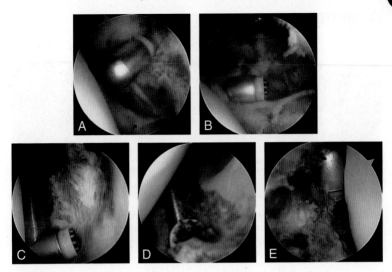

FIGURE 2 Arthroscopic views show capsular release for frozen shoulder.
A, The electrocautery is inserted through the anterior portal. The ArthroWand (ArthroCare Sports Medicine) allows the surgeon to cut into the capsule directly adjacent to where the electrocautery device enters the joint. **B,** The release begins just below the long head of the biceps and proceeds inferiorly to the superior edge of the subscapularis, including the coracohumeral ligament and the superior glenohumeral ligament. **C,** Inferior to the subscapularis tendon, the lower region of the middle glenohumeral ligament and the anterior band of the inferior glenohumeral ligaments are released as part of the capsular release. **D,** Once the 5-o'clock position is reached, the orientation of the electrocautery is changed such that the head points superiorly and the angle points inferiorly, to prevent axillary nerve damage. **E,** Similar to the anterior release, the posterior release proceeds from superiorly at the posterior border of the long head of the biceps tendon to inferiorly meet the anterior release.

- Posterior release proceeds from superior to inferior; posterior release is indicated for the limitation of internal rotation
- After release, the joint is gently ranged sequentially through abduction, elevation, external rotation in adduction, external rotation in abduction, and internal rotation (**Figure 3**)
- Can also translate the humeral head parallel to the glenoid joint surface in the posterior, anterior, and inferior directions
- Joint is reentered with the arthroscope to assess the results of the capsular release
- Evaluation of the subacromial space is critical because of persistent impingement pathology
- If subacromial involvement is present, then adhesiolysis, bursectomy, and acromioplasty are commonly required

---

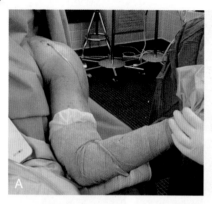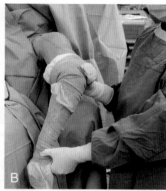

FIGURE 3 Intraoperative photographs demonstrate range of motion performed at the completion of capsular release. This examination demonstrates improvements in external rotation in adduction (**A**) and in internal rotation in abduction (**B**).

COMPLICATIONS

- Complications are rare
- Approximately 20% of patients will develop transient decrease in motion 3 to 5 weeks after the procedure
- A theoretical risk to the axillary nerve, posterior circumflex humeral artery, and brachial artery exists but is not commonly encountered
- Instability, although possible, has not been described
- Outcomes following arthroscopic release are generally excellent
    - Significant improvement in Constant and American Shoulder and Elbow Surgeons scores
    - Visual analog scale pain scores improve
    - Elevation, internal rotation, and external rotation all improve
    - Diabetes may confer worse outcomes
    - Average time to pain-free ROM is 6 to 10 weeks

POSTOPERATIVE CARE AND REHABILITATION

- Sling with derotational wedge to avoid internal rotation
- Physical therapy begins 1 to 2 days after surgery
- Patients with profound stiffness can also be admitted to hospital for aggressive physical therapy on the day of surgery
- Authors provide oral ketorolac for 4 days and oral narcotics to be taken as needed
- Home continuous passive motion machines are reserved for patients who have required repeat capsular release, patients with diabetes, and others in whom the risk of failure is high

- Home exercises include pendulums, pulleys, elevation, and passive external and internal rotation done for 15 to 20 minutes three or four times per day
- Even light resistance exercise is discouraged until 6 to 8 weeks, or until the patient achieves pain-free, flexible, and ROM

VIDEO 25.1 Arthroscopic Management of the Frozen Shoulder. Peter N. Chalmers, MD; Seth L. Sherman, MD; Neil Ghodadra, MD; Gregory P. Nicholson, MD (4 min)

PEARLS

- Arthroscopic capsular release for frozen shoulder is a challenging procedure requiring patience on the part of the surgeon.
- The beach-chair position, a pump system with which the surgeon is well acquainted with independent control of flow and pressure, and a 90° 3.5-mm bipolar electrocautery can all increase the likelihood of success.
- Selective capsular resection of the rotator interval or of the anterior capsule alone should be reserved for patients with solitary deficits of external rotation and with documented full ROM intraoperatively after selective capsular resection. Most patients need completion of inferior and posterior capsular release to regain ROM comparable with the contralateral shoulder.
- Release of the intra-articular portion of the subscapularis tendon should be reserved for cases in which global capsular release does not provide sufficient external rotation.
- Aggressive shoulder manipulation before arthroscopic capsular release should be avoided because the ensuing hemorrhage can compromise intra-articular visibility.

26 Arthroscopic Rotator Cuff Repair

INTRODUCTION

- Many causative factors for rotator cuff disorders have been implicated, but pathogenesis remains controversial
- Most common factors include age-related tendon degenerations, mechanical impingement, and changes in tendon vascularity
- Natural history is recognized as a continuum, progressing from simple tendinopathy to partial- and full-thickness rotator cuff tears

PATIENT SELECTION

- Patients must undergo thorough history and physical examination
- Initial management consists of activity modification, NSAIDs, physical therapy, and possible corticosteroid injection (**Figure 1**)
- Lack of improvement after 4 to 6 weeks indicates further investigation, including MRI

PREOPERATIVE SURGICAL DECISION MAKING

- Full-thickness or high-grade partial-thickness tears with associated pain and limited function despite an appropriate interval of nonsurgical management are candidates for arthroscopic repair
- Primary indication is pain relief; improved strength and mobility are secondary

Contraindications

- Absolute—Acute infections, significant glenohumeral arthritis, acromiohumeral arthropathy with fixed superior migration of the humeral head, inability to tolerate anesthesia, or inability to comply with postoperative rehabilitation
- Relative—Chronic or recurrent tears, tears with massive size and/or significant retraction, poor tendon quality, poor muscle quality, profound motor dysfunction (clinical anterosuperior escape, chronic elevation or external rotation pseudoparalysis), multiple corticosteroid injections, medical comorbidities (diabetes mellitus, obesity), social factors (smoking status, Workers' compensation claim), and advanced patient age

---

Based on Duquin TR, Hohman DW Jr, Hartzler RU: Arthroscopic rotator cuff repair, in Colvin AC, Flatow E, eds: Atlas of Essential Orthopaedic Procedures, ed 2. Rosemont, IL, American Academy of Orthopaedic Surgeons, 2020, pp 205-217.

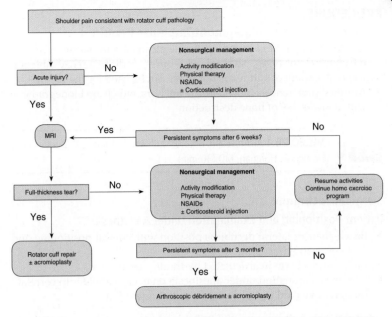

FIGURE 1 Diagram depicts the treatment algorithm for shoulder pain consistent with rotator cuff pathology. (Adapted with permission from Duquin TR, Sperling JW: Rotator cuff disorders, in Margheritini F, Rossi R, eds: *Orthopaedic Sports Medicine: Principles and Practice.* Milan, Italy, Springer-Verlag, 2011, pp 211-225.)

PREOPERATIVE IMAGING

Radiography

- True AP, scapular Y, and axillary views
- Radiographic signs of large/massive tears include superior head migration and decreased acromiohumeral distance

Magnetic Resonance Imaging

- T1- and T2-weighted images in coronal, sagittal, and oblique planes
- Must include entire scapula on MRI to assess atrophy and fatty infiltration of rotator cuff
- The tangent sign is used to quantify degree of supraspinatus atrophy

Ultrasonography

- Acceptable alternative to MRI with near equivalent sensitivity and specificity
- Extremely operator dependent

PROCEDURE

Special Instruments/Equipment/Implants Required

- 30° arthroscope, fluid pump system, instruments for suture passing/retrieving/knot-tying, shavers and burrs, radiofrequency ablation wand. A variety of suture anchor types can be used for the repair
- Authors' preference—Biocomposite anchors, which are biodegradable with a lower risk of bone destruction

 VIDEO 26.1 Arthroscopic Rotator Cuff Repair. Thomas R. Duquin, MD; Donald W. Hohman, MD (30 min)

Surgical Technique

Patient Positioning and Examination Under Anesthesia

- Beach-chair or lateral decubitus position with careful positioning and wide prep and draping
- Place surgical arm in articulated hydraulic arm holder
- Perform examination under anesthesia on every shoulder to correlate preoperative pain and physical examination findings

Intra-articular Arthroscopy and Débridement

- Identify and outline
  - The acromion, distal clavicle, and coracoid processes
  - Mark standard anterior, posterior, and lateral portals (**Figure 2, Table 1**)

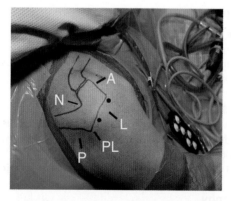

FIGURE 2 Anatomic landmarks and the location of arthroscopic portals are marked on the skin. The circles represent stab incision locations for anchor introduction. A = anterior portal, L = lateral portal, N = Neviaser portal, P = posterior portal, PL = posterolateral portal.

TABLE 1 Tips for Portal Placement for Arthroscopic Rotator Cuff Repair

Portal	Tip/Pearl	Location
Posterior portal	Provides best visualization of the shoulder joint; placement too far lateral should be avoided or joint visualization will be difficult	1-3 cm distal and 1-2 cm medial to the posterolateral tip of the acromion
Anterior portal	Working portal for instruments and suture management; placed using the outside-in technique under arthroscopic visualization and spinal needle localization into the triangle formed by the labrum (medial border), biceps tendon (superior border), and subscapularis (inferior border)	Halfway between the acromioclavicular joint and the lateral aspect of the coracoid; pierces the anterior fibers of the deltoid and enters the joint in the interval between the supraspinatus and subscapularis
Lateral portal	Working portal for the subacromial space; used to visualize the subacromial space; if placed too posteriorly in a large or muscular patient, it will be difficult for the instruments to "turn the corner" to reach the anterior acromion.	Placed laterally, in line with the midclavicle and 2-3 cm lateral to its lateral edge
Posterolateral portal	Visualization of the subacromial space during rotator cuff repair	1 cm distal to the posterolateral corner of the acromion
Neviaser	Working portal for the subacromial space; useful for suture passage in rotator cuff repair	Superomedial portal bordered by the clavicle, the acromioclavicular joint, and the spine of the scapula

- Enter posterior portal with arm in 15° abduction and 30° forward flexion
- Perform diagnostic arthroscopy
- Use 4.5-mm shaver for débridement as indicated through an anterior portal
- Treat biceps tendon pathology as indicated with tenotomy, tenodesis, and débridement
- Perform initial débridement of rotator cuff

Subacromial Bursectomy and Acromioplasty
- Move arthroscope to the subacromial space
- Identify coracoacromial ligament

- Create lateral working portal through the deltoid muscle in line with the posterior aspect of the distal clavicle and 2 to 3 cm lateral to the edge of the acromion
  - If evidence of impingement is present or if the subacromial space is too small to allow arthroscopic rotator cuff repair, then an acromioplasty is performed

Rotator Cuff Tear Characterization and Mobilization

- Make posterolateral portal 2 cm distal to posterolateral corner of acromion
- Using tendon-grasping instrument or traction suture helps assess tear pattern and tendon mobility
- For tension-free repair, bursal and/or articular releases may be required
- Coracohumeral ligament release can enhance mobility of rotator cuff tear

Tuberosity and Tendon Preparation

- Débride tendon to healthy tissue and create bleeding bone surface, which is essential for healing
- Clear tuberosity of soft tissue with ablation wand; use burr to create a bleeding surface

Margin Convergence Sutures

- These are tendon-to-tendon sutures not included in the anchor; meant to reduce longitudinal tears (**Figure 3**)
- Tear types most amenable are the L-, reverse L-, and U-shaped tears
- The passage of margin convergence sutures can be performed using sharp suture-passing instruments, suture shuttle devices, or antegrade suture-passing devices

Anchor Placement and Suture Passage

- Accessory transdeltoid portal facilitates anchor insertion
- Several methods of anchor placement and suture passage have been described
  - There are biomechanical data indicating superior fixation and increased surface area contact/compression using double-row repairs; however, no studies have shown clear superior clinical outcomes associated with double-row repairs
  - Systematic reviews and meta-analyses demonstrate superior healing rates for double-row over single-row repairs, and healed repairs result in improved strength over nonhealed repairs
  - Author's preference is to perform double-row repairs for all tears greater than 1 cm in size
- For single-row repairs, place suture anchors more towards the lateral aspect of tuberosity; one limb of anchor is placed in horizontal mattress configuration; pass other limb as simple suture

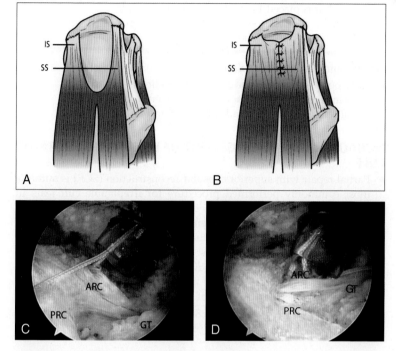

FIGURE 3 Images depict the use of margin convergence sutures to repair a rotator cuff tear. Illustrations show a U-shaped rotator cuff tear pattern amenable to marginal convergence suture placement before (**A**) and after (**B**) placement of the sutures. **C**, Arthroscopic view depicts marginal convergence suture placement viewed from the posterolateral portal. A free suture is passed through the anterior and posterior margins of the longitudinal portion of the tear. **D**, Knot tying results in closure of the longitudinal split in the tendon, reducing the tendon defect. ARC = anterior rotator cuff leaflet, GT = greater tuberosity, IS = infraspinatus, PRC = posterior rotator cuff leaflet, SS = supraspinatus.

- For double-row repairs, place medial row at medial aspect of tuberosity
- Pass sutures in horizontal mattress fashion, and tie to secure tendon

Knot Tying

- Knots can be simple, sliding, or sliding-locking
- Authors' preference—Sliding-locking, followed by three alternating half hitches

Lateral-Row Fixation

- In suture-bridge repair, the sutures from the medial row, usually one from each medial knot, are retrieved through the lateral portal and then passed into a knotless anchor

- The anchor is placed 1 cm lateral to the tuberosity
- Compression of tendon tissue is important, but overtightening can compromise tendon blood supply

Closure and Perioperative Care
- After portal closure an abduction pillow sling is applied
- Dressings removed at 72 hours and showering is permitted
- Initial follow-up and wound check at 10 to 14 days post repair

INTRAOPERATIVE MANAGEMENT OF IRREPARABLE ROTATOR CUFF
- Partial repair with superior capsular reconstruction (SCR) is author's most commonly performed procedure for irreparable cuff tears in younger patients
- SCR has a growing body of evidence for its use, including anatomical, biomechanical, and short-term clinical studies
- Subscapularis repair (if torn) must precede SCR. Irreparable subscapularis tear is a contraindication to SCR
- SCR is an adjunctive procedure and should accompany partial cuff repair when possible, treatment of the biceps, subacromial decompression, and margin convergence of graft to remnant cuff
- See full text for detailed procedural description

COMPLICATIONS
- Overall rate of 10% (**Table 2**)
- Stiffness, failure of tendon repair and rerupture
  - Risk factors for stiffness: preoperative joint contracture and history of arthrofibrosis
  - Risk factors for failure of repair: larger tear size, poor tendon quality, fatty muscle atrophy
- Superficial infection has a very low incidence

POSTOPERATIVE CARE AND REHABILITATION
- Tend to be surgeon-specific
- Accelerated protocols show no differences in range of motion (ROM), but show higher rates of recurrent tear at 1 year
- Authors suggest three-phase plan
  - Healing phase (weeks 0 to 5)—Hand/wrist/elbow ROM, pendulums of shoulder, gentle passive ROM
  - Recovery of motion phase (weeks 6 to 12)—Discontinue sling; arm can be used for activities of daily living, active and active-assisted ROM; patient should have full motion at end of this phase
  - Strengthening phase (weeks 12 and later)—Formal rotator cuff strengthening

TABLE 2 Reported Complications of Rotator Cuff Repair

Complication	No. of Shoulders (%)
Failed tendon repair	182 (6.2)
Nerve injury	33 (1.1)
Infection	31 (1.1)
Deltoid avulsion	16 (0.5)
Frozen shoulder	16 (0.5)
Suture granuloma	14 (0.5)
Wound hematoma	11 (0.4)
Dislocation	3 (0.1)
Reflex dystrophy	2 (0.1)
Greater tuberosity fracture	1 (0.1)
Acromion fracture	1 (0.1)
Total	310 (10.5)

Reproduced with permission from Mansat P, Cofield RH, Kersten TE, Rowland CM: Complications of rotator cuff repair. *Orthop Clin North Am* 1997;28(2):205-213.

PEARLS

- Minimize swelling and fluid extravasation and facilitate visualization
  - Keep total arthroscopy time under 2 hours.
  - Use cannulas for all working portals.
  - Maintain low fluid pressure and flow (40 to 50 mm Hg).
  - Use retractors to improve visualization in presence of significant swelling or fluid extravasation.
  - Can use hypotensive anesthesia (a systolic blood pressure of 100 to 110 mm Hg).
- To facilitate accurate assessment of tear pattern and a plan for method of repair
  - Place traction sutures in tendon to facilitate mobilization and reduction.
  - Release of adhesions on the bursal and articular sides of tendon and rotator interval may be required in retracted tears.
  - When placing multiple anchors, start with the most anterior anchor and work in posterior direction.
  - Pass and dock the sutures from each anchor in anterior portal before inserting next anchor.
  - Perform knot tying once all sutures have been passed, starting with the most posterior suture and proceeding anteriorly.
  - For single-row repairs, each suture is cut following knot tying; in suture-bridge repairs, sutures are docked in posterior portal.

27

Percutaneous Pinning of Proximal Humerus Fractures

PATIENT SELECTION
Indications
- For select two-, three-, and four-part fractures
  - ▶ Displaced surgical neck fractures without calcar or medial comminution
  - ▶ Three-part fractures where height and version can be restored
  - ▶ Valgus-impacted four-part fracture
- Timing of surgery affects success; reduction performed more than 1 week from injury may be difficult due to hematoma and scarring

Contraindications
- Osteopenic bone is a relative contraindication
- Extensive comminution of the tuberosities, medial calcar, or head segment
- Varus-displaced fractures with loss of medial bone integrity
- Three- and four-part fracture-dislocations or head-split fractures

PREOPERATIVE IMAGING
- True AP, scapular lateral, and axillary lateral radiographs (**Figure 1**)
- CT helps assess fragment positioning, angulation, and comminution
- MRI usually not indicated

 VIDEO 27.1 Percutaneous Pinning: When and How to Do It. Jonathan P. Braman, MD; Evan L. Flatow, MD (7 min)

PROCEDURE
Room Setup/Patient Positioning
- Beach-chair position
- Articulating arm positioner is routinely used
- Must be able to obtain high-quality multiplanar fluoroscopic imaging

---

Based on Parsons BO: Percutaneous pinning of proximal humerus fractures, in Colvin AC, Flatow E, eds: Atlas of Essential Orthopaedic Procedures, ed 2. Rosemont, IL, American Academy of Orthopaedic Surgeons, 2020, pp 218-225.

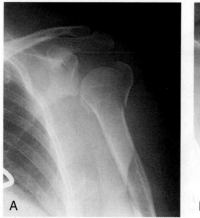
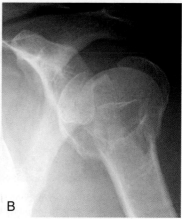

FIGURE 1 Grashey (**A**) and AP (**B**) views of the shoulder demonstrate a valgus-impacted four-part proximal humerus fracture.

Special Instruments/Equipment/Implants

- Small elevators, bone tamps, small skin hooks, surgical clamps
- 3.5-/4.0-mm partially threaded cannulated screws to fix tuberosity fragments
- Rigid, terminally threaded 2.4- or 2.8-mm pins used for shaft-to-head fixation

Surgical Technique

- After preparation and draping of extremity, mark osseous landmarks
- Mark portals for fracture reduction and proximal screw fixation; position reduction portal 2 to 3 cm distal to the anterolateral acromial corner (**Figure 2**)
- Establish reduction portal with arm in neutral to slight external rotation
- Place small elevator in fracture site to develop the fracture plane
- Use small tamp to elevate the humeral head (**Figure 3**)
- After reduction, pin head segment with 2.8-mm terminally threaded pin (**Figure 4**)
- Once through the cortex, advance pins by hand to prevent articular penetration
- Using a soft-tissue sleeve prevents soft-tissue injury during pin passage
- Confirm length of pin on multiplanar fluoroscopy
- Place a second pin parallel to the first, usually 2 to 3 cm apart
- Turn attention to fixation of the tuberosity fragments, if present (**Figure 5**)

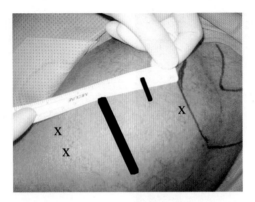

FIGURE 2 Photograph shows markings (X) for placement of portals for fracture reduction and pin placement, including the distal portals for placement of 2.8-mm pins into the shaft and head. The tuberosity Kirschner wire portal, next to the lateral acromion, is denoted by the purple line. The short black line denotes placement of the reduction portal, usually 2 to 3 cm distal to the anterolateral acromial corner. The long black line denotes the typical course of the axillary nerve, approximately 5 cm distal to the lateral edge of the acromion.

▸ Reduce greater tuberosity by placing skin hooks through fracture reduction portal deep to the deltoid in the subacromial space
  – Make provisional fixation with two percutaneously placed 1.6-mm Kirschner wires

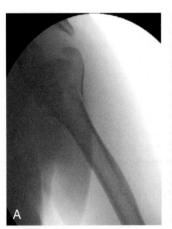
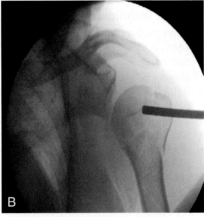

FIGURE 3 Fluoroscopic images show a valgus-impacted fracture. **A,** Preoperative image demonstrates tuberosity malposition. **B,** A small bone tamp is placed into the fracture plane beneath the humeral head, and impaction is used to anatomically reduce the humeral head into appropriate inclination and version.

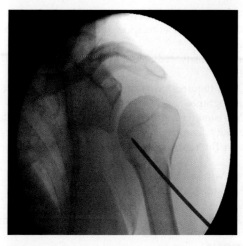

FIGURE 4 Fluoroscopic image shows placement of a 2.8-mm terminally threaded pin via the distal skin portals into the shaft and humeral head in a retrograde fashion. Once appropriate angulation into the head is confirmed by fluoroscopy, pins are advanced by hand with care to prevent penetration through the subchondral bone into the joint.

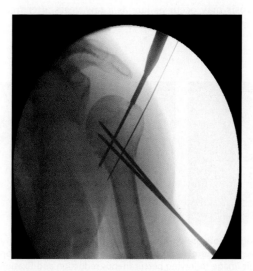

FIGURE 5 Fluoroscopic image shows placement of two Kirschner wires (K-wires) for provisional fixation after tuberosity reduction. K-wires are routinely placed distally into the humeral medial calcar for optimal fixation.

  – Place cannulated screws after overdrilling
  – Bicortical screw fixation is necessary for maintenance of reduction.
  ▸ Lesser tuberosity reduction is achieved through the reduction portal
    – Often requires visualization on scapular lateral and axillary radiographs
    – Provisional fixation is similar to that of the greater tuberosity.
- After tuberosity fixation, bring shoulder through a range of motion (ROM) under fluoroscopy; carefully examine for joint penetration by hardware
- Any crepitus with motion should be appreciated
- Hardware is most likely to penetrate posterosuperior quadrant of humeral head
- Remove Kirschner wires and cut the 2.8-mm pins beneath the skin

COMPLICATIONS

- Reported series indicate nearly 100% union rate and low complication rate
- Complications include loss of reduction, malunion, hardware failure, and late osteonecrosis
- Tuberosity failure is often secondary to screw pullout (**Figure 6**)
- Pins may penetrate into the joint
- Osteonecrosis may occur as late as a few years after treatment; more common in four-part fractures

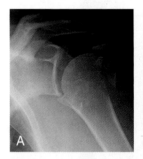 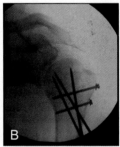 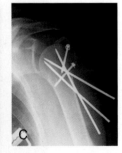

FIGURE 6 Images show the shoulder of a patient with a displaced three-part proximal humerus fracture. **A**, Preoperative AP radiograph. **B**, Intraoperative AP fluoroscopic image following percutaneous reduction and fixation. Note the questionable lack of bicortical fixation of the tuberosity screws into the humeral calcar distally. This patient fell postoperatively at 7 days and presented with loss of fixation and tuberosity redisplacement at 9 days postoperatively (**C**). Critical to success is stout fixation of the greater tuberosity with bicortical screw fixation into the humeral calcar.

POSTOPERATIVE CARE AND REHABILITATION

- Immobilize surgical arm in sling for 4 weeks
- At 4 weeks, remove 2.8-mm pins under sedation and local anesthesia in the operating room
- Examination under anesthesia assesses fracture stability and guides therapy goals
- Begin active-assisted and passive ROM after pin removal
- Start active ROM at 6 to 8 weeks

PEARLS

- Should operate within 5 to 7 days after injury.
- Some fracture patterns are more amenable to percutaneous treatment, including two-part fractures without varus displacement or medial calcar comminution.
- Place reduction portal directly off anterolateral corner of acromion.
- Place elevator within the fracture plane and beneath the humeral head to lift the head out of valgus.
- Take care to critically assess hardware placement.

VIDEO REFERENCE

 Video 27.1 Braman JP, Flatow EL: *Percutaneous Pinning of Proximal Humerus Fractures: When and How to Do It* [video]. Rosemont, IL, American Academy of Orthopaedic Surgeons, 2006.

28 Fixation of Proximal Humerus Fractures

INTRODUCTION
- Increased interest in fixation of proximal humerus fractures for several reasons:
  - Humeral head replacement has an unpredictable outcome
  - Osteonecrosis is no longer seen as a clinical disaster
  - More accurate preoperative imaging
  - Improvements in fluoroscopy
  - Refined reduction maneuvers
  - Improved implants
- Clinical results remain inconsistent

PATIENT SELECTION
Indications
- Neer guidelines remain useful
- Treat minimally displaced fractures nonsurgically; treat most displaced fractures surgically
- Most two- and three-part fractures are amenable to fixation.

Contraindications
- Very few absolute contraindications
- Low-demand and infirm patients are likely nonsurgical candidates
- Four-part fracture-dislocations and most head-split fractures
- Rotator cuff tear arthropathy
- Severe glenohumeral arthritis

PREOPERATIVE IMAGING
- Rely on intraoperative fluoroscopic imaging to assess quality of reduction
- Use comparison radiograph of contralateral shoulder to assess reduction
- Well-centered AP view of scapula with arm in external rotation demonstrates greater tuberosity relative to the head

Based on Torchia ME, Obermeyer TS: Fixation of proximal humerus fractures, in Colvin AC, Flatow E, eds: Atlas of Essential Orthopaedic Procedures, *ed 2. Rosemont, IL, American Academy of Orthopaedic Surgeons, 2020, pp 226-236.*

- Two-dimensional CT reveals extent of bone loss
- Three-dimensional CT shows tuberosity attachment

PROCEDURE

Room Setup for Fluoroscopic Imaging/Patient Positioning

- Need unrestricted access to shoulder for fluoroscopic imaging (**Figure 1**)
- Supine or beach-chair position
- Table is rotated 90° to allow C-arm to enter
- Verify access to imaging before starting the case

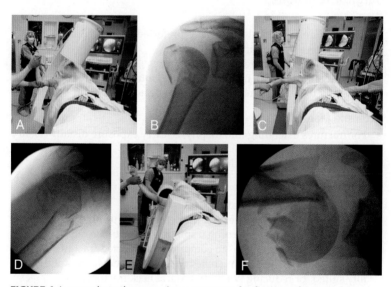

FIGURE 1 Images show the operating room setup for fixation of a proximal humerus fracture. **A,** Photograph shows positioning of the fluoroscopic imaging device to direct the fluoroscopic beam perpendicular to the scapula, with the patient's arm held in external rotation. **B,** Preoperative AP external rotation fluoroscopic view shows the relationship among the humeral shaft, the humeral head, and the greater tuberosity. **C,** Photograph shows patient positioning for the Velpeau axillary view taken with the arm held in internal rotation and slight longitudinal traction. Gentle traction lateralizes the scapula away from the operating room table and the patient's head and allows unobstructed imaging of the proximal humerus and glenoid. **D,** Preoperative Velpeau axillary internal rotation fluoroscopic view depicts the typical apex anterior angulation between the shaft and head segment. **E,** Photograph shows patient positioning for the standard axillary view taken with the arm held in neutral rotation and longitudinal traction. **F,** Preoperative fluoroscopic axillary view shows the position of the lesser tuberosity and the relationship of the humeral head to the glenoid. (Reproduced from Torchia ME: Technical tips for fixation of proximal humeral fractures in elderly patients. *Instr Course Lect* 2010;59:553-561.)

Special Instruments/Equipment/Implants

- Intraoperative fluoroscopy
- Large Weber clamp
- Precontoured low-profile locking plate
- Kirschner wires and Steinmann pins
- Cobb or periosteal elevator
- Miniature malleable retractor
- Bone void filler
- Possible allograft fibular strut, possible fracture prosthesis

Surgical Technique

Exposure

- Extended deltopectoral approach is preferred
- Use "tug test" to identify axillary nerve
- Abduction of the arm relaxes the deltoid.
- Incise rotator interval, tenotomize biceps intra-articularly, and deliver it distally to be later tenodesed to top of pectoralis tendon

Extensile Maneuvers

- For fractures extending into diaphysis, carry exposure distally (Henry approach)
- Release anterior fibers of deltoid

Reduction Maneuvers

- Determined by fracture pattern
- In impacted fracture, elevate humeral head using square-tipped impactor placed through coronal split in greater tuberosity (**Figure 2**)
- Use "parachute technique" to compress unimpacted fractures
- Valgus impaction osteotomy relies on tension-band sutures and is ideally suited for reducing two-part surgical neck fractures
- Parachute technique requires intact rotator cuff and cannot be used in fractures with displaced tuberosity fragments (**Figure 3**)
- Can use intramedullary fibular allograft for excessive humeral shortening and inferior instability

Humeral Head Support

- In mild bone loss, the humeral head can be supported by the shaft of the humerus
- In moderate bone loss, use bone graft or a bone graft substitute
- In severe bone loss, use an intramedullary fibular allograft

Provisional Fixation

- Place Steinmann pin or pins posterior to the long head of the biceps tendon
- Tension the traction sutures and tie them to the pin (**Figure 4**)

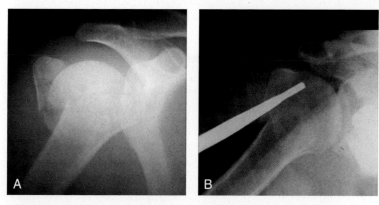

FIGURE 2 Valgus-impacted four-part fracture of the proximal humerus. **A,** Preoperative AP radiograph. **B,** Intraoperative fluoroscopic image shows elevation of the humeral head using a square-tipped impactor placed through a coronal split in the greater tuberosity. (Reproduced from Torchia ME: Technical tips for fixation of proximal humeral fractures in elderly patients. *Instr Course Lect* 2010;59:553-561.)

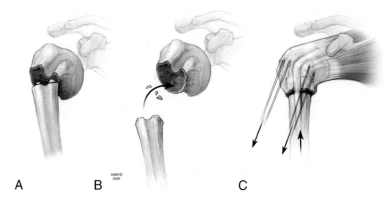

FIGURE 3 Illustrations show the Banco parachute technique for valgus impaction osteotomy. **A,** The transverse line delineates the intended level of the osteotomy. Prominent edges of the shaft anteriorly and laterally are trimmed with a rongeur to create a relatively flat surface that will allow balanced compression of the head segment. **B,** The "trimmings" are placed into the head segment and function as local bone graft. **C,** The head segment is supported by upward impaction of the shaft. The position of the head segment is adjusted with traction sutures placed at the bone-tendon junction of the subscapularis and supraspinatus tendons. (Reproduced with permission from the Mayo Foundation of Medical Education and Research, Rochester, MN.)

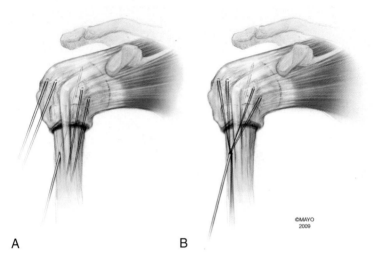

A   B

©MAYO
2009

FIGURE 4 Illustrations show a method of provisional fixation of proximal humerus fractures using pin and tension-band suture fixation. This form of robust provisional fixation allows rotation of the arm for high-quality fluoroscopic imaging to assess the reduction in multiple planes. **A,** A long Steinmann pin is placed from the shaft into the head segment. **B,** Traction sutures are tensioned and tied to the pin. Tensioning the sutures pulls the head segment out of varus. (Reproduced with permission from the Mayo Foundation of Medical Education and Research, Rochester, MN.)

Assessment of Reduction

- The shaft of the humerus should be under the humeral head, greater tuberosity should be 5 to 10 mm below top of the head, and articular surface should point toward upper portion of the glenoid
- Attempt to match the tuberosity height and neck-shaft angle of opposite shoulder
- Use long head of biceps tendon to confirm the rotational accuracy of the reduction

Definitive Fixation

- Apply precontoured locking plate laterally and hold with a push-pull device
- Assess hardware from the external rotation view
- Gaps between the plate and bone in the metadiaphysis are acceptable
- When position is optimal, place screws into the humeral head
- Drill only the outer cortex
- Insert depth gauge and advance under fluoroscopic control
- Following pin applications, place tension band sutures (**Figure 4**)

COMPLICATIONS

- Most common complication is inadequate reduction
- Avoid fixing fractures with residual varus by referencing a comparison radiograph
- Screw penetration most commonly occurs in posterosuperior humeral head; avoid by checking intraoperative Velpeau axillary radiograph
- Surgeon may place finger through rent in rotator interval to check for screw penetration
- Nerve palsy may occur with fracture-dislocations
- Inadequate protection of hardware construct

POSTOPERATIVE CARE AND REHABILITATION

- Avoid aggressive range-of-motion and strengthening exercises before fracture union
- Sling for the first 6 weeks after surgery
- Supine active-assisted range of motion initiated after 6 weeks
- After 12 weeks, discontinue sling; encourage light activities of daily living

PEARLS

- Good intraoperative radiographs/fluoroscopic images are essential.
- Temporary traction sutures placed at the bone-tendon junction of the rotator cuff facilitate mobilization and reduction of the tuberosities.
- Support of the osteoporotic humeral head is essential; can be achieved with the proximal humeral shaft or with a structural bone graft in cases with metaphyseal comminution.
- Varus malreduction of the humeral head leads to malunion and loss of motion postoperatively.
- Placing the plate too proximally leads to subacromial impingement and should be avoided.
- Apply the plate after the fracture has been reduced, compressed, and provisionally fixed with pins and tension-band sutures.
- Appropriate screw length is critical.
- Achieve improved screw purchase in the osteoporotic head segment by drilling only the lateral cortex and pushing the depth gauge to the desired screw length with fluoroscopic control.
- Tension-band sutures neutralize the deforming forces of the rotator cuff and should be used liberally.
- In the elderly, protect hardware with a 6-week period of immobilization, which in the authors' experience has not led to disabling stiffness.

PATIENT SELECTION

Indications

- Severely displaced four-part fractures
- Fracture-dislocations
- Head-splitting fractures
- Impression articular fractures involving over 40% of the articular surface
- Dislocation present for more than 6 months
- Humeral head devoid of soft-tissue attachment
- Selected three-part fractures not amenable to surgical fixation

Contraindications

- Nondisplaced fractures
- Fractures amenable to open reduction and internal fixation
- Active infection
- Chronic osteomyelitis
- Relative contraindications—Massive rotator cuff tears, uncontrolled shoulder spasticity, poor general health

HISTORY AND PHYSICAL EXAMINATION

- Note history of antecedent shoulder problems
- Limit physical examination in setting of acute fracture
- Pay specific attention to sensory and motor functions of the axillary nerve
- Motor function assessment is difficult because pain may inhibit deltoid contraction

PREOPERATIVE IMAGING

Radiography

- AP view of glenohumeral joint in neutral rotation, axillary view, scapular outlet view

Based on Rodriguez Santiago AI, Edwards TB: Hemiarthroplasty for proximal humerus fractures, in Colvin AC, Flatow E, eds: Atlas of Essential Orthopaedic Procedures, *ed 2. Rosemont, IL, American Academy of Orthopaedic Surgeons, 2020, pp 237-245.*

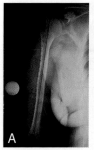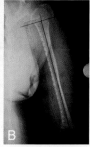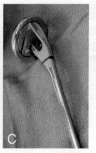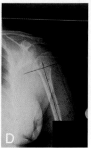

FIGURE 1 Images used in preoperative planning for the Gothic arch technique of determining proper humeral component position. **A,** From a full-length AP radiograph of the unaffected humerus, the length of the humerus from the superior aspect of the humeral head to the transepicondylar axis is measured and normalized for magnification. **B,** On the AP radiograph of the affected extremity, a line perpendicular to the prosthetic axis is drawn at the level of the fracture medially. The distance between the medial fracture line and the transepicondylar axis (residual humeral length) is measured. The difference between the humeral length measured on the unaffected radiograph and the residual humeral length measured on the affected radiograph is calculated. **C,** This difference is marked on the humeral implant to establish the height at which the humeral stem should be positioned with respect to the medial fracture line. **D,** The length of the greater tuberosity, when available, is used as a checkrein.

- Obtain humeral head height from full-length AP radiographs of ipsilateral and contralateral humerus; authors' preference—Gothic arch technique (**Figure 1**)

CT
- Perform CT in all patients with significant displacement
    - Allows evaluation of fracture pattern and degree of displacement
    - Helps determine relationship of humeral head to tuberosities
- Placement of the prosthesis at the correct height remains a significant challenge

PROCEDURE
Room Setup/Patient Positioning/Instruments
- Standard operating table with patient positioned off table enough to allow full extension
- Place rolled sheet between scapulae
- Modified beach-chair position; back of table elevated 45° to 60° relative to floor
- Check head and neck for neutral alignment
- Instruments used during the procedure are listed in **Table 1**

TABLE 1	Instruments Used in Hemiarthroplasty for Proximal Humerus Fractures

Instrument (Quantity)	Use
Vascular forceps (2)	Dissection
Ferris-Smith forceps (2)	Dissection
Adson forceps with teeth (1)	Skin closure
Long curved Metzenbaum scissors (1)	Dissection
Long curved Mayo scissors (1)	Dissection
Straight Mayo scissors (1)	Cutting suture
Bandage scissors (1)	Removal of draping
Medium skin rake (2)	Skin retraction
Army-Navy retractor (2)	Deltopectoral retraction
Cerebellar retractor (1)	Deltopectoral retraction
Hohmann retractor (4)	Proximal retraction; humeral retraction
Narrow Richardson retractor (1)	Conjoined tendon retraction
Standard hemostat (6)	Tagging stay sutures
Lahey forceps (1)	Handling of the tuberosities
Battery-powered drill (1)	Humeral drill hole preparation for suture
Long No. 3 knife handle (2)	Skin incision, biceps tenotomy
8-inch Mayo needle holder (2)	Suture passage
1-inch osteotome (1)	Tuberosity osteotomy when required
Mallet (1)	Insertion of implants; tuberosity osteotomy
Freer elevator (1)	Removal of excess cement
Small bone tamp (1)	Impaction of bone graft
Large bone tamp (1)	Impaction of bone graft
Cobb elevator (2)	Blunt dissection; tuberosity identification
No. 0 Vicryl (taper needle)[a] (3)	Hemostasis; wound closure
No. 2 Ethibond (taper needle)[a] (2)	Subscapularis stay suture; biceps tendon
No. 2 FiberWire (taper needle)[b] (6)	Tuberosity fixation
2-0 Vicryl[a] (1)	Wound closure
3-0 PDS (polydioxanone suture)[a] (1)	Wound closure
Electrocautery with needle tip (1)	Hemostasis; dissection
Suction tip with tubing (1) bulb syringe (1)	Visualization irrigation

[a]Ethicon.

[b]Arthrex.

Surgical Technique

Surgical Approach and Tuberosity Handling

- Use standard deltopectoral approach for exposure
- Start skin incision at tip of coracoid and extend distally and laterally 10 to 15 cm
- Interval between deltoid and pectoralis is developed by locating cephalic vein
- The authors prefer to retract the vein laterally
- Identify conjoined tendon and trace to coracoid insertion
- With arm abducted and externally rotated, identify interval between the coracoacromial ligament and conjoined tendon
- Use Cobb elevator to define tuberosities
- Place stay sutures through the subscapularis tendon
- Identify and remove humeral head with locking forceps
- Obtain control of greater tuberosity and posterosuperior rotator cuff by passing No. 2 braided permanent suture through rotator cuff tendons medial to their insertion on the tuberosity (**Figure 2**)

Humeral Prosthesis Positioning

- Humeral shaft is identified and sequentially reamed
- Locate bicipital groove and place two 2-mm drill holes 1 cm distal to fracture site, one on each side of groove
- The biceps tendon stump is tenodesed to the pectoralis tendon with No. 1 nonabsorbable braided suture
- Insert trial humeral implant (**Figure 3**)
- Base prosthesis height on preoperative calculations
- Set humeral retroversion between 20° and 30°

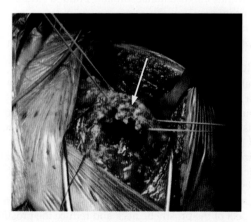

FIGURE 2 Intraoperative photograph demonstrates mobilization of the greater tuberosity (arrow) with sutures through the posterior rotator cuff.

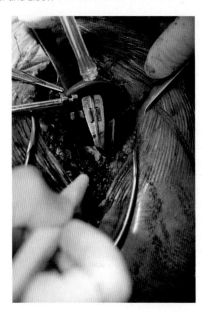

FIGURE 3 Intraoperative photograph demonstrates insertion of the trial humeral component to the desired level.

- Reduce the trial and use electrocautery to mark the position of the fin of the prosthesis
- Place a cement restrictor in the humeral canal to create a 1-cm distal cement mantle
- Pass two strands of No. 2 nonabsorbable braided suture in an outside-to-inside technique
- Mix cement and place within canal
- Insert implant, continuously checking height and version

Tuberosity Reduction and Fixation
- Two key elements of tuberosity fixation—Reliable suture fixation and bone graft to assist tuberosity healing
- Autologous bone graft is obtained from the humeral head fragment
- Fixation is achieved with reproducible suture fixation techniques as described by Boileau (**Figure 4**)
- Four horizontal cerclage sutures previously placed in rotator cuff
- Two vertical cerclage sutures made of the two strands of No. 2 braided suture previously placed in the humeral diaphysis
- Pass sutures controlling greater tuberosity around the smooth-polish medial aspect of the prosthetic neck and reduce the prosthesis
- Place second of the two bone graft plugs lateral to the neck to accommodate greater tuberosity bone loss

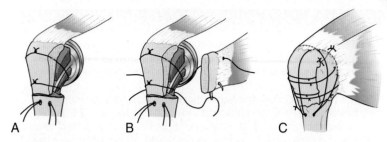

FIGURE 4 Illustrations show the Boileau technique of tuberosity fixation. **A,** Horizontal cerclage sutures secure the greater tuberosity. **B,** Passage of two additional horizontal cerclage sutures for fixation of the greater and lesser tuberosities. **C,** Completed construct with four horizontal and two vertical cerclage sutures.

- Place one of the vertical sutures in the diaphysis through the subscapularis and supraspinatus tendons medial to their insertion and then tie
- Pass second suture through the infraspinatus and supraspinatus tendons just medial to their osseous insertion and tie

COMPLICATIONS
Intraoperative
- Intraoperative complications are uncommon
- Many patients have preoperative axillary nerve neurapraxia, and this fact should be documented; less than 2% of patients have permanent dysfunction
- Vascular injuries can involve the axillary artery
- Intraoperative fractures can occur within the diaphysis

Postoperative
- Nonunion and malunion of the tuberosities are most common
- Glenoid erosion can occur
- Aseptic loosening occurs more frequently in cases involving trauma
- Periprosthetic fractures often result from low-impact trauma
- Instability is related to tuberosity malunion or nonunion
- Stiffness is a common problem; attempt physical therapy to improve mobility; revision surgery indicated if no improvement within 6 months
- Infections most commonly caused by *Cutibacterium acnes* or *Staphylococcus aureus*
- Treat early infections with multiple irrigation and débridement, with retention of components

POSTOPERATIVE CARE AND REHABILITATION
- Maintain sling for 4 to 6 weeks to protect tuberosity healing
- Can initiate hydrotherapy 4 to 6 weeks after surgery

PEARLS

- If locating the cephalic vein is difficult, the deltopectoral interval can be readily detected proximally by identifying a small triangular area devoid of muscle tissue between the proximal portions of the deltoid and pectoralis major muscles.

- Use the largest diaphyseal reamer that can be advanced down the humeral canal without difficulty to avoid selecting too small a diameter humeral implant, which can inadvertently be positioned in varus or valgus.

- If the humeral head fragment is between humeral head component head sizes, select the smaller size to avoid insertion of too large a component, which can lead to nonunion of the tuberosities.

- After glenohumeral reduction, direct the humeral head into the center of the glenoid fossa with the arm held in neutral rotation.

- Autologous bone graft, taken from the humeral head fragment, serves two purposes. First, it enhances healing between the greater and lesser tuberosities and between the tuberosities and the humeral diaphysis. Second, because the greater tuberosity is often no more than a thin shell of bone, the bone graft positions the greater tuberosity laterally in a more anatomic position.

- The tuberosities and the humeral head implant should move as one unit at the termination of the procedure.

Reverse Shoulder Arthroplasty for Proximal Humeral Fractures

PATIENT SELECTION AND INDICATIONS
- Reverse shoulder arthroplasty is used for proximal humerus fractures not amenable to internal fixation or hemiarthroplasty
  - This is determined based on fracture pattern and displacement and patient characteristics, as summarized in **Tables 1** and **2** and **Figure 1**
- Hemiarthroplasty is preferred in the following 2 cases:
  - Head impaction fractures involving more than 40% of the articular surface with intact tuberosities
  - Varus posteromedial or valgus fractures with a single large greater tuberosity fragment
- Contraindications
  - Active infection
  - Severely compromised glenoid bone stock. This may be encountered with concomitant fracture of the proximal humerus and the glenoid or in those with preexisting glenoid bone loss secondary to arthritis or old trauma
  - Relative contraindications include:
    - Dysfunction of the axillary nerve or brachial plexus
    - Prior deltoid insufficiency
    - Fractures of the scapular spine or acromion

PREOPERATIVE (DIAGNOSTIC) IMAGING
- Radiographs including anterior-posterior and axillary views
- CT scan with three-dimensional reconstruction

PROCEDURE
- Room setup/patient positioning
  - Beach-chair position
  - Deltopectoral approach

Based on Sanchez-Sotelo J: Reverse shoulder arthroplasty for proximal humeral fractures, in Colvin AC, Flatow E, eds: Atlas of Essential Orthopaedic Procedures, *ed 2. Rosemont, IL, American Academy of Orthopaedic Surgeons, 2020, pp 246-255.

TABLE 1 **The Mayo Clinic-FJD Classification System for Proximal Humerus Fracture**

Surgical neck (SN)	Isolated (SN)
	With fractured tuberosities (SN-GT, SN-LT, SN-GT-LT)
Tuberosity fractures	
• Greater tuberosity (GT)	Isolated (GT)
	In the setting of anterior dislocation (GT-DI)
• Lesser tuberosity (LT)	Isolated (LT)
	In the setting of posterior dislocation (LT-DI)
Varus posteromedial (VPM)	Intact tuberosities (VPM)
	Fractured tuberosities (VPM-GT, VPM-LT, VPM-GT-LT)
Valgus (VL)	Intact tuberosities (VL)
	Fractured tuberosities (VL-GT, VL-LT, VL-GT-LT)
Head fracture or dislocation	Head splitting (HS)
	Head impaction (HI)
	Head dislocation (HD)

Surgical Technique

- Authors routinely perform biceps tenotomy and tenodesis by suturing the tendon of the long head of the biceps to short head of the biceps
- The fracture line between the tuberosities is found usually lateral to the bicipital groove. If the lesser tuberosity is not fractured off the head, a microsagittal saw may be used to "create" a lesser tuberosity fragment

TABLE 2 **Fractures Considered for Shoulder Arthroplasty**

- Complex fracture dislocations with
  - the dislocated head fractured from the shaft *and*
  - one or both tuberosities fractured
- Head splitting fractures
- Head impaction fractures involving over 40% of the articular surface
- Varus posteromedial fractures with
  - one or both tuberosities fractured *and*
  - severe comminution, poor bone quality, advanced age
- Valgus fractures with
  - one or both tuberosities fractured *and*
  - severe comminution, poor bone quality advanced age, unstable head segment

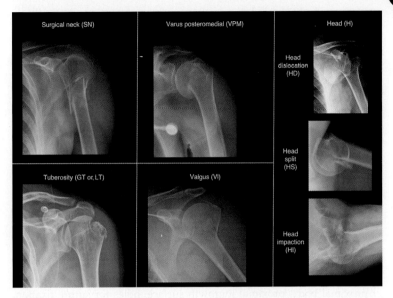

FIGURE 1 Radiographic examples of the various categories of the Mayo Clinic-FJD classification system for proximal humerus fracture patterns.

- Place a traction suture around the lesser tuberosity and subscapularis tendon
- Remove humeral head prior to attempting to gain control of the greater tuberosity
- Place arm in abduction to reduce tension of deltoid. Place two sutures at the infraspinatus and two at the infraspinatus/teres minor junction
- Place the glenoid component baseplate flush with the inferior glenoid rim and with adequate inferior tilt
- Glenosphere size selection depends on surgeon's preference and the biomechanical features of the implant selected
- Excessive lateralization of the humeral shaft may compromise tuberosity healing
- Author's preference is to place humeral component at 20° of retroversion as opposed to 30° to provide more space for the greater tuberosity to fit and heal
- To determine the height of humeral component, the author's preference is to place the trial humeral component a few millimeters deeper to the predicted location of the surgical neck in reference to the uppermost portion of the fractured shaft, and then trial to assess for deltoid tension, and at the same time confirm that the tuberosities will reach the shaft with slight overlap
- Trial with the thinnest humeral bearing available to minimize humeral lateralization

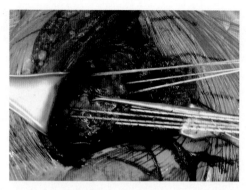

FIGURE 2 Intraoperative photograph showing four heavy nonabsorbable sutures placed through the posterosuperior rotator cuff and around the greater tuberosity, two proximal and two distal.

- The author favors a component with "fracture-specific features": small proximal body, proximal ingrowth surface, holes for suture fixation, laser marks to replicate height, and convertibility between anatomic and reverse components
- Cement the humeral component in the exact height and version
- Fixation of the tuberosities to the humeral component to each other, and to the shaft is crucial. The author's specific technique is detailed in **Figures 2** through **5**

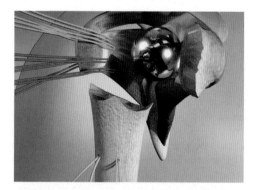

FIGURE 3 Schematic representation of the six heavy nonabsorbable sutures that will be used for tuberosity fixation, placed prior to implantation of the humeral component.

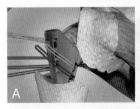
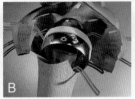
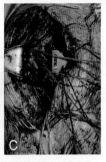

FIGURE 4 A, Illustration of two horizontal sutures being passed through the medial holes of the humeral component. **B,** Illustration of the other two horizontal sutures being passed around the lesser tuberosity. **C,** Intraoperative photograph of suture configuration once the humeral component has been implanted.

COMPLICATIONS
- Main potential complications include tuberosity resorption, nonunion or malunion, dislocation, infection, heterotopic ossification, brachial plexopathy, aseptic loosening, glenoid bone loss secondary to notching, and vascular injury

POSTOPERATIVE CARE AND REHABILITATION
- Immediately postoperatively immobilize the shoulder in some abduction and external rotation
- Postoperative day 1 begin active range of motion exercises of the elbow, wrist, and hand
- Initiate shoulder therapy at week #6

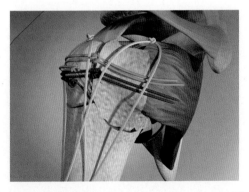

FIGURE 5 Schematic representation shows horizontal and vertical fixation of the greater and the lesser tuberosities.

- Passive and active assisted range of motion exercises in all planes start at week #6, with isometric exercises added at week #10
- Elastic band strengthening exercises at week #12

PEARLS

- Use the biceps as a landmark during fracture exposure.
- Place sutures around the greater tuberosity after removing the fractured humeral head.
- Avoid excessive glenoid reaming.
- Place the glenoid component with some inferior tilt and inferior glenosphere overhang to decrease notching.
- Avoid excessive lateralization or distalization to decrease tension on the repaired tuberosities.
- Select a humeral component with fracture features.
- Place the humeral component in slightly decreased retroversion.
- Pack bone graft on the upper portion of the humeral canal and under the tuberosities.
- Use a humeral bearing with a 135° angle to decrease notching; achieve secure horizontal and vertical fixation of both tuberosities.
- Immobilize the shoulder in some external rotation.

31 Total Shoulder Arthroplasty for Osteoarthritis

PATIENT SELECTION

- Successful outcome depends on proper patient selection, preoperative planning, surgical technique, and postoperative rehabilitation
- Most common etiologies are primary and secondary arthritis
- Pathology includes osteophytes, joint space narrowing with subchondral sclerosis, and cyst formation
- Rheumatoid and inflammatory arthritis and osteonecrosis are also indications
- Contraindications include cuff tear arthropathy, active infection, brachial plexopathy, excessive glenoid bone loss, and Charcot arthropathy

PREOPERATIVE IMAGING

- Plain radiographs, including Grashey AP in neutral/external/internal rotation, axillary, and scapular Y views (**Figure 1**)

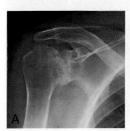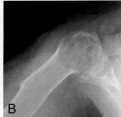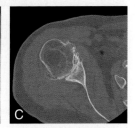

FIGURE 1 Images obtained before total shoulder arthroplasty for osteoarthritis. **A**, AP radiograph of a right shoulder demonstrates loss of glenohumeral joint space, marginal osteophyte formation, sclerosis, subchondral cysts, and maintenance of acromiohumeral distance, suggesting an intact rotator cuff. **B**, Axillary lateral radiograph demonstrates marginal osteophytes and posterior glenoid wear. **C**, Axial CT cut illustrates posterior wear of the glenoid, with good glenoid vault bone stock and glenoid version.

Based on Hsu SH, Bigliani LU: Total shoulder arthroplasty for osteoarthritis, in Colvin AC, Flatow E, eds: Atlas of Essential Orthopaedic Procedures, *ed 2. Rosemont, IL, American Academy of Orthopaedic Surgeons, 2020, pp 256-264.*

- CT scans help determine glenoid version, depth of glenoid vault, and wear pattern
- MRI is useful if there is concern regarding rotator cuff integrity

VIDEO 31.1 Total Shoulder Arthroplasty. Louis U. Bigliani, MD; Stephanie H. Hsu, MD; Howard Y. Park, BA (6 min)

PROCEDURE

Room Setup/Patient Positioning

- Authors use indwelling regional interscalene catheter block
- Give antibiotics within 1 hour of incision
- Beach-chair position with head of the bed raised 30° to 40°
- Position patient toward edge of table for full range of motion (ROM)
- Check ROM under anesthesia.
- Identify and mark relevant anatomy

Special Instruments/Equipment/Implants

- Total shoulder arthroplasty system of the surgeon's choice
- Additional instruments listed in **Table 1**

TABLE 1 **Instruments Used in Total Shoulder Arthroplasty**
Baby Richardson retractor
Darrach retractors (wide, special sharp tip)
Army-Navy retractors
High-speed drill
Drain/Hemovac
No. 1 and No. 2 nonabsorbable nylon sutures
Absorbable monofilament
Needle-tip Bovie
Fukuda posterior glenoid retractor/malleable retractors
Metal finger/elevator
Straight Adson
Flat-blade oscillating saw
Mallet
Gelpi retractors

Surgical Technique

Approach

- Deltopectoral approach is preferred (**Figure 2**)
- Start incision 2 cm inferior to clavicle, lateral to coracoid, and extend distally toward the deltoid insertion, approximately 10 to 12 cm
- Create full-thickness skin flaps
- Identify cephalic vein adjacent to fat strip in deltopectoral fascia and mobilize laterally with the deltoid
- Incise clavipectoral fascia and perform blunt dissection to mobilize strap muscles
- Identify axillary nerve under inferior border of subscapularis
- Release anterior leading edge of coracoacromial ligament to aid visualization
- Release superior third of pectoralis tendon
- Identify and cauterize anterior circumflex humeral artery and veins
- Release subscapularis from bone 1 to 1.5 cm medial to its insertion
- Tag released tendon with No. 2 braided suture
- Identify and tag biceps tendon within groove

Humeral Preparation

- Place arm in extension, adduction, and external rotation
- Identify and remove marginal osteophytes
- Identify starting position for opening reamer
- Perform reaming, increasing in 1-mm increments until cortical contact is made to the 130-mm mark
- Leave last reamer in canal and attach humeral head cutting guide
- Place guide pins for 30° of retroversion

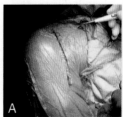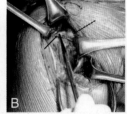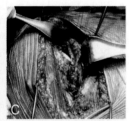

FIGURE 2 Intraoperative photographs show the deltopectoral approach for total shoulder arthroplasty. **A,** The incision. **B,** The coracoacromial ligament is resected anteriorly for superior exposure. The solid arrow indicates the coracoacromial ligament, and the dashed arrow indicates the coracoid. **C,** The subscapularis tendon is carefully taken down with a needle-tip Bovie, just medial to the bicipital groove, and marked with nonabsorbable heavy suture.

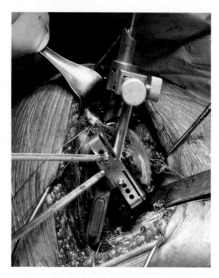

FIGURE 3 Intraoperative photograph shows placement of the humeral neck cutting guide. The guide is placed over the appropriate trial humeral shaft reamer, making sure to align the cut using the supraspinatus insertion as a guideline for appropriate cut depth. A Richardson or loop retractor is used to protect the rotator cuff, and a Darrach retractor is used to protect tissues medially.

- Cut native humeral head and measure against prosthesis size and offset (**Figure 3**)
- Test trial head against native glenoid, ensuring 30% to 50% posterior subluxation

Glenoid Exposure
- Place Fukuda or malleable retractor posterior to glenoid (**Figure 4**)
- Place Richardson retractors for medial and lateral retraction
- Place sharp-tip Darrach retractor along anterior glenoid
- Release origin of biceps with Bovie cautery
- Perform partial anterior capsulectomy
- Remove inferior labrum while protecting axillary nerve

Glenoid Component Placement
- Use scraper to remove any remaining articular cartilage
- Select glenoid centering guide for appropriate size (**Figure 5**)
- When correct, drill center hole of the guide
- Use circular reamer to prepare glenoid face
- Place pegged guide; drill and deepen superior and inferior holes
- Place and assess trial glenoid for position and stability
- Irrigate wound with pulse lavage, and insert thrombin-soaked sponges into each drill hole

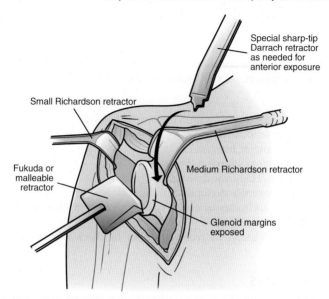

Special sharp-tip Darrach retractor as needed for anterior exposure

Small Richardson retractor

Fukuda or malleable retractor

Medium Richardson retractor

Glenoid margins exposed

FIGURE 4 Illustration shows glenoid exposure for total shoulder arthroplasty. Full exposure is attained using Richardson retractors for soft tissue, a malleable or Fukuda retractor posteriorly on the glenoid rim, and a sharp-tip special Darrach retractor if needed anteriorly.

- Remove sponges and dry holes for cement placement
- Place cement into each hole and impact
- Repeat impaction process three times, place and impact glenoid component, and hold component in place with manual pressure until cement hardens
- Trial head again and check for stability
- Place three drill holes for repair of the subscapularis to the lesser tuberosity

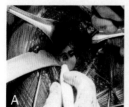
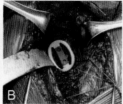
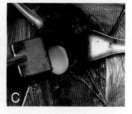

FIGURE 5 Intraoperative photographs show glenoid component placement for total shoulder arthroplasty. **A,** The glenoid is marked with the centering guide. **B,** A fenestrated trial glenoid is placed, assuring flush seating with the glenoid face and central placement. **C,** The final glenoid is cemented in place.

- Pass suture through each drill hole and then through subscapularis tendon
- Place final humeral component with appropriate version
- Use of cement is optional.
- Reduce glenohumeral joint and assess for stability

Closure
- Tenodese biceps tendon within the bicipital groove
- Reattach subscapularis to lesser tuberosity with existing drill-hole sutures; the rotator interval can be closed with the arm in the appropriate amount of external rotation
- Place medium Hemovac drain after irrigation
- Loosely approximate deltopectoral interval
- Close dermis and subcutaneous tissues with 3-0 and 4-0 monofilament absorbable suture
- Take AP radiograph in recovery room to check components and alignment

COMPLICATIONS
- Avoid infection by using sterile technique and perioperative antibiotics
- Component-related complications include glenoid loosening, periprosthetic fracture, and dislocation
- Postoperative stiffness or failure of subscapularis repair is possible

POSTOPERATIVE CARE AND REHABILITATION
- Keep interscalene catheter until afternoon of postoperative day 1
- Remove drain, swathe, and abduction pillow on postoperative day 1
- Assistive-passive ROM for first 2 weeks to ensure subscapularis healing
- Discharge patients on postoperative day 2 and see in follow-up in 10 to 12 days

PEARLS

- Preoperative planning using an axillary radiograph and CT to evaluate the glenoid vault is essential to successful surgical outcome.
- Remove the leading edge of the coracoacromial ligament to release and define the subdeltoid/subacromial space; helps exposure and ROM.
- Anterior to posterior osteophyte removal from the humeral neck aids in mobilization.
- Perform anterior capsulectomy to help glenoid exposure and subscapularis mobilization.
- Manual pressurization of the cement at the glenoid pegs creates improved bony interdigitation.

Reverse Total Shoulder Arthroplasty for Rotator Cuff Arthropathy

INTRODUCTION
- Cuff tear arthropathy is characterized by superior migration of humeral head, erosions of inferior acromion and superior glenoid, and collapse of soft, atrophic head
- Patients cannot elevate arm above 90° and have limited external rotation
- Reverse shoulder arthroplasty features a medialized center of rotation and lengthened deltoid lever arm.

PATIENT SELECTION
Indications
- Most common indication is cuff tear arthropathy
- Patients older than 65 or 70 years with irreparable cuff tear and pseudoparesis of elevation
- Must have functioning deltoid muscle and adequate glenoid bone stock

Contraindications
- Absolute—Deltoid loss, inadequate glenoid bone stock, infection
- Relative—Age younger than 65 years, rheumatoid arthritis

PREOPERATIVE IMAGING
- Plain AP and axillary radiographs (**Figure 1**)
- Characteristic findings—Area of collapse of proximal humeral surface, paucity of osteophytes, reduced acromiohumeral distance, rounding of greater tuberosity, and erosion of undersurface of acromion
- Seebauer classification is most useful; describes functional and biomechanical finding (**Figure 2**)
- Use CT to assess glenoid bone stock
- Use MRI to assess degree of cuff atrophy and fatty infiltration

---

Based on Silvero P, Wirth MA: Reverse total shoulder arthroplasty for rotator cuff arthropathy, in Colvin AC, Flatow E, eds: Atlas of Essential Orthopaedic Procedures, *ed 2. Rosemont, IL, American Academy of Orthopaedic Surgeons, 2020, pp 265-271.*

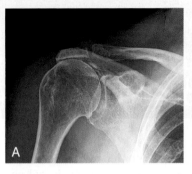
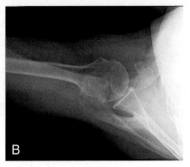

FIGURE 1 Preoperative AP (**A**) and axillary lateral (**B**) radiographs show the typical changes seen in cuff tear arthropathy. Note the rounding of the greater tuberosity, decreased acromiohumeral distance, and thinning of the acromial arch.

PROCEDURE

Room Setup/Patient Positioning

- Semi-Fowler position; head in headrest with patient on edge of table so arm can be fully extended
- True AP of the shoulder is obtained with C-arm
- Record position of machine at time of imaging for use during the case

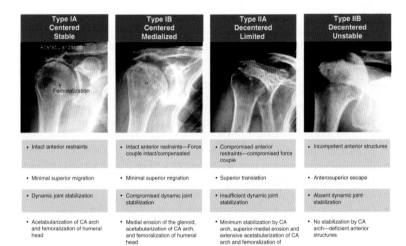

FIGURE 2 Illustration showing the Seebauer classification of cuff tear arthropathy. CA = coracoacromial. (Adapted with permission from Visotsky JL, Basamania C, Seebauer L, Rockwood CA, Jensen KL: Cuff tear arthropathy: Pathogenesis, classification, and algorithm for treatment. *J Bone Joint Surg Am* 2004;86:35-40.)

Surgical Technique

- Two approaches—Anterior deltopectoral and superior-lateral
- Authors prefer deltopectoral approach
- Incision extends from lateral to coracoid 8 to 10 cm distally along deltopectoral interval
- Elevate subcutaneous flaps
- Dissection should be medial to the cephalic vein
- Incise clavipectoral fascia from inferior border of coracoacromial ligament distally to superior border of pectoralis tendon
- Palpate and protect axillary nerve
- Identify anterior humeral circumflex vessels along lower border of subscapularis and cauterize
- Elevate subscapularis and capsule off lesser tuberosity
- Dislocate humeral head by externally rotating and extending humerus
- Identify starting point for the medullary canal reamer
- Ream sequentially until reamer begins to bite cortical bone
- Assemble cutting guide with retroversion set to 0°
- Resection level should be just below the top of the greater tuberosity
- Perform a 360° release of subscapularis
- Rotator interval is incised, and inferior capsule is dissected
- Remove labrum and biceps stump
- Use key elevator to remove any remaining articular cartilage
- Place glenoid baseplate positioner as inferior as possible (**Figure 3**)
- Drill guide pin through the center hole
- Start reamer at low speed with goal of preserving the subchondral bone

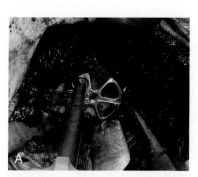
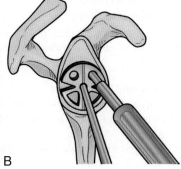

FIGURE 3 Images show correct positioning of the glenoid baseplate positioner for reverse total shoulder arthropathy. **A,** Intraoperative photograph shows the glenoid baseplate positioner in place. Note the key elevator at the inferior aspect of the glenoid and the positioner placed just above it. **B,** Corresponding diagram of the glenoid baseplate positioner illustrates proper positioning at the inferior glenoid with the central guide pin in place.

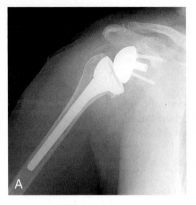
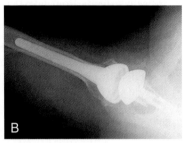

FIGURE 4 Postoperative AP (**A**) and axillary lateral (**B**) radiographs taken in the operating room show completion of reverse total shoulder arthroplasty.

- Secure glenoid baseplate with inferior and superior screws
- Place final glenosphere with inferior overlap of 3 to 5 mm
- Prepare humeral component based on manufacturer's specifications
- Perform trial reduction and assess stability and tensioning
- Resolve inadequate tension with a thicker cup, spacers, or a larger glenosphere
- Pass two or three nonabsorbable sutures through the proximal humerus near the lesser tuberosity to enable reattachment of the subscapularis
- Irrigate wound and close over a drain
- Obtain postoperative AP and axillary lateral radiographs (**Figure 4**)

COMPLICATIONS

Scapular Notching
- Occurs with frequency of 44% to 96%
- Lower Constant scores have been found with increasing levels of notching

Hematoma Formation
- Only formally described in one study
- Occurred in 20.6% of cases, with 50% requiring return to operating room
- Thought to be related to early initiation of motion

Glenoid Loosening
- Most studies show rates of 5% or less
- Can occur when baseplate is insecurely anchored or with suboptimal positioning
- Placement of inferior screw is most critical

Dislocation

- Accounts for up to 40% of all complications
- Factors include number of prior surgeries, deltopectoral approach, bone deficiency, subscapularis deficiency, component malposition, and trauma
- Irreparable subscapularis has been found to be a significant risk factor for dislocation

Infection

- Prevalence of up to 10%
- Most infections develop because of patient-related immunosuppression

POSTOPERATIVE CARE AND REHABILITATION

- Sling with abduction pillow
- Limit shoulder range of motion for first 2 weeks
- After 2 weeks, start physician-directed stretching program
- After 6 weeks, may add strengthening program

PEARLS

- Important to position the patient's arm completely free of table edge to allow full extension of the arm.
- Place a metal plate over the resected proximal humerus to prevent bone loss during glenoid preparation.
- Essential to identify axillary nerve and protect it throughout the case.
- Essential to adequately remove soft tissue from around the glenoid.
- Place glenoid baseplate low on glenoid to avoid impingement of proximal humerus on the lateral scapula and inferior neck.
- Use C-arm to verify screw position within baseplate.

INTRODUCTION

- Advantages of arthroscopy—Reduced iatrogenic insult by decreasing incision size, more thorough evaluation of the intra-articular compartments of elbow, and possibly reduced scarring and potential stiffness
- Disadvantages—Technical requirements needed to safely perform the procedure
- Need thorough knowledge of elbow anatomy to avoid neurovascular injury

ANATOMY

- Palpate superficial landmarks and mark for reference during surgery
- Identify the triceps and olecranon posteriorly
- Moving medially, palpate ulnar nerve in groove along posterior aspect of medial epicondyle
- Mark medial epicondyle
- Laterally, the lateral epicondyle, radial head, and tip of olecranon form a triangle marking the boundaries of the "soft spot" of the elbow
- Superficial nervous structures include the medial and lateral antebrachial cutaneous nerves
- Deeper neurovascular structures include the median, radial, and ulnar nerves and the brachial artery

PATIENT SELECTION

Indications

- Diagnostic arthroscopy performed for elbow arthritis with and without loose bodies
- Capsular contracture
- Osteochondritis dissecans of the capitellum
- Lateral epicondylitis
- Synovitis
- Certain intra-articular elbow fractures

Based on Giel TV III, Field LD, Savoie FH III: Arthroscopy of the elbow, in Colvin AC, Flatow E, eds: Atlas of Essential Orthopaedic Procedures, *ed 2. Rosemont, IL, American Academy of Orthopaedic Surgeons, 2020, pp 272-281.*

Contraindications
- Gross deformity of the elbow
- High risk for neurovascular injury
- Relative—Prior ulnar nerve transposition

VIDEO 33.1 Elbow Arthroscopy: Principles, Portals, and Techniques. Champ L. Baker, Jr, MD, FACS (21 min)

PROCEDURE
Equipment
- Standard 30° arthroscope
- Metal cannulas without side vents for the arthroscope; inflow as well as plastic cannulas for instruments to reduce insult to capsule
- Mechanical pump or gravity inflow
- Tourniquet

Anesthesia
- Ranges from general anesthesia to regional blocks, local anesthesia, and intravenous blocks
- Many surgeons elect to use general anesthesia when it can be safely tolerated

Patient Positioning
- Three patient positions for elbow arthroscopy are shown in **Figure 1**

Supine Position
- Advantages—Surgical side is close to table edge; ease of setup; allows use of regional blocks
- Disadvantages—Arm must be in traction device; difficulty accessing posterior compartment

Lateral Decubitus Position
- Laterally on beanbag; elbow flexed over bolster allowing forearm to hang free
- Advantages—Ease of patient positioning; access to posterior compartment
- Disadvantage—Need a specialized holder

Prone Position
- Advantages—Gravity assists traction; full range of motion of arm
- Disadvantages—Need for repositioning; limited airway access

Portal Placement
- Mark medial and lateral epicondyles, olecranon, and radial head
- Palpate ulnar nerve within the groove

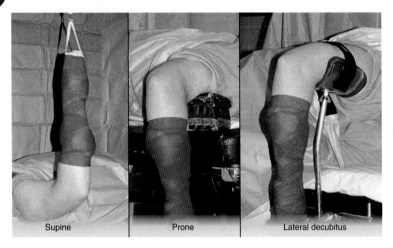

Supine | Prone | Lateral decubitus

FIGURE 1 Photographs show three patient positions for elbow arthroscopy. Each position has inherent advantages and disadvantages with respect to anesthesia options, the need for positioning or traction devices, and the ease with which conversion to open procedures can be accomplished.

- Insufflate joint with 18-gauge needle and saline at the soft spot (**Figure 2**)
- Distension improves ease of cannula passage and protects neurovascular structures

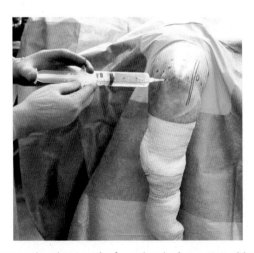

FIGURE 2 Preoperative photograph of a patient in the prone position shows pertinent landmarks marked for elbow arthroscopy, including the medial and lateral epicondyles (circles), the ulnar nerve (parallel lines), and portal sites (X marks). Insufflation of the joint is demonstrated through the lateral soft spot.

Anteromedial Portal
- Place 1 to 2 cm anterior and 2 cm distal to the medial epicondyle
- Greatest risk is to medial antebrachial cutaneous nerve, which passes 1 to 2 mm from portal site

Proximal Anteromedial Portal
- Make 2 cm proximal to medial epicondyle and anterior to intermuscular septum
- Main structure at risk is medial antebrachial cutaneous nerve, which passes 2 cm from portal site
- Portal provides visualization of entire anterior compartment from medial to lateral gutter

Anterolateral Portal
- Outside-in technique—Make portal 1 cm anterior and 3 cm distal to lateral epicondyle
- Inside-out technique—Advance arthroscope from anteromedial portal and press it against capsule lateral to the radial head
- Posterior interosseous nerve courses 1 to 1.5 cm from radial head around the radial neck
- Radial nerve passes 5 to 9 mm from this portal site

Proximal Anterolateral Portal
- Establish portal 2 cm proximal and anterior to lateral epicondyle
- Radial nerve passes between 10 and 14 mm from this portal when elbow is flexed to 90°
- Lateral antebrachial cutaneous nerve passes 6 mm from this portal site

Direct Lateral Portal
- Also known as the soft-spot portal; found in the soft spot in triangle marked by the lateral epicondyle, radial head, and tip of olecranon
- Biggest risks of this portal are fluid extravasation into soft tissues and postoperative portal drainage

Posterior Portal
- Make 3 cm proximal to the olecranon tip, through triceps tendon (**Figure 3**)
- Provides visualization of posterior aspect of ulnohumeral joint, olecranon fossa, and medial and lateral gutters
- Take care in medial gutter; ulnar nerve lies just superficial to joint capsule

Posterolateral Portal
- Make 3 cm proximal to tip of olecranon, just lateral to triceps tendon
- Sometimes helps to bring elbow to 45° of flexion to relax triceps and posterior capsule

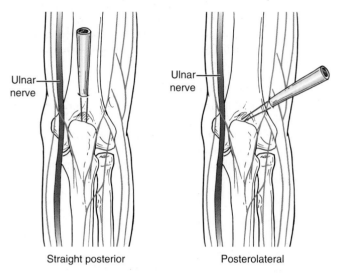

Straight posterior   Posterolateral

FIGURE 3 Illustrations show placement of the posterior and posterolateral portals. The posterior portal is established approximately 3 cm proximal to the olecranon tip, and the posterolateral portal is made 3 cm proximal to the olecranon tip and immediately lateral to the triceps tendon. These portals can be used interchangeably for working in the posterior compartment.

Accessory Posterolateral Portal
- Place portal between the straight lateral and posterolateral portals
- Main structures at risk are triceps tendon and ulnohumeral articular cartilage

Specific Surgical Techniques
Diagnostic Arthroscopy
- Insert 18-gauge needle into soft-spot portal in elbow; insufflate with sterile saline
- Perform systematic inspection of anterior structures
- Move arthroscope into proximal anterolateral portal, using metal cannulas to visualize medial joint capsule
- With the inflow in place, through one of the anterior portals, make a posterolateral portal
- Advance arthroscope into lateral gutter for visualization of radiocapitellar joint

Loose Bodies
- Patients present with elbow pain and stiffness; often report catching, snapping, popping, or locking
- Loose bodies do not cause contractures, but often are seen in patients with contractures

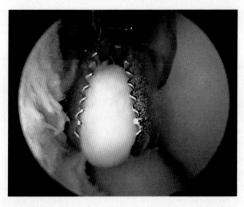

FIGURE 4 Arthroscopic view shows a grasper removing a large loose body from the anterior compartment of the elbow.

- Can be seen on AP and lateral radiographs
- Use prone or lateral decubitus position for easier visualization
- Can be removed with a variety of arthroscopic grabbers (**Figure 4**)
- Helpful to break up larger loose bodies to facilitate removal
- Débride inflammatory tissue and reactive synovitis
- Take care when using shaver near the anterior capsule
- Then turn attention to posterior compartment for loose body removal
- If loose body is too large, remove it through the posterolateral portal to avoid injuring triceps tendon
- Milking maneuver can be performed on the medial gutter; repeat maneuver in lateral gutter

Arthroscopic Synovectomy
- Allows access to anterior and posterior compartments while minimizing iatrogenic insult of open approach
- Thickened synovitis can sometimes limit visualization
- Perform complete synovectomy of lateral joint through proximal anteromedial portal
- Switch arthroscope to lateral portal and perform medial joint synovectomy
- Take care in posteromedial gutter to avoid damaging posteromedial capsule and ulnar nerve

COMPLICATIONS
- High risk of serious neurovascular injury
- Portal infections
- Fistula formation
- Heterotopic bone formation (rare but potentially serious complication)

PEARLS

- Carefully palpate and mark superficial landmarks.
- Take great care with portal placement.
- Palpate ulnar nerve to confirm its location.
- Joint distention accomplished by injecting saline into the elbow joint makes capsular penetration with blunt trocars more reliable.
- Relatively proximal anteromedial and anterolateral portals are preferred over more distally placed anterior portals; more proximal portals are farther from neurologic structures.
- Arthroscopic retractors improve visualization in the elbow joint and protect vital structures.
- Take care during arthroscopic débridement and capsular release in anterior elbow near radial head because of proximity of posterior interosseous nerve. Also take care in posteromedial gutter because of proximity of ulnar nerve.

RADIAL HEAD FRACTURES

Patient Selection

- Mason classification (**Figure 1**)
  - Type I—Nondisplaced; no mechanical block to motion.
    - Treat with sling and early range of motion (ROM)
    - Can be assessed after injection of lidocaine through the soft spot
  - Type II—More than 2 mm of displacement and more than one-third of radial head involved.
  - Type III—Comminuted, multifragmented fractures.
- Options for management—Fragment excision, *open reduction and internal fixation* (ORIF), radial head excision, or arthroplasty.
  - Consider fragment excision if elbow stability is not compromised and fragments are less than 25% of the head.
  - May perform ORIF by fixation within the safe zone or lateral area, with arm in neutral position.
  - Consider arthroplasty or radial head excision in cases with severe comminution.

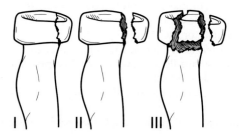

FIGURE 1 Illustration depicts the Mason classification of radial head fractures.

Based on Adams JE, Steinmann SP: Open treatment of radial head fractures and olecranon fractures, in Colvin AC, Flatow E, eds: Atlas of Essential Orthopaedic Procedures, *ed 2. Rosemont, IL, American Academy of Orthopaedic Surgeons, 2020, pp 282-291.*

Preoperative Imaging

- Include three views of elbow—Lateral, AP, and oblique.
- Obtain prereduction and postreduction images if a reduction is performed.
- CT is helpful in complex injury patterns.

Procedure

Room Setup/Patient Positioning

- Supine position with arm table or with arm over chest
- A tourniquet helps with visualization
- Mini C-arm for intraoperative imaging
- Use regional or general anesthesia
- In the presence of other bony injuries, can use universal posterior incision
- For isolated injuries, lateral incision is preferred

Special Instruments/Equipment/Implants

- For ORIF, have a radial head replacement on standby
- Kirschner wires (K-wires) and suture anchors

Surgical Technique

- Make lateral incision overlying epicondyle and extending down over radial head.
- Create full-thickness skin flaps.
- For associated lateral ulnar collateral ligament (LUCL) injury, use Kocher interval, between anconeus and extensor carpi ulnaris tendon.
- If LUCL is intact, perform exposure through the tendinous origin of extensor digitorum communis (**Figure 2**).
- Keep forearm in pronation to protect posterior interosseous nerve.
- Once radial head is exposed, determine whether to fix via ORIF, perform arthroplasty, or excise.
- Can obtain provisional fixation with small K-wires.
- Preferable to use headless screws rather than plates if the decision is made to proceed with ORIF.
- If fracture is not amendable to fixation, can perform radial head arthroplasty (**Figure 3**).
- Various implant options are available; base decision on surgeon preference.
- Critical to not overstuff joint—Sizing can be difficult; guidelines include the following:
  - Use excised head and neck as guide
  - Dish of radial head replacement should be about same size as inner dish of native radial head surface

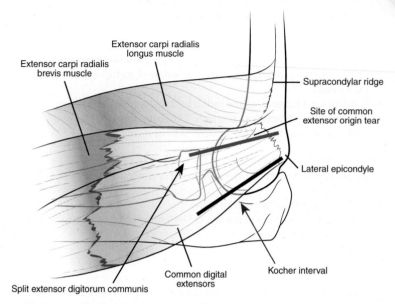

FIGURE 2 Illustration shows the muscle-splitting approach. The radial head may be approached easily through a split in the tendon origin of the extensor digitorum communis (blue line).

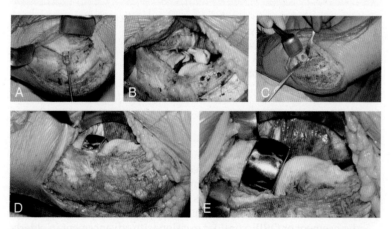

FIGURE 3 Intraoperative views show the implantation of a radial head prosthesis in an elbow with an irreparable radial head fracture. **A,** The surgical interval. **B,** Exposure. **C,** Excision of the irreparable radial head. **D,** Insertion of the radial head. **E,** Radial head implant of appropriate size in place.

‣ Radial head prosthesis should be within 2 mm of proximal radioulnar joint

‣ Use fluoroscopy to assess for joint widening after placing trial head

- Critical to rule out Essex-Lopresti lesion if radial head excision is performed.
- Can perform intraoperative radial pull test under fluoroscopy.
- Repair deep structures, reattach LUCL to epicondyle with suture anchors or bone tunnels, and close skin in layers

Complications

- Injury to the posterior interosseous nerve, infection, stiffness, and failure to heal.
- Radiocapitellar arthritis may develop.
- Hardware irritation, stiffness, or heterotopic bone formation may require second surgery.
- Residual instability

Postoperative Care

- If no ligamentous injury, encourage early range of motion (ROM).
- If LUCL was repaired, splint arm at 90° in pronation, then start early flexion-extension motion, avoiding terminal extension.

PEARLS

- Avoid excising radial head without radial head replacement in presence of elbow instability and Essex-Lopresti injury.
- "Safe zone" for hardware placement for radial head and neck is in nonarticular region.
- Do not overstuff the radial head prosthesis.

OLECRANON FRACTURES

Patient Selection

- Mayo classification (**Figure 4**)
- Treat type I nondisplaced fractures with immobilization in midflexion and neutral rotation for 7 to 10 days, followed by active ROM.
- Displaced type II and III fractures typically require surgery.
- Options for surgery include excision of the proximal piece and triceps advancement or ORIF; consider excision with advancement in elderly, low-demand patients, and those with significant comminution.
- ORIF is the most common method of treating olecranon fractures; reliable for restoring extensor power, achieving union, and restoring motion.

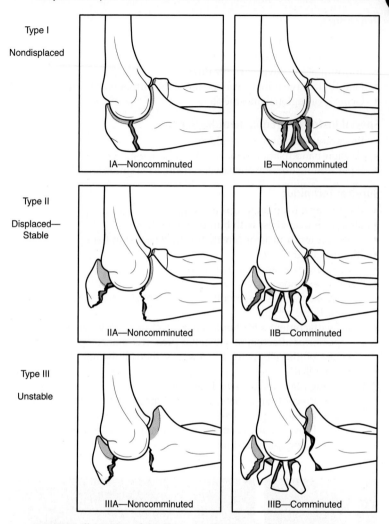

FIGURE 4 Illustration of the Mayo classification of olecranon fractures.

- Fixation options include plate-and-screw constructs, intramedullary devices, and tension-band wiring.

Preoperative Imaging
- Need three views of elbow.
- Two- and three-dimensional CT can clarify position and type of fracture fragments.

Procedure

Room Setup/Patient Positioning
- Supine position with arm table or arm over chest
- Tourniquet improves visualization
- Helpful to have mini C-arm available for intraoperative imaging
- General or regional anesthesia

Special Instrument/Equipment/Implants
- Precontoured plates are available.
- Tension-band fixation with K-wires and fine-gauge wire.
- If performing excision and advancement, have suture anchors available.

Surgical Technique
- Prepare arm from fingertips to axilla.
- Hold arm over chest with bump of towels.
- Make posterior incision; create full-thickness skin flaps.
- Identify ulnar nerve.
- Identify fracture and remove hematoma.
- Perform excision.
    - Excise fracture fragments and reattach triceps to bone with suture anchors.
    - Reattachment site should be at level of articular surface; a more posterior attachment site better preserves extension strength.
    - Immobilize elbow for 4 to 6 weeks, then allow motion.
- Perform ORIF
    - Using plate and screws (**Figure 5**)
        - Precontoured plates produce high rate of satisfactory results.
        - Locking options may be helpful in osteoporotic bone.
        - Provisionally reduce fracture and hold with K-wires.
        - Apply plate and fill with screws.

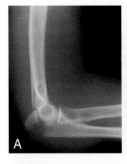 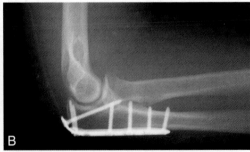

FIGURE 5 Radiographs depict an elbow treated with open reduction and internal fixation in which a plate-and-screw construct provides stable fixation. **A**, Preoperative lateral view demonstrates fracture of the olecranon. **B**, Postoperative lateral view demonstrates osteosynthesis with a plate-and-screw construct.

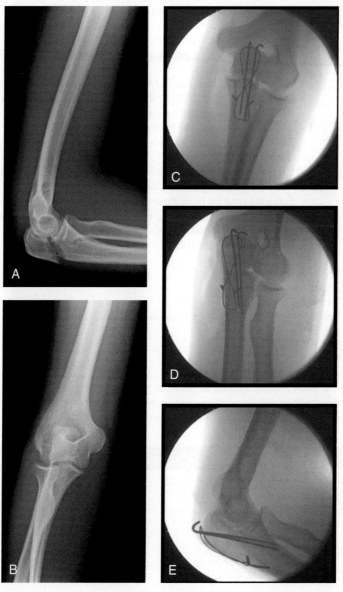

FIGURE 6 Preoperative lateral (**A**) and AP (**B**) radiographs demonstrate an olecranon fracture amenable to tension-band fixation. Intraoperative PA (**C**), oblique (**D**), and lateral (**E**) fluoroscopic views demonstrate satisfactory open reduction and internal fixation with a tension-band fixation construct.

▸ Using tension-band wiring (**Figure 6**)
  – Unsuitable for comminuted fractures or those with component distal to midpoint of olecranon.
  – Also likely to fail in presence of instability or with concomitant elbow fractures.
  – Use bone reduction clamp for provisional fixation.
  – Drive two parallel 0.045- or 0.062-in K-wires from proximal to distal, exiting the anterior cortex.
  – Withdraw K-wires 5 to 10 mm.
  – Drill transverse hole in ulna and pass single 18- or 20-gauge wire through.
  – Pass wire in figure-of-8 fashion over dorsal surface of ulna and through triceps using large angiocatheter needle.
  – Tension wires by twisting on both sides.
  – Bend K-wires to a 180° angle and cut so that crook of K-wire captures tension-band wire.
  – Impact K-wires into ulna.

Complications

- Prominent hardware
- Wound complications
- Fixation of olecranon fractures may result in joint stiffness.

Postoperative Care

- ORIF
  ▸ Splint elbow for a few days.
  ▸ Start motion as soon as possible.
- Proximal fragment excision and triceps advancement—Cast or splint elbow for 4 to 6 weeks, then allow motion.

PEARLS

- Ensure that full-thickness skin flaps are raised to avoid soft-tissue complications over the olecranon.
- Olecranon fractures are ideally fixed with sufficient stability to enable early active motion.

Open Reduction and Internal Fixation of Distal Humerus Fractures

PATIENT SELECTION

- Incidence of distal humerus fractures is 5.7 per 100,000 people per year
- Treatment is generally surgical and can be challenging
- AO/Orthopaedic Trauma Association classification
    - Type A—Nonarticular fractures
    - Type B—Partial articular fractures
    - Type C—Complete articular fractures
- Goals of treatment—To obtain anatomic reduction with adequate stability to allow early range of motion (ROM)
- Important to discuss loss of motion and possible transient ulnar nerve paresthesias with patient

Indications

- Displaced fractures
- Open or impending open fractures
- Fractures with vascular injury
- Ipsilateral upper extremity injury
- Pathologic fractures

Contraindications

- Poor health precluding tolerance of surgery
- Active infection
- Lack of appropriate soft-tissue coverage
- Poor compliance
- Extreme osteopenia
- Nonsurgical treatment best for stable, nondisplaced fractures and patients with preexisting conditions creating nonfunctional limb

PREOPERATIVE IMAGING

- AP, lateral, and oblique radiographs of elbow
- When indicated, shoulder and wrist radiographs
- Traction radiographs and CT can be helpful (**Figure 1**)

Based on McKee MD: Open reduction and internal fixation of distal humerus fractures, in Colvin AC, Flatow E, eds: Atlas of Essential Orthopaedic Procedures, *ed 2. Rosemont, IL, American Academy of Orthopaedic Surgeons, 2020, pp 292-299.*

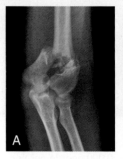
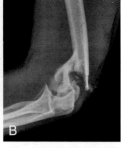
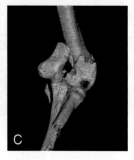

FIGURE 1 AP (**A**) and lateral (**B**) preoperative radiographs demonstrate an intra-articular distal humerus fracture. Evidence of air also is seen, because this was an open fracture. **C,** CT reconstruction of the same injury shows a proximal ulnar fracture, which is not readily evident on the radiographs. This fracture was an avulsion of the ulnar insertion of the medial collateral ligament.

PROCEDURE

Room Setup/Patient Positioning

- Lateral decubitus position with arm over bolster provides excellent access (**Figure 2**)
- Supine position for polytrauma patients
- Pad all bony prominences
- Position for ease of intraoperative imaging

Special Instruments/Equipment/Implants

- Small-fragment plates, mini-fragment plates and screws, Herbert screws, Kirschner wires
- Sterile tourniquet

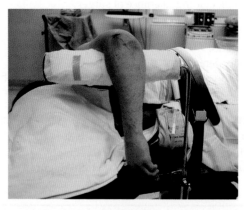

FIGURE 2 Photograph shows a patient secured in the lateral decubitus position via a beanbag and safety strap, with the affected arm placed over a padded bolster. All bony prominences are padded appropriately.

- Reduction clamps, osteotomes, oscillating saw
- Wire set, bone-graft set
- Mini C-arm fluoroscope

Surgical Technique

- Perform surgical briefing at outset
- Prepare iliac crest if bone graft will be harvested
- Apply sterile tourniquet to proximal arm
- Use a direct posterior incision (**Figure 3**); can be curved around olecranon to avoid a scar
- Essential to identify and mobilize ulnar nerve

Extensor Mechanism

- Options exist for treating the extensor mechanism
- Paratricipital approach
  - Allows visualization of fracture on either side of triceps
  - For dissection, free radial and ulnar borders of triceps
  - Elevate triceps and septum off humerus
  - Use this approach for elbow arthroplasty in presence of distal humerus fracture and for technically simpler fractures
  - Do not switch from paratricipital approach to triceps split because extensive devitalization of triceps occurs

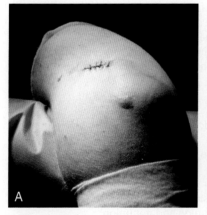 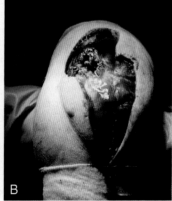

FIGURE 3 Intraoperative photographs show the straight posterior approach for open reduction and internal fixation of a distal humerus fracture. The open fracture wound (**A**) was incorporated into the incision and the skin edges were excised (**B**). The large rent in the triceps and skin was created by the humeral shaft as it protruded at the time of injury. More than 90% of open wounds in this type of injury are posterior.

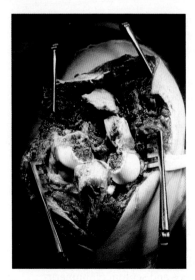

FIGURE 4 Intraoperative photograph shows a midline triceps split, in which the rent in the triceps was débrided and incorporated, exposing the fracture fragments. Preoperative imaging accurately predicted the split into the articular surface with metaphyseal comminution.

- Triceps split approach (**Figure 4**)
  - Allows adequate exposure for most intra-articular fractures
  - Involves a midline split in triceps, which continues on to olecranon, reflecting full-thickness flaps of triceps and its tendon medially and laterally
  - Radial nerve limits proximal dissection
  - To repair triceps split, use interrupted transosseous sutures in the proximal olecranon and nonabsorbable braided stitches through drill holes in olecranon
- Olecranon osteotomy
  - Provides best exposure
  - Chevron-shaped intra-articular osteotomy with apex pointing distally
  - Predrill ulna before fixation to ensure anatomic reduction of osteotomy site
  - Disadvantages
    - Need for fixation of osteotomy site
    - Potential for delayed union and nonunion
    - Hardware can be irritating
    - Conversion to arthroplasty is technically challenging
- Triceps peel
  - Affords excellent exposure and accommodates conversion to arthroplasty

▶ Extensor mechanism is reflected in full-thickness manner from the olecranon, working from ulnar side to radial

▶ Repair involves transosseous olecranon fixation using nonabsorbable suture

Reduction and Fixation

- Re-creation of the ulnar and radial columnar triangle is key to success
- After visualizing and cleaning fracture, determine extent of articular damage and loss
- Restoring relationship of trochlea to capitellum is crucial
- Surgical goals—Re-create articular surface and then securely fasten it to the humeral shaft
- Use Kirschner wires to achieve temporary fixation
- Alternatively, use tenaculum to clamp across articular surface and provide compression (**Figure 5**)
- Goal of distal screws is to traverse as many fracture fragments as possible
- Screws should be as long as possible; interdigitation is desired
- Once articular surface is reconstructed, fix plates to shaft via oblong holes

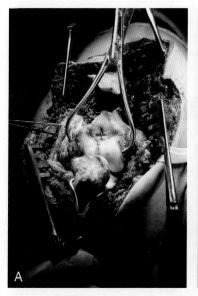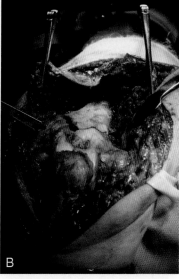

FIGURE 5 Intraoperative photographs show open reduction and internal fixation of a distal humerus fracture. **A,** With a tenaculum providing compression of the articular fragments, a compression screw is placed in the subchondral region to lag the condyles together. **B,** Kirschner wires are used to provisionally hold in the assembled articular surface to the metaphysis.

- Place a proximal screw through the plate in a compressive mode to provide additional compression
- Compression of articular surface to the shaft confers stability to overall construct
- If both columns have significant bone loss, best to shorten humerus
- Parallel plates should be of different lengths to minimize stress-riser forces
- After fixation, put elbow through ROM to assess stability
- Debate exists about need for anterior transposition of ulnar nerve; authors transpose the nerve if preoperative nerve deficit is present or if nerve directly contacts the hardware

COMPLICATIONS
- Elbow stiffness
- Hardware failure or irritation
- Triceps avulsion
- Nerve injury
- Infection
- Nonunion of olecranon osteotomy or fracture

POSTOPERATIVE CARE AND REHABILITATION
- Splint in extension for 24 to 48 hours
- Physical therapy—Active flexion with gravity-assisted extension
- If concerned about soft tissues, keep splint on for 10 days
- Authors reserve indomethacin or radiation prophylaxis for heterotopic ossification for high-risk patients only

PEARLS

- Lateral decubitus patient positioning allows gravity to aid reduction.
- If an ORIF may have to convert to an arthroplasty, avoid an olecranon osteotomy.
- Precontoured plates save surgical time dedicated to contouring straight plates.
- Interdigitating screws in the distal fragments contribute to overall construct stability.
- Long screws originating from one column and gaining purchase in contralateral humeral column are preferable.
- Can remove a sterile tourniquet to allow greater proximal exposure if needed.
- Instituting early motion after a brief period of splinting (2 to 10 days) optimizes functional results.
- Preoperative patient discussion should cover the loss of ROM typical with these injuries and the chance of ulnar nerve paresthesias.

INTRODUCTION
- Current implant designs are linked, unlinked, or hybrid linkable
- Decision to use linked or unlinked depends on underlying pathology, adequacy of bone stock, and integrity of soft-tissue envelope
- Unlinked implants require joint stability and good bone stock but provide a theoretical reduction in stress across prosthesis
- Linked implants are joined by a "sloppy hinge," allowing slight movement in varus-valgus plane
- Hybrid linkable implants permit implantation in an unlinked fashion, but can be converted to linked implant if stability cannot be established

PATIENT SELECTION
Indications
- Goals—To treat pain and improve function
- Indicated for rheumatoid arthritis, posttraumatic arthritis, acute fracture, primary osteoarthritis, and malunion/nonunion/recalcitrant instability

Contraindications
- Absolute—Infection of joint and lack of motor function
- Relative—Younger patients, particularly laborers; patients who cannot live with activity and weight restrictions; neuropathic joint (unpredictable outcomes and high complication rate)

PREOPERATIVE IMAGING
- AP, lateral, and oblique radiographs of elbow (**Figure 1**)
- Obtain stress radiographs if ligamentous instability is suspected
- CT can be useful for acute fracture, malunion/nonunion, or heterotopic ossification
- MRI plays limited role

Based on Johnston P, Ramsey ML: Total elbow arthroplasty, in Colvin AC, Flatow E, eds: Atlas of Essential Orthopaedic Procedures, *ed 2. Rosemont, IL, American Academy of Orthopaedic Surgeons, 2020, pp 300-308.*

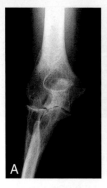 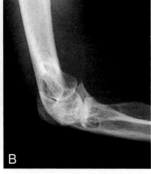 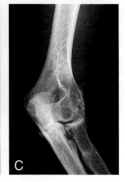

FIGURE 1 AP (**A**), lateral (**B**), and oblique (**C**) radiographs of the elbow of a patient with rheumatoid arthritis demonstrate joint destruction and cyst formation in the capitellum severe enough to consider total elbow arthroplasty.

PREOPERATIVE EVALUATION
- Important to assess overlying skin, prior incisions, contractures, limb alignment, joint stability, and flexion-extension arc
- Consider location of ulnar nerve and any ulnar nerve symptoms if prior surgery was performed

PREOPERATIVE PLANNING
- Radiographs, underlying pathology, and surgeon experience guide selection of implant type
- If choosing unlinked system, have linked system at hand in case elbow cannot be stabilized

PROCEDURE
Room Setup/Patient Positioning
- Supine position, with bump under ipsilateral scapula and arm on bolster across chest
- Place well-padded tourniquet on upper surgical arm; increases zone of sterility

Surgical Technique
- Make straight posterior incision off tip of olecranon extending 9 cm proximal and 8 cm distal
- Create subcutaneous flaps
- Identify and transpose ulnar nerve
- Management of triceps is guided by underlying pathology, type of implant, and surgeon preference

Bryan-Morrey Triceps-Reflecting Approach

- Perform by reflecting the triceps tendon, forearm fascia, and periosteum as one unit from medial to lateral
- Elevate triceps in continuity with anconeus subperiosteally from medial to lateral (**Figure 2**)
- Release lateral collateral ligament and medial collateral ligament (MCL) from their origin
- If performing unlinked total elbow arthroplasty, tag lateral ulnar collateral ligament (LUCL) and MCL for reattachment via bone tunnels

Triceps-Sparing Approach

- Authors' preferred approach for linked implant
- Identify medial and lateral borders of triceps and completely mobilize triceps bluntly from posterior humerus to proximal ulna (**Figure 3**)
- Subperiosteally dissect flexor-pronator group and MCL from medial epicondyle

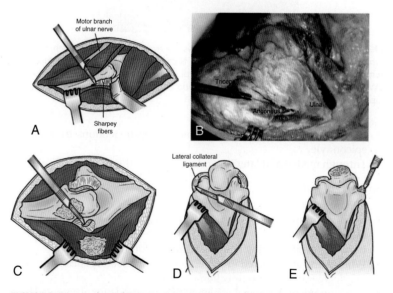

FIGURE 2 Images show the Bryan-Morrey triceps-reflecting approach.
A, Illustration shows the triceps in continuity with the anconeus reflected from the ulna. **B**, Intraoperative photograph demonstrates the Bryan-Morrey approach. **C**, Further elevation laterally allows identification of the radiocapitellar joint. The lateral (**D**) and medial (**E**) collateral ligaments are released, allowing dislocation of the joint. (Panel B adapted with permission from Morrey BM: Semiconstrained total elbow arthroplasty, in Morrey BF, ed: *Master Techniques in Orthopaedic Surgery: The Elbow*. Philadelphia, PA, Lippincott Williams & Wilkins, 2002, p 317.)

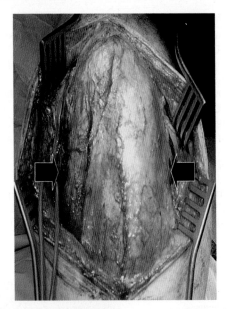

FIGURE 3 Intraoperative photograph shows the triceps-sparing approach, in which the medial and lateral aspects of the triceps are developed. (Reproduced with permission from Kamineni S: Elbow replacement for acute trauma, in Wiesel SW, ed: *Operative Techniques in Shoulder and Elbow Surgery*. Philadelphia, PA, Lippincott Williams & Wilkins, 2011, p 395.)

- Similarly, release LUCL and common extensor tendons from lateral epicondyle
- Through medial and lateral windows, release the anterior capsule

Bone Preparation

- Remove central portion of trochlea
- Identify intramedullary canal of the humerus by opening a window in roof of olecranon
- Implant-specific cutting jigs guide the resection
- When using an unlinked implant, must balance soft tissues with varying degrees of humeral resection
- Enter intramedullary canal of ulna with high-speed burr at coronoid base
- Pass broaches parallel to the subcutaneous border of ulna
- Radial head is important stabilizer but may be sacrificed if necessary when using a linked implant and with some unlinked designs
- With a linked implant, obtain full flexion-extension arc
- Must evaluate soft tissue for possible contracture
- In severe comminution, can resect up to 2 cm of distal humerus without compromising triceps strength
- Perform cementing with antibiotic cement

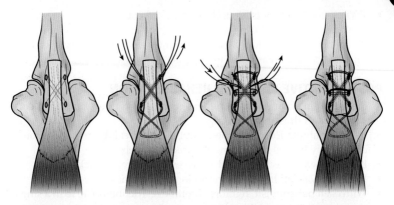

FIGURE 4 Illustration shows reattachment of the triceps in a total elbow arthroplasty via cruciate drill holes supplemented by a transverse "cinch" suture.

- Add methylene blue to cement for visualization in case revision is needed
- It is critical to maintain appropriate axis of rotation during insertion of components
- After cement has hardened, reattach triceps to ulna through cruciate tunnels
- Tie all knots with elbow at 90° of flexion (**Figure 4**)

COMPLICATIONS

- Deep infection is the worst complication, with rates of 2% to 11%
- Inflammatory arthritides are risk factor for infection
- With well-fixed implants, make attempt to preserve the implants
  - Repeated irrigation and débridement often needed to eradicate infection
  - *Staphylococcus epidermidis* and gram-negative infections respond poorly to irrigation and débridement alone
- Treat prosthetic infection that has gross loosening of implants with component removal, antibiotic spacer placement, intravenous antibiotics, and staged reimplantation
- Instability almost always is associated with unlinked implants
- Immediate instability is due to component malposition
- Early instability occurs within 6 weeks and may be due to soft-tissue insufficiency
- Late instability usually results from trauma, limb malalignment, component malposition, or polyethylene wear
- Instability in linked implants is due to disruption of linking mechanism from bushing wear or axis-pin disengagement
- Loosening is typically associated with linked constructs
- Rate of periprosthetic fracture is as high as 23%; critical to assess for component loosening

- Triceps insufficiency is an underrecognized complication; can present as elbow weakness during overhead activity and posterior elbow pain
- Ulnar neuropathy—Rates of permanent deficit are as high as 10%; transient paresthesias occur in up to 26% of cases

POSTOPERATIVE CARE AND REHABILITATION

- Place arm in volar splint in full extension for 48 hours, and then convert to a soft dressing and sling
- Begin rehabilitation only when wound looks healthy; rehabilitation is dictated by triceps management intraoperatively
- If triceps was reflected, avoid active extension for 6 weeks
- If triceps was left intact, begin motion in all planes
- With each patient visit, reinforce lifetime restrictions of 10 lb in a single event and 5 lb in repetitive lifting

PEARLS

- Perform careful history, physical examination, and radiographic evaluation; attend to underlying pathology, associated deformities, previous surgery, and immunosuppressive therapies.
- Patient selection is critical. Compliant patients with realistic expectations who understand postoperative activity limitations do best.
- Attention to bone quality/architecture and ligamentous integrity is key to selecting appropriate linked or unlinked implant.
- Carefully identify, dissect, and protect the ulnar nerve throughout the procedure.
- Select the approach—triceps-reflecting versus triceps sparing—based on surgeon experience and underlying pathology.
- Complete releases of the capsule, excision of scar tissue in the olecranon/coronoid fossa, and release of triceps from posterior cortex of the humerus are essential to optimize exposure and ROM.
- Tag the LUCL and the MCL for anatomic repair to the humerus for an unlinked implant.
- Using trial components—with close attention to soft-tissue tensioning, ROM, and implant stability—is helpful, particularly with an unlinked implant.
- Bony impingement can occur posteriorly between the olecranon and the humerus and anteriorly between the coronoid and the anterior humeral flange of a linked prosthesis.
- Use antibiotic cement with intramedullary cement restrictors in the humerus and ulna.
- Components should be seated to re-create the axis of rotation of the distal humerus and ulna.
- Use a postoperative extension splint for 48 hours with a subcutaneous drain.
- A conservative postoperative course reinforces functional limitations.

Hand and Wrist

3

Section Editor
Julie E. Adams, MD, MS

PATIENT SELECTION

Indications

- Failed nonsurgical treatment (activity modification, wrist splint, corticosteroid injection)
- Carpal tunnel release (CTR) produces good to excellent results in 95% of cases

Contraindications

- Consider delaying surgery until other local diagnoses/conditions (eg, tendinitis of wrist, forearm, or elbow) improve
- Discuss with patient in advance how these conditions may affect surgical outcomes

ELECTRODIAGNOSTIC TESTING

- Helps support diagnosis or eliminate secondary diagnoses
- Interpret in context of clinical signs and symptoms
  - Carpal tunnel syndrome is a constellation of symptoms
  - Median neuropathy at the wrist (an electrodiagnostic diagnosis) is sometimes seen in the absence of carpal tunnel syndrome (and vice versa)
- Median motor latency of >4.5 ms and or sensory study >3.5 ms generally indicative of median neuropathy at the level of the wrist
- Nerve conduction velocity—Change from normal (50 to 60 m/s) to 30 m/s is highly suggestive of peripheral neuropathy
- Electromyography or EMG portion may reveal denervation patterns can be seen in median nerve–innervated thenar muscles

PROCEDURE

Patient Positioning

- Supine position with arm on hand table
- Generally, local or local anesthesia with sedation is most commonly used

---

Based on Diao E: Carpal tunnel release, in Colvin AC, Flatow E, eds: Atlas of Essential Orthopaedic Procedures, *ed 2. Rosemont, IL, American Academy of Orthopaedic Surgeons, 2020, pp 309-318.*

- Nonsterile tourniquet may be applied to the forearm or upper arm or may be avoided especially with the use of local anesthesia with epinephrine

Special Equipment
- Loupe magnification may be helpful
- Specialized equipment may be required for endoscopic techniques

Surgical Technique
- Goal of CTR surgery is decompression of median nerve by complete division of transverse carpal ligament (TCL)

 VIDEO 37.1 Carpal Tunnel Release. Edward Diao, MD (3 min)

Open Carpal Tunnel Release
- The intended incision may be represented by the intersection of the Kaplan cardinal line and line along radial border of fourth ray, ending at wrist flexion crease; alternatively, the incision may be parallel or on the thenar crease in line with the radial aspect of the fourth ray (**Figure 1**)
- If the wrist crease is crossed, it should be crossed in an oblique fashion

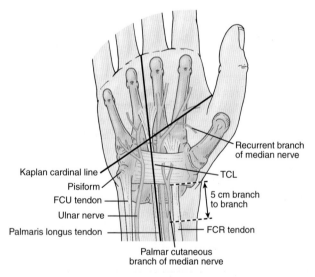

FIGURE 1 Illustration shows surface landmarks and critical deep structures to be considered when contemplating surgical release of the median nerve. FCR = flexor carpi radialis, FCU = flexor carpi ulnaris, TCL = transverse carpal ligament.

- Incise skin, and then dissect through subcutaneous fat. The palmar fascia is then incised, exposing the transverse fibers of the TCL
- If palmaris brevis muscle is present superficial to TCL, incise and release from ligament
- Incise TCL over a small segment, avoiding injury to deep structures
- One may place a small hemostat or Freer elevator into canal to define undersurface of ligament and direction of release. It is helpful to use a right-angle or Meyerding loupe retractor superficially from the radial and ulnar sides to expose the TCL and (on the ulnar side) to protect the ulnar neurovascular bundle
- Release TCL leaving a radially based TCL leaflet over median nerve
- Release distal forearm fascia proximally
- Inspect median nerve and canal contents for rare space-occupying lesion; in general, the literature does not support routine internal neurolysis or tenosynovectomy
- Close wound and apply sterile dressing

Single-Incision Endoscopic Carpal Tunnel Release (Modified Agee)

- Mark palmaris longus (PL), flexor carpi radialis, and flexor carpi ulnaris (**Figure 2**)
- Make transverse 1- to 2-cm incision in wrist flexion crease centered over or just ulnar to PL; if PL not present, make incision halfway between flexor carpi radialis and flexor carpi ulnaris
- Expose PL and retract radially with Ragnell retractor; identify flexor retinaculum deep
- Incise flexor retinaculum and create 1-cm–wide distally based U-shaped flap; elevate flap and retract using mosquito clamp
- Pass small and large hamate finders antegrade down the carpal canal; instrument tip should be palpable subcutaneously distal to TCL at Kaplan cardinal line (**Figure 3**)

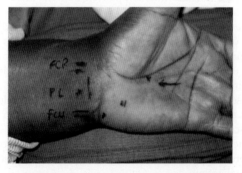

FIGURE 2 Photograph shows the key landmarks for endoscopic carpal tunnel release: the flexor carpi radialis (FCR), the palmaris longus (PL), and the flexor carpi ulnaris (FCU). The arrow indicates the palpated landmark for the distal end of the transverse carpal ligament. The transverse wrist incision is inscribed.

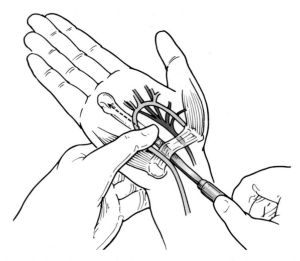

FIGURE 3 Illustration shows a synovial elevator used to reflect the synovial tissue from the undersurface of the transverse carpal ligament.

- Pass tenosynovial elevator proximally and distally 12 times along axis of fourth ray; feel for "washboard" effect. Introduce endoscopic CTR device into carpal canal with endoscope palmar; visualize undersurface of TCL (has characteristic transverse striations)
- Watch monitor while advancing instrument to distal margin of TCL (identify change from white transverse fibers to yellow fat); use the nondominant hand to perform ballottement maneuver on palm to distinguish transition
- Palpate tip of CTR device in palm as it emerges subcutaneously distal to TCL; the transillumination pattern from the device changes as it passes distal to TCL
- Elevate blade and withdraw device slowly, cutting TCL distal to proximal; keep device pressed against undersurface of TCL so only the TCL is cut (**Figure 4**)
- Cut only under excellent visualization; if needed, withdraw device and redefine undersurface of TCL as described above
- Full release prevents visualization of radial and ulnar leaflets simultaneously and permits device to be placed in trough to visualize the thenar fascia
- Reintroduce hamate finder to confirm increased volume of carpal canal
- Release proximal antebrachial fascia with tenotomy scissors under direct visualization
- Close incision and apply soft dressing
- Inability to safely visualize structures with the endoscopic CTR device warrants conversion to two-incision or open CTR

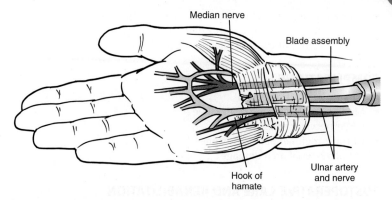

FIGURE 4 Illustration demonstrates how the endoscopic carpal tunnel release device is inserted into the carpal canal until the distal end of the ligament is visualized.

Two-Incision Endoscopic Carpal Tunnel Release (Chow)

- Make proximal incision and create distally based U-shaped flap of antebrachial fascia as in single-incision endoscopic technique
- Pass clamp, elevator, or trocar under TCL until palpable in palm subcutaneously distal to TCL; make second small incision to expose instrument tip at junction of proximal and middle thirds of palm
- May use open or endoscope-assisted technique; keep wrist hyperextended; complete distal TCL release may be verified by direct visualization
- Pitfalls of two-incision techniques are incomplete release of the TCL distally and the potential for injury to the palmar arterial arch and/or branches of the median or ulnar nerve

Revision Carpal Tunnel Release

- If recurrent carpal tunnel syndrome is from a prior incomplete release, may revise with endoscopic CTR if surgeon is experienced; otherwise, use open technique
- Make generous skin incision; technique similar to that for primary open CTR
- Use scalpel to dissect scarring; carefully separate TCL from median nerve (expect dense adhesion); completely release TCL and median nerve, taking care to protect median nerve motor branch
- Use operating microscope to inspect median nerve for damage or scarring; perform external epineurotomy to expose bands of Fontana if significant nerve scarring is present
- If minimal scarring is present, close wound in usual manner
- If nerve injury is dramatic and rescarring is likely, consider covering the median nerve with hypothenar fat-pad flap; dissect fat to ulnar nerve and artery, advance radial edge to cover nerve, and sew edge to radial flap of TCL; may also use palmaris brevis flap by releasing its insertion subcutaneously and transposing over nerve

- Vein wrapping and neural conduit are other options
- May create TCL flap through Z-lengthening if flexor tendon prolapse or palmar migration of median nerve are likely

COMPLICATIONS

- Incomplete TCL release
- Median nerve scarring or damage
- Ulnar nerve or artery damage
- Chronic regional pain syndrome
- Palmar arterial arch damage

POSTOPERATIVE CARE AND REHABILITATION

- Splinting is not necessary
- Hand therapy is helpful, if patient has difficulty with full digital active and passive motion
- Grip and pinch strength, subjective symptoms, and functional evaluations are helpful
- Prolonged tenderness under TCL or pillar pain may require extended hand therapy and time to regain strength and endurance

CURRENT TRENDS

- Establishment of AAOS Appropriate Use Criteria (AUC) for the management of carpal tunnel syndrome, which is a recent update of a pre-existing clinical practice guideline from September 2008
- Current clinical practice guideline altered recommendation for using electrodiagnostic studies to aid in diagnoses to using it only for specific situations
- Studies now support the use of office ultrasonography examination to confirm clinical diagnosis of carpal tunnel syndrome; comparable to electrodiagnostic testing in terms of specificity and sensitivity
- Wide-awake local anesthesia and no tourniquet (WALANT) approach is becoming more popular for carpal tunnel surgery and other hand and wrist procedures
- Advantages include no sedation, no tourniquet use during surgery, no need for anesthesiologist to be present during procedure, and ability of surgeon to see active components regarding motion intraoperatively
- Anesthetic needs to be administered about 30 minutes before actual procedure
- Higher trend in WALANT approach in Canada in a local procedure room compared with the general operating room, but it this will likely increase in the United States going forward

PEARLS

- Full history and physical examination, consideration of all differential diagnoses, prevent poor patient selection.
- Release TCL with technically proficient manner and confirm release, especially distally.
- Must be able to identify and distinguish anatomic structures. Protect the median nerve. When the median nerve is visualized, inspect it after TCL release.

38 Surgical Treatment of Cubital Tunnel Syndrome

INTRODUCTION

- Occurs at elbow as a compressive neuropathy of the ulnar nerve
- Second most common peripheral nerve compression syndrome after carpal tunnel syndrome

PATIENT SELECTION

Physical Examination

- Inspect for muscle atrophy/weakness, sensory deficits, Tinel sign at the cubital tunnel, results of elbow flexion test and cubital tunnel compression test. The ulnar nerve is evaluated for any subluxation or instability
- Examine ulnar innervated muscles, particularly FDP to the ipsilateral small finger. M4 motor strength indicates early compression of the ulnar nerve in the cubital tunnel
- Finally, document the range of motion of the elbow joint and examine the ulnar nerve for subluxation

ELECTRODIAGNOSTIC TESTING AND PREOPERATIVE IMAGING

- Electrodiagnostic testing (electromyography and nerve conduction velocity tests) is often obtained to support the diagnosis, exclude alternative diagnoses, or determine the extent of nerve changes; however, these studies are not always abnormal in early cases
- Radiographs in at least two projections may be obtained in some cases
- Ultrasonography and MRI are gaining importance in detecting morphologic changes in select cases, but are generally not necessary for most patients as cubital tunnel syndrome is a clinical diagnosis
- CT is recommended only in the setting of skeletal deformity (**Figure 1**)

INDICATIONS AND CONTRAINDICATIONS

- Regardless of technique, a few principles are important and common for each technique: complete decompression of compressive structures, assuring the nerve is in hospitable environment, avoiding iatrogenic

Based on Hoffmann R, Lubahn JD: Surgical treatment of cubital tunnel syndrome, in Colvin AC, Flatow E, eds: Atlas of Essential Orthopaedic Procedures, ed 2. Rosemont, IL, American Academy of Orthopaedic Surgeons, 2020, pp 319-327.

The authors wish to recognize the work of John Dupaix, MD and Wayne Chen, MD for their contributions to this chapter.

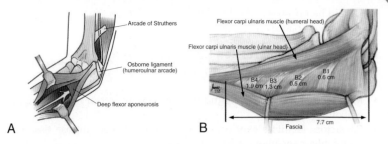

FIGURE 1 Illustrations depict the anatomy of the cubital tunnel. **A,** The most common sites of ulnar nerve compression are labeled. **B,** Additional potential sites of compression of the ulnar nerve located in the submuscular membrane of the flexor-pronator muscle. (Panel B copyright Joe Kanasz, the Cleveland Clinic Foundation, Cleveland, OH.)

injury to medial antebrachial cutaneous nerve, and assessing for nerve instability following end of procedure
- Recent studies in the literature suggest that endoscopic cubital tunnel release procedures compare favorably to open in situ decompression
- Cubital tunnel decompression may be indicated in patients with failure of nonsurgical treatment

IN SITU DECOMPRESSION
Room Setup/Patient Positioning
- Outpatient setting
- General anesthesia preferred
- Supine position with shoulder abducted 90°, elbow flexed, forearm supinated
- Apply well-padded tourniquet around upper arm

Special Instruments/Equipment/Implants
- Karl Storz endoscopy set for endoscopic decompression; includes illuminated speculum, 30° endoscope, endoscopic bipolar forceps
- Other commercial systems are also available

Open Decompression
- Exsanguinate limb and elevate tourniquet
- Make a longitudinal incision centered over the medial aspect of the elbow posterior to the medial epicondyle
- Protect branches of medial and posterior cutaneous nerves
- Expose the ulnar nerve and divide arcuate ligament (Osborne ligament)
- Decompress the nerve through the two heads of the flexor carpi ulnaris (FCU) fascia
- Divide the fascia proximally in similar fashion
- Identify intermuscular septum; consider resection especially if anterior transposition of the ulnar nerve is planned or if impingement upon the nerve is noted

- Obtain hemostasis and close skin in usual fashion
- Apply well-padded bandage

Endoscopic Decompression (Hoffmann Technique)

- Raise hand table to nearly eye level of the seated surgeon
- Palpate ulnar nerve
- Make 1.5- to 2.5-cm longitudinal incision posterior to the medial epicondyle
- Retractors facilitate exposure of the nerve; dissect adipose tissue or epitrochlear anconeus muscle as needed
- Divide arcuate ligament under direct vision while keeping epifascial layer in view
- Introduce tunneling forceps into space between subcutaneous tissue and fascia—not into the cubital tunnel, that is, not beneath the arcuate ligament adjacent to the nerve
- Spread forceps distally, then proximally, to create workspace cavity; work gently
- Insert illuminated speculum with 9- to 11-cm blade and divide remaining arcuate ligament under direct vision; up to 5 cm of ulnar nerve may be decompressed or fascia excised to muscle fibers of the FCU (**Figure 2, A**). Introduce 4-mm, 30° endoscope with blunt dissector at tip and advance distally to lift up soft-tissue envelope
- While watching the monitor, blunt tipped scissors measuring 17 to 23 cm in length are used to divide the forearm fascia 10 to 15 cm distal to the epicondyle
- Protect cutaneous nerve branches or veins that cross fascia (**Figure 2, B** and C)
- Pull back endoscope and further dissect close to the ulnar nerve
- Divide the two muscular heads of the FCU distally from the arcuate ligament; the first fibrous bands are located and divided at 3 cm distal to the epicondyle, then the fibrous raphe is transected and all constricting elements up to 9 to 14 cm distal are divided; include the submuscular membrane in this dissection (**Figure 2, D**). Most muscle vessel branches can be protected rather than cauterized or clipped; if necessary, use long bipolar forceps or endoscopic bipolar forceps from instrument set
- Proximally, the tunnel roof is decompressed similarly; divide fascia, but not intermuscular septum, 8 to 14 cm proximal from retrocondylar groove; constricting elements are not regularly observed here
- Close skin in usual fashion
- Apply bulky cotton compression dressing, then deflate tourniquet

---

VIDEO 38.1 Endoscopic Management of Cubital Tunnel Syndrome. Reimer Hoffmann, MD; John D. Lubahn, MD (7 min)

© 2021 American Academy of Orthopaedic Surgeons

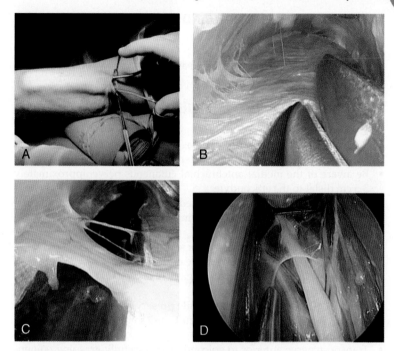

FIGURE 2 Images show endoscopic in situ decompression of the ulnar nerve. **A,** Intraoperative photograph shows the creation of a workspace for a soft-tissue endoscope using a special blunt-tipped tunneling forceps. **B,** Endoscopic view shows the soft-tissue endoscope maintaining a well-visualized workspace while the forearm fascia is released. **C,** Endoscopic view shows the forearm fascia released beneath a crossing branch of the medial antebrachial cutaneous nerve, which must be preserved. **D,** Endoscopic view shows excellent visualization of the muscle branches.

POSTOPERATIVE CARE AND REHABILITATION

- Early range of motion (ROM) of elbow is allowed. Remove dressing 24 to 72 hours postoperatively, and apply elastic bandage, which is worn for 4 weeks
- Avoid resting elbow in flexion for 4 weeks
- Light work is allowed within 3 to 5 days; heavy labor in 3 weeks
- Increased loading is allowed over 4 to 8 weeks

COMPLICATIONS

- Extremely rare
- Profuse subcutaneous hematoma occurs in 4% to 5% of patients
- Recurrence rate is 1%

TRANSPOSITION TECHNIQUES AND MEDIAL EPICONDYLECTOMY

- Choice of anterior transposition technique based on surgeon preferences
- Recommended if after in situ release, ulnar nerve subluxates with elbow flexion

Subcutaneous Anterior Transposition

Surgical Technique

- Same preparation and positioning as that for in situ decompression
- Make incision 15 cm in length, centered over medial epicondyle
- Be aware of the medial antebrachial cutaneous nerve approximately 3.5 cm distal to the epicondyle
- Identify ulnar nerve posterior to medial epicondyle, and continue dissection proximally to the medial intermuscular septum; release the arcade of Struthers
- Incise the edge of the intermuscular septum generously to avoid kinking of nerve; if resecting, protect the perforating vessels
- Dissect distally to release arcuate ligament and FCU fascia; stop at first and second nerve branches to FCU
- Mobilize ulnar nerve from bed while preserving as much blood supply as possible; this step is difficult and sometimes impossible to achieve
- Transpose nerve anterior to epicondyle by carefully grasping epineurium; loosely suture the 2-cm flap of forearm fascia over the nerve Close wound with interrupted sutures; a small drain can be used
- Apply dressing and splint (**Figure 3**)

Postoperative Care and Rehabilitation

- Sutures are removed at 1 week
- Splint is worn for 2 to 3 weeks

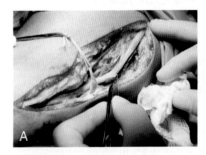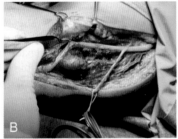

FIGURE 3 Intraoperative photographs show subcutaneous transposition of the ulnar nerve. **A,** Incision and dissection of the ulnar nerve before subcutaneous transposition. **B,** Subcutaneous.

- After splint removal, gentle active ROM is allowed under supervision of a therapist or independently in a trustworthy patient
- Return to work 6 to 12 weeks or more postoperatively
- In cases of motor palsy, therapy for strengthening paretic muscles is recommended

Anterior Submuscular Transposition

Surgical Technique

- Same preparation and positioning as that for in situ decompression
- Make 15-cm incision centered posterior to the medial epicondyle
- Be aware of medial antebrachial cutaneous nerve crossing the incision approximately 3.5 cm distal to epicondyle; preserve throughout the dissection
- Identify ulnar nerve posterior to medial epicondyle and continue dissection proximally to medial intermuscular septum; divide arcade of Struthers
- Incise intermuscular septum generously to avoid kinking of the nerve
- Dissect distally to release arcuate ligament and FCU fascia; stop at first and second nerve branches to FCU
- Elevate flexor pronator origin from epicondyle to create submuscular bed for ulnar nerve; do not divide medial collateral ligament
- Mobilize nerve from behind epicondyle while preserving as much blood supply as possible; this step is difficult and sometimes impossible to achieve
- Transpose the nerve anterior to the epicondyle by carefully grasping the epineurium; place nerve beneath muscle without excess tension
- Reattach the flexor pronator origin to the epicondyle with heavy nonabsorbable sutures; place sutures sequentially, then tie them, ensuring that the nerve is free
- Close wound with interrupted nonabsorbable suture; a small drain is often used
- Apply dressing and a posterior splint

Postoperative Care and Rehabilitation

- Arm supported in posterior splint for 3 weeks
- Return to work 6 to 12 weeks or more postoperatively
- In cases of motor palsy, therapy for strengthening paretic muscles is recommended

Intramuscular Transposition

Surgical Technique

- Same preparation and positioning as that for subcutaneous decompression
- Same incision as that for subcutaneous transposition
- Upon deep dissection, make the incision in the flexor forearm musculature; gently separate muscle fibers to create a bed for the nerve

- Transpose ulnar nerve in similar fashion as in previous procedure; place nerve into intramuscular bed
- Loosely close fascia over the nerve for protection
- Close wound in the usual fashion
- Apply dressing and a posterior splint

Postoperative Care and Rehabilitation
- Complete immobility for 3 weeks followed by restricted activity for 10 weeks
- Return to work 6 to 12 weeks or more postoperatively
- In cases of motor palsy, therapy for strengthening paretic muscles is recommended

Medial Epicondylectomy
Indications
- Severe deformity of the medial epicondyle
- Valgus deformation
- Revision surgery cases with intraoperative findings of perineurial scarring

Surgical Technique
- Same preparation and positioning as transposition procedures
- Surgical exposure is also the same
- After identifying the ulnar nerve, expose the medial epicondyle with subperiosteal dissection
- Use a small osteotome to score epicondyle at planned depth of resection (<20% of total depth of the epicondyle)
- Resect only enough bone to allow free gliding of the ulnar nerve during elbow arc of motion
- Remove chosen depth of epicondyle while avoiding damage to the anteromedial band of the medial collateral ligament; avoid incidental arthrotomy
- Smooth edges of bone with a file or rasp; suture together periosteal flaps to prevent nerve scarring to the exposed bone
- Close wound with 4-0 nylon suture; consider placement of a small drain
- Apply dressing

Postoperative Care and Rehabilitation
- Gentle ROM begins at 1 week
- Resistance exercises must be avoided for 10 to 12 weeks
- Return to work 6 to 12 weeks or more postoperatively
- In cases of motor palsy, therapy for strengthening paretic muscles is recommended

COMPLICATIONS
- Hematoma
- Injury to medial antebrachial cutaneous nerve

- Injury to or kinking of the ulnar nerve
- Recurrence
- Joint contraction after postoperative immobilization
- Elbow joint instability after medial epicondylectomy
- Complex regional pain syndrome

PEARLS

- Decompression of the ulnar nerve should extend at least 5 to 7 cm distal and proximal from the retrocondylar groove. Avoid circumferential dissection.
- Epineurolysis is rarely indicated.
- Cubital tunnel is differentiated from distal compression by hypoesthesia on the dorsoulnar area of the hand.
- In primary cubital tunnel syndrome, the ulnar nerve can always be located posterior to the medial epicondyle and can be recognized by longitudinally running vasa nervorum..
- In situ neuroplasty carries less risk than transposition, if decompression is adequately achieved by either technique.
- Patients with cubital tunnel syndrome sometimes have difficulty describing both the onset of symptoms and postoperative improvement. Carefully document objective findings.
- One of the best objective measures is the motor strength of the FDP to the small finger. Patients with cubital tunnel almost always are grade 4, meaning the examiner can overcome the patient. In cubital tunnel syndrome diagnosed early, this converts immediately to grade 5 when the patient is examined in the recovery room.
- If electrodiagnostic testing is negative, check which muscles were tested. Needle placement into the first dorsal interosseous muscle is more reliable than placement into the hypothenar muscles.
- Always visualize the entire cutting edge of the scissors when dissecting to avoid damaging tissue outside the field of vision.

First Dorsal Extensor Compartment Release

PATIENT SELECTION
- Patients present with radial-side wrist pain, worse with radial-ulnar deviation and thumb motion
- Indications for surgery include failure of nonsurgical treatment (splinting, injections, activity modulation)

PHYSICAL EXAMINATION
- Patients have pain with resisted thumb abduction
- Localized swelling and tenderness over first dorsal compartment may be obvious or more subtle
- Finkelstein test is pathognomonic for de Quervain syndrome

DIAGNOSTIC IMAGING
- Radiographs—Wrist PA and lateral; hyperpronated view of thumb (Roberts view) to differentiate de Quervain from other pathology
- Exclude thumb arthritis, scaphoid fracture, and radiocarpal arthrosis

PROCEDURE
Room Setup/Patient Positioning
- Supine position with hand table
- Apply tourniquet around arm and set to 250 mm Hg if using general anesthesia or local with sedation
- Perform procedure without tourniquet with WALANT method; total of 10 mL of 1% lidocaine with 1:100,000 epinephrine and 1 mL of 8.4% bicarbonate is injected into the area where dissection will occur, preferably 20 to 30 minutes before procedure

Special Instruments/Equipment/Implants
- Loupe magnification may be helpful
- Soft-tissue set with fine hand instruments

Based on Papatheodorou LK, Venouziou AI, Giannoulis FS, Sotereanos DG: First dorsal extensor compartment release, in Colvin AC, Flatow E, eds: Atlas of Essential Orthopaedic Procedures, *ed 2. Rosemont, IL, American Academy of Orthopaedic Surgeons, 2020, pp 328-333.*

Surgical Technique

- Protect superficial radial nerve and its branches
  - ▶ Make longitudinal incision from tip of radial styloid distally 1.5 cm
  - ▶ Sharply dissect just through dermis
  - ▶ Retract skin edges and bluntly dissect subcutaneous fat down to retinaculum of first dorsal compartment with tenotomy scissors
  - ▶ Protect superficial branches of radial nerve
  - ▶ Identify extensor pollicis brevis (EPB) and abductor pollicis longus (APL) tendons distal to compartment (**Figure 1**)
  - ▶ Place retractors to visualize entire sheath
- Release first dorsal compartment on dorsal margin with blade or tenotomy scissors, leaving thick volar-based flap which serves as a barrier to tendon subluxation
  - ▶ Avoid injury to the EPB tendon while releasing compartment in cases where the retinaculum is extremely thick
- Ensure complete release of stenosing compartment
  - ▶ First dorsal compartment is divided into two fibro-osseous tunnels in 40% to 60% of population; EPB subcompartment may be subtle
  - ▶ Release both subcompartments and examine floor for anomalous tunnels with aberrant tendons
  - ▶ Must identify EPB and APL tendons to ensure complete release
  - ▶ EPB tendon is more dorsal and is rounder and smaller than APL and absent in 5% to 7%; muscle fibers in compartment associated with EPB (**Figure 2**)

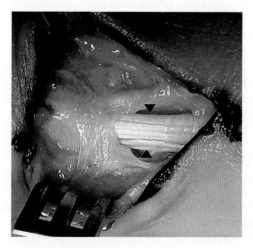

FIGURE 1 Intraoperative photograph shows the extensor pollicis brevis and abductor pollicis longus tendons (between the black arrowheads).

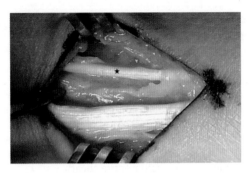

FIGURE 2 Intraoperative photograph shows the extensor pollicis brevis (EPB) tendon (star) released from its separate compartment and the intracompartmental septum excised. The EPB tendon is rounder and smaller than the abductor pollicis longus tendon.

- Traction on EPB tendon should elicit thumb metacarpophalangeal joint extension; if no extension occurs, look for subcompartment
- APL tendon usually has two or more slips; traction on APL tendon should elicit thumb ray abduction
- Flex and extend wrist following release to check for tendon subluxation
- If using WALANT method, patient can actively move wrist and thumb to identify separate subcompartments and/or tendon subluxation
- Release tourniquet, ensure hemostasis, irrigate wound
- Close skin in the usual fashion
- A thumb spica splint may be considered postoperatively to prevent volar tendon subluxation

VIDEO 39.1 First Dorsal Extensor Compartment Release. Filippos Giannoulis, MD; Douglas S. Musgrave, MD; Alexander H. Payatakes, MD; Dean Sotereanos, MD (3 min)

COMPLICATIONS

- Iatrogenic radial sensory nerve injury or radial sensory neuritis
- Fibrosis and adhesions
- Incomplete release of first dorsal compartment or inadequate release of subcompartments
- Tendon subluxation
- Wound infection
- Hypertrophic scarring

POSTOPERATIVE CARE

- In patients in whom splinting is used, generally it is discontinued by 10 to 14 days
- Encourage immediate thumb and hand motion as tolerated
- Formal hand therapy rarely necessary
- Address local soreness with wound massage
- Restrict heavy activities until wound healing has occurred

PEARLS

- Longitudinal dissection minimizes opportunity for injury to superficial radial sensory nerve.
- Perform blunt dissection of subcutaneous fat parallel to incision.
- Incise sheath on dorsal margin to prevent volar tendon subluxation.
- Traction on one released tendon must cause metacarpophalangeal joint extension; otherwise look for separate EPB subcompartment and excise any intracompartmental septa.
- Postoperative splinting may be considered to help prevent volar tendon subluxation.

40 Trigger Finger Release

INTRODUCTION
- Trigger finger most commonly results from painful catching of flexor tendons at A1 pulley
- Pathologic changes include stenosis of sheath due to inflammation and reactive nodule in flexor digitorum superficialis (FDS) tendon
- Surgery can be performed using WALANT method (wide-awake local anesthesia no tourniquet)

PATIENT SELECTION
Special Populations/Situations
Children
- Usually trigger thumb with inability to straighten interphalangeal joint
- Spontaneous resolution possible; one may consider observation for 6 months in children younger than 3 years
- Persistent triggering may require surgical release to prevent joint contractures

Diabetes
- Lower success rate of nonsurgical treatment
- Potential temporary hyperglycemic effect from steroid injection
- In patients who have a preoperative proximal interphalangeal (PIP) joint contracture, this will likely persist even after success trigger digit release and may result in decreased patient postoperative satisfaction

Rheumatoid Arthritis
- Primary pathology is synovitis within sheath, not stenosis of A1 pulley
- Recommend early surgery with flexor synovectomy with or without release of ulnar slip of FDS; avoid A1 pulley release because it may result in more ulnar drift of digit
- In patients in whom the inflammatory disease is well controlled and in whom there is no overt active synovitis or MCP deformity, most surgeons treat as idiopathic trigger finger and incise the A1 pulley alone

---

Based on Bindra R: Trigger finger release, in Colvin AC, Flatow E, eds: Atlas of Essential Orthopaedic Procedures, *ed 2. Rosemont, IL, American Academy of Orthopaedic Surgeons, 2020, pp 334-339.*

Distal Triggering

- Rare triggering at A3 pulley with pain at PIP joint; flexor digitorum profundus is involved
- Recommend A3 pulley excision

Proximal Interphalangeal Contracture

- Typically this accompanies trigger digits that have been of long-standing duration. It may also be seen in the setting of those with concomitant diabetes mellitus
- Before surgery, advise patient about residual contracture after A1 pulley release, and the possible need for excision of part of the superficialis tendon

Indications

- Failed nonsurgical treatment with one to three steroid injections
- Chronic triggering which has been present for >6 months
- Those who decline corticosteroid injection but have bothersome triggering
- Locked trigger digits

Contraindications

- None

PREOPERATIVE IMAGING

- Ultrasonography and radiography are rarely indicated, but in select cases may be indicated only if diagnosis unclear (eg, arthritis, tumors)
- Ultrasonography may show thickened A1 pulley or abnormality of flexor tendons

RELEVANT SURGICAL ANATOMY

- Surface anatomy—Measured distance between digital palmar crease and PIP crease can be used to locate A1 pulley
- Neurovascular anatomy
  - Neurovascular bundles for each digit run parallel to flexor sheath immediately radial and ulnar to the sheath
  - Identify and preserve radial digital nerve during trigger thumb release
- Flexor tendon sheath anatomy is illustrated in **Figure 1**.

 VIDEO 40.1 Management of Trigger Finger: From Injection to Surgery. Randy R. Bindra, MD (15 min)

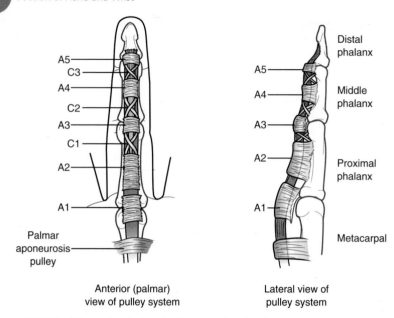

FIGURE 1 Illustration depicts the flexor tendon sheath/pulley system anatomy.

PROCEDURE

Room Setup/Patient Positioning

- WALANT method can be performed in most cases
- Local anesthesia with sedation as necessary. Supine position with arm on arm board
- Apply well-padded tourniquet on upper arm

Surgical Technique

Release of Central Digits (Ring or Long Finger Release)

- Surface anatomy—Proximal edge of A1 pulley lies at level of distal palmar crease in ring and small fingers, at proximal palmar crease in index finger, and halfway between both creases in long finger
- Draw midline of finger and A1 pulley landmarks on skin (**Figure 2, A**)
- Local anesthetic is administered at the incision site by subcutaneous infiltration of 5 cc of 0.5% Marcaine with 1:100,000 epinephrine mixed with sodium bicarbonate (10:1)
- Incise skin and place skin hooks for initial retraction
- Dissect subcutaneous tissue with tenotomy scissors gently
- Maintain dissection along midline; neurovascular structures run along sides of flexor sheath; identify, but do not dissect out

- Place 90° angled retractors and continue spreading dissection until flexor sheath is identified and clearly visualized; place self-retaining retractor
- Use sharp No. 15 scalpel to incise center of A1 pulley
- Release distal and proximal ends of A1 pulley with tenotomy scissors; pulley usually generates grating sensation when cut
- A1 pulley measures 10 mm in length, and A2 pulley is immediately distal; may differentiate by several millimeters of thinned retinacular tissue
- May release palmar aponeurosis proximally if also tight (**Figure 2, B**)
- To confirm adequate release of triggering, ask patient to actively flex and extend finger several times
- If patient continues to trigger after A1 pulley release, one of the slips of the FDS tendon may be excised
- May inspect tendons and floor of sheath by delivering tendons into wound; débridement or synovectomy of tendon not usually required
- Release tourniquet and ensure hemostasis
- Close skin with 4-0 or 5-0 nonabsorbable suture
- Place nonadherent dressing and low-profile compression bandage; leave digits free for mobilization

Trigger Thumb Release

- Surface anatomy—Proximal edge of A1 pulley lies at metacarpophalangeal (MP) crease
- Draw course of radial and ulnar digital nerve; radial digital nerve crosses flexor sheath just proximal to A1 pulley
- Exsanguinate limb and elevate tourniquet

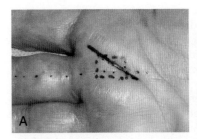 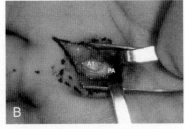

FIGURE 2 Intraoperative photographs demonstrate trigger finger release. **A,** The skin incision is marked. **B,** The anatomic relationship between the A1 pulley, which has been released, and the palmar aponeurosis pulley is visualized. PA = palmar aponeurosis

- Incise skin along oblique line centered on MP crease; parallels course of radial digital nerve to avoid injury to nerve
- Carefully dissect subcutaneous tissue with tenotomy scissors parallel to neurovascular bundles
- Always protect radial digital nerve
- Identify and clearly visualize flexor sheath
- Use sharp No. 15 scalpel to incise center of A1 pulley at level of MP crease; release distal and proximal ends of A1 pulley with tenotomy scissors
- Be aware of radial digital nerve during proximal retraction and release
- Confirm adequate release of triggering by asking patient to actively flex and extend thumb
- May inspect tendon and floor of sheath by delivering tendons into wound
- Release tourniquet and ensure hemostasis
- Close skin with nonabsorbable sutures and apply nonadherent dressing without obstructing thumb motion

COMPLICATIONS
- Incomplete release
- Digital nerve injury
- Scar tenderness
- Postoperative stiffness
- Bowstringing
- Residual triggering

POSTOPERATIVE CARE AND REHABILITATION
- Start active motion of fingers and use of hand for light activities immediately
- Use elevation and ice for first 2 days
- See patient in office 2 days after surgery
  - Evaluate wound and reduce dressing to adhesive bandage
  - Evaluate motion and encourage active exercises
  - Allow return to light work if desired
- See patient again 2 weeks after surgery
  - Remove sutures
  - Instruct in strengthening exercises and scar management, which involves taping silicone sheet on scar overnight and massaging lotion into scar several times a day for 6 to 10 weeks
- Encourage home program of active motion isolating proximal and distal interphalangeal joints
- May use dynamic splint (eg, Capener) for persistent PIP joint contracture

---

PEARLS

- Surgery is easily performed with patient wide-awake using local anesthetic with epinephrine to allow intraoperative evaluation of complete release.
- Oblique incision along a skin crease allows safe exposure, easy incision of sheath, and extension as needed; transverse or longitudinal incisions are also appropriate.
- Dissect along midline of finger to prevent damage to neurovascular structures.
- Identify and protect radial digital nerve and accompanying artery in trigger thumbs.
- Ask patient to actively move finger after pulley release to verify adequate release.
- If triggering not completely relieved after A1 pulley release, consider palmar aponeurosis pulley release, A3 pulley release, reduction flexor tenoplasty, or ulnar FDS release.

Open Reduction and Internal Fixation of the Distal Radius With a Volar Locking Plate

PATIENT SELECTION

- Indication for surgical treatment is an unstable fracture resulting from
  - ▶ Inadequate alignment after closed reduction
  - ▶ Loss of adequate alignment after manipulative reduction
  - ▶ High likelihood of healing with inadequate alignment with cast alone
    - – Fracture displacement, comminution, age, and functional level are related to probability of losing reduction
  - ▶ Inadequate alignment defined as more than 10° of dorsal tilt, more than 3 to 5 mm of ulnar positive variance, or 2 mm or greater articular step-off
- Surgery involves closed or open reduction and internal fixation
- An alternative is closed reduction (or repeat closed reduction)

PREOPERATIVE IMAGING

Plain Radiography

- PA and lateral radiographs before and after manipulative reduction (**Figure 1**)
- Traction radiographs may be helpful

Computed Tomography

- Not always indicated, but for certain fracture patterns they may provide further details about number, size, location, and displacement of articular fractures
- Three-dimensional reconstructions are easy to interpret

Based on Jupiter JB, Ring D: Open reduction and internal fixation of the distal radius with a volar locking plate, in Colvin AC, Flatow E, eds: Atlas of Essential Orthopaedic Procedures, *ed 2. Rosemont, IL, American Academy of Orthopaedic Surgeons, 2020, pp 340-344.*

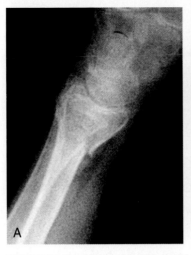 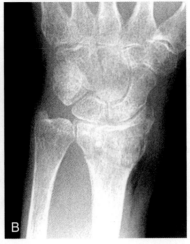

FIGURE 1 Lateral (**A**) and PA (**B**) image-intensifier views show a fracture of the distal radius.

PROCEDURE
Surgical Technique

- Make longitudinal incision over flexor carpi radialis (FCR)
- Incision may be extended obliquely across wrist crease if needed
- Incise volar and dorsal FCR sheath; leave radial artery undissected radially
- Avoid palmar cutaneous branch of median nerve
- The FCR is retracted ulnarly to protect the median nerve
- Bluntly dissect fat in space of Parona; retract flexor pollicis longus ulnarward
- Incise pronator quadratus longitudinally and elevate subperiosteally off volar surface of radius
- Identify and mobilize fracture fragments
- Reduce fracture; may be helpful to lever distal fragments away from shaft
  - Use thumb to apply dorsal counterpressure during reduction of osteoporotic bone
- Apply plate centered over shaft proximally and metaphysis distally; avoid placing plate more distal than watershed region of distal radius
- Hold reduction using provisional Kirschner wires or can place fixed-angle drill guide through some implants
- Place fixed-angle screws distally and use standard (or rarely locking screws) proximally, depending on bone quality and preference

---

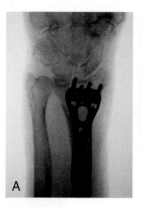
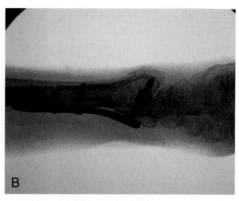

FIGURE 2 Intraoperative PA (**A**) and lateral (**B**) image-intensifier views show plate position and fracture alignment.

- Use fluoroscopy to evaluate reduction and hardware placement; be aware of anatomy of distal radius
- The pronator quadratus may be repaired
- The skin is closed
- Splinting depends on fracture stability and fracture pattern
- Final images of the patient are shown in **Figure 2**

COMPLICATIONS
- Infection
- Wound complications
- Nerve injury
- Misplaced screws
- Prominent implants
- Tendon rupture
- Malunion

POSTOPERATIVE CARE AND REHABILITATION
- Emphasize finger motion, then forearm rotation, then wrist flexion and extension; start exercises immediately if fracture fixation stability allows
- Wean from splint as patient tolerates
- Encourage functional use of hand for light tasks
- Instruct patient in proper stretching techniques
- Demonstrate empathy and normalize patient's pain; help change patient's mindset from pain as a reminder of injury to pain as a result of healthy stretching exercises and recovery
- Some forceful activities may start around 6 weeks, with full activity at 3 months

PEARLS

- The volar ulnar cortex is the strongest bone in the distal radius. Use it to facilitate reduction.
- After volar cortex is realigned, the length and ulnarward inclination of distal radius are restored, leaving only palmar tilt to correct.
- Keep implants proximal to the watershed area and check for prominent screws dorsally.
- Patient confidence about stretching pain is key to effectiveness of exercises, not how soon exercises are begun.

External Fixation of Distal Radius Fractures

INTRODUCTION
- External fixation is an option for fixation of distal radius fractures alone or in conjunction with other fixation techniques
- External fixation may be applied in a spanning fashion, crossing the radiocarpal joint; or a nonspanning construct, in which the entire construct is placed on the radius and does not span the radiocarpal joint
- One advantage of external fixators is that they can easily be removed after bony healing in the office without a second surgical procedure

PATIENT SELECTION
Indications
- Failed closed reduction—More than 2 to 3 mm loss of radial length, articular tilt >5° to 10°, radial inclination <10°
- Unstable distal radius—Patient older than 60 years, dorsal tilt greater than 20°, dorsal cortex comminution, intra-articular extension, ulna fracture, metaphyseal comminution, ulnar variance
- Radiocarpal incongruity greater than 1 to 2 mm
- At least 1 cm intact volar cortex for pin purchase
- High-grade open distal radius fractures
- Initial treatment of polytrauma patient
- Always consider patient hand dominance, occupational requirements, medical comorbidities, and expectations

Contraindications
- Volar or volar shear displacement pattern
- Dorsal shear displacement pattern

DIAGNOSTIC IMAGING
Radiography
- AP, lateral, oblique (**Figure 1**)
- Obtain before and after reduction

Based on Freibott CE, Rosenwasser MP: External fixation of distal radius fractures, in Colvin AC, Flatow E, eds: Atlas of Essential Orthopaedic Procedures, ed 2. Rosemont, IL, American Academy of Orthopaedic Surgeons, 2020, pp 345-353.

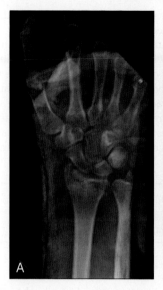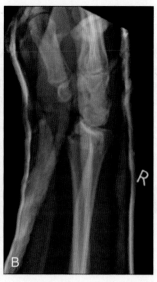

FIGURE 1 AP (**A**) and lateral (**B**) radiographs show an AO 23-C2.1 distal radius fracture before reduction. (Courtesy of Columbia University Medical Center, New York, NY.)

- Imaging of contralateral wrist helps determine normal anatomy
- Traction views can clarify fracture fragments

Computed Tomography
- Delineates bony anatomy
- Cost and lack of traction limit utility

PROCEDURE
Room Setup/Patient Positioning
- Supine position with arm on hand table
- Regional or general anesthesia
- Nonsterile tourniquet to upper arm set to 250 mm Hg
- Prophylactic antibiotics
- C-arm or mini C-arm fluoroscopy

Surgical Technique
- Perform closed reduction with manipulation as well as traction and countertraction
- Choose spanning or nonspanning fixator
- If large distal fragment (>10 mm) present, may use nonspanning fixator; articular comminution not absolute contraindication, but half-pins must be centered in fragments; otherwise, use spanning fixator

- May use Kirschner wires (K-wires) as joysticks for fragment manipulation
- Percutaneous or limited open reduction is possible through 3-cm dorsal incision (between third and fourth compartments); enhance reduction quality and stability with K-wires, impaction grafting of metaphyseal void, arthroscopy or other tools as indicated
- Place K-wires in radial styloid subchondrally, to support articular facets, or intramedullary, to realign radial inclination and length
- Wrist arthroscopy may improve reduction; helps visualize ligament and intercarpal ligament injuries; use vertical traction and start in 3-4 portal. Dry arthroscopy is generally favored in the setting of fractures

VIDEO 42.1 External Fixation of Distal Radius Fractures.
Jonathan R. Danoff, MD; Michael V. Birman, MD;
Neil J. White, MD, FRCS; Melvin P. Rosenwasser, MD (7 min)

Placement of Proximal Fixator Pins

- Place proximal fixator pins in radius first, 10 cm proximal to tip of radial styloid or at least 5 cm outside zone of injury; place in palpable bare area between brachioradialis and extensor carpi radialis longus muscles; may use in spanning or nonspanning frame
- Use limited open approach to protect branches of superficial radial and lateral antebrachial cutaneous nerves; plan incision to allow skin closure without tension
- Place pins at 45° to long axis of forearm for spanning fixator, or dorsal to volar for nonspanning frame; avoid drilling across interosseous membrane to prevent heterotopic ossification
- Use fixator clamp to space pins properly; check placement with fluoroscopy

Placement of Distal Fixator Pins

- Place distal fixator pins for spanning frame in proximal 60% of second metacarpal, oriented 45° to long axis of shaft; place through longitudinal incision over proximal third of second metacarpal in bare area between first dorsal interosseous muscle and extensor tendon
- Center pins in the index metacarpal shaft to avoid stress fracture, using fixator clamp to space pins properly; terminal threads must engage far cortex for maximum purchase; proximal pin may be advanced through third metacarpal to obtain four cortices
- Insert distal fixator pins for nonspanning frame through 2-cm longitudinal incisions between dorsal compartments 2-3 and 4-5; at least 6 to 10 mm of intact volar cortex proximal to subchondral plate is required for 3-mm threaded half-pins

- Place pins on either side of Lister tubercle while protecting extensor pollicis longus tendon; insert ulnar pin first, parallel to subchondral surface of lunate facet; radial pin need not be parallel if fixator clamps are modular
- Check all pin placements with fluoroscopy; terminal threads must engage volar cortex when manipulating fragments

Assembly of Fixator Frame

- Close skin incisions without tension
- Assemble frame with clamps placed one fingerbreadth away from skin; ensure range of motion is not blocked
- Connect first rod proximally, then distally, after making adjustments and verifying fluoroscopically; may use second rod to increase frame stiffness
- Apply only gentle traction during frame assembly for spanning frame, then restore length, translation, angulation, and rotation; avoid over-pronation of distal fragment
- Apply nonspanning frame loosely; reduce with thumb pressure on half-pins at skin entry, verify with fluoroscopy, then lock frame; avoid overreduction and pin pullout from osteopenic bone
- Overreduction can be prevented by placement of an intramedullary K-wire through the radial styloid first
- Obtain final images and perform final tightening of frame
- Assess distal radioulnar joint (DRUJ) stability by comparing with contralateral side; if translation is increased, consider procedures or immobilization to stabilize the DRUJ
- Cover pin sites with petroleum gauze and bulky dressing; may use splint for comfort, especially with nonspanning fixator

COMPLICATIONS

- Pin-site infection
- Nerve injury
- Nonunion
- Stiffness
- Complex regional pain syndrome
- Malunion

POSTOPERATIVE CARE AND REHABILITATION

- Most patients are treated as an outpatient
- A splint may be used for comfort, especially for patients without a non–joint spanning fixator
- Pin-site care is controversial; with some surgeons advocating for no specific care, and others having a detailed routine. There is no clear evidence in the literature regarding the optimal technique for pin care
- The patient should commence immediate digital range of motion with the goal of making a composite full fist. A supervised therapy program may be helpful in some patients

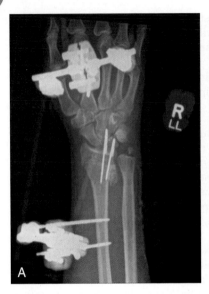 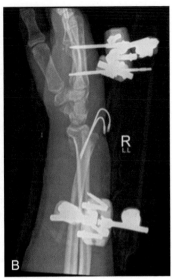

FIGURE 2 Postoperative AP (**A**) and lateral (**B**) radiographs obtained at 3-week follow-up show the final frame assembled. (Courtesy of Columbia University Medical Center, New York, NY.)

- Routine follow-up in office at around 10 to 14 days for suture removal and radiographs (**Figure 2**) and consideration of a supervised or unsupervised home exercise program
- Retighten pin clamp screws at each visit; monitor for unrestricted finger motion
- Union at 6 to 8 weeks judged by radiographs and absence of fracture pain; remove fixator pins under local anesthesia in office; advance hand therapy

OUTCOMES
- Clinical results similar between external and internal fixation
- Good subjective and objective long-term outcomes should be anticipated, although subjective outcomes may be better early (6 weeks) with volar plate versus spanning external fixation

PEARLS

- Use injury, postreduction, and traction radiographs to develop treatment plan.
- Ligamentotaxis will not achieve and maintain reduction alone except in simplest fractures.
- Protect sensory nerves to avoid painful neuromas or complex regional pain syndrome.

- Use sleeve when drilling to protect soft tissues.
- Avoid overpronating distal fragment when locking frame to prevent loss of supination.
- Tensionless closure of limited incisions reduces pin-tract complications.
- Assess DRUJ stability with translation shuck test.
- Not all fractures are amenable to internal fixation with plates and certain fracture types may be ideal for external fixation:
  - Very distal fractures may have inadequate room for adequate stabilization with any type of volar locking plate.
  - Poor bone quality may lead to inadequate purchase of dorsal rim fragments leading to dorsal facet escape and loss of reduction.
  - Die punch injuries are suited to elevation and joint spanning external fixation.
- External fixator application is relatively easy to master and does not require a second trip to operating room for hardware removal.

Open Reduction and Internal Fixation of Scaphoid Fractures

PATIENT SELECTION
- Scaphoid fractures represent 11% of all hand fractures; occur mainly in men between the ages of 20 and 30 years
- Unrecognized injury and/or inadequate treatment can result in non-union, which can lead to chronic pain, functional loss, and arthritis

Indications
- Displacement
- Carpal collapse
- Comminution
- Desire to avoid prolonged immobilization
- Risk factors for delayed union, including delay to diagnosis, proximal fracture type, or other patient factors

Contraindications
- Comorbidities (relative)
- Inability to tolerate anesthesia (relative)

PREOPERATIVE IMAGING
Radiography
- PA, lateral, and oblique and navicular view radiographs of wrist; look for loss of carpal height, intercarpal widening, carpal malalignment, associated fractures
- Navicular view (30° extension with ulnar deviation) demonstrates long axis of scaphoid (**Figure 1**)
- Nondisplaced fractures may not appear on initial radiographs

Bone Scan
- Technetium methylene diphosphonate (MDP)-99 has high sensitivity and specificity
- Must wait 48 to 72 hours after injury
- Mostly of historical interest

Based on Matullo KS, Shin AY: Open reduction and internal fixation of scaphoid fractures, in Colvin AC, Flatow E, eds: Atlas of Essential Orthopaedic Procedures, *ed 2. Rosemont, IL, American Academy of Orthopaedic Surgeons, 2020, pp 354-363.*

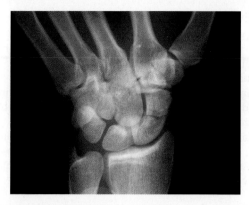

FIGURE 1 Scaphoid view radiograph, taken with the wrist in extension and ulnar deviation, demonstrates a scaphoid waist fracture.

Magnetic Resonance Imaging

- High sensitivity and specificity reported (**Figure 2**)
- May perform as early as 24 hours after injury
- False-positive results exist because of marrow edema

CT Scanning

- May be used for diagnostic purposes or for preoperative planning
- More commonly used for evaluation and treatment planning in the chronic setting to evaluate for bone loss or bone healing than in the acute setting for diagnosis

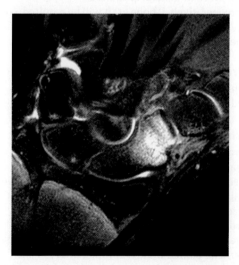

FIGURE 2 A coronal T2-weighted MRI of the wrist demonstrates increased signal intensity of the distal portion of the scaphoid, consistent with an occult fracture.

Preferred Evaluation Sequence

- Radiographic series
- If fracture not demonstrated but high suspicion exists, consider immobilization in a thumb spica cast
- High-demand patients may undergo MRI
- Low-demand patients or those who prefer watchful waiting may have repeat radiographs and clinical examination after 10 to 14 days of immobilization
- Nondisplaced fractures particularly of the distal scaphoid or even of the waist, or those that are visible only on MRI, are most commonly amenable to nonsurgical treatment; surgical treatment may be chosen to allow return to activity sooner

PROCEDURE

VIDEO 43.1 Open Reduction and Internal Fixation of Scaphoid Fractures. Kristofer S. Matullo, MD; Alexander Y. Shin, MD (2 min)

Room Setup/Patient Positioning

- Supine position with radiolucent hand table
- Obtain preoperative C-arm fluoroscopy images to guarantee visualization
- Apply tourniquet around upper extremity
- Use regional block or general anesthesia
- Consider preoperatively if bone graft will be required; consider obtaining consent and positioning should iliac crest, olecranon, or distal radius bone grafting be needed

Special Instruments/Equipment/Implants

- C-arm (mini or standard)
- Cannulated headless compression screws

Surgical Technique for Volar Approach

- Used for waist and distal pole fractures
- Percutaneous or open techniques may be used
- For open surgery, make a hockey-stick–shaped incision along flexor carpi radialis tendon and angle toward thumb at wrist crease; center distal incision over distal pole of scaphoid
- Dissect through subcutaneous tissue
- Identify branches of radial artery or superficial radial sensory nerve; ligate superficial palmar branch of radial artery
- Open flexor carpi radialis sheath and retract tendon radially or ulnarly

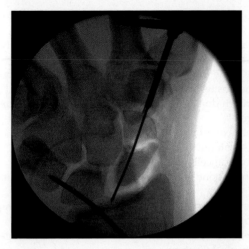

FIGURE 3 Intraoperative fluoroscopic image demonstrates the guidewire along the central axis of the scaphoid. (Reproduced with permission from the Mayo Foundation for Medical Education and Research, Rochester, MN.)

- Incise floor of sheath and volar carpal ligaments longitudinally; long radiolunate and radioscaphocapitate ligaments also are divided with incision
- Elevate capsule distally to expose distal pole of scaphoid at scaphotrapezium joint
- To improve exposure for guidewire, may remove portion of trapezium with rongeur or osteotome
- Extend wrist over bolster to further aid visualization
- If required, insert two Kirschner wires (K-wires) into proximal and distal fracture fragments as joysticks to aid reduction
- Reduce fracture; verify with visualization of midcarpal and radiocarpal regions of scaphoid
- Insert guidewire (at least 1 mm) down central axis of scaphoid from distal to proximal; confirm with multiple C-arm views and live rotation view (**Figure 3**)
- Advance guidewire to proximal pole articular margin; measure length for screw
- Subtract 4 to 6 mm from original measured screw length to prevent articular penetration
- Use cannulated drill over guidewire; drill to depth of original screw measurement, otherwise screw will be prominent or fracture distracted; check with C-arm
- Younger patients or those with sclerotic bone may need distal scaphoid overdrilled to insert screw without distraction of fracture

- Comminuted fractures may benefit from second parallel guidewire to prevent rotation or displacement
- Use bone grafting for comminution, humpback deformity, postreduction defect; use cancellous bone for central void
- Bone may come from distal radius, olecranon, tibial tubercle, or iliac crest (or other sites)
  - ◗ Approach dorsal distal radius through small incision over Lister tubercle
  - ◗ Protect extensor pollicis longus tendon
  - ◗ Use osteotome to elevate tubercle
  - ◗ Remove cancellous bone from metaphysis of radius
- Use structural bone graft if scaphoid has humpback deformity greater than 30°
- Insert screw and remove guidewire; obtain final radiographic images with C-arm
- Irrigate wound with saline; repair volar radiocarpal ligaments with nonabsorbable 2-0 suture
- Deflate tourniquet and obtain hemostasis
- Close skin in standard technique and apply sterile dressing
- Place well-padded thumb spica splint

Surgical Technique for Dorsal Approach

- Percutaneous, mini-open, or open approaches may be used
- For an open approach, make 1- to 2-cm incision ulnar and distal to Lister tubercle; used for wrist and proximal pole fractures
- Sharply dissect subcutaneous tissue; preserve veins
- Incise distal extensor retinaculum; retract extensor pollicis longus and radial wrist extensors radially
- Open distal wrist capsule transversely; protect scapholunate interosseous ligament
- Limit dissection of capsule to scaphoid waist to avoid injuring scaphoid vasculature
- Expose scaphoid with wrist flexed, pronated, and ulnarly deviated
- Insert K-wire at most proximal point of scaphoid, radial to scapholunate interosseous ligament insertion (**Figure 4**)
- Advance guidewire along plane of thumb down center axis of scaphoid; confirm with C-arm imaging; must elevate entire arm to obtain true PA of wrist
- Measure depth with guidewire tip at subchondral margin
- Subtract at least 4 to 6 mm from measured length; advance guidewire distally to avoid inadvertent removal while drilling
- Use cannulated drill over guidewire; drill to depth of original screw measurement, otherwise screw will be prominent or fracture distracted; check with C-arm
- Younger patients or those with sclerotic bone may need distal scaphoid overdrilled to insert screw without distraction of fracture

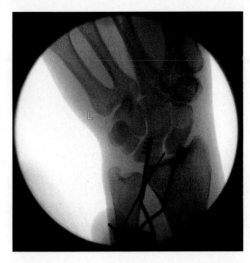

FIGURE 4 Fluoroscopic image shows the starting point of a dorsal K-wire, just radial to the scapholunate interosseous ligament. The K-wire is aimed up the central axis of the scaphoid. (Reproduced with permission from the Mayo Foundation for Medical Education and Research, Rochester, MN.)

- Comminuted fractures may benefit from second parallel guidewire to prevent rotation or displacement
- Insert screw and remove guidewire; use C-arm to obtain final fluoroscopic images (**Figure 5**). Irrigate wound with saline; repair volar radiocarpal ligaments with nonabsorbable 2-0 suture
- Deflate tourniquet and obtain hemostasis
- Relocate extensor tendons and repair retinaculum
- Close skin in standard technique; apply sterile dressing
- Place well-padded thumb spica splint

Extensile Dorsal Approach
- Extensile approach allows full exposure of the scaphoid and carpus
- Incision centered about the third metacarpal base extending proximally to the distal radius
- Excellent for addressing scaphoid fractures that occur as part of transscaphoid perilunate-type injury
- After skin incision, create flaps and protect superficial branch of radial nerve; open third extensor compartment and create ulnarly based retinacular flap by dividing septations between 3 to 4 and 4 to 5 extensor compartments
- Spare the ligaments when making capsulotomy

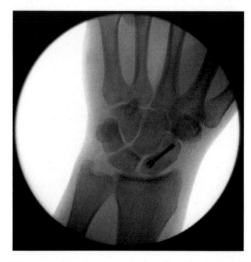

FIGURE 5 Final fluoroscopic image shows a dorsally placed scaphoid screw. (Reproduced with permission from the Mayo Foundation for Medical Education and Research, Rochester, MN.)

- The radiocarpal and midcarpal joints are now exposed and a derotational wire can be inserted across the fracture from the proximal to distal pole of scaphoid followed by placement of a headless compression screw as previously described

COMPLICATIONS
- Malunion
- Nonunion
- Prominent hardware
- Retained hardware (guidewire breakage)
- Iatrogenic neurovascular or neurologic injury
- Iatrogenic tendon injury

POSTOPERATIVE CARE AND REHABILITATION
- First postoperative visit in 10 to 14 days for suture removal and radiographs
- Length of immobilization depends on fracture type, fixation, and surgeon preference
- Ultimate goal—Full wrist and thumb range of motion at fracture union
- Second postoperative visit at 6 to 8 weeks, with new radiographs
  - If fracture united, start strengthening exercises; if not, splint until union
  - CT may help visualize union
    - The CT should be obtained in the plane of the scaphoid and examined for visualization of bridging bone

PEARLS

- It may be helpful to remove proximal volar portion of trapezium for access to the scaphoid with the guide pin and screw.
- It may be helpful to use K-wires in proximal and distal fragments to aid reduction. Place guidewire in scaphoid up to fracture line, and then advance across fracture after reduction.
- If using antirotational K-wire, it must be placed parallel to guidewire.
- Use bone graft for comminution or fracture gap.
- Measure screw length and subtract no less than 4 to 6 mm to allow the screw to be confined to the scaphoid and allow for fracture compression across the site.
- It may be helpful to advance the guidewire out of skin on the opposite side of the wrist and clamp; this allows for easy removal of both ends of the wire if the guidewire is broken during drilling.
- Maintain drill collinear with guidewire when drilling screw path. Intermittently pull back on drill to prevent binding. Check integrity of K-wire with C-arm if concerned.
- Insert compression screw at least 2 mm below articular surface and confirm with direct visualization and/or fluoroscopy.
- Multiple fluoroscopic views should be obtained to ensure that the screw is not in the radiocarpal or scaphotrapezial joint.

Open Reduction and Internal Fixation of Phalangeal Fractures

INTRODUCTION
- Goal is stable anatomic reduction with early functional recovery
- "Less is more" in terms of fixation, because of propensity for stiffness from close association of flexor and extensor tendons. It is therefore desirable to avoid open incisions, excessive hardware, or bulky hardware whenever possible

PATIENT SELECTION
Indications
- Displaced unstable fractures
- Multiple phalangeal or metacarpal fractures
- Open fractures
- No contraindications

PREOPERATIVE IMAGING
- AP, lateral, and oblique radiographs

PROCEDURE
Special Equipment
- Mini C-arm fluoroscopy

Surgical Technique

 VIDEO 44.1 Lateral Approach for Plate Fixation of a Phalangeal Fracture. William B. Geissler, MD (4 min)

Percutaneous Screws for Condylar Fractures of Phalanx
- Closed reduction possible within 7 to 10 days of injury (**Figure 1**)
- Attempt closed reduction under fluoroscopic guidance
- If unsuccessful, use dental pick, Kirschner wire (K-wire), or hypodermic needle to assist in anatomically reducing fracture

Based on Geissler WB, Barber JA: Open reduction and internal fixation of phalangeal fractures, in Colvin AC, Flatow E, eds: Atlas of Essential Orthopaedic Procedures, *ed 2. Rosemont, IL, American Academy of Orthopaedic Surgeons, 2020, pp 364-372.*

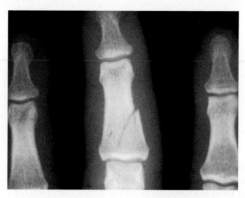

FIGURE 1 PA radiograph shows a phalangeal condylar fracture. Note the displaced fracture angulation from the base of the middle phalanx of the long finger.

- Provisionally fix the fracture with a pointed bone reduction clamp
- Verify reduction with fluoroscopy; the condyles should align on lateral view—if not anatomically reduced, the condyles appear as double convexity (touchy sign)
- Once anatomically reduced, insert one K-wire for the cannulated screw in center of fragment parallel to articular surface and distal to origin of collateral ligament
- Place second K-wire eccentrically into condylar fragment to prevent rotation of the fracture fragment during screw insertion
- It is important to pass both K-wires through the far cortex and skin for easy removal if they break (**Figure 2**)

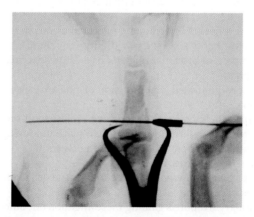

FIGURE 2 PA fluoroscopic view shows reduction of a phalangeal condylar fracture. The anatomic reduction of the fracture with placement of the guidewire through the reduction clamp is shown.

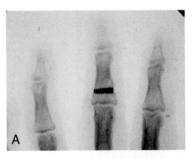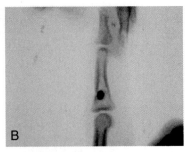

FIGURE 3 PA (**A**) and lateral (**B**) fluoroscopic views show fixation of a phalangeal condylar fracture. The headless cannulated screw is placed within the bone, and the fracture has been anatomically restored.

- Incise skin over central guidewire; bluntly dissect to bone
- Drill over guidewire but only near cortex for unicondylar fracture; fractures with diaphyseal extension need bicortical drilling
- Insert 8- to 10-mm headless screw over guidewire
- Use fluoroscopy to verify screw is entirely inside bone (**Figure 3**)
- Use second headless screw used for diaphyseal extension; insert from opposite side to avoid fragmentation
- Test stability with range of motion of digit under fluoroscopy
- Apply adhesive bandage

Plate Fixation for Phalangeal Shaft Fractures

- Percutaneous K-wires or limited open reduction and internal fixation with lag screws is preferred for most; consider plate fixation for multiple fractures, comminution, malunion/nonunion, or athletes
- Make incision in midaxial line of phalanx; ulnar side avoids lumbrical insertion
- Perform blunt dissection to bone; protect cutaneous nerves dorsally
- Retract lateral band and extensor digitorum communis tendon dorsally; if fracture of proximal phalanx base is present, may excise part of lateral band
- Place low-profile locked plate on side of phalanx; insert nonlocking screws first
- For long oblique fracture, also may use headless mini-screws; pointed clamp to reduce under fluoroscopy, then place guidewires; drill both cortices and insert screws. Close wound in layers
- Apply dressing (**Figures 4** and **5**)
- A review of plate fixation location, either dorsal or lateral, showed no differences in outcome
- Intramedullary fixation is gaining more attention but outcomes are the same as plate fixation after 6 months postoperatively, and it is associated with an increased incidence of complications

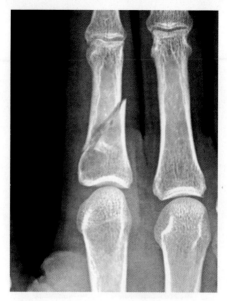

FIGURE 4 PA radiograph shows an unstable oblique fracture of the proximal phalanx of the index finger in a college athlete who desired to return to play as soon as possible.

COMPLICATIONS

Condylar Fractures of Phalanx

- Loss of motion (increased risk with open reduction and internal fixation) common in unicondylar fractures given intra-articular involvement
- Displacement (increased risk with single K-wire fixation)

Phalangeal Shaft Fractures

- Stiffness
- Extensor lag
- Joint contracture
- Delayed union
- Plate prominence

POSTOPERATIVE CARE

- Start immediate range of motion
- Strengthening begins at 4 to 6 weeks postoperatively
- Athletes may return to play within 1 week with buddy tape for unicondylar fractures or shaft fractures managed with plate

---

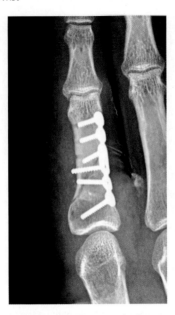

FIGURE 5 PA radiograph shows stable fixation of a fracture of the proximal phalanx of the index finger. The fracture has been anatomically reduced and stabilized with a series of locking and nonlocking screws.

PEARLS

- Unicondylar fractures inherently unstable; only rarely can be managed by closed treatment.
- Single K-wire for definitive fixation is rarely sufficient for unicondylar fractures.
- Percutaneous headless screw fixation offers some advantages compared with traditional mini-screws or K-wires alone.
- Most shaft fractures can be treated with K-wires to minimize scarring.
- Plate fixation of shaft fractures is recommended only for special cases; the plate should be placed on the ulnar or radial side to reduce scarring in the extensor tendon mechanism.

45 Surgical Fixation of Metacarpal Fractures

PATIENT SELECTION

- Metacarpal fractures most commonly result from an axial load transmitted from metacarpophalangeal (MCP) joint proximally down shaft of metacarpal (**Figure 1**)
- Most metacarpal fractures are treated nonsurgically
- Indications—Extensive soft-tissue injury, multiple metacarpal fractures, isolated metacarpal fractures with rotational deformity, angular deformity, or excessive shortening
- Contraindications—None

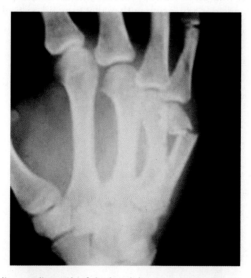

FIGURE 1 Oblique radiograph of the hand demonstrates a metacarpal neck fracture of the small finger (boxer's fracture). These fractures typically are seen in a patient who has punched a solid object.

Based on Geissler WB, Keen CA, Barber JA: Surgical fixation of metacarpal fractures, in Colvin AC, Flatow E, eds: Atlas of Essential Orthopaedic Procedures, *ed 2. Rosemont, IL, American Academy of Orthopaedic Surgeons, 2020, pp 373-381.*

PREOPERATIVE IMAGING

- AP, lateral, and oblique radiographs of the hand
- Use Brewerton radiographic view to assess metacarpal head fractures

PROCEDURE

Special Equipment

- Mini C-arm fluoroscopy
- Kirschner wires (K-wires) plates may be helpful (2.0-2.7 mm size)

Surgical Technique

Metacarpal Neck Fractures

- Many methods of fixation are recommended
- May place K-wires transversely across metacarpal neck into adjacent metacarpal; easier for border digits (**Figure 2**)
- May place K-wires longitudinally down metacarpal
    - ▹ When pinning distal to proximal, flex MCP joint to control distal fragment; use smooth 0.045- or 0.054-in K-wires; start on radial or ulnar collateral recess
    - ▹ Reduce fracture as wire approaches fracture site; advance wire into base; consider advancing with mallet to avoid cortical penetration

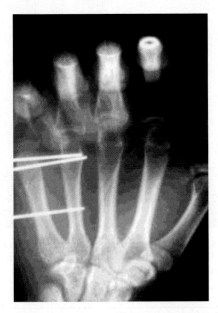

FIGURE 2 Fluoroscopic PA image shows a fifth metacarpal neck fracture that has undergone closed reduction and stabilization with cross-pinning of the proximal and distal fragments to the fourth metacarpal.

- Place K-wires with bouquet technique for index or small digit
  - For index, make 2-cm skin incision on radial side of second metacarpal base
  - For small digit, make incision on ulnar side
  - Elevate extensor tendon insertion
  - Cut off tip of 0.045-in K-wire; bend gently along length
  - Under fluoroscopy, identify proximal part of metaphysis; penetrate through canal with 2-mm drill; enlarge to 5 mm as needed
  - Place precontoured K-wire into metacarpal base and advance across fracture; place multiple K-wires similarly to enter distal fragment at various sites and create bouquet
- Metacarpal fractures can also be treated with intramedullary cannulated headless compressions screws
  - A 0.5 to 1 cm transverse incision is made and the extensor tendon is opened longitudinally
  - A 1.0 mm guidewire is placed within the longitudinal axis of the metacarpal with fluoroscopic guidance
  - The screw is long enough to engage in leading threads in the endosteal canal where the screw gains fixation
- May also be treated with intramedullary fixation with proximal locking
- Consider plate fixation for extensive comminution
  - Place low-profile locking plate dorsally
  - Use meticulous dissection; close periosteum over plate, reducing risk of adhesion and tendon irritation

Metacarpal Shaft Fractures

- Many fixation options are available including K-wires, interosseous wires, lag screws when appropriate, and plate fixation
- Base implant choice on amount of comminution, number of metacarpal fractures, fracture configuration, and surgeon preference and experience
- For plate fixation, use 2-mm plates along the dorsal aspect (**Figure 3**)
  - Useful for comminuted fracture and neutralization of lag screw in short oblique fracture
  - Verify rotation with passive wrist flexion and extension
  - Consider plate fixation in border digits of contact athletes (**Figure 4**)
- For lag screw fixation, oblique fracture must be three times diameter of screw
  - During open reduction, screw better than K-wire for initial stabilization; 0.045-in K-wire equals diameter of 1.1-mm drill bit
  - Lag screws recommended for spiral fractures; fracture line must be at least two times diameter of bone for lag screw alone; use at least two 2.0- or 1.5-mm screws
  - Place one screw perpendicular to shaft, one to fracture line

---

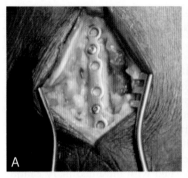 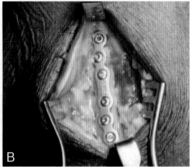

FIGURE 3 Intraoperative photographs show fixation of a fifth metacarpal shaft fracture. **A,** The fracture has been reduced and initially stabilized with a locking plate and nonlocking screws in the proximal and distal fragments. **B,** After rotational alignment is confirmed, the remaining screw holes are filled with locking and nonlocking screws to enhance fracture stability.

- Intramedullary fixation of displaced fractures has recently been considered
  - Biomechanical studies show that intramedullary fixation of unstable metacarpal shaft fractures offers less stability compared with plating

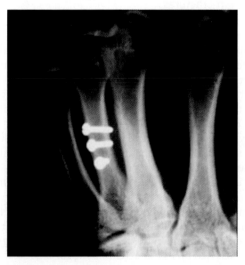

FIGURE 4 Postoperative oblique radiograph shows a spiral fracture to the fourth metacarpal shaft that has been stabilized with three lag screws.

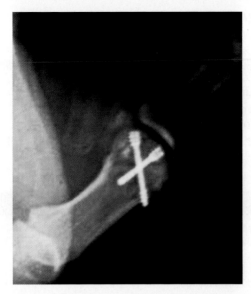

FIGURE 5 AP radiograph shows a comminuted thumb metacarpal head fracture that has been reduced and stabilized with headless screws.

- A separate study comparing intramedullary fixation versus plating showed that intramedullary fixation had improved clinical outcomes compared with plate fixation until 6 months post-op, where the difference was no longer clinically significant. Intramedullary fixation had significantly more complications compared with plate fixation

Metacarpal Head Fractures
- Usually in coronal plane
- Split extensor tendon in midline; incise capsule longitudinally
- Flex MCP joint to expose fracture
- Reduce fracture with clamp or stabilize with K-wire
- Insert headless cannulated screws (**Figure 5**)

COMPLICATIONS
- Stiffness
- Malrotation
- Tendon irritation
- Complex regional pain syndrome
- Hardware failure
- Nonunion

POSTOPERATIVE CARE AND REHABILITATION

Kirschner Wire Fixation

- Immobilize for 3 weeks in intrinsic position
- Remove pins in clinic; place removable splint; start motion

Plate Fixation

- Place soft dressing; start motion immediately
- Close follow-up necessary
- If stiffness develops, start aggressive hand therapy; supplement with dynamic and static splinting

PEARLS

- K-wire pinning is more cosmetic than plate fixation.
- Intramedullary pinning may have better range of motion than transverse pinning.
- Beware of intra-articular penetration of metacarpal head with intramedullary pinning.
- Plate fixation is better tolerated in hand than in phalanges.
- Plate fixation allows earlier return to athletics and possibly to work than do K-wires.
- Plate fixation is recommended over lag screws alone in contact athletes because of risk of refracture.

Excision of Ganglion Cysts of the Wrist and Hand

INTRODUCTION
- Most common soft-tissue mass of hand and wrist
- Usually occur along dorsal aspect of wrist (60% to 70%)
- Twenty percent occur in volar wrist

PATIENT SELECTION
Indications
- Pain
- Stiffness
- Impairment of function
- Nerve compression
- Skin necrosis

Contraindications
- Infection
- Irregular properties (eg, abnormal margins)
- Pediatric ganglions
- Avoid aspiration of volar wrist ganglions
- No steroid injections for mucous cysts of distal interphalangeal (DIP) joint

PREOPERATIVE IMAGING
Radiographs
- May show scapholunate widening or DIP joint arthritis
- Rarely change management; may not be cost-effective

Ultrasonography
- Relatively economical
- High sensitivity/specificity; diagnostic modality of choice

---

Based on Nagle DJ, Kalawadia JV: Excision of ganglion cysts of the wrist and hand, in Colvin AC, Flatow E, eds: Atlas of Essential Orthopaedic Procedures, ed 2. Rosemont, IL, American Academy of Orthopaedic Surgeons, 2020, pp 382-388.

Magnetic Resonance Imaging

- Helpful for unclear diagnosis
- Detects associated wrist pathology
- Visualizes neurovascular structures adjacent to ganglion

PROCEDURE

Room Setup/Patient Positioning

- Supine with arm on hand table
- Tourniquet on arm
- Bier, axillary, or wrist block

Instruments/Equipment

- Hand surgery instruments
- Hand holder
- Operating microscope (for open volar ganglionectomy)

Surgical Technique

Open Dorsal Wrist Ganglionectomy

- Fill ganglion with 1 to 2 mL of 0.1 mL methylene blue diluted in 5 mL of normal saline; use 25-gauge needle to inject and another to vent
- Make transverse incision centered over ganglion
- Dissect between second and fourth extensor compartments; protect nerves and tendons
- Follow pedicle with deeper dissection down to scapholunate interosseous ligament (**Figure 1**)

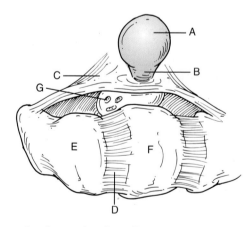

FIGURE 1 Illustration shows a dorsal ganglion cyst, which typically manifests over the scapholunate ligament. A = cyst, B = stalk of cyst at its confluence with dorsal wrist capsule and scapholunate interosseous ligament, C = dorsal wrist capsule, D = scapholunate interosseous ligament, E = scaphoid, F = lunate, G = capsular microcyst.

- Resect entire cyst from base with small rim of normal ligament; do not weaken ligament
- Do not close rent in ligament; risks postoperative stiffness
- Close dermal layer with thin absorbable braided suture; close skin with running subcuticular nonabsorbable monofilament
- Apply bulky dressing and dorsal wrist splint in mild flexion

Open Volar Wrist Ganglionectomy

- Perform Allen test preoperatively; if the ulnar artery is occluded, prepare for possible radial artery repair
- Set up operating microscope in case needed
- Fill ganglion with methylene blue solution as described previously only if neurovascular structures can be avoided
- Radial-side ganglionectomy
  - Cyst lies between radial artery and flexor carpi radialis (FCR) (**Figure 2**)
  - Make longitudinal incision radial to FCR for most cases
  - Use loupe or microscope dissection; protect superficial nerves with vessel loops
  - Dissect and mobilize radial artery; may cauterize or tie small branches
  - Open FCR sheath and retract tendon ulnarly; note palmar cutaneous nerve
  - Continue dissection down to carpus; remove cyst with cuff of normal capsule; protect ligaments
  - If cyst adheres to radial artery, resect rest of cyst and leave adherent tissue

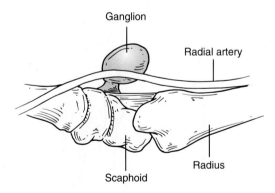

FIGURE 2 Illustration shows a volar radial-side ganglion cyst. Note the proximity to the radial artery. The cyst can be located adjacent to the radial artery or attached to it. The surgeon must be aware of this possibility and be careful during surgical dissection to avoid injury to the artery.

- Ulnar-side ganglionectomy
  - Make longitudinal incision just radial to flexor carpi ulnaris tendon
  - Use loupe or microscope dissection
  - Mobilize ulnar neurovascular bundle radially; protect during deeper dissection
  - Mobilize flexor carpi ulnaris tendon ulnarly; protect dorsal sensory branch of ulnar nerve
  - If cyst comes from pisotriquetral joint, consider releasing Guyon canal for exposure; may excise pisiform if it is arthritic
- For both approaches, close incision as described previously for dorsal wrist ganglionectomy

Retinacular Cyst Excision

- Apply arm tourniquet; may use Bier, wrist, or digital block
- Make transverse volar incision if cyst in digital or flexion crease; otherwise center oblique incision over cyst
- Use loupe dissection; protect neurovascular bundles
- Sharply excise cyst with small cuff of tendon sheath (**Figure 3**); if cyst lies on A2 pulley, elevate with Freer elevator to locate pedicle before excision
- Sheath defect does not need repair

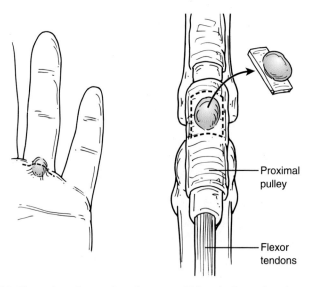

Proximal pulley

Flexor tendons

FIGURE 3 Illustrations show retinacular cysts, which typically are found attached to the tendon sheath. Dissection should be performed so that the pedicle of the cyst is identified. A cuff of retinacular tissue should be excised along with the pedicle, as depicted.

- Close incision with horizontal mattress nonabsorbable monofilament suture
- Apply dressing

Mucous Cyst Excision

- Use digital block with digital tourniquet; neurapraxia can occur after excessive tourniquet time or tightness
- Can use various incisions (H-, T-, L-, and U-shaped) (**Figure 4**); make over DIP joint
- Dissect down to joint capsule (loupes helpful)
- Excise cyst, origin, and cuff of dorsal capsule between terminal extensor tendon and collateral ligaments
- Débride osteophytes through arthrotomy; avoid injuring terminal extensor tendon
- Using rotational flaps for coverage versus leaving superficial cystic body is controversial
- Close incision with horizontal mattress nonabsorbable monofilament suture; if rotation flap used, avoid tension to protect vascular supply of flap
- Apply dressing; if body of cyst left, apply mallet finger splint for 1 week

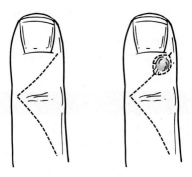

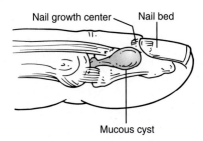

FIGURE 4 Illustrations show a dorsal zigzag incision for a mucous cyst excision. Various incisions can be used. To minimize the likelihood of a joint contracture, care must be taken to not cross the joint in a linear fashion.

COMPLICATIONS

Ganglionectomy

- Wrist stiffness
- Infection
- Scar tenderness
- Keloid
- Carpal instability
- Superficial radial nerve branch injury (dorsal wrist)
- Median nerve or radial/ulnar artery injury (volar wrist)
- Palmar cutaneous branch of median nerve injury (volar wrist)

Digital Mucous Cyst Excision

- Loss of DIP joint extension
- Nail deformity
- Terminal extensor tendon injury
- Acceleration of arthritic process (rare)

POSTOPERATIVE CARE AND REHABILITATION

- Splint wrist for 1 week in slight flexion (dorsal ganglion) or extension (volar ganglion)
- For retinacular/mucous cysts, can remove dressing 3 days postoperatively
- Splint after mucous cyst excision for 1 week if cyst body preserved; during second week remove splint daily for range-of-motion exercises

PEARLS

- Excision of ganglion root/origin most important to prevent recurrence.
- Preservation of cyst makes deeper dissection easier.
- Filling cyst with diluted methylene blue can help identify cyst origin.
- Send excised cyst to pathology per surgeon preference; limited cost-effectiveness when diagnosis is clear.

Surgical Excision of Digital Mucous Cysts

PATIENT SELECTION
- Most digital mucous cysts are asymptomatic
- Can develop suddenly or over months

Indications
- Increasing size
- Nail grooving
- Painful distal interphalangeal (DIP) joint arthrosis

Contraindications
- Excessive thinning of skin; temporize by aspirating cyst first
- Infection of cyst

PREOPERATIVE IMAGING
- Plain radiographs
  - Not diagnostic; make diagnosis with history and physical examination
  - May show nonspecific osteoarthritic changes
  - More advanced imaging usually not required
- Ultrasonography
  - Reveals rounded/lobulated hypoechoic mass adjacent to synovial compartment
  - Operator dependent
- MRI
  - Shows homogeneous low-intensity lesion on T1-weighted images
  - Increased signal intensity, sharp borders on T2-weighted images
  - Other features of cyst—Intracystic septa, satellite cysts, cyst pedicles, DIP joint osteoarthritis, subungual cysts, multiple flattened cysts
- CT
  - Shows well-defined water density mass with normal adjacent soft tissue
  - Transillumination with penlight may aid diagnosis

Based on Tomaino MM: Surgical excision of digital mucous cysts, in Colvin AC, Flatow E, eds: Atlas of Essential Orthopaedic Procedures, ed 2. Rosemont, IL, American Academy of Orthopaedic Surgeons, 2020, pp 389-391.

PROCEDURE

- Traditionally, simple or radical excision of cyst is performed
- Recently, excision and débridement of joint osteophytes advocated
- In general, aggressive dissection leads to fewer recurrences, more nail deformities
- Controversy remains regarding treatment approaches
- Asymptomatic cysts and spontaneous regression common, latter occurs in approximately 50% of cases
- Consider cost of treatment options
- Reasonable treatment plan involves multiple attempts of needling, aspiration, and injection; surgery if needed

Surgical Technique

- Use local or regional anesthetic
- Inflate tourniquet
- Elevate subdermal skin flaps using curvilinear, triradiate, or Bruner-type incisions
- Identify extensor tendon margin and excise cyst (**Figure 1**)
- Note that germinal matrix begins 1 to 2 mm distal to extensor insertion
- Remove osteophyte with small rongeur; avoid injuring extensor tendon insertion
- Close incision as preferred
- May need local rotation flap if ulcerated skin lesion is removed
- Apply compressive dressing
- Check wound 3 to 5 days later; remove sutures at 10 to 14 days
- Wound healing complete by 4 weeks

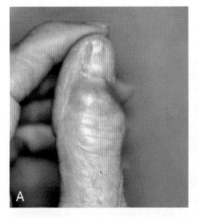 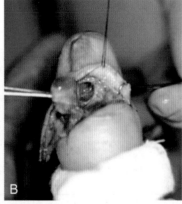

FIGURE 1 Preoperative photograph (**A**) and intraoperative photograph (**B**) of a digital mucous cyst at the thumb distal interphalangeal joint

COMPLICATIONS

- Recurrence
- Local depigmentation from steroid injection with triamcinolone
- Radial or ulnar deviation of DIP joint
- Impaired joint motion
- Nail deformity
- Tendon injury
- Mallet deformity
- Superficial infection
- DIP joint septic arthritis
- Increased arthritic symptoms
- Persistent swelling, pain, numbness, stiffness

POSTOPERATIVE CARE AND REHABILITATION

- Little special care required beyond ensuring wound healing
- Do not remove sutures prematurely
- Marginal wound necrosis usually resolves with local dressing changes and time

PEARLS

- Can usually manage digital mucous cysts nonsurgically.
- Reassure patient of benign nature of cyst.
- Resection indicated for pain, aesthetics, enlarging cyst, skin thinning.
- Skillful removal of cyst typically succeeds; high patient satisfaction.

Surgical Treatment of Basal Joint Arthritis of the Thumb

INTRODUCTION

- Arthritis of the thumb carpometacarpal joint is common, and with advancing age is present in a high percentage of patients
- Although symptomatic thumb CMC joint arthritis is common, there are many patients who are asymptomatic or who find adequate treatment with nonsurgical care
- Multiple surgical options are available with no clear evidence for a superior procedure; the author uses variation of Thompson's abductor pollicis longus (APL) suspensionplasty

PATIENT SELECTION

- Painful Eaton stage II, III, or IV basal joint arthritis
- Symptoms that persist despite nonsurgical management such as splints, NSAIDs, cortisone injections, activity modifications, or therapy programs

DIAGNOSTIC IMAGING

- Radiographs useful for preoperative planning, assessment
- Radiographic staging does not correlate well with symptoms

PROCEDURE

Room Setup/Patient Positioning

- Most commonly, general anesthesia or regional anesthesia is used
- Supine position; hand on table/arm board
- Apply well-padded tourniquet around upper arm

Surgical Technique

Abductor Pollicis Longus Suspensionplasty

- Make Wagner incision transversely over flexor carpi radialis (FCR) tendon curving to glabrous skin junction at radial border of thumb metacarpal distally

---

Based on Diao E: Surgical treatment of basal joint arthritis of the thumb, in Colvin AC, Flatow E, eds: Atlas of Essential Orthopaedic Procedures, *ed 2. Rosemont, IL, American Academy of Orthopaedic Surgeons, 2020, pp 392-403.*

- Raise skin, subcutaneous flaps and retract; preserve branches of radial sensory nerve
- Dissect dorsally to expose extensor mechanism over metacarpal and APL insertion at base
- Perform subperiosteal dissection between extensor pollicis longus (EPL) and extensor pollicis brevis (EPB) 1 cm distal to APL insertion
- Reflect thenar muscles off radial aspect of metacarpal, including accessory APL
- Distract thumb to expose scaphotrapezial (ST) and trapeziometacarpal (TMC) joints; expose trapezium subperiosteally and remove in pieces; remove osteophytes from capsule
- Expose base of thumb metacarpal; Carroll elevator is helpful
- Pierce center of articular surface with awl, Kirschner wire (K-wire), or drill; make second hole dorsally 1 cm distal to articular surface
- Use curet to expand holes and join them with intramedullary tunnel; avoid fracturing bone
- Harvest APL at musculotendinous junction with tendon stripper; use rotating action while holding stripper; trim free end of tendon as needed
- Pass APL retrograde through dorsal metacarpal hole and out articular hole using tendon passer or loop of wire (**Figure 1**)
- Inspect ST joint for significant wear; if present, remove abnormal cartilage, subchondral bone with curet

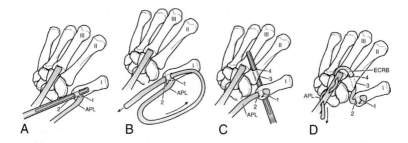

FIGURE 1 Illustrations demonstrate the surgical technique for abductor pollicis longus (APL) suspensionplasty. **A,** Creation of a bone tunnel in the thumb metacarpal. The bone tunnel is carefully created to connect hole 2, which is located in the articular center of the metacarpal base, and hole 1, which is located at the dorsal surface of the proximal metacarpal metaphysis 1 cm distal to the articular surface. **B,** After division of the APL at the proximal musculotendinous junction, the free end of the APL tendon is passed through the bone tunnel from hole 1 to hole 2. **C,** A bone tunnel is created from palmar (3) to dorsal (4) in the index metacarpal at the metaphyseal-diaphyseal junction. **D,** The APL tendon is passed through both bone tunnels at the thumb and index metacarpal (from 1 through 2 and from 3 through 4), emerging dorsally from the index metacarpal tunnel with a weave through the extensor carpi radialis brevis (ECRB) tendon to anchor the ligament reconstruction and tension the tendon transfer. I = thumb metacarpal; II = index finger metacarpal; III = long finger metacarpal.

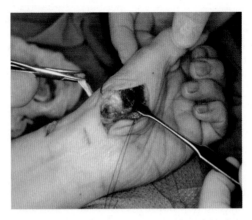

FIGURE 2 Intraoperative photograph shows assessment of the ligamentous reconstruction in APL suspensionplasty. The APL has been passed through the second bone tunnel, which is a palmar-to-dorsal transverse bone tunnel at the metaphyseal-diaphyseal junction of the proximal index metacarpal. The tendon is being tensioned by the clamp on the upper left. By applying this tension, the thumb is suspended into a position that maintains the space that the trapezium had once occupied and the overall thumb ray length is maintained.

- Expose base of index metacarpal; make palmar hole with awl at meta-diaphyseal junction; create tunnel dorsally though cortex; make 2-cm incision dorsally over exit point of awl; dissect to expose subcutaneous tissue
- Expand tunnel with curet or gouge to accept tendon graft; pass graft in palmar-to-dorsal direction; assess stability of reconstruction
- Expose extensor carpi radialis brevis just ulnar to dorsal bone tunnel in index metacarpal; use tendon weaver to pierce extensor carpi radialis brevis; pass APL graft
- Tension graft and secure junction with 4-0 nonabsorbable synthetic suture; perform process three times (**Figure 2**)
- Remove any remnant of APL; no need for tendon interposition when using whole APL for reconstruction; if using half of APL, pin thumb metacarpal with 0.045-in K-wire
- Reattach thenar muscles with 4-0 Vicryl suture (Ethicon); close skin with 5-0 plain absorbable suture
- Apply sterile dressing, radial gutter splint

Ligament Reconstruction Tendon Interposition Arthroplasty
- Make Wagner incision; protect branch of superficial radial nerve (**Figure 3**)
- Develop plane between extensor pollicis longus/EPB tendons to expose TMC joint capsule

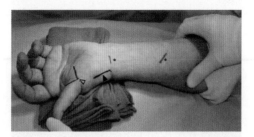

FIGURE 3 Photograph shows skin markings of surgical incisions for ligament reconstruction tendon interposition arthroplasty. A straight longitudinal incision in the interval between the volar glabrous and dorsal nonglabrous skin is indicated by the solid arrowhead. A zigzag incision over the thumb metacarpophalangeal joint (open arrowhead) facilitates exposure to perform a volar capsulodesis if adaptive hyperextension is present. Incisions at the radial wrist crease and proximally at the musculotendinous junction of the flexor carpi radialis (FCR, asterisks) facilitate the harvest of the FCR tendon.

- Make longitudinal arthrotomy perpendicular to long axis of TMC joint and parallel to midline of trapezium; continue incision to ST joint
- Elevate periosteum; remove osteophytes; excise trapezium in pieces; protect underlying FCR tendon (**Figure 4**)
- If ST joint arthritic, remove 0.4-cm wafer of trapezoid articular facet
- Make oblique bone tunnel in base of thumb metacarpal; enter 1 cm distal to articular surface perpendicular to plane of thumbnail; exit just volar to center of thumb base articular surface
- Use gouge to enlarge hole (bone tunnel); use medium gouge for half of FCR, large gouge for entire FCR
- Place 28-gauge steel wire or 0 Prolene suture (Ethicon) through tunnel
- Place double-armed 3-0 braided synthetic figure-of-8 suture in capsule at base of arthroplasty space

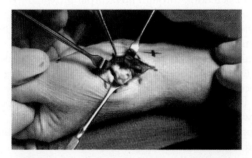

FIGURE 4 Intraoperative photograph shows trapezium exposure for ligament reconstruction tendon interposition arthroplasty. The trapezium is exposed after the capsule is incised and the periosteum is elevated. The probe demonstrates a large osteophyte off the trapezium.

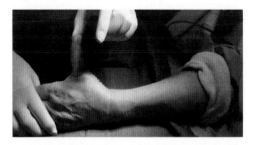

FIGURE 5 Intraoperative photograph shows adaptive hyperextension of the metacarpophalangeal joint during tendon harvest and delivery and capsulodesis in ligament reconstruction tendon interposition arthroplasty. The author advocates a volar capsulodesis if extreme hyperextension is present and arthrodesis if arthrosis is present.

- Harvest FCR tendon through two small transverse incisions, distally at level of wrist crease, proximally in mid forearm
- Incise sheath distally, place hemostat deep to tendon; proximally, dissect around musculotendinous junction and divide **FCR** tendon; deliver FCR tendon into distal wound
- Identify FCR at base of arthroplasty space; use hemostat to deliver it into space
- If excessive metacarpophalangeal joint hyperextension present, address now with arthrodesis (K-wire, screw, tension-band); if joint is not arthritic, author prefers volar capsulodesis with 2-0 Ethibond suture with or without bone anchor (**Figure 5**)
- To secure thumb metacarpal, place 0.045-in K-wire down canal through head to keep metacarpophalangeal joint flexed; or may pin metacarpal to scaphoid at end of procedure
- Use previously placed steel wire or Prolene suture to secure free tendon end; pass tendon through metacarpal proximal to distal; extend and abduct metacarpal and tension FCR; secure tendon to periosteum with two mattress or figure-of-8 sutures of 3-0 braided synthetic suture
- Roll remaining graft around hemostat and suture at each end with absorbable suture; place into arthroplasty space; secure with previously placed double-armed Ethibond suture
- Advance previously placed K-wire into scaphoid or trapezoid; verify position with fluoroscopy
- Close capsule over graft; mattress suture in APL insertion increases abduction force
- Cut EPB tendon distally; suture to periosteum of metacarpal base
- Close skin with 5-0 absorbable suture
- Apply sterile dressing, thumb spica cast

Thumb Trapeziometacarpal Arthroscopy

- May use regional or general anesthesia; supine position with arm on hand table; use arm tourniquet, vertical traction tower
- Mark landmarks, including course of superficial radial nerve, and 1-R (radial) and 1-U (ulnar) portals
- Create 1-U portal first with 20-gauge needle; inject 2 mL saline; incise skin and use hemostat to bluntly penetrate capsule
- Insert 1.9- or 2.7-mm arthroscope; create working portal under direct visualization
- Inspect and débride joint; may use 2.0-mm synovial resector initially
- Check integrity of superficial, deep anterior oblique ligaments with probe through radial portal and scope in ulnar portal; switch portals to check dorsoradial and posterior oblique ligaments; view ulnar collateral ligament from either portal
- If only early degenerative changes exist, use 2.0-mm full-radius shaver to débride
- If ligament laxity present, perform electrothermal capsular shrinkage; may use monopolar or bipolar probes; irrigate copiously
- If most of trapezium eburnated, resect at least half of distal bone with 2.0-mm burr
- If scaphotrapeziotrapezoid joint arthritis visible in midcarpal portal, perform complete trapeziectomy; use fluoroscopy throughout to verify burr position and remaining bone; reintroduce arthroscope to check resection
- For hemitrapeziectomy, place polyurethane urea spacer via transverse incision, connecting portals
- For complete trapeziectomy, pin joint with 0.045-in K-wire under fluoroscopic guidance
- For any trapezial resection, also can shrink capsule for tension (**Figure 6**)

COMPLICATIONS
- Fracture of bone tunnel
- Tension in tender graft is inadequate
- Residual ST joint arthritis not addressed

POSTOPERATIVE CARE AND REHABILITATION
- Postoperative care varies by surgeon and procedure, with some surgeons favoring immobilization for a minimal period and others preferring a 6-week course of immobilization. Immobilize in thumb spica splint for 2 to 4 weeks; allow interphalangeal motion
- Change to removable long opponens splint; start active range of motion (ROM)
- Grip strengthening at 2 months

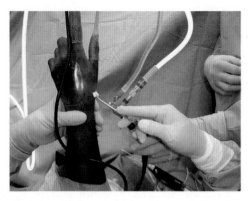

FIGURE 6 Intraoperative photograph shows an interposition arthroplasty implant being placed in the basal joint in a thumb trapeziometacarpal arthroplasty procedure.

- With arthroscopic hemitrapeziectomy, start active ROM at 4 weeks; custom splint weaned after 6 weeks postoperatively; start strengthening at 8 weeks
- If pin placed for total trapeziectomy, remove at 6 weeks postoperatively; start active ROM at 6 weeks, strengthening at 8 weeks

PEARLS

- Although symptomatic thumb CMC joint arthritis is common, asymptomatic thumb CMC joint arthritis is also common.
- Many patients may "burn out" and gradually become asymptomatic.
- Nonsurgical treatment commonly is all that is needed and can include activity modification, splinting, injections, therapy.
- When surgical treatment is considered, a number of treatment alternatives exist with no one procedure having a clear advantage over another. For arthroscopy, distal trapezial preparation and resection of medial osteophytes near the second metacarpal are critical.
- Fluoroscopy can be helpful intraoperatively.
- Tailor postoperative plan to intraoperative findings and patient compliance.
- Although 90% good to excellent results are achievable, counsel patients about potential for revision surgery. Cochrane review in 2017 concluded that there was no distinctive advantage of "one treatment over another."

49 Partial Palmar Fasciectomy for Dupuytren Disease

INTRODUCTION
- Dupuytren disease is a benign fibroproliferative disorder of the palmar fascia
- Differentiate from non-Dupuytren disease fascial proliferation secondary to trauma

PATIENT SELECTION

Indications for Treatment for Dupuytren Disease Include the Following
- Metacarpophalangeal joint contracture of at least 30°
- Proximal interphalangeal joint contracture of 15°
- Limitation of function due to prominent cords or nodules
- The "table top test" is a useful way to counsel patients regarding treatment—if patients cannot place the hand flat on table, intervention may be considered

Contraindications
- Non-Dupuytren disease
- Open hand wound
- Infection
- Low functional demands; no benefit from surgery
- Psychologically unfit for surgical procedure
- Caution with patients on anticoagulation that cannot be stopped; risk of hematoma

Alternatives to Surgical Treatment
- Needle aponeurotomy
- Collagenase injection

PREOPERATIVE IMAGING
- Not routinely obtained
- Plain radiographs of the hand may be considered in those with underlying degenerative disease

---

Based on Lehman TP, Peterson SL, Rayan GM: Partial palmar fasciectomy for Dupuytren disease, in Colvin AC, Flatow E, eds: Atlas of Essential Orthopaedic Procedures, *ed 2. Rosemont, IL, American Academy of Orthopaedic Surgeons, 2020, pp 404-411.*

PROCEDURE

Room Setup/Patient Positioning

- Supine position with arm on hand table
- Nonsterile padded tourniquet to upper arm
- Prepare volar forearm in case graft needed
- Position body to allow access to flaps as needed
- Anesthesia may be general, regional, or local

Special Instruments/Equipment

- Lead hand can help with exposure
- No. 15C Bard-Parker surgical blade
- Small Beaver blade scalpels
- Microscope available in case of injury to nerves or arteries

Surgical Technique

Preoperative Planning

- Plan selective removal of cords causing contracture
- Multiple cords may be present—Pretendinous, spiral, lateral, central, abductor digiti minimi, natatory, and proximal and distal commissural cords (**Figure 1**)
- Make Bruner (volar zigzag) incision from palm into digit; alternatively, can use longitudinal midline incision in digit; close with multiple Z-plasties
- May combine both incisions with transverse palm incisions, which are closed, grafted, or left open to heal

Initial Dissection

- After superficial incision, elevate skin flaps carefully from adherent tissue; avoid buttonholing flap
- Identify neurovascular bundles displaced superficially and toward midline; protect throughout procedure

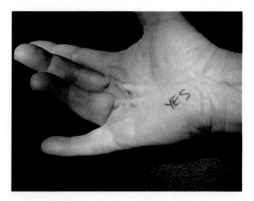

FIGURE 1 Photograph depicts metacarpophalangeal joint flexion contracture due to pretendinous cords in the palm.

- If cannot separate skin flaps, consider dermofasciectomy and skin grafting
- Retract skin flaps with stay sutures
- In severe contracture, divide proximal portion of cord to increase digit extension

Tissue Excision
- Excise diseased tissue only after identifying important neurovascular structures; begin proximally, move distally
- Limited fasciectomy, release of contractures usually sufficient; remove diseased fascia en bloc or in pieces; multiple cords may require more release
- If cannot separate diseased tissue from skin or if skin is scarred from previous surgery, consider dermofasciectomy
- Pay attention to palmodigital region, where risk to neurovascular structures is highest

Assessing Joint Contracture
- Residual proximal interphalangeal joint contracture greater than 30° not correctable by manipulation requires release of checkrein ligament component of volar plate, possibly portion of collateral ligaments
- Check tension on digital neurovascular bundle; place postoperative splint in flexion to relieve tension if necessary
- Deflate tourniquet; ensure hemostasis; apply gentle pressure as needed
- Ensure adequate digital circulation; correct arterial spasm with topical vasodilator such as lidocaine, flexion, and warming of digit; repair or graft any arterial laceration

Wound Closure
- Close Bruner skin incisions primarily, with corners approximated in Y-V fashion as necessary; close midline incision with multiple Z-plasties (**Figure 2**)
- For dermofasciectomy, harvest full-thickness skin graft, and apply to defect; donor site may be volar wrist, antecubital fossa, glabrous skin of foot, or groin
- May leave palmar wound open
- Apply bulky dressing with splint in extension, without causing vasospasm; fingertips should be visible to assess circulation

COMPLICATIONS
- Infection
- Neurovascular injury
- Complex regional pain syndrome
- Recurrence and extension of disease
- Stiffness

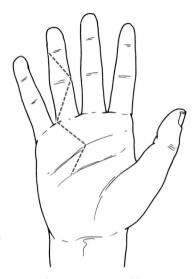

FIGURE 2 Illustration shows the Bruner incision (dashed line) for fasciectomy of the ring finger and palm.

POSTOPERATIVE CARE

- Keep hand in splint 7 to 10 days
- Remove sutures at 10 to 15 days; may discontinue splint or keep for 2 more weeks, depending on initial contracture severity; patient may remove splint two to three times per day for passive range-of-motion exercises
- At 4 weeks, discontinue splint during day; continue nocturnal use of splint for at least 6 weeks

PEARLS

- Consider dermofasciectomy and skin grafting if skin flaps cannot be safely elevated.
- Identify digital arteries and nerves and protect throughout procedure.
- Divide proximal portion of cord in cases of severe flexion contracture to allow sufficient extension of digit for visualization.
- Confirm circulation to all digits after fasciectomy. Flexion and warming of digits or topical vasodilator may help if circulation is not adequate. Repair or graft lacerated vessels.
- Obtain hemostasis before wound closure to minimize risk of hematoma formation and subsequent flap necrosis.
- Risk of neurovascular injury is increased in revision cases where there is more scarring.
- Alternatives include needle aponeurotomy and collagenase injection.
- Recurrence or inability to maintain PIP extension is common; MCP contractures are much more forgiving than are PIP joint contractures.

INTRODUCTION

- Dupuytren disease is a benign fibromatosis of the fascia of the hand and fingers
- Starts as nodule or palpable mass and enlarges and leads to development of pathologic cords which thicken and contract (**Figures 1** through **3**)
- Most commonly affected digits are the ring and little finger (50% to 60%)

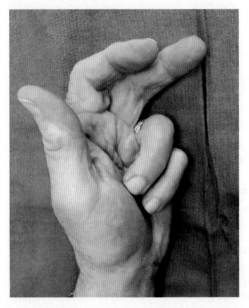

FIGURE 1 Photograph of severe untreated Dupuytren disease.

Based on Pess GM: Needle aponeurotomy, in Colvin AC, Flatow E, eds: Atlas of Essential Orthopaedic Procedures, *ed 2. Rosemont, IL, American Academy of Orthopaedic Surgeons, 2020, pp 412-420.*

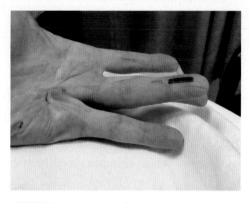

FIGURE 2 Photograph of mild Dupuytren disease.

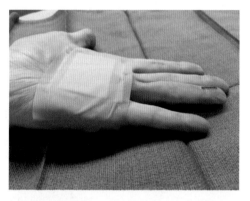

FIGURE 3 Photograph of complete correction of mild Dupuytren disease with needle aponeurotomy (NA).

PATIENT SELECTION

Indications

- Palpable cords causing contracture (**Figure 4**)

Contraindications

- Contracted skin, skin grafts, and scar tissue from prior fasciectomy (**Figure 5**)
- Contractures secondary to spasticity or ulnar nerve palsy

Surgical Anatomy

- Pretendinous cord—originates from pretendinous band, begins proximal to the proximal finger crease, contracts the MP joint of fingers or thumb
- Central cord—located midline between neurovascular bundles and distal to the proximal finger crease, is a continuation of the pretendinous cord, contracts the PIP joint

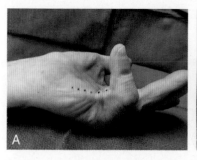 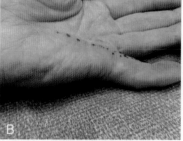

FIGURE 4 Photographs showing that the area of maximum bowstringing is the best location for needle aponeurotomy (NA) portals. **A,** Before. **B,** After.

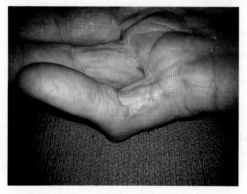

FIGURE 5 Photograph shows that needle aponeurotomy (NA) can be performed as long as a palpable cord is present and the contracture is not just due to scar.

- Lateral cord—composed of diseased lateral digital fascia, located superficial to neurovascular bundle, contracts PIP joint
- Retrovascular cord—located deep to neurovascular bundle, can contract both the PIP and DIP joints
- Natatory cord—contracts the second, third, and fourth web spaces
- Commissural cords (proximal and distal)—contracts the first web space, may be rope-like in consistency
- Abductor digiti minimi cord—contracts the little finger MP and PIP joints. Can displace the neurovascular bundle in a volar, midline, and distal direction
- Spiral cord—contracts PIP joint—usually a combination of pretendinous cord, diseased lateral digital fascia, and Grayson's ligament. Can displace neurovascular bundle in a volar, midline, and distal direction (**Figure 6**)

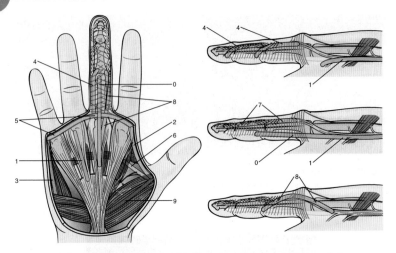

FIGURE 6 Illustration of anatomy of pathologic cords. 0 = central cord; 1 = pre-pretendinous cord; 2 = distal commissural cord; 3 = abductor digiti minimi cord; 4 = lateral cord; 5 = natatory cord; 6 = proximal commissural cord; 7 = retrovascular cord; 8 = spiral cord; 9 = thumb pretendinous cord. (Redrawn from an illustration provided courtesy of Charles Eaton, MD.)

PREOPERATIVE IMAGING
- No special imaging necessary
- Plain radiographs useful to evaluate articular surfaces for long-standing severe contractures
- Radiographs required in setting of old injury or dislocation

PROCEDURE
Room Setup/Patient Positioning
- Performed usually in outpatient treatment room under local anesthesia
- For patients with low pain tolerance, sedation can be used in surgery center or hospital setting; patient must remain responsive to stimuli and communication
- Recumbent or sitting position
- No tourniquet
- No prophylactic antibiotics

Special Instruments/Equipment
- 5 mL syringe filled with 3 mL lidocaine 1% plan and 1 mL methylprednisolone acetate injectable suspension 40 mg
- Short 25-gauge needle, 16 mm (5/8 inch) length needles (**Figure 7**)
- 18-gauge, 40 mm (1.5 inch) needle can be bent to 90° for subcision
- Clamp/needle holder

Surgical Technique

 VIDEO 50.1 Treatment of Dupuytren Disease With Needle Aponeurotomy. Gary M. Pess, MD (2 min 30 s)

 VIDEO 50.2 Treatment of Dupuytren Disease of PIP Joint With Needle Aponeurotomy. Gary M. Pess, MD (2 min 25 s)

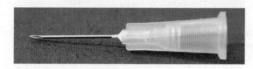

FIGURE 7 Photograph of a short 25-gauge, 16-mm (5/8-inch) needle with which needle aponeurotomy is performed.

Preoperative Planning

- Abnormal cords are identified by palpation and marked with surgical marker
- Portal sites chosen in areas of definite cords where the cord is maximally bowstringed
- Needle insertion into supple and mobile skin is to avoid skin tear
- Skin creases, clefts, and pits should be avoided
- Avoid neurovascular bundle when spiral or abductor digiti minimi cord is present

Portal Sites and Anesthesia

- Apply traction to skin and look for blanching
  - If diseased cord is tighter than skin, the skin will not blanch with traction
  - Blanching indicates that skin is contracted and there may not be an underlying cord present to release
  - Blanching will advance distally when the underlying cord has been adequately released
- Center of cord used as a single needle entrance site (**Figure 8**)
  - Can also use two needle insertion sites, radial and ulnar, if cord is >5 mm (**Figure 9**)
- Modify injection sites after releasing the MP joint
- Intradermal anesthesia is performed with 0.1 to 0.5 mL lidocaine 1% plain injected into the area of the palmar portals before release
- Only penetrate the dermis; inject as the needle is withdrawn

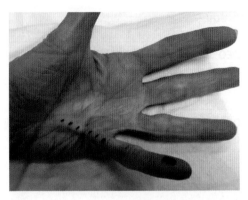

FIGURE 8 Photograph showing the portal sites marked out before release with needle aponeurotomy (NA).

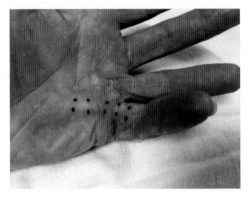

FIGURE 9 Photograph showing the two parallel insertion sites that are used for wide cords > 5 mm.

- Each time the portal is entered, inject 0.1 mL of lidocaine/corticosteroid mix
- Identify neurovascular bundles displaced superficially and toward midline; protect throughout procedure

Cord Release Technique
- Cords can be released proximally to distally or vice versa; however releasing proximal to distal is easier and safer
  - ▶ Release of the MP joint frequently leads to partial release of the PIP joint, making it easier to complete the release of PIP joint
- Use a "pinch and poke" technique
  - ▶ Palpate cord and pinch between fingertips (**Figure 10**)
- Align bevel of needle perpendicular to the cord

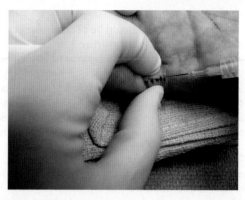

FIGURE 10 Photograph demonstrating pinch and poke technique for needle aponeurotomy (NA).

- Flex and extend the finger after each needle insertion to confirm that the needle is not in the flexor tendon
- Create portal at area of maximum bowstringing and area furthest away from the neurovascular bundle
- Continuously ask if patient feels electric shocks during the procedure
- Three maneuvers are used to release cords: perforate, slice, and subcision
    - Can use an up and down motion to perforate the cord with the needle oriented vertically
    - A gentle pendulum side-to-side slicing motion can be used with needle tip perpendicular to the cord's longitudinal axis
    - In areas of pitting, a tangential clearing motion or subcision is used with an 18 or 22 gauge needle bent to a 90° angle horizontally in the subdermal layer to release vertical fibers separating adherent skin from the cord (**Figure 11, A** through C)

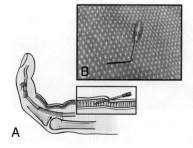
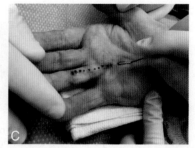

FIGURE 11 Subcision technique. **A,** Line drawing. **B,** Photograph of the subcision needle. **C,** Photograph of the technique.

- Divide cords from superficial to deep
- Resistance and crackly sound should be heard as the cord is cut
- Push the cord against needle while slicing
- Frequently change needles (can use from 6 to 20 needles per finger depending on severity)
- Place gentle extension tension on the cord during release and use passive extension to rupture the cord (pop may be felt or heard); manipulate finger in abduction, adduction, pronation, and supination to release all cords
- Manipulate unaffected fingers as this can help release any residual cords

Natatory Cord Release

- Orient needle parallel to longitudinal axis of finger and perpendicular to the transverse axis of the cord
- Release with a slicing motion, moving proximally to distally
- Massage the released cord to help disrupt remaining deep fibers; can also be useful when releasing narrow lateral and retrovascular cords (**Figure 12, A through C**)
- Assess for residual cords after completing release, and release remaining cords if necessary
- May often be nonpalpable central cord that results in PIP joint contracture even after release of all cords
  - ▷ Palmar release of this cord can be performed in the midline, proximal to the middle finger crease
  - ▷ Stay superficial to avoid entering the flexor tendon sheath (**Figure 13**)

Resistant and PIP Joint Contractures

- Transverse retinacular ligament is released by entering dorsal to the midaxial line and orienting the needle horizontally
- Ligament is released in a proximal-to-distal or distal-to-proximal direction
- Collateral ligament can be released deep to the transverse retinacular ligament just superficial to the head of the proximal phalanx and PIP joint
- Can release both radial and ulnar sides of PIP joint to correct contracture (**Figure 14**)

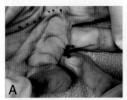 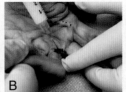 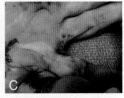

FIGURE 12 Photographs demonstrating natatory cord release by aligning needle parallel to the longitudinal axis of the finger. **A,** Before. **B,** Needle aponeurotomy (NA) procedure. **C,** After.

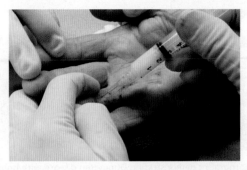

FIGURE 13 Photograph demonstrating the release of residual nonpalpable central cord, contributing to proximal interphalangeal (PIP) joint contracture.

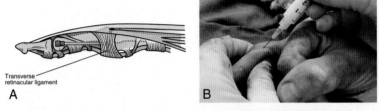

Transverse
retinacular ligament

A   B

FIGURE 14 Release of the transverse retinacular ligament. **A,** Line drawing.
B, Photograph of the technique. (**A,** Courtesy of Keith A. Denker, MD.)

Severe PIP Joint Contractures

- In severe PIP joint contractures, can use a wrist or digital block for supplementary anesthesia after the needle aponeurotomy procedure for postprocedure analgesia
- After all cords are released, inject nodules with a mixture of lidocaine and corticosteroid to reduce inflammatory reaction and ease postoperative recovery
- A significant boutonniere deformity may be present when there is a severe contracture of the PIP joint, usually >65°
- These digits are hyperextended at DIP joint and cannot be passively flexed to neutral
- Treat with Fowler or Dolphin tenotomy, cutting the terminal extensor tendon percutaneously with a 25 gauge needle
- Insert needle radially and ulnarly over the head of the middle phalanx, cutting the tendon in a lateral to central direction (**Figure 15**)

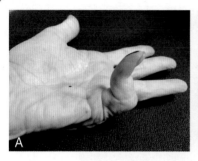 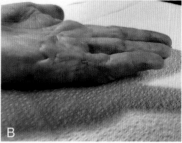

FIGURE 15 Photographs demonstrating Dupuytren disease with boutonnière deformity. **A**, Before. **B**, After.

COMPLICATIONS

- Pain
- Swelling
- Ecchymosis
- Skin tears (~3% to 5%)
- Infection
- Transient neurapraxia
- Nerve laceration
- Tendon rupture
- Arterial laceration
- Complex regional pain syndrome

POSTOPERATIVE CARE

- Apply light dressing with gauze bandage—can remove that evening or next morning
- Can wash hand and use hand routinely
- Fit extension splint immediately postprocedure
- Night splint for 3 to 4 months
- Exercise at home 5 to 10 minutes twice a day for 4 weeks
- Avoid heavy grasping for 1 to 2 weeks, especially after treatment of PIP joint contractures
- Therapy not required in most instances

PEARLS

- Flex and extend finger after each needle insertion to confirm that it is not in the flexor tendon.
- Maintain tension on the cord.
- Align needle bevel perpendicular to the cord.
- Release perpendicular to longitudinal axis of the cord.
- Change needles frequently.

- Choose area of maximum bowstring for insertion.
- Select areas farthest from neurovascular bundle.
- Communicate with patient frequently and ask if they feel electric shock.
- Usually insert needle in the center of the cord but side by side portals for thick portals >5 mm can be used.
- Manipulate finger in all planes (**Figure 16**).
- Manipulate unaffected fingers.
- Massage cords to disrupt the cord.
- Release nonpalpable central cord for residual PIP joint contractures.
- Release transverse retinacular ligament for resistant PIP joint contractures.
- Inject PIP joint for anesthesia before manipulating severe contractures.
- Treat boutonniere deformity with a release of the terminal extensor tendon.

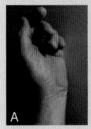 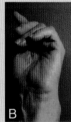 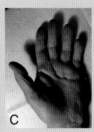 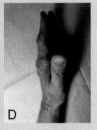

FIGURE 16 Photographs of successful treatment with needle aponeurotomy (NA). **A** and **B**, Before. **C** and **D**, After.

51

Thumb Metacarpophalangeal Joint Ulnar Collateral Ligament Repair

INTRODUCTIONS
- Common in active population
- Partial UCL tears can be treated nonsurgically in a cast for 4 weeks

PATIENT SELECTION

Indications for Surgery
- Complete injury to the UCL as evidenced by instability to radial deviation stress testing with no firm end point
  - \>30° of deviation with radial stress
  - \>15° to 20° of deviation with radial stress compared with contralateral side
- Stener lesion (adductor aponeurosis interposition blocking reduction of UCL)
- Failure of nonsurgical management (**Figures 1** and **2**) which can include continued pain or instability despite an adequate period of immobilization

---

VIDEO 51.1 Radial Deviation Instability. Preoperative examination of a patient with ulnar collateral ligament injury demonstrating more than 30° radial deviation at MCP joint with radial stress. Blake K. Montgomery, MD; Jeffrey Yao, MD (5 s)

Contraindications
- Articular cartilage changes or frank osteoarthritis of the MCP joint

PREOPERATIVE IMAGING
- Plain radiographs of thumb including three views to evaluate for subluxation, deformity, fracture, and arthritis
- MRI if examiner unable to determine if UCL is completely torn
- Stress radiographs compared with those of contralateral thumb

---

Based on Montgomery BK, Yao J: Thumb metacarpophalangeal joint ulnar collateral ligament repair, in Colvin AC, Flatow E, eds: Atlas of Essential Orthopaedic Procedures, *ed 2. Rosemont, IL, American Academy of Orthopaedic Surgeons, 2020, pp 421-427.*

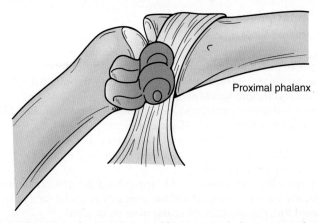

Proximal phalanx

FIGURE 1 Illustration of a Stener lesion. Adductor aponeurosis prevents avulsed ulnar collateral ligament (UCL) from reaching the UCL insertion on the proximal phalanx.

PROCEDURE

Room Setup/Patient Positioning

- Standard patient positioning with hand table with brachial tourniquet inflated to 250 mmHg
- Regional, general, or local anesthesia

Special Instruments/Equipment

- Sutures anchors of the surgeon's choice should be available before the start of the procedure (size of anchor should be <3 mm)
- Bone gouges, suture passer, and interference screw should be available in the event of the need for reconstruction

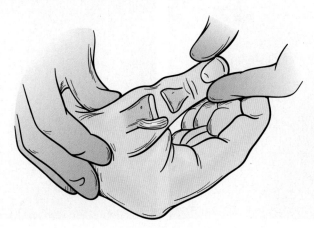

FIGURE 2 Illustration of radial deviation instability. Examiner provides radial stress onto MCP joint causing radial deviation beyond 30°.

Surgical Technique

Approach and Dissection

- Examine thumb under anesthesia before start of procedure to assess degree of instability compared with contralateral side
- 5 cm curvilinear incision along ulnar aspect of thumb MCP joint over the ulnar collateral ligament (**Figure 3**)
- Protect and identify the dorsal radial sensory nerve over the adductor aponeurosis; retract volarly (**Figure 4**)
- Dissect subcutaneous tissue until adductor aponeurosis
- Incise adductor aponeurosis and leave 2 mm cuff adjacent to the EPL for later repair (**Figure 5**)
- Perform dorsal capsulotomy and inspect MCP for chondral injury
- Typically the UCL avulses from the proximal phalanx; rarely can they disrupt the midsubstance or avulse from metacarpal

Repair

- For midsubstance tear, repair with vertical mattress, nonabsorbable sutures
- For avulsion of proximal phalanx, attempt reduction to ensure adequate ligament for repair
    - Identify UCL attachment at ulnar aspect of base of proximal phalanx
    - Decorticate to healthy cancellous bone
    - Insert suture anchor into base of proximal phalanx (**Figure 6**)

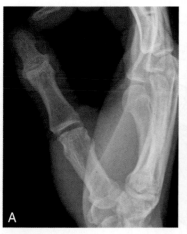 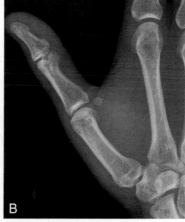

FIGURE 3 Preoperative radiographs. **A** and **B**, AP and lateral radiographs of a right thumb with ulnar collateral ligament injury.

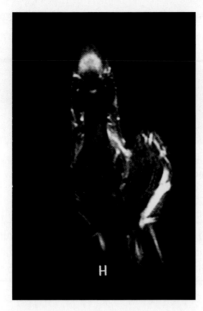

FIGURE 4 T2-weighted magnetic resonance image, coronal view, demonstrating complete thickness rupture of ulnar collateral ligament.

- Sutures from the anchor are placed with horizontal mattress suture as the thumb is ulnarly deviated for appropriate tensioning (**Figure 7**)
- Stress the thumb gently after sutures are tied (**Figure 8**)
- Can stabilize with K-wire in patients with poor ligament quality or patients with questionable compliance
- Can augment repair and reconstructive procedures with internal brace (Arthrex, Naples FL) to allow earlier motion or short immobilization

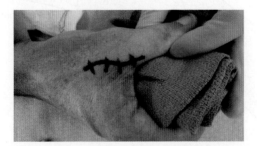

FIGURE 5 Photograph of an incision. Curvilinear incision along the ulnar aspect of the thumb MCP joint overlying the ulnar collateral ligament.

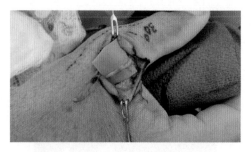

FIGURE 6 Intraoperative photograph showing dorsal radial sensory nerve, highlighted with blue background.

 VIDEO 51.2 Intraoperative Stability Assessment. After repair of UCL, gentle intraoperative radial stress testing demonstrates stable MCP joint. Blake K. Montgomery, MD; Jeffrey Yao, MD (5 s)

Reconstruction

- Consider reconstruction with tendon autograft if UCL is insufficient
- Harvest palmaris longus; if not present, use half of FCR
- Create bone tunnel in proximal phalanx using gouge holes; gouge angles should be angled 45° to the bone and directed at each other to facilitate bone tunnel creation

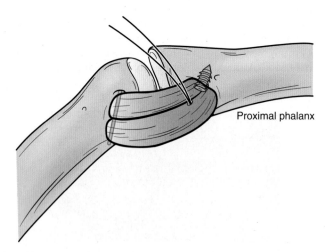

Proximal phalanx

FIGURE 7 Illustration of ulnar collateral ligament (UCL) repair with bone anchor sutured to UCL ligament.

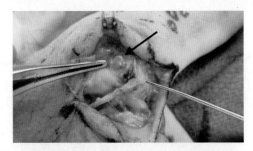

FIGURE 8 Intraoperative photograph of a stener lesion. Complete tear of the ulnar collateral ligament with displacement superficial to the adductor aponeurosis (arrow).

- Position first hole at the 7 o'clock position just distal to joint and subchondral bone (for right thumb); ensure adequate bone bridge to avoid fracture
- Connect the two holes and insert wire into tunnel to pass autograft (**Figure 9**)
- Create a proximal bone tunnel in the metacarpal by making gouge hole at the origin of the UCL; angle tunnel obliquely and proximally to exit radial aspect of first metacarpal
- Make small skin incision over gouge and pass wire through the bone tunnel
- Pass graft through proximal phalanx and suture tails of graft together (**Figure 10**)
- Pass tail into hole created in the metacarpal neck
- Ulnarly deviate thumb and tension graft
- Use suture button with nonabsorbable suture on the radial aspect of thumb or interference screw may be placed on the proximal/dorsal aspect of graft (**Figures 11** and **12**)
- Stress collateral ligament
- Can use K-wire to protect repair

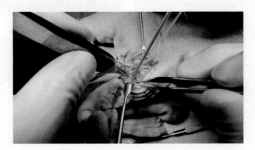

FIGURE 9 Intraoperative photograph showing bone anchor being inserted into the proximal phalanx.

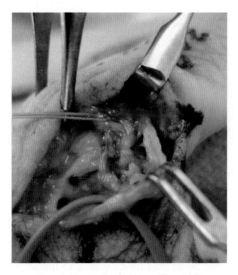

FIGURE 10 Intraoperative photograph of ulnar collateral ligament repair. Suture securing ulnar collateral ligament to bone anchor in proximal phalanx.

Closure

- Irrigate
- Close capsule and adductor aponeurosis with 4-0 nonabsorbable suture
- Take fluoroscopic images of the MCP joint to assess location of anchor
- Take stress fluoroscopy of the thumb MCP through full ROM
- Close skin and apply forearm based thumb spica splint

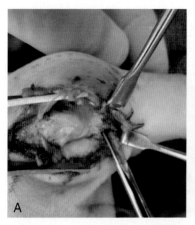 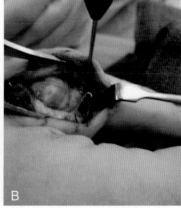

FIGURE 11 Intraoperative photographs showing bone tunnel. **A,** Bone gouge in bone tunnel in proximal phalanx. **B,** Wire in bone tunnel in proximal phalanx.

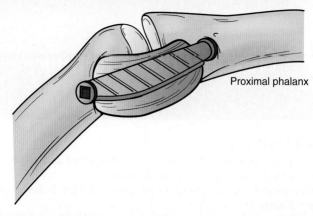

Proximal phalanx

FIGURE 12 Illustration of ulnar collateral ligament (UCL) reconstruction with graft in tunnels and secured with interference screw.

COMPLICATIONS

- MCP joint stiffness
- Dorsal radial sensory nerve neurapraxia
- Progression of osteoarthritis
- Recurrent or residual instability

POSTOPERATIVE CARE

- 4 to 6 weeks of immobilization is usually routine. This is often first with a thumb spica splint for 2 weeks, followed by a thumb spica cast
- At 4 to 6 weeks, full time immobilization is discontinued. A removable thumb spica splint may be used for 2 to 4 weeks during lifting activity and sleep; start occupational therapy at this time
- Strengthening starts 6 to 8 weeks postop
- Protect thumb for 4 to 6 months after surgery
- If internal brace is used in repair or reconstruction, immobilize for 1 to 2 weeks and provide thumb spica splint for activity and sleep; allow strengthening at 3 to 4 weeks postop and unrestricted activities at 4 to 6 weeks

PEARLS

- Appropriately tension UCL ligament repair or reconstruction.
- Prefer to tension the repair with the thumb MCP in slight ulnar deviation because the repair or reconstruction can stretch out postoperatively.
- Consider augmentation of the repair or reconstruction with an internal brace or similar construct in high-level athletes.

PATIENT SELECTION

- Suture techniques have become more sophisticated and rehab protocols have kept pace with surgical advances
- Flexion cascade of the hand will be altered if there is flexor tendon injury (**Figure 1**)
- Test FDS by holding uninvolved digits at the MCP Joints in hyperextension and IP joints in extension and ask patient to flex PIP joints at the level of the middle phalanx
- Test FDP by holding involved digit at the middle phalanx level and ask patient to flex the DIP joint
- Use wrist flexion/extension tenodesis effect to indirectly enhance examination

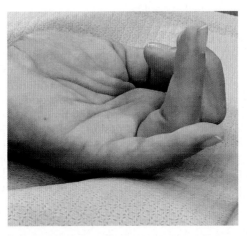

FIGURE 1 Photograph shows demonstration of flexor tendon cascade with ring finger FDP disruption and little finger FDP and FDS disruption.

Based on Weiss LE, Patricia Fox M, Sweet S: Flexor tendon repair, in Colvin AC, Flatow E, eds: Atlas of Essential Orthopaedic Procedures, *ed 2. Rosemont, IL, American Academy of Orthopaedic Surgeons, 2020, pp 428-434.*

- Assess FPL laceration by compression of the muscle belly proximal to the wrist by looking for IP joint flexion of the thumb; beware of "pseudotendon" which can mimic an intact tendon when the injured tendon retracts
- Level of volar skin laceration may not represent true level of tendon injury, especially if digits were flexed
- Palpate palm to reveal level of retracted stump
- Observe for presence/absence of palmaris tendon; may need for graft during repair of staged reconstructive procedure
  - Alternative grafts include plantaris tendon, extensor digitorum longus (toe extensors)
  - Discuss with patient preoperatively regarding possibility of requiring graft

Special Populations/Situations
Complex Injuries
- Challenging to balance immobilization requirements and rehabilitation in cases of complex open injuries with tendon lacerations and fractures
  - Must modify therapy protocols to balance combination of soft-tissue, nerve, artery, tendon, and osseous injury
  - Precedence given to neurovascular status and skeletal stabilization to the detriment of early tendon mobilization protocols

Patients With Delayed Presentation
- Some cases when patients present in delayed fashion
- MCP, PIP, and DIP joints must be passively supple to have surgery
- Level of retraction and compliance of tendon is critical to determine if it can be repaired
- Debatable whether it is necessary to fuse or tenodese DIP joint after FDP excision
- Primary grafting of tendon is rarely indicated; rare exceptions where sheath remains open and both FDP and FDS tendons are rupture

Patients With Carpal Fractures
- Attritional rupture of flexor tendons can be secondary to prior carpal fracture
- A hook of the hamate fracture or nonunion can cause abrasive surface leading to flexor rupture of the ring and/or little finger
- Treatment consists of hook of hamate excision and tendon reconstruction or adjacent tendon transfers

Flexor Injuries in Children
- Same techniques for direct repair and tendon graft in children as it is in adults
- Repair will require smaller caliber sutures

- Avoid the physis with suture passage if using transosseous sutures
- Casting in young children who are unable to participate therapy program yields satisfactory outcomes
- Use absorbable skin sutures

Patients With Rheumatoid Arthritis
- FPL is most commonly ruptured flexor tendon in the RA population (Mannerfelt lesion)
- Also consider AIN dysfunction as a cause for lost ability to actively flex the thumb IP joint
- FPL ruptures can be secondary to volar osteophyte on the scaphoid or other volar radial location; management includes osteophyte removal and tendon transfer, interposition graft, or IP joint fusion

Indications
- Medically fit patient who can demonstrate compliance with rehab protocol
- Emergent repairs indicated in compromised perfusion requiring microvascular repair

Contraindications
- Medically unstable patient
- Active infection
- Noncompliant patient

PREOPERATIVE IMAGING
Radiography
- Plain radiographs of the affected digit and hand to evaluate for avulsion injury or presence of foreign body (**Figure 2**)
- MRI or ultrasonography to evaluate continuity of tendon and assess gap distance (**Figure 3**)

PROCEDURE
Room Setup/Patient Positioning
- Supine with arm on radiolucent hand table
- Regional or local anesthesia in unsedated patient to allow intraoperative assessment of quality of repair
- Tourniquet

Special Instruments/Equipment/Implants
- Hand stabilization device (eg, Alumni-hand, Tupper hand retractor set, lead hand, and ASSI table)
- 3-0 or 4-0 nonabsorbable braided suture
- 5-0 or 6-0 monofilament suture for epitendinous suture (with tapered needle)

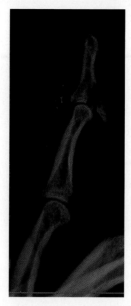

FIGURE 2 Appearance of an FDP avulsion, which in this case includes an intra-articular distal phalanx fracture as noted on radiograph. There was a fracture combined with an FDP avulsion that was retracted to the A-2 pulley that is not visible on plain radiographs (making this a type IV injury).

- Tendon retrieval in pulley system with single skin hook; can use Toby or similar device to pass tendon underneath pulley
- Keith needle and padded button for zone 1 repairs
- 25 gauge needle to help capture and maintain proximal tendon section to prevent retraction
- Autologous tendon grafting for subacute and chronic injuries
- Tendon stripper and/or passer
- Silicone implants for pulley reconstruction

Surgical Technique

- Ideal repair includes easy suture placement, secure knots, smooth end-to-end tendon apposition, minimal to no gapping at the repair site, avoiding injury to tendon vasculature, early postoperative motion
- Strength of repair proportional to number of core sutures that cross repair site (**Figure 4**)
- Minimum of four-strand core suture repair should be performed with possible addition of epitendinous suture
- Venting pulley, such as the A4 pulley, is acceptable

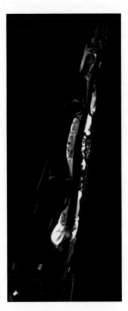

FIGURE 3 Magnetic resonance image demonstrating an intact FDP and FDS but surrounding flexor tenosynovitis throughout the flexor sheath.

Zone I Injuries
- Region distal to FDS insertion
- Repair is based on distal stump length—if >1 cm, primary end-to-end tendon repair is preferred; if <1 cm, alternative options include pull-out sutures technique or suture anchor into bone
- For acute avulsions, treatment guided by Leddy-Packer classification
  - Type I, FDP retracts into palm (vincular blood supply disrupted)
    - Treat <7 days from injury for optimal outcomes
  - Type II, tendon retracts to level of the PIP joint (vincular blood supply partially intact)
  - Type III, FDP is avulsed with portion of volar distal phalanx
    - Type II and III injuries can be addressed <6 weeks from injury given intact blood supply

Step by Step Zone I Repair
- Bruner incision distally first to confirm tendon is injured; extend proximally as required
- Identify proximal tendon stump and milk retracted tendon from proximal to distal
- Retrieve with single tine skin hook or a sheath retractor and suture retriever

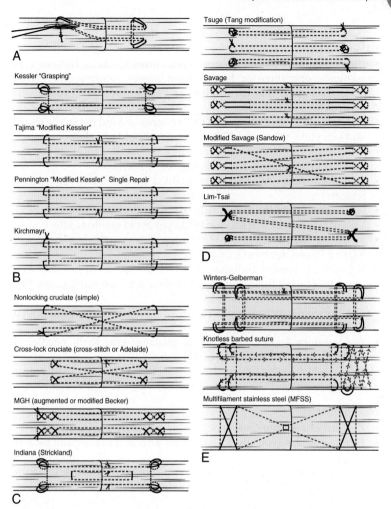

FIGURE 4 **A** through **E**, Illustration showing examples of various described flexor tendon core suture repair techniques. **A**, Kessler-Tsuge technique. **B**, Two-stranded flexor tendon repairs. **C**, Four-stranded flexor tendon repairs. **D**, Six-stranded flexor tendon repairs. **E**, Eight-stranded repair (Winters-Gelberman) and alternative suture repair options. (Part A redrawn from Renner C, Corella F, Fischer N: Biomechanical evaluation of 4-strand flexor tendon repair techniques, including a combined Kessler–Tsuge approach. *J Hand Surg* 2015;40(2):229-235, Figure 8, with permission from Elsevier. doi:10.1016/j.jhsa.2014.10.055. Parts B through E redrawn from Chauhan A, Palmer BA, Merrell GA: Flexor tendon repairs: techniques, eponyms, and evidence. *J Hand Surg* 2014;39(9):1846-1853, with permission from Elsevier. doi:10.1016/j.jhsa.2014.06.025.)

- Secure proximal tendon with a 25 gauge needle transversely through the tendon, avoiding neurovascular bundles
- Vent A4 pulley if needed before or after repair
- Place 3-0 monofilament suture (eg, prolene) in a Bunnell-type fashion using three or four crossed passes; confirm that suture is not locked so that it can glide and be removed at 6 to 8 weeks postoperatively
- Pass two Keith needles parallel to each other and out the sterile matrix and nail plate; the rupture FDP foot print should be visible
- Bring suture through needles and pull the needles together through nail bed to deliver the sutures through a padded button
- Tie suture limbs together over padded button while maintaining tension
- Suture anchors in the distal phalanx are an alternative method
- Do not overadvance or shorten tendon to avoid quadriga effect
- Suture residual intact distal FDP stump, if any, to the repair site with 5-0 or 6-0 monofilament suture
- If fracture is present and attached to the tendon stump, modify technique by placing Bunnell-type suture first and then stabilize the fracture with two 1.0 or 1.3 mm screws
- Can use dental pick, or temporary K-wire (0.28 mm) can be helpful to hold fracture in correct position
- Bring suture limbs around distal phalanx with Keith needles or through distal phalanx as described above
- Routine skin closure followed by dorsal blocking splint past finger tips to include PIP and DIP joints with wrist in 15° to 20° of flexion

Zone II Injuries

- Region between proximal aspect of the A1 pulley to FDS insertion
- FDP lacerations typically do not retract proximal to midpalm because they are held by lumbricals
  - Evaluate tendons for partial versus complete tears after exposure
  - Partial tears <50% can be trimmed or repaired with a small caliber suture
- Assess bulk of two-tendon repair with selective repair of one slip of FDS or repair of FDP in isolation

Step by Step Zone II Repair

- Retrieve proximal tendon stumps as descried above
- Milking tendon from proximal to distal may assist in delivery of the tendon
- Avoid obtaining proximal tendon stump through palmar incision using proximal tendon delivery because it can disrupt vincular blood supply; if the tendon is already in the palm, then this approach is necessary to advance tendon into sheath

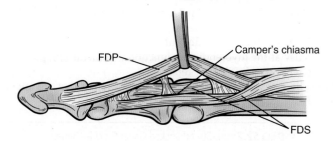

FIGURE 5 Illustration showing Camper's chiasm anatomy. (Redrawn with permission from Wolfe SW, et al, eds: *Green's Operative Hand Surgery*, ed 6.Philadelphia, Elsevier, Churchill Livingstone, 2011. ISBN:9781416052791.)

- Pulley windows can be created to retrieve tendon but preserve as much possible (especially if A4 pulley is vented)
- Flex distal part of digit to deliver the distal stump proximally
- When FDS laceration is distal to Camper's chiasm, this tendon is selectively repaired first because it is the deepest
- The tendon is quite flat at this location, so interrupted or running nonabsorbable 5-0 or 6-0 monofilament suture is used
- Consider sacrificing a slip of FDS to avoid bulk
- The entire FDS in little finger may be sacrificed if it is small and insufficient (**Figure 5**)
- Carry out four-strand repair with epitendinous suture; repair of traumatic/intentional sheath laceration is optional
- Closure and splinting as per zone I

VIDEO 52.1 FDS Repair Distal to Camper's Chiasm.
Lawrence E. Weiss, MD; M. Patricia Fox, MD;
Stephanie Sweet, MD (2 min 30 s)

Zone III, IV, and V Injuries

- Zone III located distal to transverse carpal ligament to start of flexor sheath at A1 pulley
  - May occur with midpalmar vascular arch injury
  - Must perform Allen's test to asses vascular injury
  - Vascular ultrasonography or arteriography may be appropriate preoperatively
- Zone IV tendon injuries occur under transverse carpal ligament
  - May have additional median or ulnar nerve injury and ulnar artery injury

- Zone V injuries located proximal to transverse carpal ligament to forearm
  - ▶ May require opening the carpal tunnel
  - ▶ Distal stumps may be difficult to retrieve at this level
  - ▶ Injury at the myotendinous junction is difficult to repair, leading to tendon gapping after repair
- Zones III-V treated with same principles of repair that are applied to zone II

VIDEO 52.2 Four-Strand Locked Grasp Cruciate Repair. Lawrence E. Weiss, MD; M. Patricia Fox, MD; Stephanie Sweet, MD (7 min 10 s)

VIDEO 52.3 Four-Strand Modified Kessler Using Accessory Horizontal Mattress Suture. Lawrence E. Weiss, MD; M. Patricia Fox, MD; Stephanie Sweet, MD (5 min 15 s)

VIDEO 52.4 Kirchmayr-Zechner Flexor Tendon Repair. Lawrence E. Weiss, MD; M. Patricia Fox, MD; Stephanie Sweet, MD (5 min 53 s)

COMPLICATIONS

- Flexor tendon adhesions
- Repair rupture
- Bowstringing if pulleys are compromised or insufficient
- Neurapraxia of digital nerves
- Wound dehiscence
- Flap necrosis
- Infection
- IP joint contracture
- Quadriga

POSTOPERATIVE CARE AND REHABILITATION

- High-quality postoperative rehabilitation is important to achieve successful outcome
- Goal of protocol is to promote excursion of tendon while being mindful of forces along the repair site
- Communication between surgeon and therapist is critical; should contact therapist and advise them of quality of repair, severity of injury, and expectations
- Should have ongoing assessment of prospective perceived patient compliance with postoperative therapy protocol

PEARLS

- Wide awake surgery has brought flexor tendon repair into new area to manage tension, assess gliding of repair, and checking for gapping with much greater ease compared with patient who is sedated and not actively participating in surgery.
- Respect soft tissues with minimal to no touch technique.
- Assess repair gap at time of surgery; there should be zero tolerance of any gapping; if not wide awake, stress with antagonistic passive extension to confirm that repair is sound.
- Must perform intraoperative hemostasis; higher risk of edema, wound dehiscence, and flap necrosis without control of bleeding.
- With flexor tendon repair in setting of fracture management, it is critical to achieve stable skeletal construct to allow for early active motion protocol; anatomical reduction within digital fibro-osseous canal is requirement for flexor tendon recovery.

INTRODUCTION

- Extensor tendon injuries are more common than flexor tendon injuries because of the subcutaneous location and the vulnerability of the hand to penetrating trauma
- Extrinsic system originates proximal at the elbow or forearm and tendons cross the dorsal wrist through six fibro-osseous tunnels which hold the tendons in close apposition to the radius
- Extensor tendon injuries classified into eight zones by Kleinert and Verdan
  - ▹ Odd numbers describe injuries at the joint level beginning with zone 1 at the DIP joint
  - ▹ Thumb extensor injuries are similarly classified into five zones (**Figure 1**)

PATIENT SELECTION

Contraindications

- Closed extensor tendon injury amenable to splint treatment
- Extensive comorbid conditions or neurologic dysfunction

PREOPERATIVE IMAGING

- Plain radiographs to assess bony avulsion type disruptions, joint subluxation, or other associated injuries
- MRI or CT rarely indicated
- Occasionally ultrasonography may be helpful
- Physical examination remains the mainstay of diagnosis

PROCEDURE

Zone I—Type 1 Mallet Injuries

- Terminal extensor tendon disruption is common that can occur with an open laceration or closed injury from a flexion force to an extended finger

Based on Jemison DM: Extensor tendon repair, in Colvin AC, Flatow E, eds: Atlas of Essential Orthopaedic Procedures, *ed 2. Rosemont, IL, American Academy of Orthopaedic Surgeons, 2020, pp 435-445.*

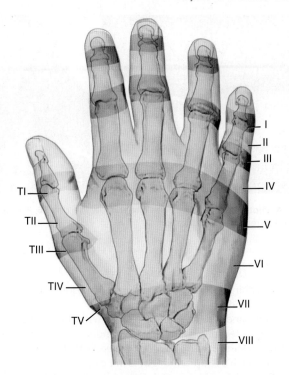

FIGURE 1 Illustration of the eight extensor tendon zones. T = thumb. (Reproduced with permission from Hunt TR, Wiesel SW: *Operative Techniques in Hand, Wrist, and Forearm Surgery*, ed 1. Philadelphia, PA, Wolters Kluwer Health, 2010.)

- Treat with full-time extension splinting for 6 to 8 weeks followed by weaning period of part-time splinting for additional 4 to 6 weeks
- Surgical pinning may rarely be indicated for patients who are unable to comply with splinting

Surgical Technique: Closed Pin Fixation of the DIPJ

- Perform under local anesthesia with fluoroscopy
- K-wires (0.045″ or 0.035″ diameter) in an axial or oblique direction across the joint
- For axial direction, start wire at the distal tuft, just under nail plate
- Wire should be in the intramedullary canal and stop just at the subchondral bone of the base of the middle phalanx to avoid PIP joint penetration
- Withdraw wire a few millimeters and cut at the skin level; tap into position just below the skin

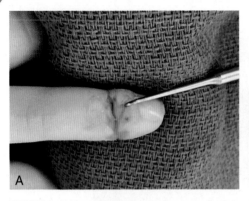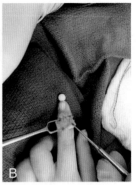

FIGURE 2 A, Photograph showing open mallet injury in a child. **B,** Photograph showing suture repair and pin fixation.

Zone I—Type II Open Mallet Injury

- Sharp or crushing laceration to the dorsal distal joint frequently injures the terminal tendon
- Débride joint and repair extensor tendon with direct suturing or dermatotenodesis technique suturing skin and tendon as one layer
- Use 4-0 or 5-0 suture with a small taper needle that will not cut through thin tendon such as Supramid that is not dyed
- Immobilize with K-wire across the joint in a buried fashion as described above or cut outside finger with a pin protector
- Apply Mallet-type splint with pin removal at 6 weeks (**Figure 2**)

Surgical Technique: Suture Techniques

- Extensor mechanism is thin and does not tolerate shortening or lengthening
- Recent evidence supports use of dorsal epitendinous suture called the running-interlocking horizontal mattress (RIHM) suture technique (**Figure 3**)
- Core sutures techniques such as modified Kessler and Bunnell are appropriate for tubular and substantial extensor anatomy in Zone V-VII

Zone I—Type III Open Mallet Injury With Soft Tissues Loss

- More complex open injury with multiple structure damaged
- May require tendon graft, or if the joint is significantly injured, an arthrodesis may be required

Zone I—Type IV B Mallet Injury

- Injury involves <50% of joint surface
- No volar subluxation

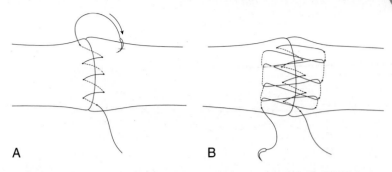

FIGURE 3 Illustration of RIHM (running-interlocking horizontal mattress) technique. **A,** How to perform the new extensor tendon running-interlocking horizontal mattress repair technique: Begin the simple running suture at the near end. **B,** How to perform the new extensor tendon running-interlocking horizontal mattress repair technique: Run the interlocking horizontal mattress suture by starting at the far end. The suture needle passes underneath the prior crossing suture to lock each throw. Finish the suture and tie at the near end. (Reproduced with permission from Lee SK, Dubey A, Kim BH, et al: A biomechanical study of extensor tendon repair methods: Introduction to the running-interlocking horizontal mattress extensor tendon repair technique. *J Hand Surg Am* 2010;35[1]:19-23.)

- Mallet splint or a closed pin fixation will result in satisfactory result in most cases
- Recommend radiograph of the finger if a volar splint is applied, because this can produce distal phalanx subluxation dorsally

Zone I–Type IV C Mallet Injury With Subluxation

- Management is controversial
- Small study suggested that these patients with subluxated DIPJ can be treated satisfactorily with splinting only
- Results of closed pin techniques have been satisfactory such as extension block pinning with low rates of complication
- Open reduction techniques have a higher complication rate and should be reserved for painful nonunions or young patients with chronic injury

Surgical Technique: Extension Block Pin Fixation—Mallet Fracture

- Local anesthesia and fluoroscopy
- DIPJ is flexed and single smooth K-wire (0.045″) drilled into head of middle phalanx at a 45° angle
- Drill similar wire from distal tuft retrograde and stop at the joint surface
- Translate distal phalanx to reduce subluxation
- The angular pin will push the fragment into a reduced position
- While reduce, drill the axial pin across the middle phalanx

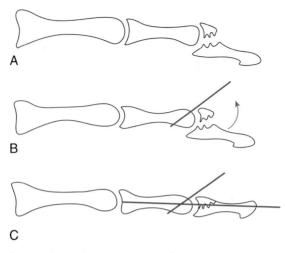

FIGURE 4 Illustration of extension block pinning. **A,** Significant mallet fracture with distal phalanx volar subluxation. **B,** Smooth K-wire placement (0.045″ diameter) at a 45° angle to the middle phalangeal shaft at the dorsal articular surface. **C,** Extend and dorsally translate the distal phalanx, thereby reducing the fragment and the joint. The transarticular wire is then drilled into middle phalanx. (Drawing courtesy of Chase Kluemper, MD.)

- Apply splint postoperatively; remove oblique pin by 4 weeks and the axial pin at 6 weeks (**Figure 4**)
- Complications include pin tract infection, stiffness, and loss of fracture reduction

Chronic Mallet Finger—Swan Neck Deformity

- Can present late with a chronic deformity consisting of distal joint flexion
  - Splinting is generally partially effective but open repair often necessary
  - Open treatment may require tendon graft or DIPJ arthrodesis
- Swan neck deformity is more often present with chronic presentation
  - Proximal migration of the terminal extensor tendon with elongated healing and dorsal shifting of the lateral bands from transverse retinacular ligament attenuation results in PIPJ hyperextension and DIPJ flexion
  - Must also have laxity at the volar plate of the PIPJ to result in this deformity

Surgical Technique: Fowler Central Slip Tenotomy

- Perform under local anesthesia to allow patient to demonstrate intraoperative improvement
- Consider use of digital tourniquet

- Mid lateral incision and protect dorsal sensory branch of the digital nerve
- Release transverse retinacular ligament and elevate the lateral band and central slip
- Identify the insertion of the central slip descending toward the dorsal ridge of the middle phalanx and release with a #11 blade
- Take care to protect lateral bands and triangular ligament distally
- Should demonstrate correction of deformity intraoperatively
- Variable recommendations for postoperative splinting but can be no immobilization to a month-long regimen of blocking full PIPJ extension and splinting the DIPJ in extension
- Complications for this procedure include insufficient correction, stiffness, or conversion of deformity to a boutonniere deformity if the triangular ligament is attenuated

Zone II Lateral Bands—Triangular Ligament

- Often from a laceration and should be repaired as described above
- Use running-interlocking horizontal mattress to avoid shortening and to provide strength
- Immobilize the DIPJ, usually with K-wire fixation

Zone III Central Slip—PIPJ Level

- Repair open injuries with joint arthrotomy and oblique K-wire for fixation
    - Use 3-0 or 4-0 braided nylon or monofilament suture
    - Reattach the central slip with a suture anchor or drill hole
    - Maintain K-wire for 4 to 6 weeks along with a PIPJ extension splint, and active DIPJ and MCPJ motion should be encouraged
- Closed injuries generally result from volar dislocation; late development can lead to boutonniere deformity
    - Deformity results from central slip rupture and the lateral bands subluxate volarly resulting in a flexion force at the PIPJ; as lateral band tightens, DIPJ hyperextension results
    - Diagnose a boutonniere deformity with Elson test; patient should not be able to extend the DIPJ with the PIPJ held in flexion with an intact central slip
    - Managed best with a static PIPJ extension splint for 6 weeks and a dynamic spring loaded splint afterward
    - With fixed a deformity, restore passive extension with splinting or serial casting
    - Perform stepwise release as described by Curtis
    - If deformity is still present, perform rebalancing procedure such as the distal Fowler or Dolphin tenotomy, which is a near-complete distal tendon release

---

Zone IV Proximal Phalanx

- Open injuries at the level are often partial because extensor mechanism surrounds the phalanx
- Repair indicated if there is >50% involvement
- Test repair by moving PIPJ and MCPJ to see which exerts more force on repair, which should direct splint management

Zone V Metacarpophalangeal Joint

- Almost always requires surgical repair; débride and close capsule if wound is not significantly contaminated
- Human bite injuries require multiple, early débridements
- Central extensor tendon is tubular and amenable to core suture placement and epitendinous suture to allow early active motion rehabilitation protocols

Closed Radial Sagittal Band Rupture

- Sagittal hood stabilizes EDC tendon over top of the MCPJ
- Attenuation of the radial sagittal band occurs causing the tendon to dislocate to the ulnar side
- Damage to sagittal band can also be from trauma, with forced ulnar deviation of the fingers; long and ring fingers often affected
- Patients present with swollen MCPJ, which is frequently ulnarly deviated and possibly locked in flexion
- Visible reduction of the tendon over the MCPJ when joint is extended
- For acute injuries, a trial of MCPJ splinting with the joint in extension can result in complete healing
- Relative motion splinting is also an option, with the affected MCPJ held in 15° to 20° more extended position than neighboring joints (**Figure 5**)
- Chronic injuries require surgical repair or reconstruction of the radial sagittal hood to centralize the tendon (**Figure 6**)

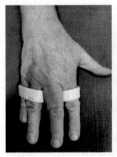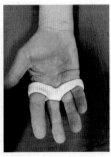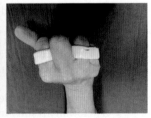

FIGURE 5 Photograph showing immediate controlled active motion splinting—note the good interphalangeal motion allowed by the splint.

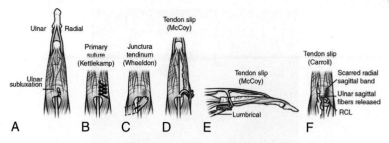

FIGURE 6 A, Illustration of ulnar subluxation of the extensor digitorum communis (EDC) tendon caused by a torn or lacerated sagittal band. **B** through **F,** Illustrations of several methods of sagittal band reconstruction. **B,** Primary suture of the radial sagittal band to center the EDC tendon. **C,** The ulnar juncturae tendinum is released from the adjacent tendon and sutured to the palmar radial sagittal band remnant of the deep intermetacarpal ligament. **D** and **E,** The distal tendon is splinted on the radial side and wrapped around the lumbrical muscle. **F,** The ulnar, distally based slip of EDC is looped around the radial collateral ligament (RCL). (Reproduced with permission from Kleinhenz BP, Adams BD: Closed sagittal band injury of the metacarpophalangeal joint. *J Am Acad Orthop Surg* 2015;23:415-423.)

Surgical Technique: Radial Sagittal Band Reconstruction

- Perform under general or regional anesthesia with arm board
- Curved incision over the injured MCPJ
- Explore dorsal hood mechanism
- EDC tendon is usually dislocated into ulnar sulcus between metacarpal heads
- Mobilize EDC tendon, usually requiring release of the ulnar sagittal band
- Create a distally based strip of EDC and sometimes juncturae is created from the radial or ulnar side of the tendon, stopping at the distal MCPJ
- Pass tendon strip through or under main tendon
- Use Carroll tendon passer to pass the strip through the volar radial hood and around the radial collateral ligament or lumbrical and then back to the EDC
- Suture with nonabsorbable braided nylon (aim toward overcorrection) **(Figures 7** and **8)**
- Close skin in standard fashion
- Immobilize with splint holding the MCPJs in some flexion and the IPJs free
- Follow up postop in 12 to 14 days for suture removal and apply relative motion splint for 8 weeks of use
- Complications include loss of correction, adhesion, stiffness, and EDC rupture

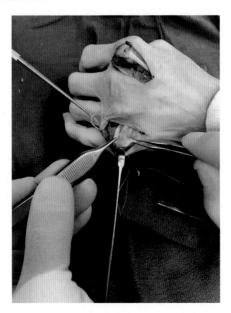

FIGURE 7 Intraoperative photograph showing radial sagittal band reconstruction. Zone V reconstruction using a distally based extensor tendon strip in a rheumatoid patient following synovectomy—note the centralized tendon at the index MCPJ.

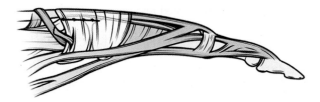

FIGURE 8 Illustration of the lateral aspect of the finger demonstrating the transfer of the ulnar-sided juncturae through the repaired radial sagittal band. This will prevent ulnar subluxation of the extensor tendon. (Reproduced with permission from Kleinhenz BP, Adams BD: Closed sagittal band injury of the metacarpophalangeal joint. *J Am Acad Orthop Surg* 2015;23:415-423.)

Zone VI—Metacarpal Level

- Lacerations at this level typically involve multiple structures and likely multiple extensor tendons
- Good prognosis for repair at this level
- Tendons are more tubular, allowing core suture placement and augmentation with epitendinous repair

- Tendons more forgiving of length changes because of the extrinsic extensor muscles
- Accurately align tendons to EIP and EDM, which are both on the ulnar side of the MCPJ

Zone VII Wrist—Extensor Retinaculum Level
- Retinaculum can be partially opened but >50% of the retinaculum needs to be preserved to prevent bowstringing
- These tendons tendon to retract as muscles shorten; advisable to repair these as quick as possible

Zone VIII Distal Forearm
- This is at the level of the musculotendinous junction, making repair difficult
- Use 3-0 or 4-0 kevlar type suture with a taper needle
- Avoid injury to dorsal radial sensory nerve

Zone IX Proximal Forearm
- Frequently involve neurovascular injury if deep
- Repair generally only consists of fascia repair
- Static splinting for 6 weeks is best option after Zones VIII because of the tenuous strength of repair at these levels

COMPLICATIONS
- Wound or pin tract infection
- Repair rupture
- Tendon adhesions

POSTOPERATIVE CARE
- Rehabilitation protocols recommended under guidance of certified hand therapist guidance

PEARLS

- Anatomic restoration for extensor tendon repairs should be goal; avoid shortening or lengthening the tendon.
- Avoid including other tissue layers such as adjacent periosteum or joint capsule with repair.
- Intraoperatively, passively move adjacent joints to assess tension at repair site.
- Zone V wrist extensor repairs should not be delayed because musculotendinous retraction occurs, making repair more difficult.

PATIENT SELECTION AND INDICATIONS

- Patients who may benefit from wide-awake hand surgery include the following:
  - ▶ Those who have procedures in which patient participation can optimize outcomes (such as tendon transfers, tendon repairs, or other such procedures)
  - ▶ Patients in whom medical comorbidities preclude use of traditional systemic or regional anesthetics
  - ▶ Patients who require anticoagulation that must continue in the perioperative period
  - ▶ Patients who can tolerate sitting or lying awake during the procedure
  - ▶ Advantages include the ability to perform surgery outside of the operating room and without a tourniquet
  - ▶ No need for preoperative medical testing, preoperative medical clearance, or placement of an IV, and no need for the patient to refrain from eating or drinking before the procedure
  - ▶ Location, procedure, and surgical site amenable to field block

Contraindications

- Excessive anxiety, unwillingness, or inability to tolerate being awake during procedure
- One of the requirements for wide-awake hand surgery is ability to provide a field block sufficient to provide anesthesia for completion of the procedure; thus certain procedures may be less amenable to this technique
- Poorly vascularized digits or substantial cardiovascular history can represent a relative contraindication in some circumstances

PROCEDURE

Room Setup/Patient Positioning

- Critical to the technique is infiltration of local anesthesia with sufficient time for epinephrine to exert its hemostatic effect (>30 min before incision)

Based on Adams JE: Wide-awake hand surgery, in Colvin AC, Flatow E, eds: Atlas of Essential Orthopaedic Procedures, *ed 2. Rosemont, IL, American Academy of Orthopaedic Surgeons, 2020, pp 446-450.*

Special Instruments/Equipment/Implants

- Local anesthesia with epinephrine (often used is 1% lidocaine 1:100,000 with epinephrine), bicarbonate solution to buffer local anesthesia (**Figure 1**)

Surgical Technique

- Tips for minimizing pain associated with local injection:
  - Buffer solution to neutralize the pH; 1 mL of 8.4% bicarbonate is mixed with 10 mL of lidocaine
  - Warm local anesthetic is less painful than colder temperatures
  - Use smaller bore needle (25, 27, or 30 gauge)
  - Inject perpendicular to skin rather than oblique angle
  - Inject slowly and advance the needle slowly
  - Steady hand to limit the movement of the needle (**Figure 2**)
- Other helpful tips
  - Use high volumes of local anesthetic (dilute the local anesthetic with saline to increase volume of the injection)
    - Maximum dose is generally 7 mg/kg of 1% lidocaine 1:100,000 with epinephrine (for a 70 kg individual, nearly 50 mL of this solution can be used, which is adequate for most cases)
    - If larger field of epinephrine is required, dilute the local anesthesia with saline; 0.25% lidocaine with 1:400,000 epinephrine is still effective and provides hemostatic effect

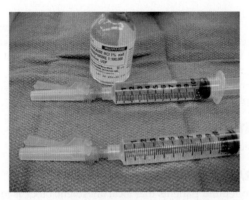

FIGURE 1 Photograph of buffered lidocaine 1:100,000 with epinephrine being drawn up and prepared to be injected. The volume used depends upon the location of surgery and procedure type. Usually 20 mL is used for a carpal tunnel release.

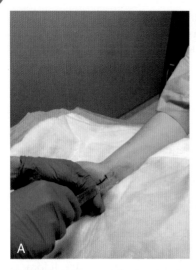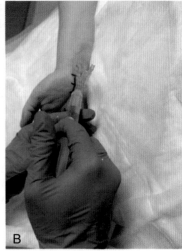

FIGURE 2 A, Photographs showing the needle being introduced just proximal to the wrist crease, perpendicular (or nearly so) to the skin, and a small wheal of anesthetic being injected subcutaneously and slowly. Pause and ask when the patient cannot feel the needle before (**B**) continuing to advance the needle obliquely and inject more medication. Inject 10 mL, and introduce second syringe, this time, advancing distally in the palm, injecting slowly and ensuring adequate local medication is ahead of the advancing needle to provide anesthetic.

▹ Inject local anesthetic as field block when used proximal to the metacarpal head level dorsally or proximal to the carpal tunnel level volarly; proximal to this level, use local anesthesia such as "extravascular Bier block"

▹ Optimal wait time is >30 minutes after injection for maximum hemostatic effect

COMPLICATIONS
• Digital necrosis

POSTOPERATIVE CARE AND REHABILITATION
• Helpful to remind patients that local anesthetic block is long lasting
• Patients should avoid situations that might cause injury to anesthetized digit

PEARLS

- For surgeons starting out with this technique, perform these procedures in operating room with light sedation and transition to local anesthesia in the office or other facility as the surgeon gains confidence in his/her ability to obtain adequate hemostasis and anesthesia.
- Inject the patient in a supine or reclining position in case the patient has a vasovagal response.
- No evidence that intraoperative monitoring of blood pressure, pulse oximetry, or other parameters is necessary.
- Use of this technique is helpful for patient education and assessing intraoperative tension of repair of injured structures such as tendon repairs or reconstructions (**Figure 3**)

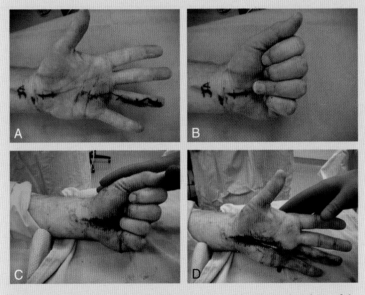

FIGURE 3 **A** and **B**, Photographs showing the case demonstrating the usefulness of having wide-awake anesthesia to assess motion and repair of a flexor tendon. This patient had an intrasubstance tendon rupture, and underwent repair. Preoperatively, he had no active flexion at the distal interphalangeal joint, indicating absent flexor digitorum profundus (FDP) function. **C** and **D**, Postoperatively, he had restoration of FDP function and could fully extend his digits without contracture or gapping of the repair.

VIDEO 54.1 This video demonstrates the capacity for the surgeon and patient to assess quality of repair (in this instance for a flexor tendon, any evidence of gapping of the repair), and motion intraoperatively. If needed, adjustments may be made before the completion of the procedure. Julie Adams, MD (17 s)

VIDEO 54.2 Wide-awake surgery is helpful to assess adequate tension for tendon transfers, as in this patient who underwent an EIP (extensor indicis proprius) to EPL (extensor pollicis longus) transfer for a ruptured EPL tendon. Julie Adams, MD (18 s)

Adult
Reconstruction

4

Section Editor
Stephen J. Incavo, MD

Hip Arthroplasty via Small-Incision Enhanced Posterior Soft-Tissue Repair

INTRODUCTION

- Small-incision enhanced posterior soft-tissue repair (SIEPSTR) is performed through a limited incision compared with the standard posterior approach
- Involves meticulous reconstruction of posterior structures to reduce dislocation risk
- No absolute contraindications; relative contraindications are the same as those for the posterior approach, including Parkinson disease, dementia, and inability to follow posterior hip precautions

PREOPERATIVE IMAGING AND PLANNING

- AP pelvis
- AP hip
- Cross-table lateral hip
- Preoperative templating and clinical examination determine the plan for leg length and offset

PROCEDURE

Room Setup/Patient Positioning

- Operating room table modified for posterior approach total hip arthroplasty (THA)
- Lateral decubitus position using well-padded lateral hip positioner
- Use an axillary roll
- Pad all bony prominences
- Test range of motion (ROM) to ensure that hip positioner does not interfere
- Place bump under the knee
- Palpate and mark greater trochanter

Based on Lee JH, Macaulay W, Orio A: Hip arthroplasty via small-incision enhanced posterior soft-tissue repair, in Colvin AC, Flatow E, eds: Atlas of Essential Orthopaedic Procedures, *ed 2. Rosemont, IL, American Academy of Orthopaedic Surgeons, 2020, pp 451-457.*

Surgical Technique: Total Hip Arthroplasty

 VIDEO 55.1 Noncemented Total Hip Arthroplasty via a Posterior Approach Using Enhanced Posterior Soft-Tissue Repair. William Macaulay, MD (16 min)

Incision

- Draw a curvilinear incision with the distal portion centered over the lateral femur and curving posteriorly in line with the fibers of the gluteus medius once the incision reaches the tip of the greater trochanter. Approximately 2/3 of the incision should be distal to the tip of the greater trochanter, with 1/3 of the incision extending proximal (**Figure 1**)

Dissection

- Sharply incise skin; coagulate bleeding vessels
- Sharply dissect down to fascia lata
- Incise tensor fascia over most prominent lateral aspect of greater trochanter
- Use Mayo scissors to extend fascial incision distally and bluntly divide gluteus maximus muscle proximally using a finger
- Identify short external rotators and place thin bent Hohmann "over the top" of piriformis to separate it from gluteus medius

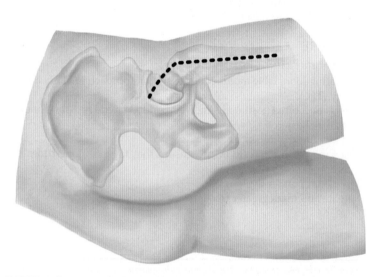

FIGURE 1 Illustration shows the position of the planned incision for hip arthroplasty using the small-incision enhanced posterior soft-tissue repair (SIEPSTR) approach.

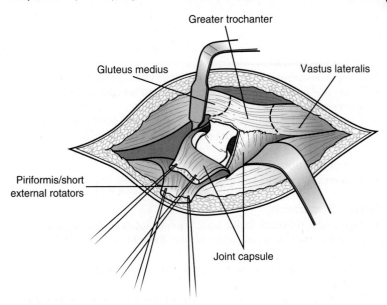

FIGURE 2 Illustration shows the exposure for total hip arthroplasty using the small-incision enhanced posterior soft-tissue repair (SIEPSTR) approach. The piriformis tendon and the conjoined tendons, which have been detached as a tendinous sleeve from their insertions, are tagged superiorly and inferiorly using nonabsorbable sutures and then reflected posteriorly. Arthrotomy of the posterior capsule has created a posteriorly based trapezoid-shaped capsular sleeve that is likewise tagged twice with sutures and reflected posteriorly.

- Place Aufranc retractor on the capsule beneath the femoral neck
- Internally rotate leg, and release short external rotator tendons from femur
- Tag tendons with two No. 2 nonabsorbable colored braided sutures
- Use Cobb elevator to sweep gluteus minimus off of capsule
- Incise capsule in "U" fashion superiorly along former inferior border of gluteus minimus and inferiorly at the trochanteric fossa
- Tag capsule superiorly and inferiorly with No. 2 braided nonabsorbable suture (**Figure 2**)
- Divide the quadratus with electrocautery to expose the lesser trochanter
- Dislocate femoral head by flexing, adducting, and internally rotating the leg
- Cut femoral neck with reciprocating saw at templated level above lesser trochanter

Acetabular Preparation
- Place anterior retractor over anterior rim of acetabulum
- Incise inferior capsule to level of the transverse acetabular ligament (TAL)

- Impact posterior retractor posteroinferiorly between labrum and capsule into ischium
- Place Steinmann pin into superior ilium beneath the minimus to enhance exposure
- Remove acetabular labrum and pulvinar while preserving the TAL
- Ream the acetabulum in approximately 40° of abduction and 20° of anteversion
- Align the trial with the anterior rim of the acetabulum and TAL. If it is too tight increase the reamer one size and gently widen the opening of the acetabulum
- Impact final acetabular shell and insert liner
- Remove any marginal or impinging osteophytes

Femoral Preparation
- Expose the proximal femur with internal rotation, a femoral elevator, and a thin bent Hohmann retractor over the anterior aspect of the greater trochanter
- Remove any remaining soft tissue in the shoulder region of the greater trochanter
- Access the proximal femoral canal using a box osteotome entering posterolaterally and in slight anteversion followed by a canal finder
- Femoral preparation with reaming if indicated and sequential broaching to appropriate fit

Trialing and Final Implant Insertion
- Trial head and neck are placed, and lesser trochanter to center of head distance is measured using a ruler and is compared with the preoperative template
- The hip is reduced and brought through a ROM to test stability
  - Combined version of the acetabulum and femoral implant is measured (goal 35° to 45°)
  - Bring hip to 90° of flexion; internally rotate to 60°
  - Bring hip to full extension, and flex the knee (drop kick test) to check for overly tight anterior musculature
  - Check for posterior impingement by placing finger between greater trochanter and ischium with the leg extended and in external rotation
- The hip is dislocated, and trial implants are removed
- Final stem is impacted with a mallet, taking care to listen for pitch change
- The lesser trochanter to center of head distance is again verified
- The hip is reduced, and stability is rechecked

Closure
- SIEPSTR is initiated by drilling two holes 1.5 cm apart on posterior aspect of greater trochanter in line with capsular tag sutures
- Use suture passer to retrieve both capsular and short external rotator tag sutures

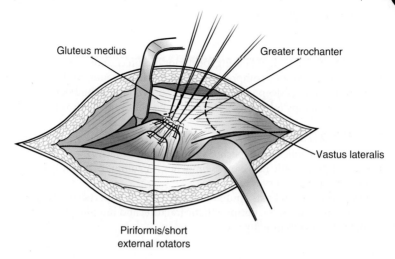

FIGURE 3 Illustration shows the reapproximation of the muscles and the hip capsule following implant placement for total hip arthroplasty using the small-incision enhanced posterior soft-tissue repair (SIEPSTR) approach. The longer superior and inferior capsular sutures are tied together first. Then the shorter external rotator sutures are tied together to restore the posterior soft-tissue envelope.

- Place leg in neutral, tie capsular tag sutures to one another, and then tie short external rotator tag sutures (**Figure 3**)
- Palpate capsule to ensure appropriate tension
- Copiously irrigate wound with pulsatile lavage
- Close fascial layer and irrigate wound again
- Final closure and drains per surgeon preference

Surgical Technique: Hemiarthroplasty

- Same approach as above but technique begins to diverge at the moment of capsulotomy
- Preserve labrum when performing capsular incision
  - ▶ Palpate edge of acetabulum before making capsulotomy
  - ▶ Make incision 10 mm away from palpated acetabular rim
- Removal of femoral head
  - ▶ Corkscrew and hip skid may be used to facilitate removal
  - ▶ Take care to keep head in one piece to allow for accurate measurement
- All bony fragments are removed from capsule and acetabulum
- Acetabulum and labrum are inspected for damage; if severe damage is noted, conversion to THA should be considered
- The femur is then prepared as described previously, trials are placed, and stability is checked
- The procedure then follows the same remaining steps as SIEPSTR THA

POSTOPERATIVE CARE

- An abduction pillow is placed
- Final radiographs are taken
- Immediate full weight bearing; posterior hip precautions for six weeks
- Early mobilization, compression devices, and chemoprophylaxis to minimize risk of deep vein thrombosis and venous thromboembolism
- Physical therapy is begun immediately and continued for 6 to 12 weeks

COMPLICATIONS

- Minimal complications specific to posterior approach
- Injury to the sciatic nerve or its branches (uncommon) possibly due to retraction of the nerve
- Deep vein thrombosis, pulmonary embolism, superficial and deep infection, dislocation, periprosthetic fracture, and limb-length discrepancy can be infrequently seen

PEARLS

- Check hip ROM after patient is positioned but before draping to ensure full ROM is achievable.
- A bolster under ipsilateral knee can relax lateral structures to make exposure easier.
- Internal rotation of leg before removal of piriformis and short external rotators allows removal of the tendons as close as possible to their bony insertions.
- "Airplane" table posteriorly during acetabular preparation to improve visualization.
- Avoid eccentric reaming leading to overreaming of the posterior acetabular wall.
- Maintain visualization of inferior femoral neck while broaching.

Hip Arthroplasty via a Traditional and Minimally Invasive Direct Lateral Approach

PATIENT SELECTION

Indications

- Primary and revision total hip arthroplasty
- Hemiarthroplasty for displaced femoral neck fractures
- Useful for patients with neuromuscular disorders, dementia, or alcoholism, because it reduces dislocation risk; also useful in those who cannot follow posterior hip precautions

Contraindications

- High hip centers or hip dysplasia requiring access to superior acetabulum and ilium
- Hardware removal or bone grafting requiring extensive dissection and exposure of the posterior wall or column

PREOPERATIVE IMAGING

- AP pelvis
- AP and lateral hip
- Cross-table lateral hip
- Judet views or CT for abnormal anatomy (ie, dysplasia)

PROCEDURE

Room Setup/Patient Positioning

- Lateral decubitus position with a lateral positioner
- Use an axillary roll and pad all bony prominences well
- Skin preparation and draping are done according to surgeon preference
- Add a sterile leg bag to final drape anteriorly to patient to maintain sterility when dislocating surgical hip (**Figure 1**)

Based on Petis S, Vasarhelyi EM: Hip arthroplasty via a traditional and minimally invasive direct lateral approach, in Colvin AC, Flatow E, eds: Atlas of Essential Orthopaedic Procedures, *ed 2. Rosemont, IL, American Academy of Orthopaedic Surgeons, 2020, pp 458-464.*

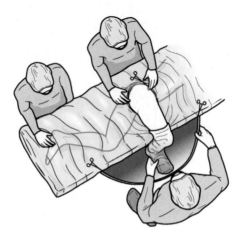

FIGURE 1 Illustration shows the use of a sterile drape bag to keep the ipsilateral leg sterile during hip arthroplasty via a direct lateral approach.

Surgical Technique: Total Hip Arthroplasty

 VIDEO 56.1 Total Hip Arthroplasty via a Direct Lateral Approach. Tahir Mahmud, BSc (Hons), MBBS, FRCS (Tr & Orth); Robert B. Bourne, MD, FRCSC (3 min)

Surgical Approach
- Mark greater trochanter on skin
- Incision centered over the greater trochanter running obliquely from posterior proximally to anterior distally (**Figure 2**)
- Dissection carried down to fascia lata using electrocautery

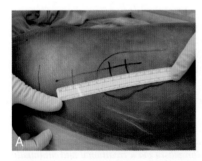
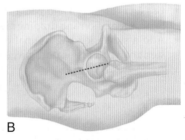

FIGURE 2 Photograph (**A**) and illustration (**B**) show the skin incision for the direct lateral approach for hip arthroplasty. The incision is centered over the tip of the greater trochanter.

- Identify and incise the fascia lata distally
- A finger is inserted to develop the plane between the fascia and deeper musculature (vastus lateralis, gluteus medius) and the fascial incision is extended
- Place Charnley retractor under anterior and posterior fascia lata to improve exposure

Exposing the Hip Joint

- Bluntly split fibers of gluteus medius longitudinally at junction of the anterior one-third and posterior two-thirds of the muscle belly
- Take care to ensure the split does not extend too far proximally (5 cm from tip of greater trochanter) to avoid damaging superior gluteal nerve (**Figure 3**)
- Reflect the gluteus medius and minimus conjoined tendons anteriorly off the greater trochanter and femoral neck

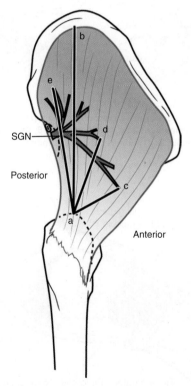

FIGURE 3 Illustration depicts the relationship of the superior gluteal nerve (SGN) to the greater trochanter. a = tip of the greater trochanter; b = gluteal ridge; c = inferior branch of the SGN; d = middle branch of the SGN; e = superior branch of the SGN

- Carry incision into the proximal anterior portion of vastus lateralis in the shape of an omega if needed for exposure (**Figure 4**)
- Insert blunt Hohmann retractor proximal to lesser trochanter to retract the anterior soft-tissue sleeve
- Sweep fat away from gluteus medius fascia, and incise tendon and capsule in line with neck
- Insert pin in iliac crest posterior to ASIS; this is used as a landmark in assessing femoral offset and leg length
- Dislocate hip by flexing, externally rotating, and adducting the leg
- Place leg into sterile bag with tibia perpendicular to floor
- Make femoral neck cut with oscillating saw at templated level (**Figure 5**)

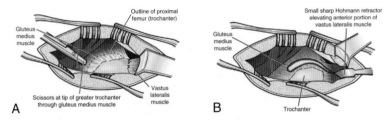

FIGURE 4 Illustrations demonstrate exposure of the hip joint for total hip arthroplasty. **A,** The gluteus medius muscle is split carefully. **B,** An anterior sleeve consisting of the gluteus medius and minimus conjoined tendons is mobilized anteriorly.

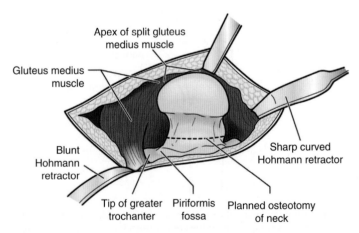

FIGURE 5 Illustration demonstrates femoral neck osteotomy for total hip arthroplasty.

Preparation of Acetabulum

- Expose acetabulum by placing blunt Hohmann retractor over the anterior rim to retract anterior tissue sleeve and a bent Hohmann over the posterior rim of the acetabulum
- Superiorly a sharp Hohmann or Hibbs retractor is used to retract the gluteus medius and minimus (**Figure 6**)
- Excise labrum and soft tissues of acetabulum
- Sequential reaming of the acetabulum to the appropriate size
- Osteophyte removal as needed

Femoral Preparation

- Insert curved Mueller retractor under posterior greater trochanter
- Flex and externally rotate leg so tibia is perpendicular to floor and place in sterile bag
- Place two straight sharp Hohmann retractors under the posteromedial femoral neck and between the trochanter and gluteus medius tendon
- The proximal femur is prepared as dictated by implant design and surgeon preference
- Trial components are placed, and the hip is taken through range of motion to ensure there is no impingement and the joint is stable both anteriorly and posteriorly
- The leg length-offset guide is used at this point to ensure appropriate restoration of offset and correction of leg lengths as templated
- Dislocate hip, remove broach and trials, and place final implants
- Reduce hip and check final stability

Wound Closure

- Layered closure using braided absorbable suture

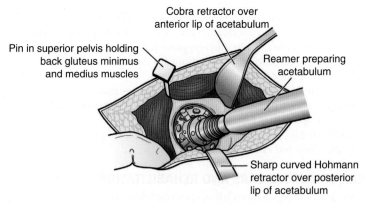

FIGURE 6 Illustration shows the exposure of the acetabulum to facilitate reaming in a total hip arthroplasty.

- Repair split in the gluteus minimus and capsule with a running suture from proximal to its distal insertion on the greater trochanter
- The gluteus medius and vastus lateralis are repaired with interrupted sutures and oversewn with a running suture. This step is critical in restoration of abductor function postoperatively
- Fascia lata closed with running suture
- Subcutaneous tissues and skin approximated with interrupted sutures and a running subcuticular suture or skin staples

Surgical Technique: Minimally Invasive Direct Lateral Approach
- Patient positioning is the same as described previously
- An 8 to 10 cm incision is sufficient for most patients
- Oblique incision centered over the midfemur proximally and the anterior femur distally
- The anterior trajectory distally allows for improved acetabular exposure, while the posterior trajectory proximally allows for in line access to the proximal femur
- The gluteus medius is split in the midline with half anterior and half posterior
- Retractor placement as described is critical for acetabular and femoral exposure. Femoral exposure may be improved with slight release of the posterior gluteus medius fibers from their insertion
- This approach is best suited for a broach only stem, as reaming may damage the soft tissues

Surgical Technique: Hemiarthroplasty
- Positioning and approach are the same as described previously
- Take care to ensure that labrum remains intact; incise capsule 10 mm away from palpated edge of acetabulum to protect labrum
- Insert deeper Charnley blade into anterior capsule to retract anterior soft-tissue sleeve more anteriorly
- Place leg into leg bag and freshen neck cut with reciprocating saw
- Place leg back onto the table and remove the femoral head with a corkscrew; take care to keep it in one piece for accurate templating
- Inspect the acetabulum and labrum for damage; may convert to total hip arthroplasty if necessary at this step
- Leave the pulvinar and acetabular soft tissues intact.
- Prepare the proximal femur as indicated by the implant system used
- Place trials, reduce hip, and check stability
- Dislocate hip, remove trials, and place final implants
- Reduce hip and check final stability

POSTOPERATIVE CARE AND REHABILITATION
- Weight bearing as tolerated on postoperative day 1
- Physical therapy should begin on postoperative day 1
- Defer abductor strengthening for four weeks postoperatively

COMPLICATIONS

- Damage to the superior gluteal nerve leading to partial denervation of the gluteus medius and tensor fascia lata
- Limp (abductor lurch) due to abductor weakness, poor repair, or superior gluteal nerve injury
- Superficial and deep infection, deep vein thrombosis, pulmonary embolism, limb-length discrepancy, dislocation, heterotopic ossification, bleeding, sciatic nerve injury, and periprosthetic fracture

PEARLS

- Avoid splitting gluteus medius more than 5 cm proximal to tip of anterior greater trochanter to prevent damage to superior gluteal nerve.
- Ensure a strong abductor repair by making the gluteus medius split at the tendinous junction just anterior to greater trochanter so a sleeve of tendon is left on both sides of split.
- When performing the minimally invasive technique, an oblique incision from slightly posterior proximally to anterior distally is preferred to facilitate exposure.

57 Direct Anterior Approach for Hip Arthroplasty

PATIENT SELECTION

Indications
- Primary total hip arthroplasty (THA)
- Hemiarthroplasty for femoral neck fractures

Relative Contraindications
- Patients who have obesity or are muscular
- Patients with short varus femoral necks
- Dysplasia or deformity
- Revision THA

PREOPERATIVE IMAGING
- AP pelvis
- AP hip
- Cross-table lateral hip

PROCEDURE

Room Setup/Patient Positioning
- Standard radiolucent table
- Supine position
- Hip flexion, adduction, and external rotation of surgical side are required
- Flexion—Place bump under pelvis and flex table 30° before femoral preparation (**Figure 1**)
- Adduction—Attach arm board distally on nonsurgical side of table; place nonsurgical leg onto arm board during femoral preparation to clear space on table for surgical extremity
- External rotation—Applied gently by second assistant when required
- Prepare and drape surgical leg free

Based on Deirmengian GK, Hozack WJ: Direct anterior approach for hip arthroplasty, in Colvin AC, Flatow E, eds: Atlas of Essential Orthopaedic Procedures, *ed 2. Rosemont, IL, American Academy of Orthopaedic Surgeons, 2020, pp 465-473.*

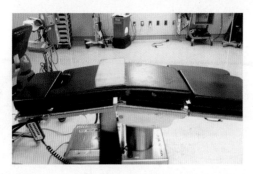

FIGURE 1 Photograph shows the room setup using a standard operating table for the direct anterior approach for total hip arthroplasty. The gel bump, 30° of table flexion, and the distal arm board on the nonsurgical side of the table facilitate the extension and adduction of the surgical lower extremity necessary for femoral exposure.

Special Instruments

- Curved or offset reamers and broaches to facilitate femoral and acetabular preparation
- Certain femoral implant design features, such as reduced lateral shoulder and contoured distal tip, facilitate femoral reconstruction

Surgical Technique: Total Hip Arthroplasty

 VIDEO 57.1 Direct Anterior Approach for Total Hip Arthroplasty. Gregory K. Deirmengian, MD; William J. Hozack, MD (23 min)

Incision Planning and Superficial Dissection

- Careful planning of skin incision is critical
- Palpate and mark borders of anterior superior iliac spine
- Mark the planned incision 2 to 3 cm distal and 2 to 3 cm lateral to the anterior superior iliac spine
- Carry planned incision 8 to 10 cm distal with a gentle lateral slope (**Figure 2, A**)
- If tensor fascia lata (TFL) is palpable, make incision in its midline and follow its course proximally and distally
- Sharply incise skin and subcutaneous fat and use electrocautery as needed for coagulation
- Incise Scarpa fascia and sweep off deep fascia encasing TFL
- Identify the TFL; its medial border is defined by a fat stripe, and its midpoint is defined by small perforating vessels
- Divide fascia overlying TFL in the midpoint of TFL; reflect fascia medially to medial border of TFL

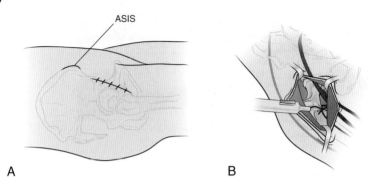

FIGURE 2 Illustrations demonstrate incision planning, dissection, and exposure for total hip arthroplasty using the direct anterior approach. **A,** The anterior superior iliac spine (ASIS) is marked as a landmark. The marking for the incision starts 2 to 3 cm distal and 2 to 3 cm lateral to the inferomedial corner of the ASIS and proceeds distally 8 to 10 cm with a gentle lateral angle. **B,** The lateral femoral circumflex vessels and their branches are cauterized.

- Insert finger posteriorly into interval between TFL and sartorius for blunt dissection to the level of anterior capsule
- Direct finger posterolaterally to reach space between abductors and capsule
- Insert blunt Hohmann retractor into this interval and place sharp angled Hohmann retractor under TFL and over vastus ridge to retract TFL laterally
- A thin layer of fascia overlying the vastus lateralis and femoral neck is now exposed
- Incise this fascia carefully, exposing lateral circumflex vessels, which are meticulously cauterized (**Figure 2, B**)
- Perform blunt dissection to access space anterior to medial femoral neck capsule; insert blunt retractor in this space
- Use Cobb elevator to develop space between anterior acetabular capsule and reflected head of rectus femoris
- Insert lighted sharp Hohmann retractor into this interval; anterior capsule should now be exposed clearly

Acetabular Exposure
- Completely excise anterior capsule by making incision starting at origin of anterior fibers of vastus lateralis and proceeding inferomedially at 45°
- Reposition blunt Hohmann retractors around the femoral neck inside capsule
- Use oscillating saw at two sites to remove a wafer of femoral neck to facilitate head removal

- Make first neck cut at head-neck junction and second at saddle of femoral neck, extending inferomedially at an angle matching proposed implant
- Remove wafer of bone, then remove femoral head with corkscrew

Acetabular Preparation

- Move lighted sharp Hohmann retractor to an intracapsular position and place double sharp angle retractor over posteroinferior lip of acetabulum
- Perform medial capsulotomy and insert angled blunt Hohmann retractor inferior to the teardrop (**Figure 3**)
- Remove all soft tissue, labrum, and osteophytes from acetabulum
- Obtain 360° view of acetabulum and medial teardrop before reaming
- Place small reamer into acetabulum and ream to a hemispherical shape; begin sequential reaming to bleeding bone using offset reamers
- Take care to avoid eccentric anterior, posterior, or lateral reaming
- Impact acetabular shell using offset handle
- If needed, screws may be placed at this time to secure shell
- Inspect rim to ensure removal of all osteophytes; also ensure that shell is completely contained within acetabulum
- Lock in final liner

Femoral Exposure and Preparation

- Remove posterior and inferior acetabular retractors, but leave anterior lighted retractor in wound
- Flex table to 30°, move nonsurgical leg to distal arm board, and have second assistant gently adduct and externally rotate surgical leg

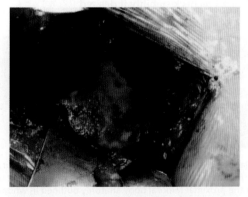

FIGURE 3 Intraoperative photograph demonstrates acetabular exposure for total hip arthroplasty using the direct anterior approach. Exposure of the acetabulum is shown after the retractors have been placed, the obscuring soft tissues have been excised, and osteophytes have been removed. Full exposure of all anatomic landmarks, including the entire rim of the acetabulum, is critical.

- Place sharp angled retractor under TFL and over vastus ridge to retract TFL laterally
- Place Muller retractor between abductors and capsule and excise lateral capsule
- Reposition Muller retractor between tip of greater trochanter and abductors
- Place bone hook into cut surface of femur; pull anteriorly to place posterolateral soft-tissue structures on tension
- Carefully excise posterolateral soft tissue to deliver proximal femur into wound (**Figure 4**)
- Remove lighted anterior retractor and place second Muller retractor along posterior cortex of remaining femoral neck
- Remove lateral femoral neck bone with box osteotome or rasp to prevent varus malpositioning of final implant
- Use curved curet as canal finder and proceed with broaching using offset broach handles
- Carefully avoid broaching from anterior to posterior to prevent perforation of posterior cortex
- After obtaining tight fit, place trial neck and head, reduce hip, and test stability including checking head-liner separation with manual traction
- Dislocate hip by pulling traction and placing anterolateral force on proximal femur with bone hook
- Remove broach and trials
- Insert final stem manually and apply insertion handle for final impaction
- Angle handle posteroinferiorly during impaction to relieve stress on calcar and reduce fracture risk
- Reduce hip and recheck stability if desired

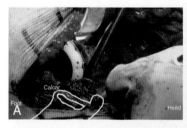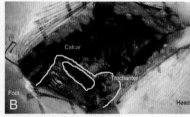

FIGURE 4 Intraoperative photographs demonstrate femoral exposure for total hip arthroplasty using the direct anterior approach. The superior aspect of the wound is shown, with the proximal femoral bony anatomy outlined in white. **A,** The anterior retractor attached to the light source rests on the anterior aspect of the acetabulum. An electrocautery instrument releases soft tissues to allow femoral elevation. **B,** A Muller-type retractor rests posterior to the trochanter, maintaining its elevated state. A second Muller-type retractor rests on the posteromedial aspect of the calcar.

Closure

- Thoroughly irrigate wound
- Reinspect lateral circumflex vessels for bleeding and recauterize as necessary
- Close fascia overlying TFL, taking care to incorporate only a few millimeters of tissue on either side to avoid incarcerating branches of lateral femoral cutaneous nerve (LFCN) in repair
- Close subcutaneous fat and skin in standard manner

Surgical Technique: Hemiarthroplasty Modification for Direct Anterior Approach

- Setup, incision planning, and surgical exposure to level of anterior capsule are identical to those of THA
- Carefully avoid damaging anterior labrum during capsulotomy
- Incise capsule from inferior to superior and place tension on anterior capsule as anterior acetabular lip is approached
- Perform remainder of capsulotomy as described previously for THA
- The femoral neck fracture may substitute for the head-neck junction cut
- Make second neck cut along saddle of neck as described previously to facilitate removal of femoral head
- Remove femoral head with corkscrew; use rongeur to remove bone on femoral neck attached to the head to create room as needed for corkscrew insertion
- Take care when elevating proximal femur out of wound; patient will likely have poor bone stock, and iatrogenic fracture needs to be avoided
- If resistance is met, perform posterolateral release to the piriformis tendon to prevent intertrochanteric fracture from excessive force
- Femoral preparation then proceeds in standard fashion used for THA

COMPLICATIONS

- Acetabular implant malpositioning resulting in excessive anteversion
- Femoral implant malpositioning resulting in excessive varus, extension, and posterior cortex perforation
- Trochanteric fracture
- Damage to femoral nerve, femoral artery, and LFCN
- Superficial and deep infection, deep vein thrombosis, pulmonary embolism, bleeding, limb-length discrepancy

POSTOPERATIVE CARE AND REHABILITATION

- Weight bearing as tolerated on postoperative day 1
- Aggressive physical therapy beginning postoperative day 1
- Adequate pain control
- Chemical deep vein thrombosis prophylaxis for 6 weeks postoperatively

PEARLS

- Careful incision placement is critical to avoid damage to the LFCN.
- Patient positioning and specialized instrumentation are essential to avoiding component malpositioning and may obviate the need for a specialized table.
- A two-step femoral neck cut obviates the need for hip dislocation to facilitate removal of femoral head.
- Adequate femoral exposure is often the limiting factor in the case, and care must be taken to perform an adequate soft-tissue release to avoid iatrogenic fracture.
- Rapid recovery depends on adequate pain control and aggressive physical therapy and mobilization.

Total Hip Arthroplasty: Direct Anterior Approach Using a Specialized Table

INTRODUCTION

- Surgical approach first described by Carl Heuter in 1881, later adapted for arthroplasty and published by Robert Judet in 1950
- Recent increase in popularity after series of anterior approach total hip arthroplasties published by Joel Matta in 2005
- Further refinement has allowed for accelerated recovery and elimination of hip precautions
- Potential downsides include steep learning curve, cost of a specialized table, and questioned benefits compared with modern posterior approach

SURGICAL TECHNIQUE

 VIDEO 58.1 Direct Anterior Approach Using a specialized table. Roy Davidovitch, MD; Dylan Lowe, BSc; Ran Schwarzkopf, MD, MSc (15 min 29 s)

Patient Positioning and Preparation

- Specialized radiolucent table that allows for sustained external rotation and extension of the surgical hip during preparation of the proximal femur
- Fluoroscopic imaging per surgeon preference
- Perineal post with no traction applied to the lower limbs
- Antiseptic (chlorhexidine) preparation of the surgical site from umbilicus to knee. Drape the surgical hip as well as image intensifier

Surgical Anatomy and Approach

- The authors prefer a vertical incision; however, a "bikini" incision may be used
- Mark the anterior superior iliac spine (ASIS) and greater trochanter and draw a line connecting the two

---

Based on Schwarzkopf R, Davidovitch R: Total hip arthroplasty: Direct anterior approach using a specialized table, in Colvin AC, Flatow E, eds: Atlas of Essential Orthopaedic Procedures, *ed 2. Rosemont, IL, American Academy of Orthopaedic Surgeons, 2020, pp 474-481.*

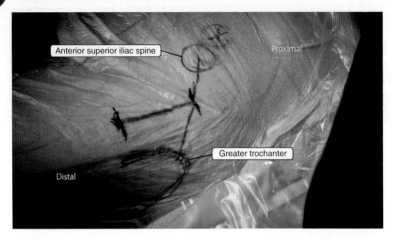

FIGURE 1 Intraoperative photograph. The surgical incision is marked by a vertical line starting 2 cm lateral and 1 cm distal to the line drawn connecting the anterior superior iliac spine and the greater trochanter and drawn toward the lateral border of the patella.

- Incision begins 2 cm lateral and 1 cm distal to the ASIS and extends distally toward the lateral border of the patella. The typical incision is 8 to 10 cm in length (**Figure 1**)
- Incision carried down to the level of the tensor fascia which is then incised
- Fascia bluntly separated from the muscle and interval between tensor and rectus developed
- Place a blunt cobra retractor over the superior femoral neck. The intermuscular interval between the tensor and sartorius can now be developed
- Identify the ascending branch of the lateral femoral circumflex and cauterize (**Figure 2**)
- Elevate the soft tissues off the anterior capsule and place a second blunt cobra retractor around the inferior neck
- The capsule is incised in line with the center of the femoral neck followed by a capsulectomy of both the superior and inferior edges at the acetabular rim
- Lateral capsule excised along the intertrochanteric line
- The superior cobra retractor is placed intra-articular along the superior femoral neck

The Lateral Femoral Cutaneous Nerve and Possible Dysasthesia

- Arises from L2-L3 nerve roots
- Anterior branch pierces fascia 8 to 10 cm below the ASIS and provides cutaneous innervation over the anterolateral thigh
- Surgical incision is lateral to the course of the nerve, but the nerve is at risk for neurapraxia

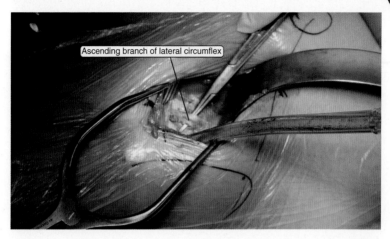

Ascending branch of lateral circumflex

FIGURE 2 Intraoperative photograph. The ascending branch of the lateral circumflex artery is identified.

Potential Pitfalls
- Note the perforating vessels on the fascia of the tensor. This can help identify the correct interval
- The correct interval will have muscle (tensor) laterally and fatty tissue medially

Femoral Neck Osteotomy
- Neck cut checked with saw blade placed on anterior neck under fluoroscopy
- The neck cut is made, and traction with external rotation of the limb will facilitate removal of the femoral head. Take care not to damage the muscle of the tensor with the cut edge of the bone

Acetabular Preparation and Cup Insertion
- Two retractors—a sharp cobra inferior to the transverse acetabular ligament (TAL) and a cerebellar retractor placed from cephalad (**Figure 3**)
- Acetabular labrum and pulvinar excised
- Reaming performed under fluoroscopic guidance. The authors prefer to use a single reamer based on the templated size
- The acetabular implant is placed under fluoroscopy with a goal anteversion of 20° and inclination of 40°
- Acetabular screws are placed as needed, and a polyethylene liner is inserted

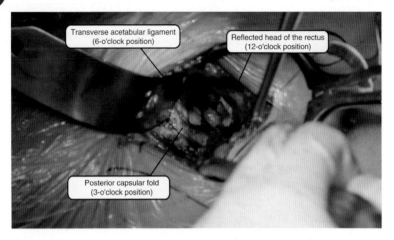

Transverse acetabular ligament
(6-o'clock position)

Reflected head of the rectus
(12-o'clock position)

Posterior capsular fold
(3-o'clock position)

FIGURE 3 Intraoperative photograph. Placement of the acetabular retractors, and final exposure is achieved before acetabular reaming.

Femoral Canal Preparation and Stem Insertion

- Femoral preparation is more challenging with the anterior approach. Proper visualization requires 90° of external rotation, 20° to 30° of extension, and visualization of the greater trochanter
- Two essential soft tissue releases
  - ▸ 6 o'clock release—vertical cut of the medial capsule (pubofemoral ligament) along the medial calcar to the level of the lesser trochanter (**Figure 4**). The limb is then externally rotated, extended, and slightly adducted
  - ▸ 12 o'clock release—vertical incision in the superior posterior capsule which allows the trochanter and proximal femur to be elevated into the field of view (**Figure 5**)
- With appropriate release, an elevating femoral hook is not necessary
- Stability is assessed both anteriorly and posteriorly.
- The trial implants are removed and the final femoral stem and head are placed.
- The fascia is closed with running absorbable suture, and the skin is closed per surgeon preference.

FLUOROSCOPY

- Advantages—visualization of the femoral neck cut, accurate reaming and implantation of the acetabular implant, assessment of femoral stem size and position, and assessment of leg lengths
- Disadvantages—radiation exposure

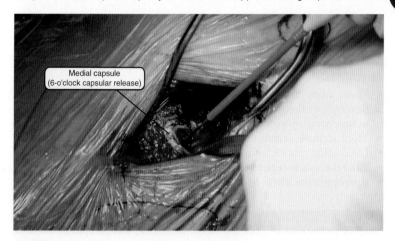

FIGURE 4 Intraoperative photograph. First femoral release referred to as the "6-o'clock release" as it is located at the level of the medial calcar.

Use of a Specialized Table

- Surgery can be performed with or without specialized table
- Authors prefer to use the table due to the ease of manipulating the leg during femoral preparation and implant position

PATIENT SELECTION

- Difficult exposure—muscular males, patients with short valgus femoral necks
- Difficult instrumentation—patients with wide iliac wing/crest, and Dorr A femurs (may have to convert to different stem geometry)

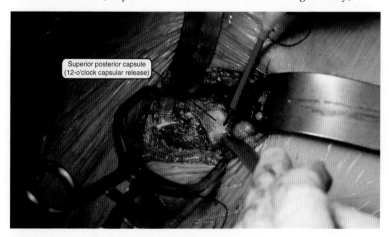

FIGURE 5 Intraoperative photograph. Second femoral release (the 12-o'clock release) where a vertical incision is made in the superior posterior capsule.

Rehabilitation

- Immediate weight bearing as tolerated without any hip precautions
- Avoid aggressive strengthening of the hip flexors

Outcomes

- Faster early recovery and rehabilitation versus posterior approach; however, in the long term, there seems to be no significant difference in functional outcomes
- More accurate acetabular cup positioning versus posterior approach
- Dislocation rate 0.6% to 1.5%
- Lateral femoral cutaneous nerve neurapraxia 7% to 30%
- Intraoperative femur fracture 2% to 3%

PEARLS

- No broaching until the trochanter and proximal femur are exposed.
- Exposure can be improved with the release of the piriformis and conjoint tendons.
- A small portion of the tensor can be released from the ASIS if additional exposure required.
- Lateral femoral neck bone removed with a rongeur and curet to prevent varus insertion of the stem.
- Sequential broaching to the templated size and placement of trial femoral implant.
- Trial reduction with gentle traction and internal rotation.
- Trial implant position is assessed under fluoroscopy as well as leg lengths. Note that the fluoroscopy can induce a parallax effect. This can be accounted for with the use of a metal rod placed across the pelvis (**Figure 6**).

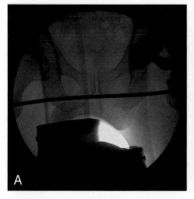 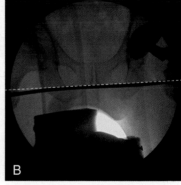

FIGURE 6 - Fluoroscopic view. When checking leg length, understanding the parallax error is important. A, Parallax error is seen and (B) parallax error corrected.

CHAPTER 59

Anterior-Based Muscle-Sparing Approach in the Lateral Position

INTRODUCTION
- Variation of Watson-Jones approach described in 1938, anterior-based muscle-sparing approach (ABMS) approach first described in 2004 by Bertin and Rottinger
- Intermuscular interval between the tensor fascia latae (TFL) and abductor muscles
- Performed in the lateral decubitus position

SURGICAL TECHNIQUE
Positioning
- Standard operating table with the patient in the lateral decubitus position and the surgical hip up
- The author prefers to use a peg board for positioning
- The hip should be able to achieve 100° of flexion, 15° of extension, and 25° to 30° of internal and external rotation without impingement
- Antiseptic prep solution and draping per surgeon preference
- Lower the foot of the bed to facilitate extension and external rotation of the surgical limb (**Figure 1**)
- A vascular roll or blankets can be used to abduct the extremity providing relaxation of the TFL and gluteus medius

Approach
- Surgeon stands on anterior side of patient
- The greater trochanter, femoral shaft, and anterior superior iliac spine (ASIS) are marked
- The incision is made longitudinally approximately 2 cm anterior and parallel to the anterior border of the femur. This incision is approximately 8 cm in length with one-third of the incision proximal and two-thirds distal to the tip of greater trochanter. (**Figure 2**)
- Incision carried down to the iliotibial band (ITB) which is sharply incised along the anterior aspect of the trochanter. Take care to avoid injury to the gluteus medius

Based on Haile NB, Kagan R, Anderson MB, Peters CL: Anterior-based muscle-sparing approach in the lateral position, in Colvin AC, Flatow E, eds: Atlas of Essential Orthopaedic Procedures, *ed 2. Rosemont, IL, American Academy of Orthopaedic Surgeons, 2020, pp 482-489.*

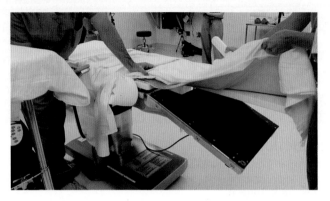

FIGURE 1 Photograph shows, after the patient is prepped and draped, the foot of the bed being dropped to allow for extension and external rotation of the surgical hip.

- "Gateway vessels" can now be identified, these are a fascial bridge between the TFL and gluteal muscles (**Figure 3**)
- Two cobra retractors are placed over the superior and inferior femoral neck
- An L-shaped capsulotomy is made (**Figure 4**), and the corner is tagged with nonabsorbable suture for later closure
- The inferior cobra is placed intra-articular over the anterior acetabulum, and the superior cobra is exchanged for a modified Hohmann retractor
- Subcapital femoral neck cut is made from an inferior to superior direction. The leg is then externally rotated and extended before the final femoral neck cut is made as previously templated (**Figure 5**)

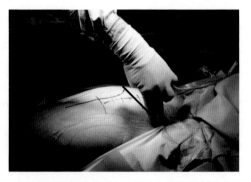

FIGURE 2 Intraoperative photograph shows that a line connecting the anterior superior iliac spine and the greater trochanter should pass through the midpoint of the incision.

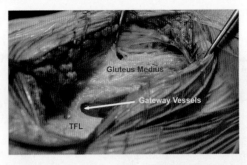

FIGURE 3 Intraoperative photograph shows that the "gateway vessels," a fascial bridge between the gluteus medius and tensor fascia lata (TFL), can be ligated to facilitate exposure.

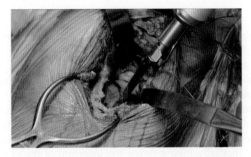

FIGURE 4 Intraoperative photograph shows the initial subcapital femoral neck osteotomy made using a reciprocating saw.

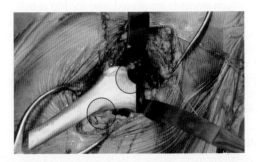

FIGURE 5 Intraoperative photograph shows the final femoral neck osteotomy made using the saddle (superior red circle) or the lesser trochanter (inferior red circle) as reference points.

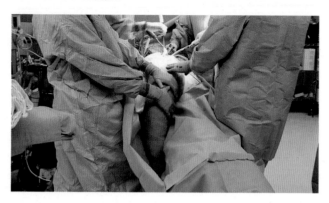

FIGURE 6 Intraoperative photograph shows the surgical hip being extended and externally rotated during exposure of the proximal femur.

- The acetabulum is exposed with a modified Hohmann placed superiorly, and the femoral head is removed
- Acetabular labrum and pulvinar are excised
- Acetabular reaming and final implantation of the acetabular implant are done according to surgeon preference
- The Hohmann retractor is now placed over the greater trochanter
- The capsule along the superior neck is released while the leg is brought into the reverse figure-of-4 position (**Figure 6**). The capsular release is continued medially taking down the insertion of the obturator internus, but the remaining external rotators are preserved
- A femoral elevator is used and preparation of the proximal femur is performed as dictated by the implant design and surgeon preference
- Trial femoral components are placed, and the hip is reduced with traction and internal rotation. Accordingly, the trial components are able to be dislocated with traction and external rotation. A bone hook is recommended to assist with this step
- The final components are inserted, and fluoroscopy or a cross-table radiograph may be obtained to assess implant positioning, leg lengths, and offset
- Wound closure is done according to surgeon preference

VIDEO 59.1 Total hip arthroplasty through the anterior-based muscle-sparing approach. Nathan B. Haile, MD; Ryland Kagan, MD; Mike B. Anderson, MSc; Christopher L. Peters, MD (13 min)

DISCUSSION

- Multiple studies have been done looking at outcomes versus a direct lateral (Hardinge) approach and minimally invasive posterior approach. Key conclusions include that the procedure is safe, allows for reliable implant positioning, and that preservation of the abductor musculature minimizes the risk for postoperative weakness or gait dysfunction
- The author's experience after transitioning from a minimally invasive posterior approach to the ABMS approach showed no difference in surgical time, estimated blood loss, patient-reported outcomes, or complications. The one significant finding noted was that there was a significantly decreased length of stay with the ABMS approach

CONCLUSIONS

- ABMS approach offers an alternative to the direct anterior approach while the patient remains in the lateral position
- Preservation of the abductor musculature limits postoperative weakness or gait abnormalities
- No specialized equipment or table is required
- The approach is extensile and can be utilized for revision procedures

PEARLS

- A sterile blanket roll can be placed under the surgical extremity to relieve tension on the ITB and abductor musculature. This will aid in exposure.
- Take care not to harm the gluteus medius muscle belly during initial fascial incision.
- The foot of the bed may be lowered to aid in femoral exposure.
- Reduction is performed by a combination of axial traction, followed by internal rotation.

60

Revision Total Hip Arthroplasty via Extended Trochanteric Osteotomy

INTRODUCTION

- Total hip arthroplasty (THA) predictably provides pain relief and improved function in patients with hip arthritis
- Despite the success of THA, several situations necessitate revision of the femoral implant
- Extended trochanteric osteotomy (ETO) is a surgical technique that allows exposure of the proximal femur using a controlled cortical fracture
- ETO facilitates the removal of well-fixed femoral implants and provides improved surgical exposure to the acetabulum and femur to allow concentric placement of a new implant through
  - Improved access
  - Concentric reaming of the distal femur
  - Appropriate abductor tensioning
  - Improved acetabular visualization
  - Predictable healing of the osteotomy
- Familiarity with ETO technique is critical for surgeons who perform revision THA or primary THA in patients with proximal femoral deformity

PATIENT SELECTION

Indications

- Removal of well-fixed cemented, proximally coated, or extensively coated femoral implant
  - Indications for removing a well-fixed implant include sepsis, recurrent dislocation due to femoral implant malposition or offset, excess corrosion or fatigue failure, and the need for improved acetabular exposure
  - Extensive bone damage can occur while attempting to remove a well-fixed implant when the bone-prosthesis interface cannot be disrupted distally with proximal exposure alone
  - A cortical window can help but will weaken the remaining host bone and require a longer stem to bypass the stress riser

---

Based on Sporer SM, Paprosky WG: Revision total hip arthroplasty via extended trochanteric osteotomy, in Colvin AC, Flatow E, eds: Atlas of Essential Orthopaedic Procedures, *ed 2. Rosemont, IL, American Academy of Orthopaedic Surgeons, 2020, pp 490-498.

- Removal of well-fixed distal cement
  - Challenging, especially when proximal femoral remodeling has occurred or a previous implant was cemented into varus position
  - Proximal exposure alone is shown to result in a higher prevalence of cortical perforations
  - ETO length can be planned to allow easy visual access to the distal cement plug such that drills, taps, and curets can disrupt the bone-cement interface and facilitate removal of retained cement
- Proximal femoral varus remodeling
  - Observed in up to 30% of patients with a loose femoral stem
  - Component extraction may be easy, but reconstruction is challenging due to the deformity
  - ETO allows concentric reaming of femoral canal
  - Attempting distal fixation in a femur with proximal deformity results in a high prevalence of cortical perforation, undersizing of the femoral implant, and/or varus malposition
- Improved acetabular exposure
  - Relative indication
  - Required because of heterotopic bone formation or the need to visualize anterior and posterior columns
  - ETO may minimize inadvertent fracture during femoral revision for severe trochanteric osteolysis
  - Rarely, ETO is used in primary THA patients with prior osteotomy, malunion, or deformity due to congenital dysplasia

Contraindications

- No absolute contraindications
- Rare indications when impaction bone grafting inside an ectatic femoral shaft is preferable to noncemented femoral fixation because of poor bone quality

PREOPERATIVE IMAGING

- Standard AP pelvis view
- AP and lateral femur views

PROCEDURE

Preoperative Planning

- Length of ETO depends on surgical indication
  - Varus remodeling—Length of ETO should extend at least to apex of deformity to account for "conflict" (inability to place femoral implant in neutral position due to varus [**Figure 1**])
  - Removal of retained distal cement—Length of ETO needs to be within a few centimeters of the distal cement plug
  - ETO can be shorter if used for improved surgical exposure or loose distal cement mantle

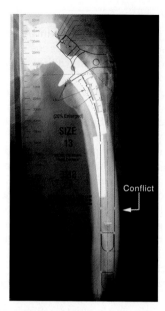

FIGURE 1 AP radiograph of a hip with a cemented total hip arthroplasty shows mechanical failure with associated proximal femoral varus remodeling, causing a "conflict." An extended trochanteric osteotomy is required for correction of the proximal deformity, as well as distal cement extraction. Note the conflict.

> Sufficient length of cortical bone below the lesser trochanter is required to securely reattach fragment
> Minimum of two cables are required to securely fix the trochanteric fragment
> ETO should be at least 14 cm below tip of the greater trochanter
- Length of ETO also depends on the implant chosen for reconstruction
  > If extensively porous-coated stem is used, a minimum of 4 to 5 cm of scratch-fit required to obtain axial and rotational stability (**Figure 2**)
  > If a tapered stem is used, ETO must not extend past the distal metaphyseal/diaphyseal flare
  > Length is measured from tip of the greater or lesser trochanter

Special Instruments/Equipment/Implants
- Small oscillating sagittal saw with a narrow blade for longitudinal limb of ETO
- Pencil-tip high-speed burr for transverse limb
- Several wide osteotomes to distribute stress along ETO fragment during osteotomy

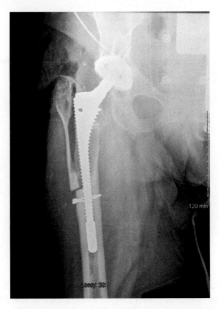

FIGURE 2 AP radiograph of a hip with a periprosthetic fracture. When determining the length of the osteotomy, it is important to consider the future femoral reconstruction.

- Metal cutting burr, Gigli saw, and cylindrical trephines may be needed to section a well-fixed extensively porous-coated stem and remove the distal portion of the stem
- Reverse hooks, cement drills, and osteotomes to remove well-fixed distal cement
- Minimum of two cerclage wires or cables

Exposure

- Posterior approach most common for ETO; several authors describe a similar technique through a direct lateral approach
- Lateral decubitus position; stabilize pelvis with positioners on sacrum and pubic symphysis
- Make lateral skin incision in line with femur over posterior one-third of greater trochanter
- Split tensor fascia lata and fascia of gluteus maximus in line with surgical incision, retract with Charnley bow
- Identify posterior border of gluteus medius tendon and retract anteriorly (**Figure 3**)
- Elevate posterior pseudocapsule and short external rotators as a posteriorly based flap to allow a later capsular repair
- Release anterior and proximal portion of gluteus maximus insertion to mobilize the femur (**Figure 4, A**)

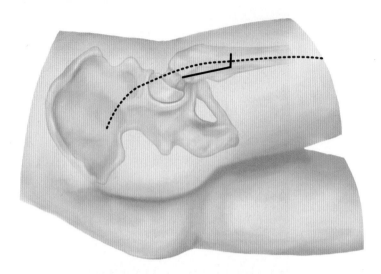

FIGURE 3 Illustration depicts the planned incision (dashed line) for a posterior approach to the hip, which allows excellent visualization of the posterolateral aspect of the proximal femur and will facilitate anterior mobilization of the vastus lateralis. The solid black line indicates the location for an extended trochanteric osteotomy.

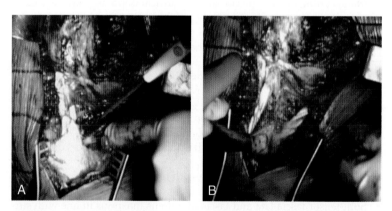

FIGURE 4 Intraoperative photographs demonstrate the initial steps in exposure for an extended trochanteric osteotomy of a left hip. **A,** The proximal and anterior portion of the gluteus maximus insertion is released to allow mobilization of the femur. Distally, the tendon remains intact unless additional exposure is required. **B,** A Hohmann retractor is placed deep to the vastus lateralis to expose the underlying femoral shaft at the level of the proposed osteotomy.

- Dislocate femoral head posteriorly; flex and internally rotate hip
- Knee remains flexed to reduce tension on sciatic nerve
- Remove soft tissue surrounding the proximal portion of the femoral stem; assess stability of the stem
- If stem is loose and greater trochanter is not preventing extrication, remove component
- If stem is well fixed or greater trochanter prevents removal, an in situ ETO should be performed
- If hip dislocation is difficult due to severe acetabular protrusio or extensive heterotopic ossification, ETO can be considered

Osteotomy

- Step 1
  - Place hip in extension and internal rotation; flex knee to minimize traction on sciatic nerve
  - Identify posterior margin of vastus lateralis, and mobilize muscle belly anteriorly off of lateral femur; minimize soft-tissue stripping
  - Place Hohmann retractor around femoral shaft at desired length of osteotomy, exposing underlying periosteum (**Figure 4, B**)
- Step 2
  - Mark position of proposed osteotomy (**Figure 5**)
  - Use tip of the greater trochanter as a landmark
  - Direct sagittal saw from posterolateral to anterolateral beginning anterior to the linea aspera (**Figure 6, A**)
  - Osteotomy fragment should encompass posterolateral one-third of proximal femur, perpendicular to anteversion of the hip
  - If femoral stem has been extracted, guide saw to far anterolateral cortex to etch the bone and facilitate a greenstick-type fracture
  - If femoral implant is retained, angle saw anterolaterally to maximize the width of the osteotomy while avoiding hitting the femoral implant
- Step 3
  - Make the distal transverse limb of osteotomy with a pencil-tipped burr
  - Round corners to eliminate stress risers and reduce risk of fracture propagation
  - Use oscillating saw or pencil-tipped burr to initiate the distal anterior limb of the osteotomy
- Step 4
  - Use multiple wide osteotomes to gently lever the osteotomy site from posterior to anterior (**Figure 6, B**)
  - Move the entire fragment as a unit to avoid fracture at the level of the vastus ridge
  - Retract the fragment anteriorly with the attached abductors and vastus lateralis

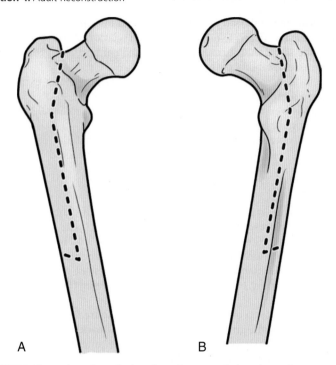

A   B

FIGURE 5 Illustrations show the location of an extended trochanteric osteotomy on the anterior (**A**) and posterior (**B**) aspects of the femur. The length of the osteotomy is measured from the tip of the greater trochanter. Depending on the indication for the osteotomy, the trochanteric fragment should allow a minimum of two cerclage wires and is generally 15 to 16 cm in length.

- ‣ Release tight pseudocapsule along the anterior aspect of greater trochanter (**Figure 6, C**)
- ‣ Minimize dissection along anterolateral limb of the osteotomy, where the blood supply and innervation to the vastus enter
- Step 5
  - ‣ If femoral implant has been extracted already, remove pseudomembrane within the femur
  - ‣ If cement is present, use a high-speed burr and cement splitters to remove the retained cement and distal plug
  - ‣ Retain cement on the trochanteric fragment until the end of the procedure to strengthen the fragment
  - ‣ If a well-fixed proximally coated stem is in place, use a pencil-tipped burr to expose the implant-bone interface, then a Gigli saw (**Figure 6, D**)

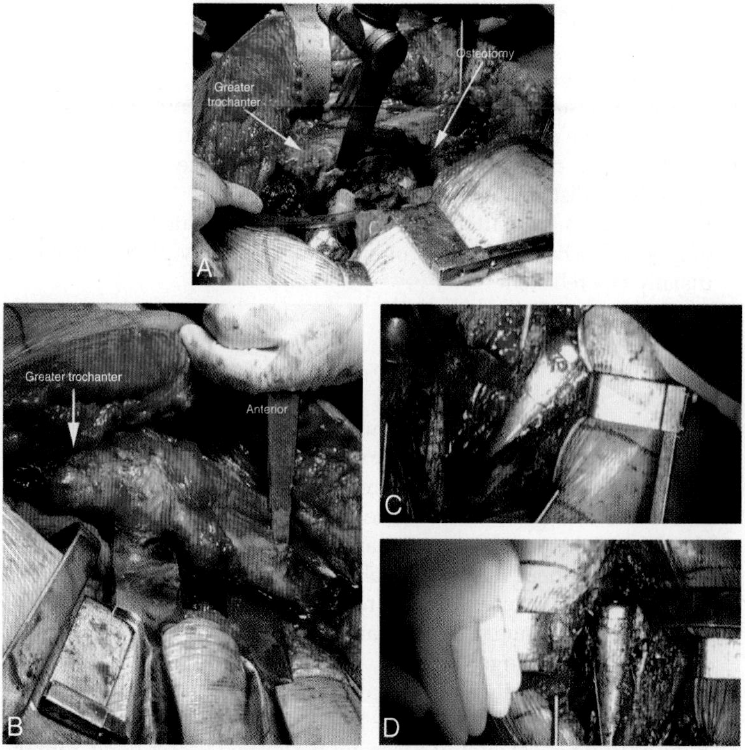

FIGURE 6 Intraoperative photographs demonstrate an extended trochanteric osteotomy. **A**, An oscillating saw with a thin blade is directed from posterior to anteromedial. Approximately one-third of the lateral femur, along with the entire greater trochanter, should be elevated. **B**, Multiple broad osteotomes are used to lever the osteotomy fragment anteriorly. Great care must be taken to avoid fracture at the level of the vastus ridge. **C**, The soft tissue along the proximal-anterior aspect of the osteotomy must be excised once the trochanteric fragment is elevated to minimize fracture of the greater trochanter. This should be performed before attempts are made to remove the femoral implant. **D**, A Gigli saw can be used to disrupt the medial interface between the prosthesis and host bone.

- If a well-fixed extensively coated stem is in place, transect the stem with a metal cutting burr; remove remaining portion of stem with cylindrical trephines 0.5 mm larger than the distal stem

VIDEO 60.1 Revision Total Hip Arthroplasty via Extended Trochanteric Osteotomy. Scott M. Sporer, MD, MS; Wayne G. Paprosky, MD, FACS (6 min)

Bone Preparation

- After removing previous femoral implant, remove any remaining pseudomembrane or cement with a reverse hook
- A distal pedestal often is observed in loose noncemented implants and should also be removed
- Most femoral revisions are performed using noncemented implants that rely on distal fixation
- Depending on the pattern of bone loss, patient anatomy, and osteotomy length, choose a bowed or straight extensively coated stem or a distally tapered stem

Wound Closure

- Remove any cement adherent to the ETO fragment once the stem is seated
- Place leg in slight abduction and internal rotation during reattachment
- A minimum of two cables or wires are needed for fixation.
- A high-speed burr may be required to shape the medial aspect of the trochanteric fragment to allow the osteotomy to rest against the lateral shoulder of the prosthesis and maximize bony apposition
- The ETO fragment may not be able to achieve apposition anteriorly and posteriorly in cases of varus remodeling
- Advance the fragment distally and posteriorly to improve stability and minimize impingement
- Tighten cables distally to proximally
- Avoid trochanteric fracture at the level of the vastus ridge
- Bone grafting of osteotomy site is not performed unless bone from the reamings is available
- Authors' preference is to repair the posterior capsule and short external rotators to the posterior aspect of gluteus medius
- Close gluteus maximus fascia and iliotibial band over a drain with nonabsorbable No. 1 suture; close subcutaneous tissue with absorbable 2.0 suture.

COMPLICATIONS

- Potential complications include proximal migration, nonunion or malunion, fracture, and recalcitrant trochanteric bursitis
- Authors report a low incidence of nonunion (1.2%) and malunion (0.6%); similar results by other authors
- Proximal migration of the ETO fragment is rare because vastus lateralis prevents migration
- Nonunion is rare because dense fibrous tissue forms
- Fracture of osteotomy fragment at the greater trochanter can lead to trochanteric escape and abductor weakness (**Figure 7**)

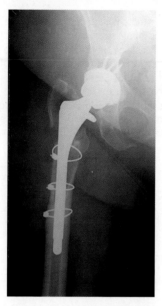

FIGURE 7 AP radiograph depicts a fracture of the osteotomy fragment at the greater trochanter following an extended trochanteric osteotomy. Such a fracture can occur during the postoperative period, frequently at the vastus ridge.

POSTOPERATIVE CARE AND REHABILITATION

- Abduction orthosis for 6 to 8 weeks postoperatively to minimize risk of instability
- Allow 30% weight bearing on surgical leg with a walker or crutch for 6 to 8 weeks
- After 6 weeks, convert to a cane and advance to weight bearing as tolerated
- Avoid abduction for 6 to 12 weeks until radiographic evidence shows healing of the ETO site

PEARLS

- ETO should be considered for the removal of well-fixed implants, removal of retained distal cement, and varus femoral remodeling.
- Use the shortest femoral revision stem possible, yet select one long enough to bypass the apex of the femoral remodeling, facilitate component and cement removal, and allow two cables to be placed for fixation.

- When levering the osteotomy anteriorly, use multiple wide osteotomes simultaneously to distribute stress along the greatest distance.
- Place a prophylactic cerclage cable distal to the osteotomy before femoral preparation and stem insertion to minimize the risk of fracture.
- Retain any cement along the ETO fragment until the time of reattachment to provide additional structural support.
- The ETO fragment should be advanced distally and posteriorly before securing to the femoral shaft to provide appropriate abductor tension and minimize the risk of impingement.

Triflange Acetabular Components for Complex Revision Cases

PATIENT SELECTION

- Revision hip arthroplasty in the setting of massive acetabular bone loss. Most of these patients will have already undergone two or more acetabular revisions
- Physical examination should include prior surgical incisions and a thorough neurovascular examination
- Infection should always be ruled out using inflammatory markers and aspiration of the hip
- Other patient-specific factors that should be evaluated include nutrition status and an anemia workup if the hematocrit is less than 30. Two particular subsets of patients have been noted to have higher complication rates
  - Elderly patients with malnutrition
  - Untreated or undiagnosed patients with anemia
- Triflange acetabular components are commonly used as a salvage type procedure. Classic indications include Paprosky type 3B defects, pelvic discontinuity, and salvage of prior failed porous metal augments, structural allografts, or cup/cage constructs

PREOPERATIVE IMAGING

- AP pelvis—the majority of information can be obtained from this radiograph
- Judet views of the pelvis—improves visualization of the anterior and posterior columns
- CT scan with 3D reconstructions—this is used to create a 1:1 bone model
- It is important to note that bone adjacent to osteolytic lesions and prior structural allografts may appear functional on imaging but lack structural viability

---

Based on DeBoer D, Christie MJ: Triflange acetabular components for complex revision cases, in Colvin AC, Flatow E, eds: Atlas of Essential Orthopaedic Procedures, *ed 2. Rosemont, IL, American Academy of Orthopaedic Surgeons, 2020, pp 499-506.*

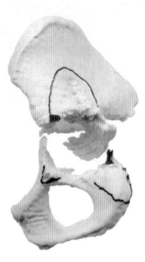

FIGURE 1 Photograph showing an actual CT model of a patient with a pelvic discontinuity. The red marking are areas of bone removal. The flange locations are marked by the surgeon.

THE DESIGN AND PRODUCTION PROCESS

- The total process from start to finish for the construction of a triflange component takes approximately 8 to 16 weeks
- Thin slice CT scan is done per implant manufacturer protocol, typically 2 mm slices
- The CT scan is then used to create a 1:1 hemipelvis model (**Figure 1**)
- The surgeon marks the regions on the model for flange placement. The minimum flange thickness is 6 mm
- Iliac flange provides the majority of the surface area for support of the implant. In general, a larger iliac flange is required in cases with greater bone loss. Most implants include two rows of 3 to 4 screws each in the iliac flange
- Ischial flange has a lateral and posterior surface for flange orientation. Ischial screw pullout is a known complication and can be minimized by using 3 to 4 screws, locking screws, or bone cement in lytic lesions to improve fixation. The ischial flange must be rounded to avoid damage to the sciatic nerve
- Pubic flange acts as a reference point. The author prefers to not use any screw fixation in the iliac flange
- The hip center of rotation and cup face orientation must be selected as well

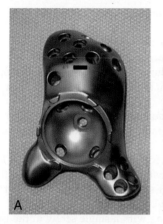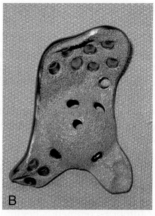

FIGURE 2 **A** and **B**, Photographs showing the front and back of a triflange component. Note the ingrowth surface.

- A prototype implant is produced and verified before final implant production
- The final components are milled from a solid bar of titanium, and the flanges are coated with a plasma sprayed ingrowth surface (**Figure 2**)

PROCEDURE

Room Setup and Instrumentation

- The team should be prepared for complex revision hip surgery with an extensile approach and prolonged exposure of the acetabulum
- Revision instrument sets including broken screw removal set, cement removal instruments if necessary, high-speed burr, and reamers
- The bone model and prototype implant should be sterilized to allow for in vivo comparison intraoperatively

Surgical Technique

- The posterolateral approach allows wide exposure of relevant anatomy
- Intraoperative cultures should be obtained
- An extended intertrochanteric osteotomy (ETO) may be used to facilitate exposure, especially of the ilium. When using implants with a large iliac flange, an ETO may be required to prevent injury to the superior gluteal nerve

---

- After removal of the acetabular implants, a subperiosteal exposure of the ilium, ischium, and pubis is performed. A portion of the hamstring origin is often released to allow for placement of the ischial flange
- The bone model and prototype should be compared with intraoperative findings to assess if additional bone needs to be removed, and the overall fit of the implant
- Any central or contained acetabular defects should be filled with freeze-dried particulate allograft and shaped with a 1-2mm undersized reamer on reverse
- The implant is placed beginning with the iliac flange with the leg in abduction, followed by the pubic flange, and lastly the ischial flange with the leg in extension. A soft tissue sleeve should be kept between the ischial flange and sciatic nerve
- The author recommends beginning with a single screw in the ischial flange, followed by the iliac flange. The remaining three to four ischial screws are placed, and four to six iliac screws are placed
- A trial reduction is performed with modular liners and the motion and stability are assessed. Radiographs should be taken to assess implant positioning and leg lengths
- Full restoration of the hip center of rotation may not be possible in patients with superior migration due to soft tissue tension. If this is not recognized in the design phase, the femoral implant may need to be revised

POSTOPERATIVE CARE
- Weight bearing as tolerated except in cases of pelvic discontinuity, in which case patients are partial weight bearing for 6 weeks
- Posterior hip precautions for 2 to 3 months
- Postoperative rehabilitation should focus on abductor strengthening, which may take up to 1 year to show noticeable improvement

COMPLICATIONS
- Relatively high complication rate as expected with complex revision surgery
- Up to 30% revision rate; however, the majority of these cases do not require revision of the triflange component
- Most common complication is instability in 8% to 26% of cases. This risk may be reduced with the use of constrained liners at the time of the index triflange procedure
- Additional complications—infection (2% to 10%), sciatic nerve palsy, ischial screw migration, heterotopic ossification, and aseptic loosening

RESULTS

- The author reports overall implant survival of 91% with 10 to 21 year follow-up
- In cases of Paprosky 3B defects, failure rates between 5% to 13.5%
- In cases of pelvic discontinuity, stable implants were obtained in 80% to 90% of cases (**Figure 3**)

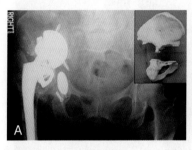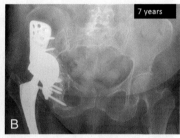

FIGURE 3 Preoperative plain radiograph (**A**) and photograph of bone model (inset) of a patient with a pelvic discontinuity. **B**, Seven-year follow-up radiograph after triflange reconstruction.

PEARLS

- The cup portion of the triflange does not need to have complete contact with host bone. In other words, the socket does not have to match the defect which makes component insertion easier.
- The iliac flange is the primary support for component and should be solidly secured during surgery.
- The hip center should not be lateralized greater than 1 cm during the design phase because of higher reported failure rates.
- The pelvis is loaded after triflange implantation, and bony remodeling of the medial wall is observed rather than stress shielding (**Figure 4**).
- Cup face orientation is critical during the design phase. Face-changing liners are helpful during surgery in some patients.
- Protect the superior gluteal nerve (SGN) during exposure. An extended trochanteric osteotomy and limb positioning are important to reduce injury to the SGN during cup insertion.
- When in doubt, use a constrained liner in the multiply operated patient.
- Ischial bone is typically the worst for screw fixation. Use locking screws or augment with bone cement if fixation is poor.
- The surgical approach is no more complicated than other complex revision cases, and excellent long-term results have been achieved (**Figure 5**).
- The design phase requires an upfront investment in time and effort. There are usually three or four design iterations before final approval is achieved.

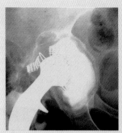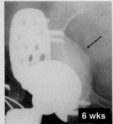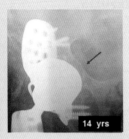

FIGURE 4 Preoperative, 6-week, and 14-year postoperative radiographs of a patient undergoing acetabular reconstruction using a triflange cup. Red arrows denote the remodeling of the medial wall.

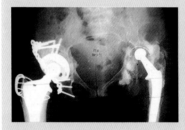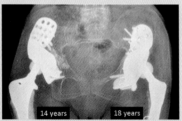

FIGURE 5 Preoperative and long-term follow-up radiographs of a triflange cup.

PATIENT SELECTION

Indications

- Primary and revision total knee arthroplasty
- Particularly well suited for shorter or obese patients and those with muscular lower extremities
- Easily modified intraoperatively for more extensile exposure as needed

Contraindications

- Narrow skin bridges of 4 cm or less may lead to skin necrosis
- Previous incisions lateral to patella may lead to compromise of the patellar blood supply with a standard midline incision

ALTERNATIVE APPROACHES

- Subvastus approach—Theoretical advantages of decreased patellar subluxation postoperatively and preserved patellar blood supply. Technically difficult especially in shorter or muscular patients
- Midvastus approach—The quadriceps tendon is preserved and the vastus medialis obliquus is split in line with its fibers. Lateral subluxation of the patella is more difficult than a standard medial parapatellar approach, but easier than a subvastus approach
- Lateral parapatellar—Most commonly used for valgus deformity as the lateral dissection avoids the risk of further attenuation of the medial soft tissues. This is a technically demanding exposure and medial retraction of the extensor mechanism can be difficult

TECHNIQUE

Medial Parapatellar

Room Setup/Patient Positioning

- Supine position on standard table with bump under ipsilateral hip if needed
- Tourniquet placed on the proximal thigh
- Draping of leg should allow full exposure of relevant anatomy

---

Based on Dayton MR, Scuderi GR: Total knee arthroplasty: Medial parapatellar and extensile approaches, in Colvin AC, Flatow E, eds: Atlas of Essential Orthopaedic Procedures, *ed 2. Rosemont, IL, American Academy of Orthopaedic Surgeons, 2020, pp 507-517.*

Instruments/Equipment/Implants

- A device to hold the knee in flexion and extension per surgeon preference
- Retractors per surgeon preference

Surgical Technique

- Mark midline incision from 4 cm proximal to the superior pole of the patella and 1 cm distal to the tibial tubercle (**Figure 1**)
- The knee is placed in flexion for the skin incision
- The incisions is carried down to the level of the retinaculum and medial and smaller lateral full-thickness flaps are developed
- Make arthrotomy 2 cm proximal to patella, curving along medial patella and then parallel to patellar ligament to the tibial tubercle, leaving a 5-mm cuff of soft tissue to facilitate repair (**Figure 2**)
- Extend knee and medial soft tissue release performed along proximal tibia to midcoronal level
- The patella can be either subluxated laterally or everted. The lateral patellofemoral ligament can be transected to assist with lateral retraction of the extensor mechanism

Wound Closure

- Begin with closing the arthrotomy at the level of the superior and inferior patella. Remaining arthrotomy may be closed with running or interrupted absorbable suture

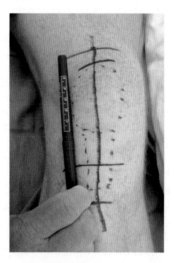

FIGURE 1 Photograph demonstrating that the incision has been marked 4 cm proximal to the superior pole of the patella and 2 cm distal to the tibial tubercle. The incision initially begins from the pole of the superior patella to just proximal to the tibial tubercle and is extended as needed to prevent skin tension during exposure.

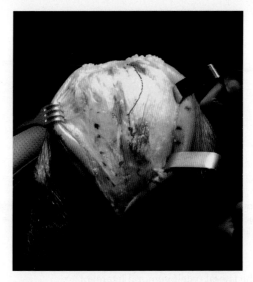

FIGURE 2 Intraoperative photograph shows a medial patellar arthrotomy. This should leave a 5-mm cuff of soft-tissue attachment medial to the patella and to the patellar ligament.

- Medial advancement can be performed in "pants-over-vest fashion" if needed

 VIDEO 62.1 Exposure for Revision Total Knee Arthroplasty via Quadriceps Snip. Ari Seidenstein, MD; Scott Scuderi, BS.

Extensile Exposure/Quadriceps Snip

Room Setup/Patient Positioning

- Standard setup and patient positioning as described above
- Consider use of a sterile tourniquet as more proximal exposure will be needed

Surgical Technique

- If a prior midline incision exists, it should be used and extended slightly proximally to establish normal tissue planes
- Obtain visualization of entire extensor mechanism, and a long medial parapatellar arthrotomy is performed
- The medial and lateral gutters are débrided and excess distal femur synovium excised
- The patellar fat pad can be split or excised, and any adhesions between the lateral tibial plateau and patellar tendon can be released

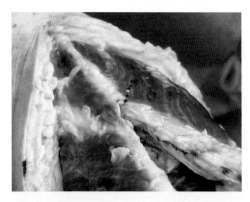

FIGURE 3 Photograph showing a close-up view of the apex of the quadriceps tendon in a cadaver specimen. The tendon is transected in an oblique fashion (blue dots) in line with the fibers of the vastus lateralis.

- Release the lateral patellofemoral ligament
- More aggressive medial release including the semimembranosus posteriorly allows for external rotation of the tibia
- At this point if 90° of flexion cannot be obtained, a quadriceps snip is indicated
- Extend the arthrotomy proximally at a 45° angle crossing the quadriceps tendon and splitting the vastus lateralis fibers (**Figure 3**)
- The exit point of the quadriceps snip should be distal to the musculotendinous junction of the rectus femoris

Wound Closure
- The arthrotomy including the oblique portion proximally are closed side to side as with a standard parapatellar approach

POSTOPERATIVE REGIMEN
- Full weight bearing with early range of motion
- No alteration in therapy protocol needed for patients who undergo a quadriceps snip unless dictated by other factors associated with the joint reconstruction

COMPLICATIONS
- Avoid malalignment of the arthrotomy closure, as it may lead to patellar maltracking, stiffness, or patella infera
- Avulsion of patellar tendon—higher risk with patellar eversion and patella infera
- Quadriceps snip—proximal extension of arthrotomy beyond the quadriceps tendon will transect a portion of the rectus femoris fibers

CLINICAL RESULTS

TABLE 1 Results for Various Arthrotomy Techniques Versus Medial Parapatellar Approach

Author(s)/Year	Number of Knees	Procedure or Approach	Mean Patient Age (Range)	Mean Follow-Up (Range)	Results
Dalury DF & Jiranek WA (1999)	48 (24 knees on each group)	Bilateral TKA: midvastus vs paramedian	70	12 wk	Decreased early pain, time to straight leg raise, increased strength in midvastus No differences in releases, range of motion (ROM)
White RE, Allman JK, Trauger JA et al (1999)	218 (109 knees each group)	Bilateral TKA: midvastus vs medial parapatellar	68 (44-87)	6 mo	Decreased time to straight leg raise at 8 d, decreased pain up to 6 wk with midvastus; increase in releases with medial parapatellar. No differences in ROM, estimated blood loss (EBL), tourniquet time, straight leg raise at 6 mo
Parentis MA, Rumi MN, Deol GS et al (1999)	51 (22 midvastus, 29 medial parapatellar)	Vastus splitting (midvastus) vs medial parapatellar	68.2 (midvastus) 65.5 (medial parapatellar)	5.8 mo	Increased lateral release, EBL with medial parapatellar. 43% abnormal electromyogram with midvastus ONLY. No differences in ROM, knee scores, tourniquet time, proprioception, or patellar tracking
Matsueda M, Gustilo RB (2000)	336: 169 medial parapatellar (1988-1992); 167 subvastus (1992-1996)	Medial parapatellar vs subvastus	67 (30-88) for medial parapatellar 69 (32-86) for subvastus	6 mo	Decreased lateral release, increased central patellar tracking with subvastus. No difference in ROM, stairclimbing, knee scores. Note: Groups done in different time periods

(Continued)

TABLE 1 Results for Various Arthrotomy Techniques Versus Medial Parapatellar Approach (Continued)

Author(s)/Year	Number of Knees	Procedure or Approach	Mean Patient Age (Range)	Mean Follow-Up (Range)	Results
Keating EM, Faris PM, Meding JB et al (1999)	200 (100 knees in each group)	Bilateral TKA: midvastus vs medial parapatellar	70.23 (42-86)	Postop day 3 (discharge)	No differences in lateral release, postop day 2 ROM, discharge day ROM, day able to do straight leg raise, leg circumference, extensor lag
Lin WP, Chang SM, et al (2008)	60 patients (80 knees, 40 in each group)	Minimal incision medial parapatellar vs quadriceps sparing (QS)	MP: 70.2 QS: 69.6	2 mo	With QS TKA, tourniquet and surgical times were lengthened, varus postoperative alignment tended to increase. Muscle strength, postop pain and functional outcomes did not differ
Liu HW, et al (2014)	Meta-analysis: 2,451 TKAs in 32 RCTs	Midvastus vs subvastus vs medial parapatellar	Mean age range: 62.5-75	1 wk to 3 yr	Midvastus better in pain and ROM at 2 wk, subvastus better ROM, straight leg raise, and absence of retinacular release at one week. Midvastus associated with longer surgical time
Berstock JR, et al. EFORT Open Rev. (2018)	Meta-analysis: 1893 primary TKAs in 20 RCTs	Medial subvastus vs medial parapatellar	Range: 57-76	Day 0 to 78 mo	Superior results for subvastus for straight leg raise, pain day 1, ROM at 1 wk, and decreased lateral release, perioperative blood loss, longer surgical time. No technique difference in long-term follow-up

PEARLS

- Multiple approaches provide adequate exposure for total knee arthroplasty.
- Create sufficient full-thickness skin flaps.
- Mark the retinaculum prior to performing the arthrotomy to ensure accurate closure.
- Quadriceps snip indicated when knee cannot be flexed greater than 90° after releases performed.
- Postoperative therapy protocol is not altered for any of the approaches discussed above.

Total Knee Arthroplasty via Small-Incision Midvastus Approach

INTRODUCTION

- Total knee arthroplasty (TKA) is highly successful in managing symptomatic end-stage knee arthritis
- Traditionally performed through standard medial parapatellar arthrotomy with eversion of patella
- TKA is now possible using smaller incision, less disruption of extensor mechanism
- Benefits—Earlier return of quadriceps function and motion, improved flexion, less postoperative narcotic use, and improved cosmesis
- Safe and accurate use of small-incision midvastus approach depends on understanding of anatomy, gentle soft-tissue handling, use of mobile window through accurate retractor placement, and minimally invasive surgery instrument use

PATIENT SELECTION

Indications

- Same as those for standard TKA—Disability from knee arthritis, refractory to nonsurgical measures
- Should first try course of activity modification, anti-inflammatory medication, physical therapy, and weight reduction

Contraindications

- No absolute contraindications
- Relative contraindications listed in **Table 1**.

PREOPERATIVE IMAGING

- Standing AP, lateral, 45° flexed PA, Merchant view radiographs
- Interpret radiographs for deformity, bone loss, presence of patella baja, and bone quality
- For deformity, useful to anticipate appropriate distal femoral cut angle and height of tibial resection

---

Based on Haas SB, Kim S: Total knee arthroplasty via small-incision midvastus approach, in Colvin AC, Flatow E, eds: Atlas of Essential Orthopaedic Procedures, *ed 2. Rosemont, IL, American Academy of Orthopaedic Surgeons, 2020, pp 518-525.*

TABLE 1	Relative Contraindications to the Small-Incision Midvastus Approach
Substantial quadriceps muscle mass in men	
Significant obesity (body mass index >40 kg/m²)	
Severe coronal plane deformity	
Flexion contracture >25°	
Passive flexion <80°	
Severe patella baja	
Significant scarring of the quadriceps mechanism	
Revision surgery	

PROCEDURE

Patient Positioning

- Same as for standard TKA
- Bolstered sandbag under drapes at level of opposite angle so knee can flex at 70° to 90° (**Figure 1**)
- Use lateral support so leg sits without being held by assistant

Special Instruments

- Specialized instrumentation is critical
- Smaller cutting blocks and guides with rounded edges for smaller incisions
- Side-specific instruments and cutting guides

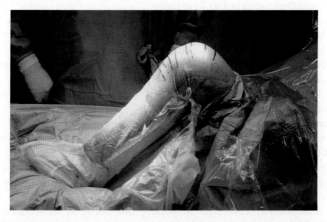

FIGURE 1 Photograph shows a patient positioned on the operating table with a bump placed across from the opposite ankle to hold the leg at 70° to 90°.

- Rigid saw blade with narrow body that fans out at distal tip
- Some systems have implants specifically for use with minimally invasive technique, such as short keel or modular stem tibial components and asymmetric tibial trays

Surgical Technique

VIDEO 63.1 Mini-Midvastus Approach. Steven B. Haas, MD, MPH; Stephen Kim, MD (16 min)

Anesthesia
- Authors prefer combined spinal/epidural anesthetic with indwelling epidural patient-controlled anesthesia for 48 hours
- Bupivacaine femoral nerve block
- Intravenous cefazolin; vancomycin for penicillin allergy

Exposure
- Exsanguinate leg with Esmarch bandage; inflate tourniquet to 250 to 300 mm Hg
- Make longitudinal incision at junction of middle and medial thirds of patella, 1 cm above proximal half of medial tibial tubercle, 8.5 to 12 cm long (**Figure 2**)
- Perform medial arthrotomy from superior pole of patella to level of tibial tubercle; leave 5-mm cuff of tissue adjacent to tubercle
- Split vastus medialis obliquus (VMO) in line with its fibers at level of superior pole of patella (**Figure 3**)
- Initiate first centimeter of VMO muscle split sharply and finish with blunt finger dissection; prevents injury to distal innervation of vastus musculature; split is 2 to 4 cm long
- Preserve suprapatellar pouch except in severe inflammatory disease
- Extend knee and carry subperiosteal dissection around medial pretibial border, releasing meniscotibial attachments
- Retract and subluxate patella laterally, do not evert; partially excise infrapatellar fat pad
- Release tibial attachment of anterior cruciate ligament and anterior horn of lateral meniscus
- Place thin bent Hohmann retractor laterally to retract patella
- Create small synovial window over anterolateral femoral cortex to aid initial anterior femoral resection
- Can cut patella first to facilitate subluxation, especially in large patellae, tight extensor mechanisms, abundant patellar osteophytes, and men
- Initial patellar resection is usually not required in women and should be avoided in older osteoporotic patients; retractors can injure patella

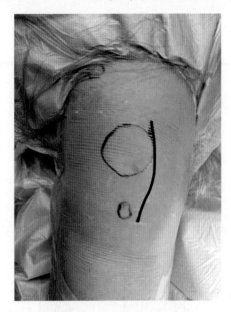

FIGURE 2 Photograph shows the incision for the small-incision midvastus approach for total knee arthroplasty. The incision extends from 1 cm above the superior pole of the patella to the proximal half of the tibial tubercle on its medial side.

Distal Femoral Resection

- Perform distal femoral cut first with knee in 70° to 90° of flexion; limiting knee flexion allows soft-tissue window to be mobile and enables visualization of distal and anterior femur through the small incision
- Full visualization of anterior femoral cortex is necessary; avoid hyperflexion, which tightens extensor mechanism and limits exposure
- Place thin bent Hohmann laterally to retract patella, placed most easily in extension; hold in place as knee is flexed up
- Place second thin bent Hohmann medially
- Mark AP axis (Whiteside line) on distal femur
- Use 9.5-mm drill to enter femoral canal in notch just anterior to posterior cruciate ligament insertion on femur
- Insert intramedullary (IM) alignment guide set to 5° valgus relative to anatomic axis, rotation determined by Whiteside line (**Figure 4**); secure in place with pins
- Insert preliminary anterior resection guide with stylus under quadriceps mechanism, set where stylus makes contact with anterolateral femoral cortex; visualization of stylus is important to prevent anterior femoral notching (**Figure 5**)

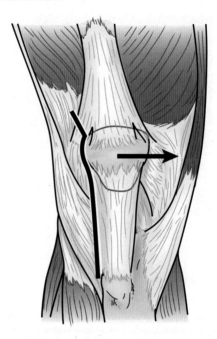

FIGURE 3 Illustration shows the arthrotomy with the mini-midvastus approach, which extends from the tibial tubercle to the superior patella and then to the muscle of the vastus medialis obliquus. The muscle fibers are not cut. The arrow indicates lateral subluxation of the patella.

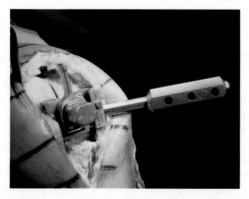

FIGURE 4 Intraoperative photograph demonstrates the use of an intramedullary (IM) alignment guide in the femur. Alignment is determined using this IM guide with the appropriate valgus angle bushing. Rotation is set by aligning the guide with the AP or epicondylar axis.

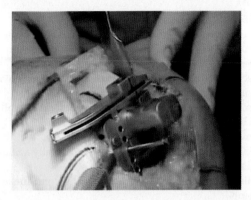

FIGURE 5 Intraoperative photograph shows a cutting guide used on the femur. A preliminary anterior resection is made to place the implant flush with the anterior cortex. This resection also aligns the implant rotation.

- Perform preliminary anterior cut, protecting proximal skin and soft tissues
- Alternatively, may use distal-cut–first instrumentation (**Figure 6**)
- Secure distal femoral cutting guide with pins
- Remove IM rod and alignment guide; assess level of distal femoral resection
- Make cut, protecting patella and soft tissues

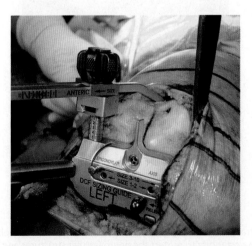

FIGURE 6 Intraoperative photograph shows the use of a distal-cut–first instrument. This guide measures implant size and rotation. Rotation can be set by the AP axis, the posterior condyles, or the epicondylar axis.

Tibial Preparation

- Can use extramedullary or IM guides; guides designed for minimally invasive approach allow accurate positioning through limited exposure
- Place knee in 90° of flexion; avoid excessive external rotation, which reduces visualization
- Place thin bent Hohmann retractors medially and laterally to protect collateral ligaments and extensor mechanism
- Remove overhanging anteromedial osteophytes
- Place tibial guide parallel to tibial crest proximally with appropriate rotational alignment
- Use tibialis anterior tendon over ankle and second metatarsal as reference points
- Adjust posterior slope in standard fashion, determine appropriate measured resection level; amount of desired resection determined by implant system as well as preoperative deformity and bone loss
- Place Aufranc retractor posteriorly to protect posterior neurovascular structures (**Figure 7**)
- Perform proximal tibial resection
- Complete medial resection by directing blade from anterior to posterior

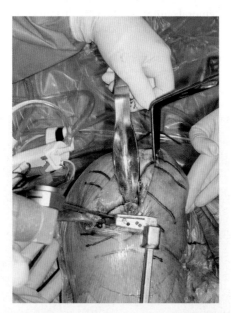

FIGURE 7 Intraoperative photograph shows an Aufranc retractor being placed in the midline posteriorly to protect the neurovascular structures and hold the tibia in an anteriorly subluxated position. The tibia cutting guide is placed on the anteromedial tibia.

- Direct blade laterally to complete resection
- Leave small rim of bone on posterolateral cortex to avoid damaging ligaments and neurovascular bundle
- Remove tibial cut surface; remove remaining rim of bone later
- Check alignment with spacer block and alignment rod
- Place knee into full extension; open extension with laminar spreader
- Now can safely remove remaining rim of posterior bone
- Check extension gap and ligament balance again

Femoral Sizing and AP Resection

- Use AP axis and posterior condyles to set rotation.
- Pin appropriately sized femoral finishing guide in place
- Identify transepicondylar axis; reference position of finishing guide to this landmark before making cuts
- Make posterior condylar, posterior and anterior chamfer, and anterior femoral cuts
- Place thin bent Hohmann retractors to protect collateral ligaments during cuts
- With knee at 90° flexion, use laminar spreaders to assess posterior condyles for retained osteophytes, which are removed with curved osteotome; also remove meniscal remnants along with posterior cruciate ligament if using posterior-stabilized system
- Insert spacer blocks in full extension and 90° flexion to assess extension and flexion spaces
- Knee should be well balanced on medial and lateral sides in flexion and extension; if asymmetric, perform soft-tissue releases or bony resections to achieve balance

Patellar Preparation

- Prepare patella after femur and tibia are cut, but before placing trial implants
- Use freehand or milled technique
- After sizing and drilling patella, insert trial patellar component
- Remove remaining osteophytes or uncovered patella, especially laterally, to minimize impingement

Final Preparation

- Flex knee to 120°; expose tibia with medial, lateral retractors; insert posterior retractor to anteriorly subluxate tibia
- Size proximal tibia with trial trays; correct size maximizes coverage without overhang
- Pin trial tray in place; ream and broach proximal tibia (**Figure 8**)
- Remove tibial osteophytes (commonly found posteromedially)
- Flex knee to 90°; perform final femoral preparation
- After femoral trial is aligned medial-lateral, prepare posterior-stabilized box by reaming through trial with guide; insert box/cam trial

---

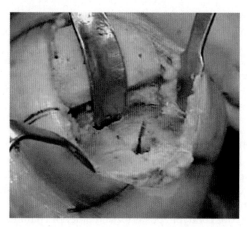

FIGURE 8 Intraoperative photograph shows the tibia is exposed by placing an Aufranc retractor posteriorly and thin bent Hohmann retractors medially and laterally.

- Hyperflex knee to allow insertion of trial liner
- Reduce trial liner into place; bring knee into full extension
- Assess stability in extension and 90° flexion
- If multiple trial liner designs available, use design with least constraint to allow assessment of stability and balance
- Perform additional soft-tissue releases or bony resections if necessary to achieve balance
- Check patellar tracking through range of motion (ROM)
- If maltracking is present with well-aligned components, recheck tracking with tourniquet deflated
- If tracking still suboptimal, perform lateral retinacular release

Component Insertion
- Authors prefer cemented implants; noncemented devices may be used
- Remove trials; clean bone surfaces using pulsatile lavage
- Fashion bone plug and impact into distal femur
- If sclerotic bone present, use 2.5-mm drill to make multiple perforations and allow cement interdigitation
- Insert tibial component first
- Obtain tibial exposure using previous trial component technique
- Impact final tibia into place and remove excess cement
- Pay careful attention to ensure appropriate rotation during insertion
- Asymmetric tibial component is preferred; easier to insert with a limited exposure
- Flex knee to 90°; firmly impact femur into place and remove excess cement

- Insert appropriately sized trial liner; reduce knee into full extension for further cement compression
- Cement patellar component into place
- Remove additional cement from suprapatellar pouch and gutters
- After cement is cured, place knee in hyperextension to expose tibia
- Clear tibial locking mechanism of debris; irrigate posterior knee and clear of cement
- Insert final polyethylene liner and engage into locking mechanism
- Reduce knee into extension; take knee through full ROM

Closure
- Deflate tourniquet; control bleeding
- Copiously lavage knee with normal saline
- Insert two deep drains
- Close capsular layer with 0-Vicryl (Ethicon) sutures into VMO tendon and perimuscular fascia; close arthrotomy with interrupted sutures
- Use 3-0 Vicryl for subcutaneous layers
- Use clips to oppose skin edges
- Place sterile dressing, bulky Jones dressing

COMPLICATIONS
- Soft-tissue trauma secondary to small incision approach
- Injury to patellar tendon, posterior neurovascular structures

POSTOPERATIVE CARE AND REHABILITATION
- Start continuous passive motion machine in recovery room; increase flexion as pain allows
- Start weight bearing on first postoperative day
- Immediately start thromboembolic prophylaxis (foot compression devices, mobilization); begin chemoprophylaxis as soon as surgeon and anesthesiologist feel comfortable, depending on type of anticoagulation and anesthesia
- Give adequate pain control without oversedation to allow aggressive early ROM

PEARLS
- Minimize dissection in suprapatellar pouch to reduce formation of local heterotopic ossification and fibrosis.
- After preserving quadriceps tendon above patella and synovium, create small window in anterior distal femoral synovium to expose cortex and judge anterior bony resection; prevents arthrofibrosis and poor flexion.

- Prepare patella before cutting tibia to enhance exposure, enable proper retractor placement; carefully avoid damaging patella, which is weakened by the cut.
- If using posterior-stabilized TKA design, cut the box later; more efficient than doing so immediately after making anterior, posterior, and chamfer cuts.
- Tension on extensor mechanism and sequence of bony cuts described above place patella at more risk than during standard TKA; mitigate risk by extending incision when necessary, placing retractor optimally, changing sequence of bony cuts, and keeping patellar trial in place.

VIDEO REFERENCE

 Video 63.1 Stuchin SA: *Surgical Techniques in Orthopaedics: Minimally Invasive Total Knee Arthroplasty* [DVD]. Rosemont, IL, American Academy of Orthopaedic Surgeons, 2005.

INTRODUCTION

- Mini-subvastus approach uses anterior incision and evolved from Hofmann subvastus technique
- Incision shorter than traditional medial parapatellar approach, but incision length does not define mini-subvastus
- Approach tries to improve functional recovery from total knee arthroplasty (TKA) by avoiding quadriceps arthrotomy and patellar eversion
- Follows standard surgical sequence
- Surgical guides are scaled-down versions of traditional TKA instruments
- Same steps, with slight adjustments
- Benefit—More rapid recovery without increased risk of complication

PATIENT SELECTION

Indications

- Approach can work for nearly all primary TKA patients
- Permits extension of subvastus release even in obese and muscular patients

Contraindications

- Knees requiring removal of significant hardware from prior fixation
- TKA requiring augments or stems due to severe deformity

PROCEDURE

Room Setup/Patient Positioning

- Supine position
- For significant external hip rotation, can tilt table away from surgical side
- Use mechanical leg holder
- Suggest more than one assistant to handle multiple retractors

Based on Schroer WC: Total knee arthroplasty via the mini-subvastus approach, in Colvin AC, Flatow E, eds: Atlas of Essential Orthopaedic Procedures, ed 2. Rosemont, IL, American Academy of Orthopaedic Surgeons, 2020, pp 526-534.

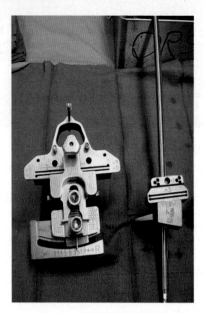

FIGURE 1 Photograph depicts distal femoral cutting guides for total knee arthroplasty. The large instrument is for traditional total knee arthroplasty, and the smaller one is used in minimally invasive surgery.

- Use tourniquet, except in patients with history of vascular surgery
  - ▶ Deflate following final bone preparation, coagulate significant bleeding
  - ▶ Reinflate before implant cementation

Special Instruments/Equipment/Implants
- Instruments are lower-profile versions of standard TKA instruments (**Figure 1**)
- Use drill pins, not push pins, which can deflect
- Full-thickness, thin retractors to protect skin and ligaments, minimize skin trauma

VIDEO 64.1 Total Knee Arthroplasty via the Mini-Subvastus Approach. William C. Schroer, MD (12 min)

Surgical Technique
Incision and Arthrotomy
- Make 10- to 16-cm midline incision from superior pole of patella to tibial tubercle (**Figure 2**)

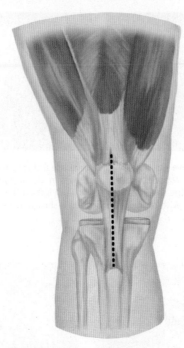

FIGURE 2 Illustration shows the skin incision (dashed line) for the mini-subvastus approach for total knee arthroplasty.

- Perform subcutaneous mobilization medially and superiorly for patella mobility
- Make horizontal arthrotomy along inferior aspect of vastus medialis obliquus (VMO), leaving cuff of retinaculum on VMO for closure (**Figure 3, A**)
- Complete arthrotomy in standard manner along medial patellar tendon
- Tag reflected retinaculum containing medial patellofemoral ligament for protection and retraction (**Figure 3, B**)

Patellar Mobilization
- Mobilize extensor mechanism to allow patellar subluxation
- Incise just through retinacular cuff of VMO on its medial border (**Figure 4, A**)
  - Allows significant lateral mobility of VMO
  - In large muscular patients, VMO will self-release a few centimeters above joint line
- Release synovial capsular reflection underneath VMO (**Figure 4, B**)
- Excise patellar fat pad (**Figure 4, C**)

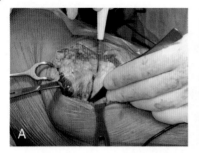 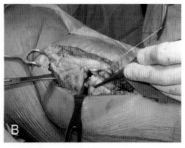

FIGURE 3 Intraoperative photographs demonstrate arthrotomy in the mini-subvastus approach. **A,** A horizontal arthrotomy is made along the vastus medialis obliquus (VMO). Note the small cuff of retinaculum left on the VMO. **B,** The completed arthrotomy with tagged retinaculum is shown. Note that the VMO is still tethered medially.

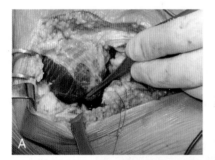 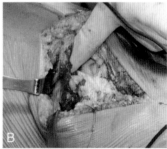

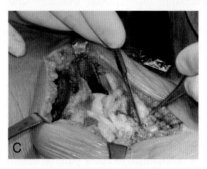

FIGURE 4 Intraoperative photographs show subvastus release and patellar mobilization in total knee arthroplasty via the mini-subvastus approach. **A,** The vastus medialis obliquus (VMO) is released through the retinacular cuff. The forceps are grabbing the recently released retinacular cuff. Note that the patella has started to move laterally. **B,** The surgeon's index finger is under the capsular reflection. Note that the VMO is releasing laterally. **C,** A Z retractor has subluxated the patella laterally. Note that the entire anterior distal femur is well visualized. Excision of the fat pad as shown completes the mobilization of the patella.

- Place Z retractor under VMO laterally; flex knee to 90°; perform most of the surgery with knee at this angle to avoid hyperflexion of knee as in traditional TKA

Femoral and Tibial Preparation

- Use 9-mm drill to open the intramedullary (IM) canal of distal femur and proximal tibia
- Position IM distal femoral alignment guide on anteromedial surface of femur
- Drill two parallel threaded pins into femur; check and adjust distal resection; place third cross pin
- Distal femur cutting guide arcs around femur from anterior to medial, allowing initial cut of medial femoral condyle from anterior to posterior; angle saw laterally to complete cut
- Use IM tibial guide; it requires fewer landmarks for orientation
- After cut is made, place knee in full extension; grasp cut tibia on its anteromedial surface and rotate out, medial side first (**Figure 5**)
- As tibia rotates out, release medial meniscus, posterior cruciate ligament, and lateral meniscus attachments off cut tibia
- With knee still in extension, remove meniscal remnants from posterior capsule; check extension gap
- Place knee in 90° flexion
- Measure distal femur with posterior reference guide, determine femoral rotation; position low-profile four-in-one cutting block on distal femur
- Make saw cuts; remove bony fragments

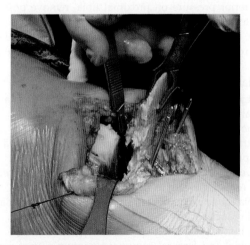

FIGURE 5 Intraoperative photograph shows tibial preparation for total knee arthroplasty via the mini-subvastus approach. The tibia is rotated out, medial side first. The cut bone is released from the medial meniscus, the posterior cruciate ligament, and the lateral meniscus.

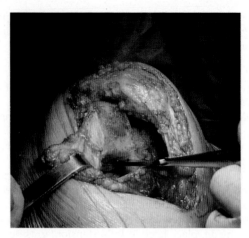

FIGURE 6 Intraoperative photograph shows posteromedial femoral osteophytes visualized through the mobile window, which affords a medial view for posterior cleanout. A view of the lateral side is obscured here but can be obtained in a subsequent step. Everything can be well visualized with the mini-subvastus surgical technique, although, unlike in a medial patellar tendon approach, not everything can be seen at once.

- If using posterior-stabilized implant, make femoral notch cut
- Allow patella to subluxate back into anatomic position; flex knee again to 90°
- With posterior pressure on proximal tibia, remove posterior medial osteophytes with curved osteotome (**Figure 6**)
- Subluxate patella laterally with Z retractor; place knee in figure-of-4 position; remove posterior lateral osteophytes with curved osteotome

Trialing, Balancing, and Final Preparation
- Position trial femoral and tibial components; perform trial reduction
- Perform and confirm final collateral ligament balancing
- Determine patellar tracking and tibial rotation
- Remove trial components; place knee in extension; tilt patella onto its side and prepare it for cemented patellar button
- Place knee in 90° flexion; position medial and lateral retractors; use posterior retractor to subluxate tibia forward
- Finish tibia for final component using previously determined rotation from trial reduction
- Clean cut bony surfaces with pulsatile irrigation
- Cement tibial and femoral components into position; remove excess cement; place trial tibial polyethylene component so cement cures under compression
- Cement patellar component with knee in extension

- Determine appropriate polyethylene thickness; make final soft-tissue balancing checks throughout flexion and extension
- Make final check for bone and cement debris
- Position polyethylene component; confirm patellar tracking
- Close arthrotomy using one figure-of-8 nonabsorbable suture placed at apex of arthrotomy, followed by double-armed running suture for rest of capsule

POSTOPERATIVE CARE AND REHABILITATION
Multimodal Pain Management
- Addresses pain before giving anesthesia; continues throughout the surgical procedure, through the postanesthesia care unit, and onto the joint arthroplasty care unit
- Give cyclooxygenase-2 inhibitors, long-acting narcotics before surgery
- Intraoperatively, give regional blocks; infiltrate soft tissues around knee with long-acting local
- Postoperatively, cyclooxygenase-2 inhibitors, oral narcotics, and cryotherapy prevent large spikes in pain
- Minimize intravenous narcotics because of nausea; give antiemetics on schedule

Mobilization
- Patient seen by physical therapy (PT) on day of surgery; assisted up to chair, encouraged to use bathroom, instructed in walker use
- Weight bearing as tolerated
- Quadriceps work while in bed; gravity-assisted knee flexion in chair
- Formal PT continues twice daily
- Use epidural, femoral nerve blocks rarely; they slow patient mobility
- Do not use continuous passive motion machines; patients need to get out of bed
- After hospital discharge, schedule home health care for 2 to 3 weeks
- Encourage stationary bicycle use for knee flexion and proprioception
- Progress patient from walker to cane to independent ambulation
- See patient in office 3 weeks after surgery; assess wounds and knee motion
- Author reports 4,500 primary cases; wound problems in less than 5% of patients, knee flexion at 3 weeks greater than 100° in more than 95%, outpatient PT necessary in less than 5%

PEARLS

- Surgical exposure involves creating subcutaneous "mobile window," in which entire knee joint is not visualized at any time.
- Skin incision length not as important as avoiding quadriceps violation and patellar eversion.

- Use drill pins, not push pins hammered into bone, to improve accuracy of cutting guide positioning; place third pin in separate plane from first pin to secure guide.
- Full-thickness retractors with fulcrum off bone minimizes skin trauma; rakes and retractors can lead to wound damage.
- Minimize soft-tissue damage by avoiding excessive and unneeded traction; avoid dislocating knee; maintain joint in anatomic position whenever possible.
- Know when and where soft tissue is at risk; protect it from saw blades and retractors.

COMPLICATIONS

- Concern exists that limited exposure will lead to increased complications
- Wound complications may develop as retractors excessively pull on skin
- Saw cuts made under poor visualization may raise risk of ligament, tendon, or neurovascular injury
- Increased soft-tissue damage; surgical time may raise perioperative infection rate
- Limited visualization may raise risk of inaccurate position and inferior long-term results
- After first 600 minimally invasive surgery (MIS) TKAs at minimum of 2 years follow-up, author reported no increase in complication rate compared with historical controls or current literature
- Recent follow-up of 875 mini-subvastus TKAs at mean 5.5 postoperative years shows major complication rate of 2.6%; 1.8% required revision (0.7% septic failure, 1.1% aseptic loosening)

CONCLUSIONS

- Author's results demonstrate rapid recovery with no increase in early or late complications
- Outcome varies with different MIS techniques and among different surgeons
- TKA outcomes can be poor with MIS or traditional technique
- Critics of MIS TKA target only short-term improvements that diminish rapidly few weeks after surgery; proponents of MIS TKA demonstrate functional differences several months after surgery
- Impact of MIS shows in surgeon awareness of soft-tissue envelope around knee and in need to optimize patient recovery after TKA
- Mini-subvastus technique can be applied to nearly all primary TKAs; complication rate compares to that of traditional TKA; has subjective and objective measures of improved functional recovery

VIDEO REFERENCE

 Video 64.1 Schroer WC: *Total Knee Arthroplasty via the Mini Subvastus Approach* [video]. Santa Barbara, CA, Copyright Video Journal Orthopaedics, 2010.

Revision Total Knee Arthroplasty via Tibial Tubercle Osteotomy

PATIENT SELECTION

- Number of total knee arthroplasties (TKAs) increased in past 20 years; projected to reach 3.5 million primary and 268,000 revision cases by 2030
- Quadriceps snip and tibial tubercle osteotomy (TTO) were developed to improve exposure in revision TKA (rTKA) as well as complex primary TKA
- Most patients are managed with quadriceps snip; surgeon may opt for a TTO early to avoid being forced into a secondary TTO after quadriceps snip fails

Indications

- Rigid, severe lack of range of motion (ROM); consider for ROM less than 90° of flexion, especially with severe fibrous block in motion
- May be necessary during rTKA for two-stage exchange for infection, stiff/painful primary TKA, and neglected aseptically loosened TKA

Contraindications

- Poor bone stock in proximal tibia
- Can be overcome by extending TTO segment further distally into tibial diaphysis

PREOPERATIVE IMAGING AND EVALUATION

- AP weight-bearing, lateral, sunrise radiographs (**Figure 1**)
- Physical examination, specifically preoperative ROM

PROCEDURE

Room Setup/Patient Positioning

- Standard supine positioning for TKA
- Excessive external rotation can be minimized with a padded bolster under the ipsilateral hip and/or a padded hip positioner placed lateral to the tourniquet

---

Based on Geller JA, Sarpong N: Revision total knee arthroplasty via tibial tubercle osteotomy, in Colvin AC, Flatow E, eds: Atlas of Essential Orthopaedic Procedures, *ed 2. Rosemont, IL, American Academy of Orthopaedic Surgeons, 2020, pp 535-539.*

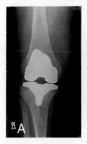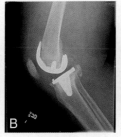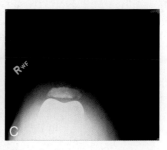

FIGURE 1 Weight-bearing AP (**A**), lateral (**B**), and sunrise (**C**) radiographs of the knee of a patient who underwent a total knee arthroplasty (TKA) 1 yr earlier. The TKA was revised for pain and stiffness.

Special Instruments/Equipment/Implants

- Full set of straight and curved osteotomes
- Motorized microsagittal saw
- 18-gauge stainless steel wires, 2.7-mm drill bit, wire tightener, or 6.5-mm cannulated screws. The authors prefer wires as they are lower profile and less likely to cause fracture through the osteotomized fragment

 VIDEO 65.1 This video segment shows a tibial tubercle osteotomy performed in an elderly patient undergoing rTKA for chronic pain and stiffness. Jeffrey A. Geller, MD. (2 min 30 s)

Surgical Technique

- Standard extensile approach for rTKA
- Follow prior skin incisions; extend enough to improve visualization and identify normal tissue; distal aspect should extend 8 to 10 cm distal to tibial tubercle (**Figure 2**)
- Lift wide, full-thickness skin flaps laterally; keep lower-leg anterior compartment intact
- Enter knee using standard medial parapatellar arthrotomy
- Perform extensive synovectomy
- With surgical marker, draw osteotomy 3 to 4 cm distal to joint line; osteotomized fragment should be 4 cm wide, 6 to 8 cm long, 2 to 4 cm deep
- Configure proximal aspect of fragment to create step cut on slight angle (**Figure 3**)
- Use microsagittal saw to perform cuts; make proximal cut first, then cut along tibial crest from medial to lateral (**Figure 4**)
- Cut should not extend across tibia; leave last few millimeters of bone and soft tissue intact to form hinge

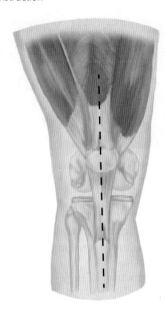

FIGURE 2 Illustration shows the incision for a revision total knee arthroplasty (TKA) via tibial tubercle osteotomy.

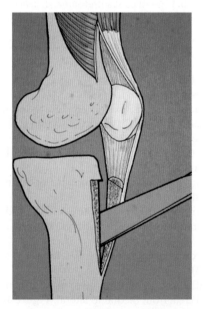

FIGURE 3 Illustration of the location of the cuts for tibial tubercle osteotomy. Lateral view.

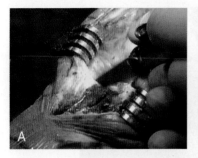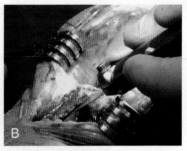

FIGURE 4 Intraoperative images demonstrate the proximal transverse step cut (**A**) and the longitudinal osteotomy cut (**B**).

- Lift osteotomized fragment up on medial side using multiple osteotomes, with the fragment hinging on soft tissues laterally (**Figure 5**); leave soft-tissue sleeve intact laterally for ease of repair and reduction, also maintains vascularity to segment
- Evert patella with TTO fragment; knee can be fully flexed up; surgeon has easy access for component removal during revision TKA
- After revision TKA prosthesis in place, reduce and fix TTO
- Prepare three to four pieces of wire, 18 inches long
- Use 2.7-mm drill bit to drill from medial aspect of intact tibia to approximately 10 mm posterior
- Pass wire through holes; repeat three to four times; space adequate distance apart
- Anatomically reduce TTO fragment into bony bed in full extension; reduce proximal segment into step cut

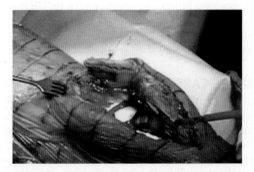

FIGURE 5 Intraoperative image demonstrates the exposure obtained after the tibial tubercle osteotomy fragment is lifted laterally.

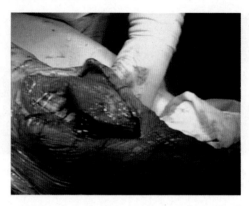

FIGURE 6 Intraoperative photograph shows the final tibial tubercle osteotomy repair, with the wire ends cut and buried beneath soft tissue.

- Bend lateral limb of wire over TTO; twist wire and tighten down; wire must be tight enough to ensure bony union
- Cut wires short; tamp down with bone tamp; bury ends under soft tissue (**Figure 6**)
- Place medium Hemovac drain to prevent hemarthrosis; close in standard fashion

COMPLICATIONS
- Proximal migration of TTO fragment
  - ▹ Occurs when the step cut in the proximal aspect of the TTO is inadequate or not done
  - ▹ If the step cut is not deep enough or too thin, the fragment may fracture removing a buttress to counteract the pull of the quadriceps
- Nonunion of TTO fragment (rare)
- Prominent hardware
- Postoperative tibia fracture

POSTOPERATIVE CARE AND REHABILITATION
- If fixation of TTO is adequate, patient begins ROM exercises without limitation and bear weight as tolerated
- Start continuous passive motion machine with standard protocol to increase ROM
- If fixation strength compromised, advance motion more conservatively; limit ROM to 45° of flexion for first 2 weeks, advance to 90° by 4 weeks, full ROM beyond 6 weeks

PEARLS

- Ensure keyed-in step cut in proximal aspect of the TTO is thick enough to prevent proximal migration of fragment; angled so that the TTO keys in upon repair
- Perform wire tightening with power drill attachment; provides more torque, can be done quicker, and with better control

66 Extensor Mechanism Reconstruction With Marlex Mesh

INTRODUCTION

- Extensor mechanism reconstruction with Marlex mesh provides durable and reliable outcomes to a catastrophic complication
- Mayo Clinic experience—65 of 77 mesh reconstructions in place at 4 years, 12 patients required a revision extensor mechanism reconstruction, extensor lag improvement of 26°, with a mean extensor lag of 9°. Knee Society scores showed a significant improvement

PATIENT SELECTION

- Patients undergoing or who have undergone total knee arthroplasty with an intraoperative or postoperative extensor mechanism injury
- Native quadriceps or patellar tendon ruptures can be treated using this technique as well
- Relative contraindication to mesh reconstruction is active infection

PREOPERATIVE (DIAGNOSTIC) IMAGING

- Standard knee radiographs
- Closely evaluate the lateral radiograph for patella alta or baja
- Less commonly, an ultrasonography or MRI may be needed

PROCEDURE

- Only a single monofilament polypropylene mesh is used (Marlex; C.R. Bard)
- Before incision, the 10 × 14-in sheet of mesh is folded onto itself 8 to 10 times and sewn together (**Figure 1**)
- The patient is then prepped and draped in the usual sterile fashion
- For both quadriceps tendon and patellar tendon disruptions, a standard medial parapatellar arthrotomy should be performed, taking care to maintain an equal amount of robust soft tissue on both the vastus lateralis and vastus medialis oblique (VMO) sides

---

Based on Abdel MP, Hanssen AD: Extensor mechanism reconstruction with Marlex mesh, in Colvin AC, Flatow E, eds: Atlas of Essential Orthopaedic Procedures, *ed 2. Rosemont, IL, American Academy of Orthopaedic Surgeons, 2020, pp 540-542.*

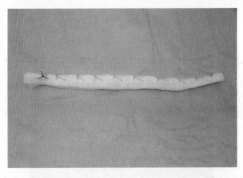

FIGURE 1 Photograph of a 10 × 14-in sheet of Marlex mesh folded on itself eight times and then unitized with a single nonabsorbable suture. (Reproduced with permission from the Mayo Foundation of Medical Education and Research, Rochester, MN.)

- If the tibia is not being revised, then a 6.5-mm round burr is used to create a trough in tibia and 5 cm of the mesh is cemented into the trough (**Figure 2**)
- After the cement has cured, a lag screw is placed across the mesh and cement and into host bone
- If the tibia is being revised, then the 5 cm of the mesh is placed in the intramedullary canal (**Figure 3**)
- It is essential to ensure that the mesh is covered with host tissue
- Next, the vastus lateralis and VMO are mobilized distally by releasing all ventral and dorsal soft-tissue adhesions.
- The mesh is then unitized to the vastus lateralis with multiple nonabsorbable sutures. The VMO is then pulled distally and laterally over the mesh and secured with multiple nonabsorbable sutures through the VMO, through the mesh, and through the vastus lateralis, unitizing the entire construct (**Figure 4**)

COMPLICATIONS
- Rerupture of the extensor mechanism or symptomatic lengthening leading to an extensor lag
- Standard complications associated with revision total knee arthroplasty

POSTOPERATIVE CARE AND REHABILITATION
- At 48 hours, the wound is evaluated and the leg placed in a long leg cast incorporating the foot with the knee in 5° of flexion
- 2 weeks to 3 months: the cast is changed every 2 to 3 weeks for a total casting time of 12 weeks

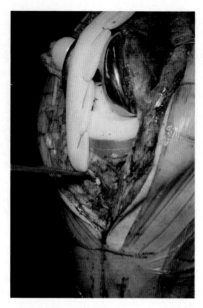

FIGURE 2 Intraoperative photograph of the aforementioned mesh placed in the tibial trough given that the tibial component was not revised. (Reproduced with permission from the Mayo Foundation of Medical Education and Research, Rochester, MN.)

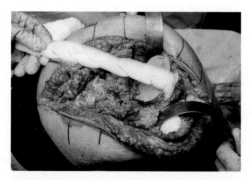

FIGURE 3 Intraoperative photograph of the Marlex mesh placed in the intramedullary canal given that the tibial component was revised at the time of the extensor mechanism reconstruction. (Reproduced with permission from the Mayo Foundation of Medical Education and Research, Rochester, MN.)

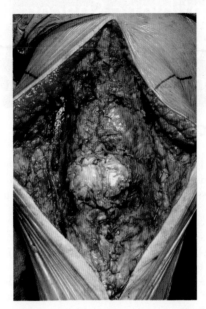

FIGURE 4 Intraoperative photograph of the pants-over-vest reconstruction where the vastus lateralis is deep, the mesh is in the middle, and the vastus medialis oblique is superficial, all unitized with multiple nonabsorbable sutures. (Reproduced with permission from the Mayo Foundation of Medical Education and Research, Rochester, MN.)

- 3 to 6 months: the cast is removed and replaced with a hinged knee brace. Active gravity flexion is permitted in the brace beginning with 45° of flexion for 1 month, 60° for the second month, and 90° for the third month. Weight bearing is permitted with the brace locked in full extension
- An ambulatory aid is recommended to help prevent falls and subsequent damage to the reconstruction

PEARLS

- Ensure the mesh is not overly wide when folding it over on itself and unitizing it. This will make insertion into the tibial trough or intramedullary canal difficult.
- Approximately 5 cm of the mesh should be cemented into the tibia.
- Mesh must be covered with native host tissue ventrally and dorsally to prevent wound compromise as well as mesh abrasion against the implant, which may lead to tearing.

PATIENT SELECTION

Introduction
- Two-stage revision first reported by John Insall in 1983
- Two-stage revision remains the benchmark in North America
- Overall success with eradication of infection in 80% to 94% of cases

Static Spacers
- Knee joint is kept in full extension or slight flexion
- Advantages—lower cost, easier implantation, joint immobilization to allow for soft-tissue healing
- Disadvantages—postoperative stiffness, spacer dissociation from bone ends resulting in further bone loss, and spacer extrusion resulting in soft-tissue damage

Articulating Spacers (Figure 1, A and B)
- Motion is allowed during the treatment period
- Advantages—prevention of extensor mechanism shortening, easier reimplantation surgery, and improved postoperative range of motion
- Disadvantages—concern for biofilm on implant surfaces
- Inexpensive or recycled components may be used to contain costs. Alternative techniques include the use of prefabricated antibiotic cement spacers or intraoperative cement molds
- Stemmed spacers deliver antibiotic to the intramedullary canal, provide additional fixation, and allow for the use of an articulating spacer in cases with bone loss
- The authors prefer the use of a preformed cement spacer with added stems

Intramedullary Static Spacer (Figure 2)
- Indicated in cases with extensor mechanism or extensive metaphyseal fracture
- Facilitates healing process before secondary reimplantation procedure

---

Based on Harper KD, Park KJ, Incavo SJ: Antibiotic spacers for the treatment of infected total knee arthroplasty cases, in Colvin AC, Flatow E, eds: Atlas of Essential Orthopaedic Procedures, ed 2. Rosemont, IL, American Academy of Orthopaedic Surgeons, 2020, pp 543-547.

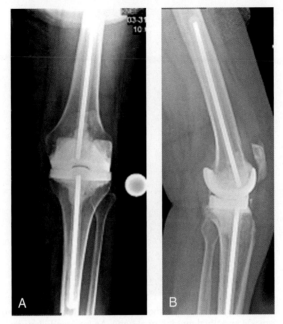

FIGURE 1 **A** and **B**, AP and lateral radiographs of an articulating spacer following an infected primary total knee arthroplasty.

PROCEDURE

Preoperative Setup

- Standard patient positioning for knee arthroplasty per surgeon preference
- Two tables are used, the first for removal of the total knee implants and the second for creation and implantation of the antibiotic spacer

Antibiotic Spacer Parameters

- Multiple recommendations exist regarding antibiotic dosing
- The authors prefer to use 3.0 to 3.3 g vancomycin, 3.6 g tobramycin per 40 g bag of cement, with most cases requiring two to three bags of cement
- Antifungal medications (amphotericin B or voriconazole) can be added in cases of fungal infection, culture negative, or immunocompromised patients
- Take care when using different cements, for example, high viscosity cement will have a higher elution rate and requires a lower dose of antibiotics

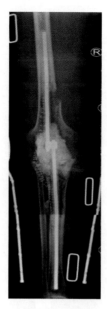

FIGURE 2 AP radiograph showing difficult component removal resulting in fracture of the femoral and tibial metaphyseal bone. An intramedullary, static spacer was placed.

Design and Assembly

- Each bag of cement (Simplex, Stryker Orthopaedics, Mahwah NJ), three vials (1.2 g each) of tobramycin, and three vials (1 g each) of vancomycin as well as a few drops of methylene blue
- The authors prefer to use preformed gentamicin-impregnated cement spacers
- Antibiotic cement–coated rods are created with 4.0 mm Steinmann pins in a plastic mold to produce a 13 mm diameter rod
- Holes are drilled in the articulating components and the rods are screwed into each spacer
- The infected implants are then removed using a saw and osteotomes, followed by a thorough irrigation and débridement to healthy, bleeding tissue. All residual cement must be removed

Spacer Insertion

- The femoral and tibial canals are reamed to 13.5 to 14 mm in diameter
- The articulating spacer implants are trialed to ensure the knee is able to achieve full extension
- The final two batches of cement are mixed and the implants are cemented in place

Static Spacer Considerations

- A static spacer will use the same intramedullary rods described above; however, the authors prefer to use a 5.5 mm spinal rod at the core
- A rod to rod connector can be used to join the stems to maintain length
- The empty joint space is then filled with cement

COMPLICATIONS

- Bone loss is a common complication, both during the treatment period as well as during removal
- The use of intramedullary stems can improve the stability of the implants and reduce the risk for spacer dislodgement

POSTOPERATIVE CARE

- Intravenous antibiotics are considered under the direction of an infectious disease consultant
- The knee is kept in extension with toe touch weight bearing for 3 weeks
- From this point weight bearing and motion is gradually progressed
- Static spacers are protected with a knee brace in full extension but allowed full weight bearing
- Two-week antibiotic holiday before consideration of reimplantation
- Before the second-stage procedure, a joint aspirate is obtained for cell count, culture, and in some cases alpha defensin

PEARLS

- The two-stage revision remains the benchmark in North America for treatment of PJI and carries with it a reported success rate of 80% to 94%.
- The articulating spacer demonstrates improved range of motion, prevention of extensor mechanism shortening, easier reimplantation surgery, and improved postoperative range of motion.
- Adding stems to a spacer will improve antibiotic delivery to the intramedullary canal, decrease risk of spacer dislodgement, and expand the indications for use of articulating spacers in cases of moderate to severe bone loss.
- Unique infective organisms may require an adjustment in antibiotics included within the cement (ie, antifungals, etc).
- Adding methylene blue to your antibiotic spacer cement will facilitate identification at subsequent surgeries and ensure complete removal of contaminated cement.

Trauma

5

Section Editor
Lawrence X. Webb, MD, MBA

68 General Principles of Surgical Débridement

INTRODUCTION

- Surgical débridement is used for wounds containing contaminated and/or devitalized tissue
- Goal—To alter the wound environment by the surgical removal of contamination and/or nonviable tissue so healing can occur free of infection
- Extending the wound outside of the initial zone of injury is often necessary to effectively evaluate and débride nonviable tissue and remove contamination
- Stabilization of bony injury is necessary to minimize osteonecrosis and thus decrease risk of infection
- Soft tissue should sufficiently cover tissues prone to infection when exposed, such as bone and tendon

PROCEDURE

 VIDEO 68.1 Surgical Débridement. Lawrence X. Webb, MD, Henry J. Dolch, DO (6 min).

Surgical Technique

- Sharply débride gross contamination and devitalized tissues. Extend the wound as needed to expose all contamination and devitalized tissue
- A tangential excision tool is useful and functions via the Bernoulli principle, whereby the surface of the wound is excised as it is pulled upward into the high-pressure saline stream
- Normal saline irrigation with a large volume of saline is an important next step. The FLOW trial shows no difference in outcome based on irrigation pressure
- Following débridement, consider use of a negative-pressure dressing at −75 mm Hg to evacuate excess edema, stabilize and moisten the soft tissues, preserve capillary blood flow, and provide sterile wound coverage

---

Based on Webb LX, Dolch HJ: General principles of surgical débridement, in Colvin AC, Flatow E, eds: Atlas of Essential Orthopaedic Procedures, ed 2. Rosemont, IL, American Academy of Orthopaedic Surgeons, 2020, pp 549-552.

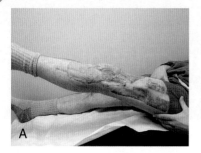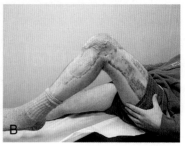

FIGURE 1 Clinical photographs of the patient shown in Video 68.1 at 12 weeks following the injury. The patient exhibits a range of motion of 0° (**A**) to 85° (**B**).

- Return patient to operating room at 48 to 72 hours for a second look, which allows a subsequent débridement of any nonviable tissue
- Change negative-pressure dressings at 48-hour intervals until the wound is appropriate for closure or until secondary closure techniques are accomplished
- If primary closure cannot be achieved, coverage options include split-thickness skin graft, local muscle flaps, or an Integra bilayer (Integra LifeSciences); following incorporation of the bilayer (typically at day 5), a split-thickness skin graft may be performed
- Bolster graft with another negative-pressure dressing at −75 mm Hg; graft should incorporate over next 7 days

POSTOPERATIVE CARE AND REHABILITATION
- Dress newly grafted tissue in sterile saline-soaked gauze; change dressing daily until epithelialization is complete
- Range of motion and mobilization should begin as soon as possible
- **Figure 1** shows the patient from Video 68.1 performing independent range of motion 12 weeks postoperatively

PRINCIPLES OF DÉBRIDEMENT
- Thoroughly evaluate the wound and potential zone of injury
- Thoroughly débride in a timely manner
- A second look at 48 hours is often necessary, particularly with highly contaminated wounds, desiccation-prone tissue, and high-energy mechanisms, to detect any demarcated nonviable tissue and débride appropriately
- Bony stability is important for soft-tissue healing
- Plan and arrange early wound coverage
- Reestablish normal musculoskeletal function early for optimal results

Fasciotomy for Compartment Syndrome of the Leg

INTRODUCTION

- Compartment syndrome arises from pressure within an osseofascial compartment high enough to compromise microvascular blood flow to tissue
- If uncorrected, tissue necrosis occurs within a few hours
- Several etiologies exist, most commonly trauma
- Cycle of tissue trauma, inflammatory response, outpouring of fluid from capillaries and cells occurs
- Results in compromised O_2 and CO_2 exchange
- Tissue pressure within compartment and its relationship to the diastolic blood pressure (within 30 mm Hg) are determining factors for compartment syndrome
- Commonly occurs in leg, but can affect the thigh, gluteal compartment, foot, forearm, hand, brachium, deltoid, and other compartments

PATIENT SELECTION

- Earliest physical examination finding is pain on passive stretch of muscle in affected compartment
- Affected compartments are tight and tender to palpation
- Over time, pain increases and is less likely to be alleviated by narcotics
- Numbness, paresthesias, diminished motor function, and pulselessness ensue; some myonecrosis has occurred if syndrome progresses to this point
- Treatment is emergent fasciotomy of all affected compartments

PROCEDURE

Surgical Technique

- Authors' method is two-incision technique for release of all four osseofascial compartments in lower leg (**Figure 1**)

VIDEO 69.1 Technique for Two-Incision Leg Fasciotomy.
Lawrence X. Webb, MD; John C.P. Floyd, MD (4 min)

Based on Webb LX, Behboudi A: Fasciotomy for compartment syndrome of the leg, in Colvin AC, Flatow E, eds: Atlas of Essential Orthopaedic Procedures, ed 2. Rosemont, IL, American Academy of Orthopaedic Surgeons, 2020, pp 553-556.

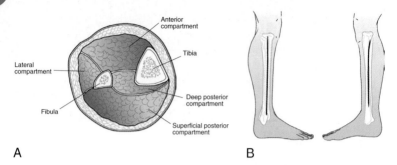

FIGURE 1 Illustrations depict a two-incision fasciotomy for compartment syndrome of the leg. **A,** Cross-sectional view shows the anatomic muscle compartments of the leg. **B,** Location of incisions on the lateral and medial aspects of the leg.

- Release anterior and lateral compartments through anterolateral incision (**Figure 2**)
  - Localize intermuscular septum proximally with short, transverse incision

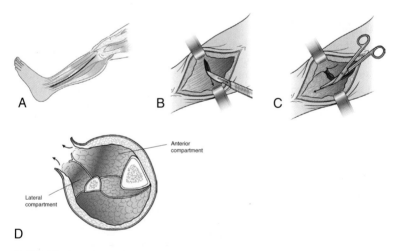

FIGURE 2 Illustrations show release of anterior and lateral leg compartments. **A,** Location of the anterolateral incision. **B,** A short transverse incision is made to localize the intermuscular septum. **C,** Release of anterior compartment fascia. The cephalad fascia has been released; the caudad portion is in the process of being released. **D,** Cross section of the leg after anterior and lateral compartment release.

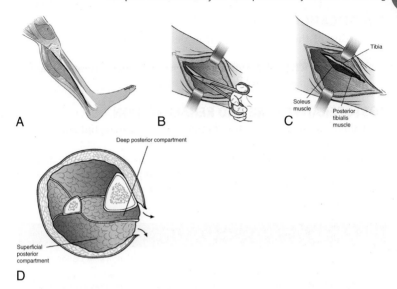

FIGURE 3 Illustrations show release of the deep and superficial posterior leg compartments. **A**, Location of the anteromedial incision. **B**, The superficial posterior compartment is released, using the same technique shown in **Figure 2**, following the creation of a small rent in the line of the fascial fibers with a scalpel. **C**, The deep posterior compartment has been released. The surgeon should be able to digitally probe the muscle space posterior to the tibia. **D**, Cross section of the leg after deep and superficial posterior compartment release.

- ▶ Make small axial incision in fascia anterior to intermuscular septum; introduce curved Mayo scissors to perform fasciotomy in a cephalad and caudad direction
- ▶ Release lateral compartment in similar fashion on other side of intermuscular septum
- ▶ Assess muscles for color, consistency, contractility, and capillary refill
- Release superficial and deep posterior compartments via anteromedial incision 2 cm medial to posteromedial tibial border (**Figure 3**)
  - ▶ Make small fascial incision to allow tips of curved Mayo scissors to release fascia of superficial posterior compartment in cephalad and caudad direction
  - ▶ Make second small fascial incision just off posteromedial tibial border to release deep posterior compartment
  - ▶ Following cephalad and caudad release, the posteromedial tibia is palpable
  - ▶ Assess viability of muscles following release
- Following fasciotomies, assess whether skin incisions need lengthening; the skin itself may tether compartments in severe cases

COMPLICATIONS

- Scarring of the skin is inherent in delayed wound closure and skin grafting
- Superficial peroneal nerve injury; nerve traverses crural fascia at a variable point on anterolateral aspect of leg

POSTOPERATIVE CARE AND REHABILITATION

- Wound can be dressed with moistened sterile gauze, but authors prefer to use negative-pressure dressing
- Return patient to operating room for staged débridement, delayed primary closure, and/or split-thickness skin grafting at 48- to 96-hour intervals depending on condition of wound

PEARLS

- Have a high index of suspicion for compartment syndrome in patients with severe unremitting limb pain and swelling.
- Most important finding is pain on passive stretch of muscles in affected compartment.
- In patients who cannot appreciate pain (eg, comatose patient, neuropathic patient), measuring compartment pressures may aid diagnosis; pressures rising within 30 mm Hg of diastolic blood pressure indicate compartment syndrome.
- After making diagnosis, perform decompressive fasciotomies emergently.

Open Reduction and Internal Fixation of Forearm Fractures

INTRODUCTION
- The forearm serves as the origin/insertion for muscle groups that control the elbow, wrist, and hand; as well as intrinsic forearm pronation and supination
- When injured, anatomic restoration is mandatory for satisfactory function
- Fracture predominant in the younger population; average age 35 years

PATIENT SELECTION
- Open reduction and internal fixation (ORIF) is the standard of care to achieve stable, rigid, anatomic fixation, and best functional outcome
- Anatomic realignment of proximal and distal radioulnar joints must be achieved to preserve pronation and supination
- Restoring radial/ulnar diaphyseal length and rotation aids restoration of articular alignment by indirect means
- ORIF enables early range of motion (ROM) and faster recovery; avoids stiffness, muscular deconditioning, skin atrophy, and potential complex regional pain syndrome
- Few contraindications to ORIF exist, but include severe contamination and burns; can use temporary stabilization with external fixator until soft tissues allow rigid fixation

EVALUATION
- Common mechanisms of injury—Direct blow, fall, gunshot injury
- Symptoms—Pain, swelling, tenderness, inability to use forearm
- Carefully examine for wounds indicating open fracture
- Thoroughly examine and document sensory, motor, and circulatory status

PREOPERATIVE IMAGING
- Obtain AP, lateral, and oblique radiographs
- Include joint above and below

Based on Varecka TF: Open reduction and internal fixation of forearm fractures, in Colvin AC, Flatow E, eds: Atlas of Essential Orthopaedic Procedures, *ed 2. Rosemont, IL, American Academy of Orthopaedic Surgeons, 2020, pp 557-570.*

- Note displacement, comminution, foreign materials, or subcutaneous air
- CT/MRI are rarely needed for diagnosis

PREOPERATIVE PLANNING

- Includes accurate drawing of fracture, details of fracture position, and location of implants; indicate screw placement
- List all needed equipment; note necessary implants and order of use to ensure procurement
- Consider dressing supplies, splint/cast material, and preoperative antibiotics

PROCEDURE

Room Setup/Patient Positioning

- Supine position; extend arm on arm table (**Figure 1**)
- Tourniquet use recommended
- Always include a time out before start of the procedure

Surgical Technique

- Exsanguinate extremity with Esmarch wrap; inflate tourniquet to 100 to 125 mm Hg above systolic blood pressure
- Fracture determines approach; authors use volar approach of Henry for radius (**Figure 2**) and ulnar midline approach for ulna; for more proximal fractures of the radius, dorsal Thompson approach may be considered
- Addressing simpler fracture first aids fixation of more complex fracture

Approach for Radial Fixation

- For volar approach of Henry, incise along length of radius as needed

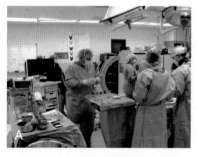 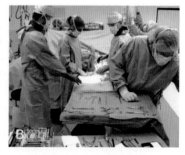

FIGURE 1 Photographs show the room setup and patient positioning for open reduction and internal fixation of a both-bone forearm fracture. **A,** The room setup, with C-arm, back table, and instruments prepared. **B,** The patient is positioned supine on the operating table with the injured arm supported on an arm table.

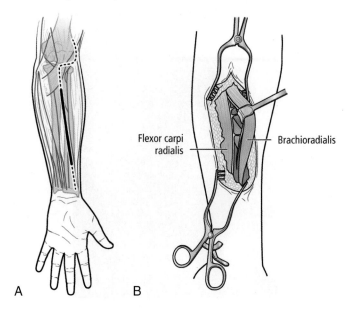

Flexor carpi radialis

Brachioradialis

A   B

FIGURE 2 Illustrations demonstrate the volar approach of Henry. **A,** The incision. The incision used in panel B is represented by the solid portion of the line. **B,** The initial exposure. A leash of vessels from the radial artery supplies the brachioradialis (BR) muscle. The vessels must be ligated to mobilize the BR muscle laterally. The superficial branch of the radial nerve is retracted with the BR muscle.

- Proximal interval is between brachioradialis (BR) muscle and flexor digitorum superficialis, with pronator teres and supinator deep; distal interval is between BR and flexor carpi radialis, with pronator quadratus deep (**Figures 2** and **3**)
- In midforearm, radial nerve is encountered along deep surface of BR; note and preemptively cauterize small perforating branches from radial artery (**Figure 4**)
- Sharply expose fracture and surrounding bone; only expose surface to which plate will be applied to avoid further bony insult (**Figure 5, A**); do not indiscriminately disrupt biology
- Preserve soft-tissue attachments to all fragments to prevent further devascularization
- Locking plate technology can be used to bypass intercalated, multi-fragmented sections of diaphysis

Provisional Reduction of the Radial Fracture

- Clean fracture ends of debris and hematoma; provisionally reduce with bone clamps or wires as necessary (**Figure 5, B**)
- Verify reduction with fluoroscopy, assuring appropriate length, rotation, and bow

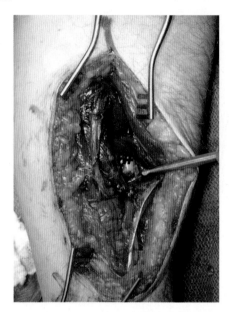

FIGURE 3 Intraoperative photograph shows proximal dissection for open reduction and internal fixation of a both-bone fracture. The brachioradialis and pronator teres muscles are retracted, exposing the fracture, which is denoted by the # sign.

Fixation of the Radial Fracture
- Use malleable aluminum templates for plate contouring (**Figure 6**)
- Use thick, rigid 3.5-mm plates for diaphyseal radius fractures; 4.5-mm plates are too large and rigid, leading to stress shielding
- Fracture pattern determines sequence of screw insertion (**Figure 7**)
- Use three bicortical screws on each side of fracture; use two bicortical screws with increased working length when bridging comminuted fracture
- Use standard, nonlocking plates; may use locking plates in multifragmentary diaphyseal fractures, metadiaphyseal fractures or pathologic bone
- Bone grafting may be indicated in cases of severe bone loss

Fixation of the Ulnar Fracture
- For ulnar fixation, make incision along ulnar midlateral border between flexor and extensor carpi ulnaris (**Figure 8, A**)
- Fixation of ulnar fracture follows principles similar to those for radial fixation (**Figure 8, B and C**)

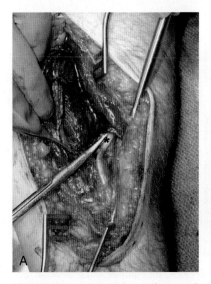 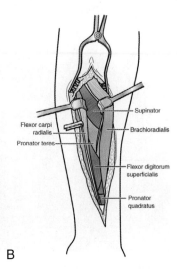

FIGURE 4 Dissection in the midforearm for open reduction and internal fixation of a both-bone fracture. **A,** Intraoperative photograph shows the brachioradialis muscle retracted. The superficial radial nerve is denoted by the asterisk. **B,** Deep to the brachioradialis and the flexor carpi radialis are the supinator muscles, the pronator teres, the flexor digitorum superficialis, and, most distally, the pronator quadratus.

Wound Closure

- Begin wound closure after fixation, tourniquet deflation, and identification and coagulation of bleeding sources
- Close wounds in layers; avoid watertight closure of deep fascial layers to permit swelling; prevents compartment syndrome
- Close subcutaneous tissue with absorbable braided or monofilament suture; close skin with absorbable or nonabsorbable sutures or staples
- Place nonadherent material under gauze bandages
- Necessity and type of splint depend on fracture pattern, fixation, and patient compliance; keep splint as small as possible and never circumferential

COMPLICATIONS

- Infection and ensuing soft-tissue damage, nonhealing, debilitation, and dysfunction
  - ▶ For persistent wound drainage or patient malaise, return to operating room for irrigation and débridement
  - ▶ Relying on laboratory tests such as C-reactive protein and erythrocyte sedimentation rate may delay incision and drainage
  - ▶ Early diagnosis and treatment is frequently successful

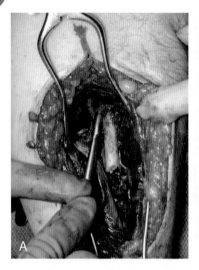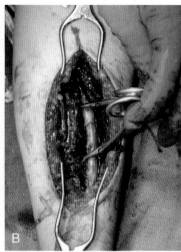

FIGURE 5 Intraoperative photographs demonstrate exposure and provisional reduction of the radial fracture in a both-bone fracture of the forearm. **A,** The fracture is exposed with a sharp periosteal elevator. **B,** Provisional reduction is achieved with bone clamps.

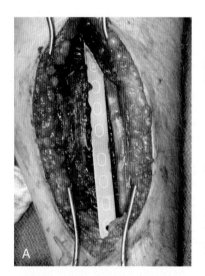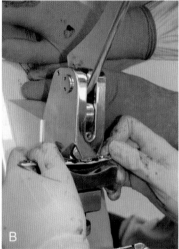

FIGURE 6 Intraoperative photographs demonstrate plate contouring. **A,** The shape and contour of the bone is determined with an aluminum template. **B,** Contouring of the plate is shown.

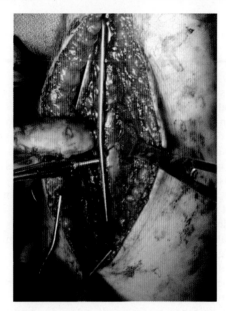

FIGURE 7 Intraoperative photograph shows the application of a plate to the radial fracture in a both-bone fracture. Note that the contour of the plate allows reestablishment of radial bow.

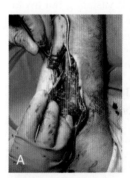
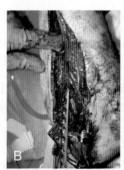
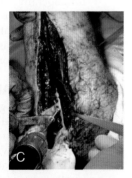

FIGURE 8 Intraoperative photographs demonstrate exposure and fixation of the ulnar fracture in a both-bone fracture. **A,** The ulna is exposed through a medial midaxial incision. **B,** The ulnar plate is inserted with limited submuscular technique. **C,** A screw hole is drilled for the ulnar plate. Note that the plate is partially covered because of the submuscular placement.

- Nonunion
  - These fractures do not create large callus; suspect nonunion in patients with persistent pain, tenderness at site, or local warmth beyond 3 to 4 months postoperatively
  - CT may help confirm nonunion or delayed union
- Radioulnar synostosis
  - Devastating complication; bony overgrowth forms bridge between radius and ulna; prevents forearm rotation
  - Highly comminuted fractures of radius at ulna at same level with prominent hardware have high risk for synostosis
  - Avoid connecting fracture sites intraoperatively, particularly when using bone graft
  - Routine prophylaxis with postoperative irradiation or indomethacin not recommended
- Loss of motion
  - Most patients have some, due to scarring and damage to interosseous ligament
  - Includes some loss of elbow and wrist motion
  - Discuss motion loss with patients before and after surgery
- Retained hardware
  - Current evidence recommends retaining hardware; hardware removal associated with more problems
  - Remove hardware when it causes discomfort, infection, or nonunion
- Iatrogenic complications
  - Intraoperative nerve or vessel damage—Devastating but avoidable with understanding of local anatomy and preoperative neurologic examination
  - "Fracture disease"—Prevent with gentle soft-tissue handling, careful dissection, solid fixation, and early rehabilitation

POSTOPERATIVE CARE AND REHABILITATION

- Elevation, ice, and gentle digit ROM help control swelling in early postoperative period
- Evaluate patient 7 to 10 days postoperatively; advance to gentle active ROM of wrist, elbow, forearm, and shoulder
  - In compliant patients, well-fitting elastic sleeve or prefabricated plastic brace provides support and reduces anxiety
  - Physical therapy reinforces need for ROM and motivates patient
- Strengthening begins about 6 weeks postoperatively; instruct patient that bone is not completely healed, so no vigorous activities
- Do not use callus formation as sign of fracture healing; instead, look for limited pain with motion and no local warmth; this occurs at 12 to 16 weeks, when patient can be released to full activity

PEARLS

- Both-bone forearm fractures disrupt the structure and function of the forearm and require meticulous restoration of the bony framework for best outcomes.
- Both-bone forearm fractures require rigid, stable, timely fixation.
- Preoperative planning is paramount and should include equipment needs, surgical tactic, fixation options and plans, and an outline of postoperative management.
- Avoid fixing both bones through a single incision.
- Postoperative rehabilitation should start early and be guided by a surgeon-therapist team.
- Some loss of motion is expected, but the functional impairment should be slight.

Open Reduction and Internal Fixation of Posterior Wall Acetabular Fractures

INTRODUCTION

Classification

- Letournel classified acetabular fractures into two fracture groups: elementary and associated (**Figure 1**)
- Each group has five types (**Figure 1**)
- Posterior wall fractures are most common type of acetabular fracture, accounting for 25% to 33%

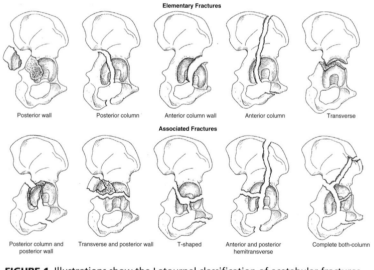

Elementary Fractures

Posterior wall   Posterior column   Anterior column wall   Anterior column   Transverse

Associated Fractures

Posterior column and posterior wall   Transverse and posterior wall   T-shaped   Anterior and posterior hemitransverse   Complete both-column

FIGURE 1 Illustrations show the Letournel classification of acetabular fractures.

Based on Webb LX: Open reduction and internal fixation of posterior wall acetabular fractures, in Colvin AC, Flatow E, eds: Atlas of Essential Orthopaedic Procedures, *ed 2. Rosemont, IL, American Academy of Orthopaedic Surgeons, 2020, pp 571-578.*

Associated Injuries

- Posterior wall fractures result from high-energy trauma; are associated with other serious injuries
- Mechanism of injury—Axial femoral loading with hip in flexed position (eg, knee strikes dashboard)
- Amount of abduction or adduction of hip at time of impact determines size of posterior wall fragment
- Upon displacement of posterior wall fragment, unconstrained femoral head subluxates or dislocates posteriorly in 78% to 86% of cases
- Marginal impaction of fractured acetabular articular surface occurs in 27% to 46% of posterior wall fractures
- Other associated injuries—Femoral head, neck, and shaft fractures; multiligamentous knee injuries

 VIDEO 71.1 Posterior Wall Fracture-Dislocation: Reduction and Traction Pin Placement. Lawrence X. Webb, MD; John M. Tabit, DO (4 min)

PREOPERATIVE IMAGING

- AP pelvic radiographs typically show fracture
- Judet oblique views, particularly obturator oblique, enable further visualization and classification
- CT helps assess femoral head, size and extent of segmentation or comminution of posterior wall fragment, and size and location of intra-articular fragments and marginal impaction fractures (**Figure 2**)

PROCEDURE

Equipment/Implants

- Self-retaining Charnley retractor
- Schanz pins (5.0-mm), hand chuck, small femoral distractor

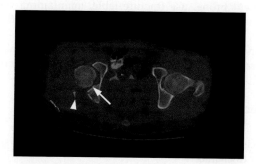

FIGURE 2 Axial CT scan of the pelvis clearly shows a marginal impaction fracture (arrow). The arrowhead indicates the edge of the posterior wall fragment.

- Sciatic nerve retractor, cobra retractor, Taylor retractor
- Adhesive plastic strips to temporarily hold retractors
- Standard and pituitary rongeurs to extract joint fragments and debris
- Cancellous bone allograft or bone graft substitute
- Ball-spike pusher
- 1.5- and 2.0-mm Kirschner wires
- Spring plates
- 3.5-mm reconstruction plates, corresponding aluminum templates, plate benders
- C-arm placed on side opposite surgeon

Early Management of Dislocation

- Timely reduction of dislocated hip important for pain relief and femoral head blood flow (dislocated longer than 12 hours has adverse effect)
- Perform reduction with conscious sedation in emergency department or with general anesthetic and muscle relaxant in operating room
- After reducing hip and verifying reduction radiographically, consider keeping knee in extension with knee immobilizer or splint if stable; use skeletal traction if reduction unstable with displaced or intra-articular fragments

Preoperative Planning and Patient Positioning

- CT can characterize nature, size, and displacement of fracture
- Use Kocher-Langenbeck approach
- Lateral decubitus or prone position; knee flexed to relax sciatic nerve (**Figure 3, A**)
- Place padded Mayo stand beneath flexed knee to achieve neutral adduction/abduction; raise or lower padded ankle using folded towels on Mayo stand to achieve internal/external hip rotation
- With patient prone, use fracture table, maintaining skeletal traction through distal femoral traction pin with knee flexed to 80° (**Figure 3, B**)
- Pad peroneal post to minimize risk of pudendal nerve palsy
- Pad contralateral foot and ankle well; place in fracture boot with knee extended

Surgical Technique

Exposure

- Direct incision obliquely between posterior superior iliac spine and tip of greater trochanter
- Cephalad extent of incision depends on necessity of posterior column exposure

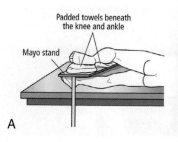
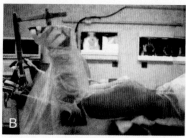

FIGURE 3 Images show patient positioning for open reduction and internal fixation of posterior wall acetabular fractures. **A,** Illustration of the lateral decubitus position. A Mayo stand, upon which the padded knee and leg rest, can be adjusted to effect hip adduction/abduction. Varying the height of a soft bump placed beneath the foot/ankle with the knee flexed is used to effect rotation. **B,** Intraoperative photograph of a patient in the prone position. Skeletal traction through a transfixing pin in the distal femur is used. The knee is maintained in the flexed position as shown. The unaffected leg is kept in extension. The thighs and the peroneal post are appropriately padded. (Panel B reproduced with permission from Siegel J, Templeman DC: Open reduction and internal fixation of the posterior wall of the acetabulum, in Tornetta P III, Williams GR, Ramsey ML, Hunt TR III, Wiesel SW, eds: *Operative Techniques in Orthopaedic Trauma Surgery.* Philadelphia, PA, Lippincott Williams & Wilkins, 2011, pp 315-325.)

- Continue incision inferiorly 45° over lateral upper femur to level of gluteal crease, which corresponds to insertion of gluteus maximus tendon
- Deepen incision to level of fascia lata, which is incised in line with skin, and carry cephalad parallel with gluteus maximus fibers, ending just short of neurovascular bundle
- At inferior portion of incision, tenotomize femoral insertion of gluteus maximus tendon 1 cm from its insertion
- Identify, tag, and tenotomize piriformis tendon, obturator internus tendon, and gemelli muscles
- Follow obturator internus tendon with finger to lesser sciatic notch and identify sciatic nerve; carefully retract obturator internus and sciatic nerve to access lesser sciatic notch and visualize lower posterior column
- Improve exposure of cephalad posterior column with sciatic nerve retractor or removal of portion of gluteus minimus origin
- Use Taylor retractor to elevate and retract lower portion of gluteus medius origin to help visualize posterior wall fragments
- Place Schanz pin in trochanter to facilitate traction on femoral head and improve visualization of joint space; can also use femoral distractor (**Figure 4**)
- After distraction, gently lavage joint and remove or deliver all incarcerated chondro-osseous fragments (**Figure 5**)

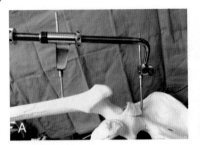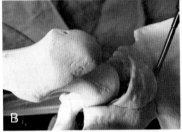

FIGURE 4 Photographs show a femoral distractor on a bone model of the hip. One pin is placed in the supra-acetabular ilium and one in the lateral proximal femur to effect traction (**A**) and enable direct visualization of the joint space (**B**).

- Address marginal impaction, if present, by hinged elevation with osteotome and by filling void with cancellous allograft or bone graft substitute (**Figure 6**)
- Use Kirschner wires to provisionally fix reduced fragments; avoid interference with definitive implant placement (**Figure 7**)

 VIDEO 71.2 Fractures of the Pelvis and Acetabulum: Kocher-Langenbeck Approach. Emile Letournel, MD; Joel M. Matta, MD (20 min)

Implant Selection

- Depends on fracture pattern; Spring or Zuelzer plates work well for small fragments, interfragmentary screws or buttress plates for larger fragments (**Figures 5, 8,** and **9**)
- Adhere to principles of anatomic reduction and secure fixation for best outcomes

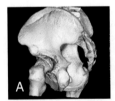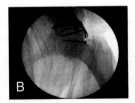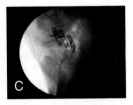

FIGURE 5 Images show an acetabular fracture with small marginal posterior wall fragments. **A,** Three-dimensional CT reconstruction shows the fracture. During surgery, the joint space was cleared of infolded debris, and three of the marginal pieces were large enough to anatomically reduce using a dental pick and narrow Kirschner-wire provisional fixation. Fixation was provided by three spring (Zuelzer) plates, as shown on the obturator oblique (**B**) and iliac oblique (**C**) fluoroscopic views.

© 2021 American Academy of Orthopaedic Surgeons

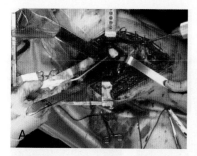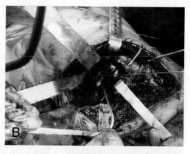

FIGURE 6 Intraoperative photographs show reduction and fixation of a posterior wall acetabular fracture with marginal impaction. **A,** The more cephalad fragment is shown, supported by the terminal end of the small suction. **B,** After the articular surface contact is concentrically restored and supported with allograft or synthetic bone, the main posterior wall fragments are reduced and provisionally fixed.

Wound Management

- Débride and thoroughly lavage wound
- Visualize and assess integrity of sciatic nerve; reattach piriformis and obturator internus tendons to their insertions
- Layered closure over medium suction drain; author uses incisional vacuum closure system; helpful in obese patients and those in intensive care unit or for wounds with high likelihood of drainage or fecal or other contamination

COMPLICATIONS

- Surgical management is challenging; complications can be significant, including infection (3%), deep vein thrombosis (7%), heterotopic ossification (37%), nerve injury (10%), femoral head osteonecrosis (7%), and hip arthrosis (10% to 33%)

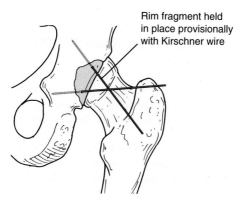

Rim fragment held in place provisionally with Kirschner wire

FIGURE 7 Illustration shows provisional fixation with Kirschner wires of the overlying and now reduced posterior wall fragment.

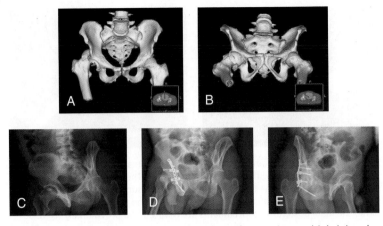

FIGURE 8 Images show posterior wall acetabular fracture in a multiply injured patient. **A** and **B**, Three-dimensional CT reconstructions obtained before reduction reveal a multifragmentary fracture. As seen on **B**, one of the fragments is nondisplaced but is situated in a position that makes it likely to fracture on reduction. This actually occurred. **C**, Fluoroscopic image shows temporary femoral traction to distract the joint and take stress off the articular cartilage of the femoral head as well as the acetabulum imposed by the incarcerated fragment. Iliac oblique (**D**) and obturator oblique (**E**) projections obtained after reduction show fixation with two spring (Zuelzer) plates and a spanning buttressing reconstruction plate.

- Initial management with closed reduction and skeletal traction must be expeditious, but definitive surgical management is best performed by a subspecialty-trained surgeon familiar with anatomy and fixation techniques

POSTOPERATIVE CARE AND REHABILITATION

- Unless contraindicated, administer chemical anticoagulant usually subcutaneously and mechanical deep vein thrombosis prophylaxis such as thromboembolic stockings; no consensus, but author continues prophylaxis for 2 weeks postoperatively followed by 81 mg aspirin daily until patient is independent, bearing full weight
- Knee immobilizer for 3 weeks to safeguard hip flexion and posterior loading if there is particular concern with posterior instability
- Restrict weight bearing to toe-touch for 10 to 12 weeks, then transition to full weight bearing

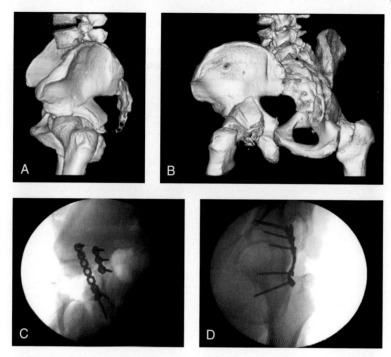

FIGURE 9 Images show a posterior wall acetabular fracture with a large fragment and an incomplete secondary fracture line. Lateral (**A**) and iliac oblique (**B**) three-dimensional CT reconstructions show the fracture. The fragment was reduced and fixed with two buttressing reconstruction plates, as shown on the iliac oblique (**C**) and obturator oblique (**D**) fluoroscopic images.

PEARLS

- Following reduction, obtain and scrutinize Judet oblique views; for loose fragments in joint, apply skeletal traction to relieve pressure on cartilage; also useful in unstable reductions.
- Keep knee flexed to at least 45° to relax sciatic nerve for prone and lateral positions.
- Tenotomize obturator internus and piriformis tendons 1 cm from their insertion to protect femoral head blood supply; tag to facilitate retraction and later repair.
- Trace acetabular portion of retracted obturator internus with gloved finger to lesser sciatic notch—good spot for seating cobra or similar type retractor.
- Use one-sided adhesive plastic strips to temporarily hold retractors.

- Acetabular rim portion of most posterior wall fracture fragments has small extended portion of labrum—good location to place suture for traction on fragment to enhance visualization of distracted joint.
- Joint distraction is aided by appropriate muscle relaxation and placement of 5-mm Schanz pin in trochanter or by placing a second supra-acetabular Schanz pin for femoral distractor use.
- Manage marginal impaction after clearing joint of loose fragments and debris, reducing head, and levering impacted fragment(s) so articular surfaces congruently "hug" each other while void is back-filled with bone graft.
- Final step in stabilization—Lock in construct by perfectly reducing and appropriately fixing rim fragment.
- Resect traumatized portion of gluteus minimus to prevent heterotopic ossification.

Open Reduction and Internal Fixation of Femoral Neck Fractures

INTRODUCTION

- Femoral neck fractures occur from low-energy mechanisms (falls) in older people
- More frequent in women than men (4:1)
- In young patients, most commonly from high-energy mechanism
- Can be intracapsular or extracapsular
- Classification systems—Garden, Pauwels, and AO/Orthopaedic Trauma Association (**Figures 1** and **2**)

PATIENT SELECTION

- Manage femoral neck fractures surgically with anatomic reduction or arthroplasty; morbidity/mortality higher with nonsurgical management
    - Immobilization without fixation increases risk of pneumonia, pulmonary embolism, skin breakdown
    - Pain from unstable fracture increases narcotic requirement
- Reserve nonsurgical management for frail patients and cases in which surgery is contraindicated
    - Consider percutaneous screw placement with local anesthetic in nonsurgical candidate with nondisplaced/incomplete fracture
    - For displaced fracture, consult pain control service to aid patients through acute phase

PREOPERATIVE IMAGING

Plain Radiography

- AP pelvis, AP/lateral hip
- Gentle traction helps characterize fracture

CT and MRI

- CT useful when open reduction and internal fixation (ORIF) planned and neck comminution present
- Three-dimensional reconstruction helps characterize fracture

Based on Webb LX, Floyd JCP: Open reduction and internal fixation of femoral neck fractures, in Colvin AC, Flatow E, eds: Atlas of Essential Orthopaedic Procedures, ed 2. Rosemont, IL, American Academy of Orthopaedic Surgeons, 2020, pp 579-587.

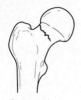 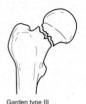 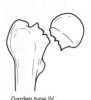

Garden type I Garden type II Garden type III Garden type IV

FIGURE 1 Illustration shows the Garden classification of femoral neck fractures. Garden I: incomplete (most often valgus-impacted). Garden II: complete, non-displaced. Garden III: complete, incompletely displaced. Garden IV: complete, completely displaced.

- MRI can be considered when history and physical findings are consistent with nondisplaced or incomplete fractures, but radiographs fail to reveal a fracture

PROCEDURE

Instruments/Equipment/Implants

- Two Gelpi retractors
- C-arm
- Small, medium, and large pointed Weber tenaculum clamps
- Two Freer elevators
- Dental pick
- Trocar-tipped terminally threaded Schanz pins (2.5 mm for femoral head fragment, 5.0 mm for distal trochanteric/femoral shaft fragment)
- 2.0-mm Kirschner wires (K-wires)
- 6.5- to 7.3-mm cannulated screws, or 130° blade plate/side plate (depends on fracture)

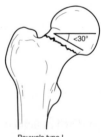 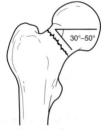 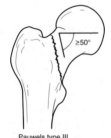

Pauwels type I Pauwels type II Pauwels type III

FIGURE 2 Illustration depicts the Pauwels classification of femoral neck fractures. Type I: The angle subtended by the horizontal and the line of the fracture on an AP radiograph is less than 30°. Type II: The angle subtended by the horizontal and the line of the fracture on an AP radiograph is between 30° and 50°. Type III: The angle subtended by the horizontal and the line of the fracture is greater than or equal to 50°.

- Bone graft if needed
- Have minifragment set with 1.5- and 2.0-mm plates available

Surgical Technique

- ORIF appropriate for patients whose physiologic age is less than 65 years with intracapsular femoral neck fractures
  - ▸ Nondisplaced/minimally displaced fractures amenable to closed reduction (Garden I and II)—Use parallel cannulated screws or sliding hip screw on radiolucent table or fracture table (**Figures 3** and **4**)

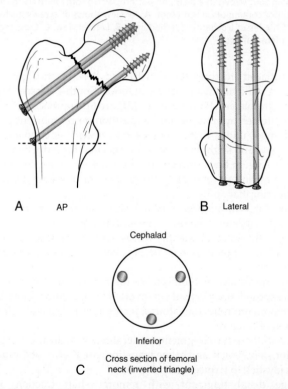

A AP

B Lateral

Cephalad

Inferior

C Cross section of femoral neck (inverted triangle)

FIGURE 3 Illustrations show correct screw placement for femoral neck fracture fixation using three screws, which usually is sufficient. The pattern of screw placement is important. **A**, The first screw is directed tangential to and contiguous with the calcar at the level of the fracture on the AP view. Starting screws below the level of the lesser trochanter (dashed line) should be avoided to minimize the likelihood of an iatrogenic subtrochanteric fracture. **B**, On the lateral view, the first screw is seen bisecting the head and neck. **C**, The spread between the screws should be maximized, as shown on the cross-sectional view of the neck.

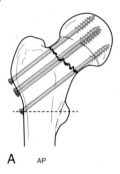
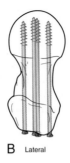
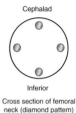

A AP   B Lateral   C Cross section of femoral neck (diamond pattern)

FIGURE 4 Illustrations show correct screw placement for femoral neck fracture fixation using four screws in a diamond pattern, which some authors recommend when posterior comminution is present. **A**, AP view shows all screws started above the level of the lesser trochanter (dashed line). **B**, Lateral view. **C**, Cross-sectional view of the femoral neck.

▶ Displaced fractures (Garden III and IV)—Fixation preceded by open reduction via modified anterior (Smith-Petersen [**Figure 5**]) or anterolateral (Watson-Jones [**Figure 6**]) approach

- Smith-Petersen approach—Supine position on radiolucent table with folded sheet under upper buttock on affected side; enables lateral C-arm view and slight hip extension if needed for reduction
- Make incision in line between anterior superior iliac spine and lateral edge of patella, approximately 15 cm long, starting 1 cm distal to anterior superior iliac spine
- Develop interval between tensor fascia lata and sartorius muscles; avoid injuring lateral femoral cutaneous nerve
- At base of this interval, identify rectus femoris and trace it proximally to its tendon; tenotomize tendon just distal to its anterior inferior iliac spine origin
- Elevate and retract tenotomized rectus femoris; underlying hip capsule is exposed; open capsule in inverted T capsulotomy and tag
- Place Hohmann retractors around femoral neck to enable direct visualization of fracture
- Anatomically reduce fragments under direct visualization, using Freer elevator, dental pick, and saline irrigation; use K-wire or 4-mm Schanz pin as joystick to reduce head fragment
- Manage distal fragment with femoral shaft traction, rotation, adduction/abduction
- Achieve provisional fixation with pointed Weber clamp, K-wire, or small plate with unicortical screws
- Assess provisional reduction with C-arm
- For definitive fixation with anterior approach, make separate lateral incision or three small incisions for cannulated screws

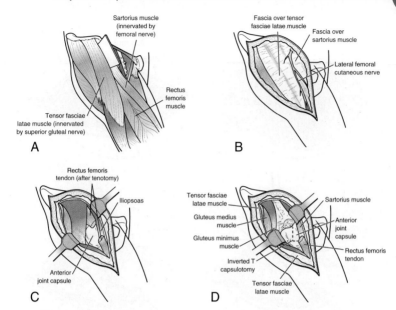

FIGURE 5 Illustrations demonstrate the modified Smith Petersen approach. **A**, The superficial plane of the approach. The rectus femoris muscle lies in the interval between the sartorius muscle, which is innervated by the femoral nerve, and the tensor fasciae latae muscle, which is innervated by the superior gluteal nerve. **B**, The surgeon must avoid injuring the lateral femoral cutaneous nerve, which pierces the fascia in the line between these muscles. **C**, The rectus femoris can be traced proximally to its tendinous attachment to the anterior inferior iliac spine. A tenotomy should be performed, with enough tendon retained on the anterior inferior iliac spine to allow a good repair at closure. **D**, The tenotomized rectus can be tagged and retracted inferiorly, exposing the underlying pericapsular tissue. An inverted T capsulotomy, with suture tagging and retraction of the capsular leaves, will enable a clear view of the fracture.

- For anterolateral Watson-Jones approach, use interval between tensor fascia lata and gluteus medius muscles
- Limit cephalad extent of approach to 5 cm cephaloanterior to greater trochanter to avoid injuring superior gluteal nerve (**Figure 6**)
- At base of interval, pericapsular fat and hip capsule are exposed
- Proceed with capsulotomy, open reduction, and provisional fixation as described previously for anterior approach
- Anterolateral approach avoids separate incision for fixation
- For highly vertical fractures (Pauwels type III), parallel screws do not address shear stress; use other fixation constructs such as nonparallel screws or a 130° blade plate (**Figure 7**)

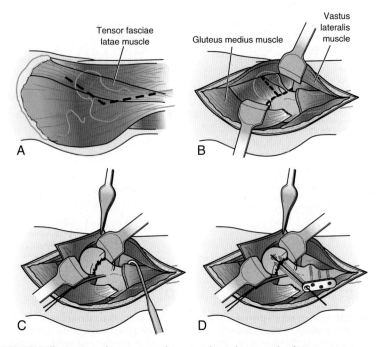

FIGURE 6 Illustrations demonstrate the anterolateral approach of Watson-Jones.
A, The skin incision extends from the standard lateral incision over the proximal femoral shaft cephalad to the level of the tip of the greater trochanter and is angled toward the anterior superior iliac spine. The interval between the tensor fasciae latae and the gluteus medius is incised no more proximally than 5 cm cephaloanterior to the greater trochanter to avoid injuring the superior gluteal nerve. This enables exposure of the anterior hip capsule. **B,** An inverted T capsulotomy is performed. **C,** Suture tagging and retraction of the capsular leaves enable direct visualization of the fracture for reduction, and provisional fixation is facilitated. **D,** Definitive fixation can be accomplished through the inferior standard lateral portion of the approach.

- For patients with femoral neck fractures and physiologic age greater than 65 years, no firm consensus exists regarding management
  - Treat incomplete, nondisplaced, or valgus impacted fractures with parallel cannulated screws or sliding hip screw
  - Manage displaced fractures with arthroplasty; revision surgery rates of ORIF are high in this population

 VIDEO 72.1 The Modified Smith Petersen Approach for Open Reduction and Internal Fixation of Femoral Neck Fractures. Lawrence X. Webb, MD; John C.P. Floyd, MD (5 min)

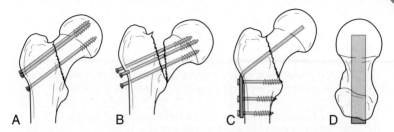

FIGURE 7 Illustrations demonstrate fixation of the highly vertical Pauwels type III fracture. **A,** A Pauwels type III fracture pattern is reduced and fixed with three parallel screws. **B,** Failure of screw fixation. Because of the poor ability of the fixation construct to negate the shear forces on this highly vertical fracture, it displaces, with offset in the neck and some backout of the screws. A more stable proposed fixation of this fracture pattern uses a 130° blade plate for fixation, shown in AP (**C**) and lateral (**D**) projections.

POSTOPERATIVE CARE AND REHABILITATION

- Following reduction and fixation, keep patient toe-touch weight bearing for 12 weeks
- Return to weight bearing depends on radiographic and clinical fracture healing

COMPLICATIONS

- Osteonecrosis and nonunion
  - ▶ Correlate with initial fracture displacement and quality of reduction, not time to fixation
  - ▶ Osteonecrosis and nonunion rates were 6% and 18%, respectively, in nondisplaced fractures and 23% and 38% in displaced fractures
  - ▶ Nonunion is associated with varus neck positioning (Pauwels valgus intertrochanteric osteotomy can effect healing in this setting)
  - ▶ Manage osteonecrosis with head collapse or precollapse with nonvascularized or vascularized fibular struts, osteotomies, or arthroplasty
- Other complications—Infection, thrombosis, heterotopic bone, periprosthetic fracture, persistent pain
- Complications specific to arthroplasty—Dislocation, loosening, wear

PEARLS

- ■ For displaced fractures in younger patients in whom ORIF is appropriate, need traction views to determine details of fracture; with comminution or segmentation, CT with three-dimensional reconstruction helpful.
- ■ Modified Smith Petersen approach affords better visualization, ease of reduction, and clamp placement but needs second incision laterally for cannulated screws or spiral blade and side plate device.

- Can carry Watson-Jones incision inferiorly over lateral thigh; can apply implants through lower extended limb of incision.
- For Pauwels type III fracture without comminution or segmentation, authors prefer Watson-Jones approach; for Pauwels type I and II fractures and all displaced femoral neck fractures with segmentation/comminution, authors prefer modified Smith Petersen approach and second lateral incision.
- Inverted T capsulotomy helps visualize and ensure reduction of inferiormost portion of Pauwels type III fracture.
- After displaced fracture clearly exposed, seat 2.5-mm trocar-tipped terminally threaded Schanz pin in femoral head fragment; seat 5.0-mm Schanz pin in femoral shaft fragment. Apply hand chuck to each pin; effect anatomic reduction and provisionally fix with K-wires, Weber clamp, or small plate with unicortical screws.

Intertrochanteric Fracture Fixation Using a Sliding Hip Screw or Cephalomedullary Nail

PATIENT SELECTION

- Approximately 340,000 patients sustain hip fractures in the United States each year
- Intertrochanteric fractures are extracapsular hip fractures occurring primarily in elderly patients or those with osteopenia or osteoporosis

Indications

- Surgical treatment is standard of care for hip fractures
- Nonsurgical management can lead to fracture displacement, pain, inability to transfer, decubitus ulcers, pulmonary complications, urinary tract infections, and deep vein thrombosis (DVT)

Contraindications

- Elderly patients with dementia who have minimal pain and were nonambulatory before fracture
- Rarely, patients with severe medical comorbidities precluding safe surgical intervention

PREOPERATIVE IMAGING

Radiography

- Good plain radiographs fully characterize fracture and enable appropriate treatment
- AP pelvis and AP and lateral hip views
- AP view with 15° internal rotation and gentle traction helps delineate fracture pattern (**Figure 1**)
- Cross-table lateral is preferred; frog-lateral uncomfortable for patient
- Two percent to ten percent of patients have negative radiographs; further imaging needed if history and examination consistent with fracture

---

Based on Schwartz AK: Intertrochanteric fracture fixation using a sliding hip screw or cephalomedullary nail, in Colvin AC, Flatow E, eds: Atlas of Essential Orthopaedic Procedures, *ed 2. Rosemont, IL, American Academy of Orthopaedic Surgeons, 2020, pp 588-594.*

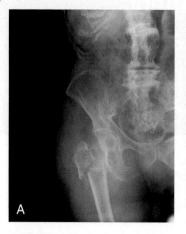 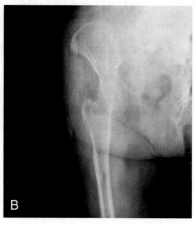

FIGURE 1 Radiographs demonstrate a comminuted proximal femur fracture. **A**, AP view of the hip. **B**, AP view obtained with the lower extremity in manual traction and internal rotation. The alignment of the hip with traction enables better understanding of the fracture pattern and its behavior with closed reduction.

- CT scan or MRI are additional modalities commonly used
- Bone scan was historically used when radiographs were negative for fracture, but it may not show positive results for up to 72 hours; may not accurately depict fracture pattern

Magnetic Resonance Imaging
- More sensitive than CT
- Completely characterizes anatomy of fracture
- Improves diagnostic speed compared with CT and bone scan
- Expensive and less available than CT

PROCEDURE
- Can treat standard obliquity intertrochanteric fractures with sliding hip screw (SHS) or cephalomedullary nail (CMN)
  - ▶ Despite regional variations and surgeon preferences, SHS considered standard treatment; CMN has higher rate of peri-implant fracture at nail tip
  - ▶ No differences in blood loss, surgical time, or recovery
- Use CMN in treatment of reverse obliquity fractures, intertrochanteric fractures with lateral wall involvement, transverse intertrochanteric fractures, and fractures with subtrochanteric extension; SHS has high rate of failure due to excessive collapse (**Figure 2**)

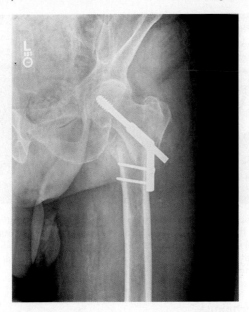

FIGURE 2 AP radiograph of the hip demonstrates an intertrochanteric fracture treated with a sliding hip screw. Excessive collapse has occurred because of a previously unrecognized lateral wall fracture.

Room Setup/Patient Positioning

- Supine position; fracture table enables easy biplanar imaging and maintains reduction
- Obtain reduction before incision; ensure C-arm can obtain AP and lateral images
- Use boot traction; pad all bony prominences well on both legs, including perineal post
- Scissor legs; surgical leg flexed, nonsurgical leg extended; avoid hyperextension and excessive traction on femoral nerve of nonsurgical leg
- Do not use leg holder for contralateral leg; reports of compartment syndrome
- Place arm on surgical side across chest; pad well, secure with silk tape (**Figure 3**)

Special Instruments/Equipment

- Implant alone will not reduce fracture
- Laterally placed, percutaneous ball-spike pusher helps correct varus proximal fragment
- Percutaneously placed Cobb elevator anteriorly or posteriorly helps correct flexion or extension deformity (**Figure 4**)
- May need reduction clamps for displaced fractures (**Figure 5**)

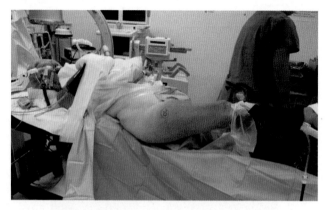

FIGURE 3 Photograph demonstrates typical setup and patient positioning on a fracture table for surgical fixation of an intertrochanteric fracture using an intramedullary (IM) nail. Note the proximal and posterior extent of draping required for IM nail fixation and the intraoperative use of a compression device on bilateral lower extremities.

Surgical Technique

Cephalomedullary Nail

- Achieve closed reduction via internal rotation and traction; assess with biplanar fluoroscopy; if unable to reduce closed, perform open reduction
- Tip of greater trochanter should be at level of center of femoral head

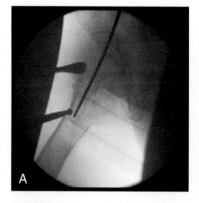
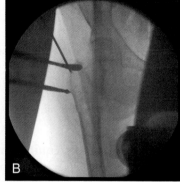

FIGURE 4 Intraoperative fluoroscopic views show reduction of an intertrochanteric fracture. **A,** Lateral view shows a Cobb elevator at the anterior neck to counteract flexion deformity of the proximal segment. A ball-spike pusher on the lateral cortex also is visualized. **B,** AP view shows a ball-spike pusher on the lateral cortex of the proximal segment, counteracting the abduction of the fragment.

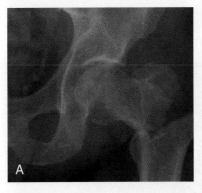
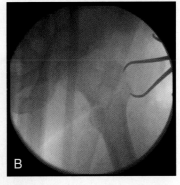

FIGURE 5 Images show a displaced intertrochanteric fracture. **A,** Preoperative AP radiograph shows the fracture, which was irreducible with traction alone. **B,** Intraoperative AP fluoroscopic view demonstrates open reduction of the fracture using a pointed reduction clamp.

- Sterile preparation performed sufficiently proximal and posterior to assure access to starting point and distally to include the knee in case a long nail is necessary
- May insert guide pin percutaneously, followed by ~3 cm incision in line with femur
- Sharply dissect through subcutaneous tissue and fascia.
- With C-arm, confirm starting point just medial to tip of greater trochanter on AP view and in line with femoral shaft on lateral view (**Figure 6**)
- Advance guide pin into metaphysis to level of lesser trochanter; advance opening reamer, then remove pin and reamer
- If using long nail, insert ball-tipped guidewire into canal and advance to distal femoral physeal scar
  - Measure nail length; ream incrementally to 1 to 1.5 mm more than chosen nail diameter
  - If using short nail, reaming not required
- Insert CMN by hand; mallet risks perforation of anterior cortex in osteopenic bone (**Figure 7**)
- Confirm final depth of nail on AP view; final placement depends solely on location of lag screw; place it "center-center"
- Advance guide pin for lag screw and confirm on AP and lateral planes
- Calculate tip-apex distance (TAD), which is sum of distances between center of femoral head and screw tip measured on AP and lateral views
- Measure screw length and insert screw
- Place set screw and tighten
- Place distal interlocking screws if fracture is rotationally or axially unstable, via jig (short nails) or using freehand technique with C-arm (long nails)

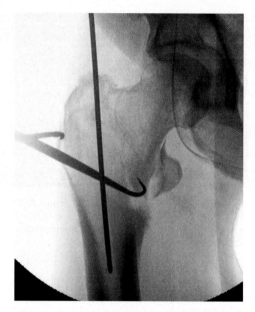

FIGURE 6 Intraoperative fluoroscopic AP view of the hip demonstrates the correct starting point for a cephalomedullary nail, just medial to the tip of the greater trochanter. This avoids accidental reaming out of the lateral cortex and minimizes the risk for varus malalignment.

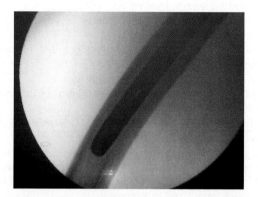

FIGURE 7 Intraoperative lateral fluoroscopic view of the femur demonstrates the potential risk of anterior cortex penetration when inserting a long cephalomedullary nail. Excessive manual force should be avoided when inserting such nails to prevent iatrogenic femur fracture during nail insertion.

- Irrigate wounds copiously and close
- Subfascial administration of TXA at the fracture site may reduce need for transfusion

Sliding Hip Screw

- If fracture is nondisplaced, a flat radiolucent table may be used
- For fracture table, position, reduce, prepare, and drape patient similarly to CMN
- May use fluoroscopy to localize appropriate start site for incision
- Incise via direct lateral approach to proximal femur through skin, subcutaneous tissue, and iliotibial band
- Preserve vastus lateralis and reflect it anteriorly from septum and retract it with Bennett retractor
- Using the correct guide, advance guidewire through lateral femur into head to obtain "center-center" position; assess position with C-arm
- Measure lag screw length over guidewire
- Ream to subchondral bone of femoral head; place lag screw, ensuring appropriate position and TAD with fluoroscopy
- Insert SHS plate, assess position, and affix with two or more screws
- May add single 6.5- or 7.3-mm cannulated screw for rotational stability
- Irrigate and close iliotibial band, subcutaneous tissues, and skin

COMPLICATIONS

- Varus malunion is most common biomechanical complication (**Figure 8**); avoid by obtaining appropriate intraoperative reduction and ensuring tip of greater trochanter is level with center of femoral head on AP view
- Screw cutout
  - Fracture displaces and collapses; screw protrudes through femoral head
  - Avoid by placing lag screw deep and central within femoral head, with TAD less than 25 mm
- Fracture at tip of CMN
  - Unique to short CMN
  - Incidence declining with newer designs

POSTOPERATIVE CARE AND REHABILITATION

- Mobilize immediately postoperatively; goal of surgery is stable fixation and anatomic alignment that allow early weight bearing
- DVT prophylaxis is essential
  - High rate of DVT and fatal pulmonary embolism without prophylaxis after hip fracture
  - Protocols controversial, but may include fondaparinux, low-molecular-weight heparin, vitamin K antagonists, or low-dose unfractionated heparin

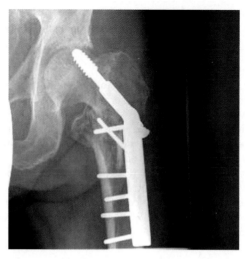

FIGURE 8 AP radiograph of the hip demonstrates failure of fixation and varus collapse following fixation of a transtrochanteric fracture treated with a sliding hip screw.

- ‣ American College of Chest Physicians recommends against using aspirin alone; advocates thromboprophylaxis for patients between time of hospital admission and surgery
- ‣ Use mechanical thromboprophylaxis in patients with high bleeding risk
- ‣ Recommended postoperative duration is up to 35 days
- Thromboprophylaxis indicated in patients of all ages who present with this injury
- Best practices for elderly patients with hip fractures
  - ‣ Postoperative antibiotics for 24 hours
  - ‣ Intermittent, not indwelling, catheterization enables earlier normal voiding.
  - ‣ Suction wound drainage has no effect on infection, revision surgery, or transfusion rates

PEARLS

- ■ Choose appropriate implant; SHS indicated for standard obliquity intertrochanteric fractures; CMN indicated for reverse obliquity fractures, transtrochanteric fractures, intertrochanteric fractures with subtrochanteric extension, and intertrochanteric fractures without intact lateral wall.
- ■ Cautiously and gently insert CMN; anterior bow of femur often is greater in elderly patients; bone is osteopenic.

- Reduce fracture before placing implant. If fracture not reducible by closed means, use percutaneous or open techniques.
- TAD is critical for SHS and CMN; take care to achieve TAD of less than 25 mm.
- Starting point for CMN is just medial to tip of greater trochanter.
- Prepare and drape adequate skin proximally and posteriorly for CMN.

74 Intramedullary Nailing of Diaphyseal Femur Fractures

PATIENT SELECTION

- Diaphyseal femur fractures necessitate surgical fixation
  - ▶ Allows earlier mobilization
  - ▶ Reduces risk of prolonged recumbency, including fat emboli syndrome, decubitus ulcers, muscle atrophy, and venous thromboembolic complications
- Intramedullary nailing (IMN) indicated for diaphyseal femur fractures in adults able to tolerate surgery
- Relative contraindications
  - ▶ Some pediatric femur fractures
  - ▶ Highly contaminated open wounds
  - ▶ Proximal or distal femoral involvement needing other fixation
- Retrograde IMN sometimes needed in patients with obesity, for bilateral femur fractures, or for ipsilateral tibia fractures

PREOPERATIVE IMAGING

- AP and lateral radiographs of entire femur, including hip and knee; evaluate femoral neck for associated fracture
- In severe comminution, image contralateral side to evaluate length and alignment; in bilateral fractures, fix simpler side first to assess length of comminuted side
- Assess rotation by comparing lesser trochanter profile on uninjured side on AP view obtained with patella straight anterior or by obtaining a perfect lateral of the knee and rotating the C-arm 90° to obtain an AP of the hip maintaining the same position of the leg
- Assess femoral anteversion by comparing angulation of proximal femur on lateral radiograph between injured and noninjured sides

PROCEDURE

Room Setup/Patient Positioning

- Author recommends supine positioning on flat Jackson table; traction table increases risk of complications

---

Based on Miller AN: Intramedullary nailing of diaphyseal femur fractures, in Colvin AC, Flatow E, eds: Atlas of Essential Orthopaedic Procedures, *ed 2. Rosemont, IL, American Academy of Orthopaedic Surgeons, 2020, pp 595-600.*

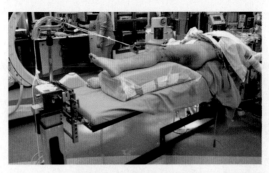

FIGURE 1 Photograph shows patient positioning and room setup for intramedullary nailing of a femoral shaft fracture. The patient is supine on a Jackson table. The injured (left) hip has been moved laterally over the edge of the table, and the leg is elevated on a ramp (encased in plastic drapes). Traction is shown in place as an example.

- Supine position at edge of table with bump under sacrum to provide complete access to the hip (**Figure 1**)
- Author uses custom device to apply intraoperative traction while keeping leg free for manipulation
- Elevate leg on ramp for lateral fluoroscopic imaging; position fluoroscopy unit on side opposite injured leg, rotated approximately 10° above horizontal to image lateral femur

Special Instruments/Equipment/Implants
- Traction setup for Jackson table
- Leg ramp and sacral bump
- Traction bow, sterile rope, 5/64-in Kirschner wire (K-wire)
- Femoral nail, reamers, appropriate insertion equipment
- Reduction devices (eg, ball-spike pusher, shoulder hook)

Surgical Technique
- Ensure drapes allow access to iliac crest and entire leg
- Place 5/64-in K-wire anteriorly in distal femur to allow room for IMN (**Figure 2, A** and **B**)
- Add approximately 10 lb traction to bow; place on opposite side of table to adduct leg
- Place starting guide pin percutaneously to medial tip of greater trochanter or piriformis fossa (**Figure 2, C**)
- Make longitudinal incision around guide pin through skin, subcutaneous tissue, and fascia; avoid cutting proximally and damaging gluteal neurovascular bundle

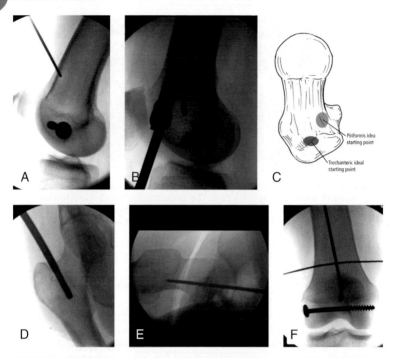

FIGURE 2 Images demonstrate the guidewire placement and starting point location for intramedullary nailing of a femoral shaft fracture. **A**, Intraoperative lateral fluoroscopic image shows the anterior starting point for the 5/64-in Kirschner wire placement. **B**, Intraoperative lateral fluoroscopic image shows the traction bow in front of the ball-tipped guidewire. Distal placement of the ball-tipped guidewire also is visible, with the wire well centered in the femur. **C**, Illustration of the axial view shows proper locations for piriformis and trochanteric entry sites. When a piriformis entry site is used, the nail should not be placed too far anteriorly because of the risk of iatrogenic fracture. When a trochanteric entry site is used, the nail should be placed medially on the trochanteric tip to avoid lateral wall blowout. **D**, Intraoperative AP fluoroscopic image of a right hip shows a dynamic hip screw reamer used to place the piriformis entry hole. **E**, Intraoperative lateral fluoroscopic image of a right hip shows proper placement of the piriformis starting point. **F**, Intraoperative AP fluoroscopic image of a right distal femur. Note the curved tip of the ball-tipped guidewire; the overall trajectory of the wire is toward the medial tibial spine.

- Place opening reamer over guide pin
  - ▸ Can use system-specific instrument or 9-mm dynamic hip screw (DHS) reamer; smaller diameter allows more flexibility (**Figure 2, D** and **E**)
  - ▸ If using DHS reamer, must subsequently use IMN manufacturer's opening reamer to ensure adequate opening for IMN

- Place ball-tipped guidewire down canal; slight bend in tip allows directionality (**Figure 2, F**)
- Place guidewire as distally as possible in femur, centrally located on AP and lateral views, aimed slightly toward medial tibial spine on AP view (**Figure 2, B** and **F**)
- Align femur appropriately before placing guidewire; can obtain alignment via external maneuvers such as pressure on skin with mallet or bump under leg
  - If external unsuccessful, traction pin or a small hook and ball spike can be used
- Use measuring device to estimate IMN length; ensure measuring device is down to starting point
- Use longest nail possible to avoid metaphyseal end point for nail; can be stress riser
- Ream sequentially in 0.5-mm increments until chatter heard in femoral diaphysis and to at least 1 mm over IMN size
- Place IMN gently over guidewire, maintaining length and rotation
- Confirm proximally and distally that IMN is well seated and of appropriate length, using fluoroscopy (**Figure 3, A** and **B**)
- With cephalomedullary nails or reconstruction nails, place proximal screws first to confirm location in femoral head (**Figure 3, C**)
- With antegrade nails that do not use screws in femoral head, may place distal screws first and backslap across fracture to compress
- Place aiming arm with sleeves for proximal interlocking screws
- Incise skin and fascia longitudinally at sites of screw entry

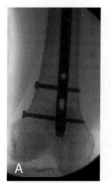 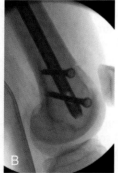 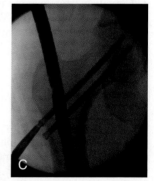

FIGURE 3 Intraoperative fluoroscopic images demonstrate correct placement of intramedullary (IM) nails. AP (**A**) and lateral (**B**) images show excellent distal placement of well-seated, long IM nails. **C,** Intraoperative AP fluoroscopic image of a right hip shows well-placed proximal screws in the femoral head in a reconstruction-style nail.

- Place trocar and sleeve down to bone; place drill through aiming sleeve; keep sleeve secured to bone to avoid aiming errors and subsequent screw misses of IMN
- For cephalomedullary nail device, place proximal screws in exact center of femoral head on lateral fluoroscopic imaging
- Measure screw length from calibrated drill bit or depth gauge, depending on system
- Place screws through aiming sleeve by hand
- Place distal interlocking screws using "perfect circle" technique; author recommends positioning leg perpendicular to fluoroscopy; having assistant hold leg can instill motion and error
- Place drill using fluoroscopic guidance; drill hole in line with C-arm
  - If resistance encountered, uncouple drill and assess drill bit trajectory
  - Correct trajectory manually as needed; lightly tap drill bit through interlocking hole with mallet; drill far cortex
- Place depth gauge for measurement and to ensure that drill hole is through IMN
- Place screw by hand
- Screws should not be overly long; can irritate patients
- Distal femur is trapezoidal; screws that appear appropriate on AP view may be too long on oblique view
- Confirm screw placement with lateral images perpendicular to each screw (**Figure 4**)
- Perform final imaging, again assessing length and rotation; check internal rotation view of femoral neck to reconfirm absence of fracture
- Copiously irrigate wounds with saline
- Close deep fascia with 0 Vicryl (Ethicon) figure-of-8 sutures; close skin with 3-0 nylon mattress sutures
- Clean and dry wounds; place sterile dressing

COMPLICATIONS

- Infection rate less than 4%
- Malunion
  - Most common in proximal or distal fractures
  - Rotational malunion common; do not underestimate patient reports of malalignment symptoms
- Limb-length discrepancy, in comminuted fractures; at end of procedure, compare limbs for length, alignment, and rotation
- Nonunion
  - Relatively uncommon; treat with dynamization, exchange nailing, or bone grafting, depending on nonunion type
  - Perform metabolic workup

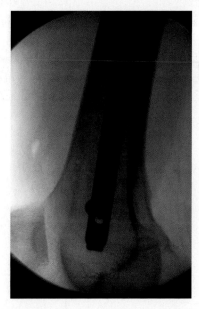

FIGURE 4 Intraoperative lateral fluoroscopic image of a distal femur after intramedullary nailing of a femoral shaft fracture shows that the distal interlocking screws are completely through the nail.

- Femoral neck fracture
  - ▶ May occur iatrogenically or during nail placement
  - ▶ Important to evaluate femoral neck before and after surgery
  - ▶ Obtain fluoroscopic image of femoral neck in full internal rotation; range hip under live fluoroscopy

POSTOPERATIVE CARE AND REHABILITATION

- Most patients can bear weight as tolerated immediately, with crutches or walker
- Begin hip range of motion and abductor strengthening immediately

---

PEARLS

- ■ In comminuted fractures, compare radiographs to uninjured side to assess length and alignment.
- ■ Position patient on flat Jackson table with bump under sacrum and hip lateralized.
- ■ Intraoperative traction and elevation on radiolucent ramp aid reduction and imaging.

© 2021 American Academy of Orthopaedic Surgeons

- For traction, place 5/64-in K-wire anteriorly in distal femur to allow IMN placement posterior to wire.
- Use 9-mm DHS reamer as starting reamer; its smaller diameter provides more flexibility in directing.
- Position leg exactly perpendicular to fluoroscopy for perfect circles.

Surgical Fixation of Fractures of the Distal Femur

INTRODUCTION

- Fixation of distal femoral metaphyseal fractures is challenging; demands anatomic axial alignment, precise reduction of articular surface
- Distal femur is defined by a square; sides same length as widest part of distal femoral epiphysis (metaphysis in adults)
  - ▶ A fracture whose center resides within this box is defined as a distal femoral fracture
  - ▶ Intra-articular fractures classified as partial or complete articular
- Factors making treatment difficult
  - ▶ High-energy distal femur fractures have soft-tissue stripping; 50% of intra-articular fractures are open; tendinous structures at distal end lead to poor environment for bone healing due to lack of extraosseous vascularity
  - ▶ High-energy fracture patterns result in articular, metaphyseal fragmentation, making reduction difficult; risk of posttraumatic arthritis; metaphyseal fragmentation contributes to delayed union, nonunion
  - ▶ Increasing incidence of osteoporosis makes these fractures more prevalent; periprosthetic fractures make management difficult

PATIENT SELECTION

Indications

- Any displaced intra-articular fracture in healthy, active, ambulatory patient
- Most displaced extra-articular fractures need surgery because long-term knee function needs alignment of distal femur

Contraindications

- Nondisplaced articular or metaphyseal fracture in healthy patient who mobilizes with cast

---

Based on Kellam JF, Warner S: Surgical fixation of fractures of the distal femur, in Colvin AC, Flatow E, eds: Atlas of Essential Orthopaedic Procedures, *ed 2. Rosemont, IL, American Academy of Orthopaedic Surgeons, 2020, pp 601-612.*

- Individuals who are unfit for surgery, nonambulatory, significantly incapacitated
- Consider total knee arthroplasty in elderly patients with multifragmented articular fracture

PREOPERATIVE IMAGING
Radiography
- AP, lateral of knee, femoral shaft; full-length femur
- If fracture significantly displaced, gentle traction may improve radiographs
- Must determine if fracture involves articular surface; rule out coronal plane fracture of medial/lateral condyle (Hoffa fracture) on lateral radiograph

Computed Tomography
- Indicated to evaluate intra-articular fracture pattern if present

PROCEDURE
Timing
- Authors recommend fixation as soon as possible when patient medically stable, appropriate staff available, and nature of injury understood
- If staff unavailable and conditions not met, consider joint-bridging external fixation to align fracture and stabilize soft tissues
- For open fractures, severe soft-tissue injury, consider joint-spanning external fixator so soft tissues can "declare" their intent (**Figure 1**)

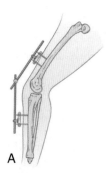
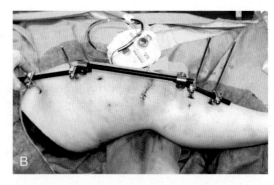

FIGURE 1 A, The illustration of the lateral aspect of the leg shows the joint-spanning external fixator. **B,** Intraoperative photograph demonstrates that it is imperative that the Schanz screws are placed outside of the proposed area for the surgical incisions for the fixation. (Courtesy of AO Archives and *AO Principles of Operative Management of Fractures.*)

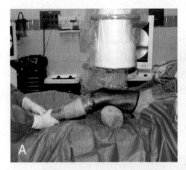 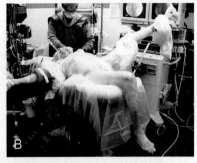

FIGURE 2 **A**, Intraoperative photograph of the lateral aspect of the leg shows the patient positioned on radiolucent table with C-arm from the side opposite the fractured limb. Note the roll under the thigh providing a force for indirect reduction along with manual traction. **B**, Intraoperative photograph of the AP aspect of the patient positioned on a regular operating table with the end flexed so as to allow access to the knee. (**A**, Courtesy of Steve Sims, MD, Charlotte, NC. **B**, Courtesy of Eric Johnson, MD, Los Angeles, CA.)

Room Setup/Patient Positioning

- Radiolucent table
- Place fluoroscopy opposite the injured leg; surgical team on side of injury
- Supine position; place sterile triangle or bump proximal to fracture to allow knee flexion up to 60° (**Figure 2, A**); also can place knee at table break to allow flexion as desired (**Figure 2, B**)
  - ▮ Placing knee at table break reduces pull of gastrocnemius and abductor magnus, preventing genu recurvatum, shortening
  - ▮ If using roll under buttock, take care to avoid malrotation of the fracture

Special Instruments/Equipment/Implants

- Periarticular reduction clamps
- Foot plates (for weak osteoporotic bone)
- Wide-throated clamps
- Kirschner wires (K-wires), used as joysticks
- Cancellous or cortical screws, sizes 2.7 to 6.5 mm; trend toward 3.5-/4.0-mm screws, which increase space for distal plate screw placement, provide good fixation
- Locking femoral condylar plate
  - ▮ Locking screws enhance angular stability of metaphyseal component
  - ▮ Shaft holes have locking or combination holes, enable axial compression with nonlocking cortical screws (**Figure 3, A** and **B**)
  - ▮ Variable angle locking plates to avoid previous implants such as TKA

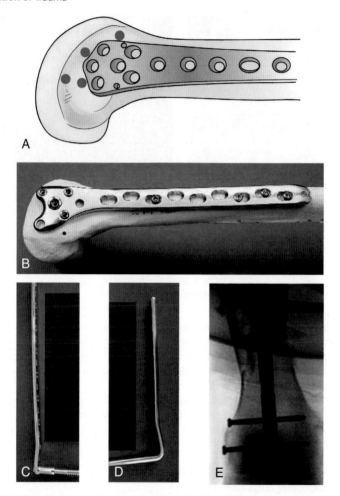

FIGURE 3 **A,** Illustration shows a round hole locking distal femoral plate on the lateral aspect of the distal femur. **B,** Photograph of the lateral aspect of a distal femoral locking plate with a combination hole allowing the insertion of locking and nonlocking screws as well as axial compression and variable screw angulation when using nonlocking screws. Other implants for stabilization of distal femoral fractures: dynamic condylar screw in the AP aspect (**C,** photograph), 95° blade plate in the AP aspect (**D,** photograph), retrograde intramedullary nail in the AP aspect (**E,** fluoroscopic view).

- Other implants include retrograde femoral nail, fixed-angle devices such as 95° blade plate and dynamic condylar screw (**Figure 3, C** through **E**); can use 3.5- or 4.5-mm T- or L-plates, standard straight plates as buttress plates for partial articular medial or lateral condylar fracture

Surgical Technique
- Preoperative planning imperative
  - Use radiographs and CT to identify fracture fragments needing reduction
  - Establish order of reduction; find main articular fracture fragment on which to build other fragments
  - Ensure screw heads do not involve footprint of plate; anterior-to-posterior screws (in coronal split fractures) must avoid screws or blade from plate
- Determine plate length
  - Requires neutralization plate providing at least four cortices above fracture for simple metaphyseal pattern; much longer plates used for multifragmentary metaphyseal-diaphyseal fractures
  - Plate length at least two to three times length of fragmented section of fracture
  - Screw fill is 50% of holes in shaft component of plate
  - Fracture-site stability determined by placing screws nearest to the fracture; can adjust by increasing plate length and proximity of screws to fracture site
  - Apply as many screws as possible in distal fragment for stability
  - In osteoporotic bone, consider plating up to greater trochanter; screws through plate into femoral neck provide splint for femoral neck in osteoporotic patient

Approaches
- Two approaches, depending on necessity of intra-articular reduction
- No intra-articular reduction needed—Make small incision centered over middle of distal lateral femoral condyle through skin, subcutaneous tissue, iliotibial tract down to distal femur
  - Dissect synovium from distal femur; avoid detaching lateral collateral ligament
  - Use periosteal elevator or plate-passing instrument to develop tunnel on lateral aspect of femur for plate insertion in submuscular fashion
  - Using muscle-splitting technique, make small 4- to 6-cm incision at proximal end of plate to ensure plate centered on bone (**Figure 4, A**); fluoroscopy helps monitor plate course
- For intra-articular reduction—Use anterolateral (Henry) or lateral parapatellar approach (**Figure 4, B** through **E**)
  - Make incision 1 cm lateral to patella, extending 4 to 5 cm suprapatellar to tibial tubercle
  - Identify lateral retinaculum and vastus lateralis insertion; detach vastus lateralis from rectus and patella

---

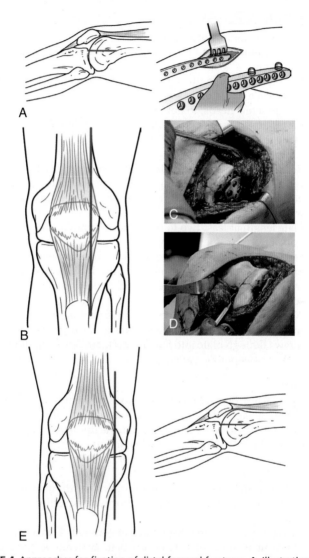

FIGURE 4 Approaches for fixation of distal femoral fractures. **A,** Illustrations show the lateral approach to the lateral distal femur for plate insertion only. **B** through **D,** The anterolateral approach to the distal femur for open reduction and internal fixation of the joint surface and plate insertion. **B,** Illustration shows the incision in the AP aspect. **C,** Intraoperative AP photograph shows joint visualization. **D,** Intraoperative AP photograph shows the patella subluxated to improve visualization. **E,** Illustrations show the two-incision technique using a medial parapatellar incision *(left)* for joint access in AP plane along with the lateral incision *(right)* for plate insertion along the lateral aspect of the femur. (Panels **C** and **D** courtesy of Steve Sims, MD, Charlotte, NC.)

▶ Dissect through joint capsule along lateral edge of patellar tendon; avoid injuring lateral meniscus

▶ Patella can then subluxate/dislocate medially, providing excellent visualization of distal femur from middle to lateral aspect of intercondylar notch (**Figure 4, B**)

- If fracture exits into medial condyle or medial coronal fracture is present, make median parapatellar incision; provides better visualization for articular reduction and fixation; use lateral approach for plate insertion (**Figure 4, C** through **E**)

Reduction Techniques

- Using joysticks and pointed clamps, align intra-articular components of fracture (**Figure 5**)
- Place K-wires across fracture lines; achieve interfragmentary compression with various screws, depending on size and location of fracture
    ▶ On AP radiograph, posterior cortical margin of medial condyle is seen; makes more anterior screws appear in bone, but they could be long

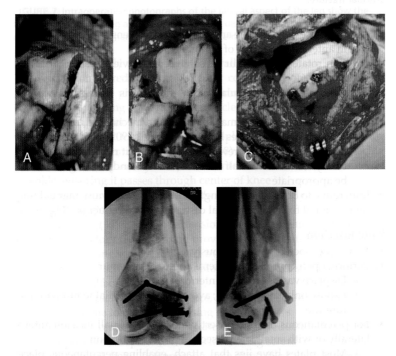

FIGURE 5 Steps in reduction and fixation of an intra-articular fracture of the distal femur. Intraoperative photographs show the unreduced fracture in the AP plane (**A**), the reduction in the AP plane (**B**), and screw placement in the lateral view (**C**). AP (**D**) and lateral (**E**) fluoroscopic views show the completed fixation.

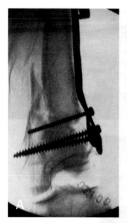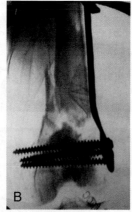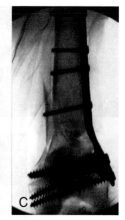

FIGURE 8 AP radiographs show the importance of length in reestablishing axial alignment. **A,** Very short; **B,** short; and **C,** correct. (Courtesy of Eric Johnson, MD, Los Angeles, CA.)

Nail Insertion

- Useful implants for extra-articular and complete articular patterns
- Medial or lateral parapatellar arthrotomy based on fracture pattern
- Provisional fixation of articular surface using clamps and/or Steinman pins
- Precise nail starting point and trajectory are critical to restoring anatomy of distal femur
- Blocking screws can be used to correct trajectory and axial malalignment
- Provisional fixation can be removed after nail inserted and replaced with 2.7 or 3.5 mm cortical screws around nail or distal interlocking screws

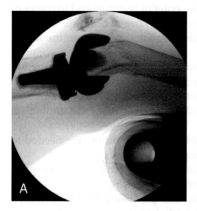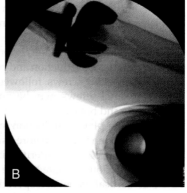

FIGURE 9 Fluoroscopic views depict the importance of knee position in the reduction of the fracture. **A,** Knee in flexion, fracture apex anterior; **B,** knee extended, fracture reduced. (Courtesy of Eric Johnson, MD, Los Angeles, CA.)

COMPLICATIONS

- Most occur from inability to obtain length, alignment, rotation; assess after plate application; revise if necessary
- Varus misalignment and malrotation, from posterior plate placement
- Early fixation failure, from too anterior or posterior plate placement; prevent by ensuring cortex present above and below plate on lateral C-arm image
- Delayed union and nonunion in high-energy, open fractures; consider acute or early bone grafting
- Joint arthrofibrosis uncommon unless knee immobilized, early active motion restricted

POSTOPERATIVE CARE AND REHABILITATION

- Place knee immobilizer for comfort for several days; encourage static isometric quadriceps exercises, straight-leg raises
- May remove knee immobilizer, begin active-assisted knee range of motion at 3 to 5 days
- Touch-down weight bearing postoperatively; permit full weight bearing with radiographic evidence of healing, between 3 and 4 months
- Recovery of knee range of motion, strengthening of thigh musculature critical; consider continuous passive motion machine, initially 0° to 45°; increase to 90° within 3 to 5 days
- Give thromboembolic prophylaxis per surgeon preference, depending on patient mobility

PEARLS

- Distal femur fractures need anatomic axial alignment, precise reduction of articular surface.
- High-energy injuries, joint damage, osteoporotic bone present problems.
- Must identify whether fracture enters joint, especially on lateral view; rule out coronal plane fractures of medial or lateral condyle (Hoffa fracture) with CT.
- Distal femur fractures are complex, require excellent preoperative planning, experienced surgical acumen.
- Surgical approach determined by need to reduce articular surface.
- After articular reduction, must reconstitute normal anatomic/mechanical axes.

Open Reduction and Internal Fixation of Tibial Plateau Fractures

INTRODUCTION

- Tibial plateau fractures involve joint surface, metaphysis of proximal tibia
- Occur from high-energy and low-energy mechanisms
- Consider severity of injury to bone and surrounding soft tissues when determining management
- Goals—Anatomic reduction, restoration of mechanical axis, stable fixation enabling early range of motion (ROM), preservation of surrounding soft tissues, avoidance of infection, ligamentous repair, or reconstruction as needed

PATIENT SELECTION

- Careful examination of injured extremity is mandatory
- Vascular injury, compartment syndrome, and open injuries should be treated emergently
- Note knee stability and soft-tissue conditions and image appropriately

Indications

- Absolute, for open treatment—Open fractures, compartment syndrome, vascular injury
- Relative—Joint instability or malalignment, medial condylar fractures, lateral plateau fractures with displacement greater than 3 mm, condylar widening greater than 5 mm, patient with multiple traumatic injuries
- Consider closed treatment for fractures with less than 2 mm of joint surface displacement, normal alignment, and stable knee in extension

Contraindications

- Consider existing comorbidities, baseline functional level
- Delay open treatment until surrounding soft tissues have time to heal, when possible

---

Based on Goulet JA, Hake ME: Open reduction and internal fixation of tibial plateau fractures, in Colvin AC, Flatow E, eds: Atlas of Essential Orthopaedic Procedures, *ed 2. Rosemont, IL, American Academy of Orthopaedic Surgeons, 2020, pp 613-621.*

- Apply temporary external fixation for gross instability, severe soft-tissue injury
- Goals—Maintain viability of soft tissues, preserve vascularity surrounding fracture

Alternative Treatments

- For bicondylar fractures—Alternative technique uses small-wire ringed external fixator
- For minimally displaced lateral split fractures with minimal joint surface comminution—Closed reduction with percutaneous fixation is an option; rule out lateral meniscus injury or incarceration preoperatively with MRI
- For some fractures with intact or restorable cortical envelope—Arthroscopically assisted reduction and fixation

CLASSIFICATION

- Two classification systems describe fracture pattern but do not consider ligamentous or soft-tissue injury or predict outcomes
- Schatzker classification
  - Six types
  - Types I, II, III—Low-energy mechanism; involve lateral plateau
  - Types IV, V, VI—Higher-energy mechanism; involve medial plateau or bicondylar injury
- AO/Orthopaedic Trauma Association classification
  - Classified as extra-articular, partial articular, and complete articular
  - Further subdivisions based on fracture severity

PREOPERATIVE IMAGING

Radiography

- AP, lateral, and internal/external oblique views of knee
- AP with beam directed 10° caudal shows articular surface displacement

Computed Tomography

- Axial with sagittal, coronal reconstructions useful in surgical planning
- Helps evaluate articular depression (**Figure 1**)

Magnetic Resonance Imaging

- Preoperative MRI helps evaluate for soft-tissue injury; meniscal, ligamentous injuries common
- Helps evaluate need for ligamentous repair before hardware placement

 VIDEO 76.1 Open Reduction and Internal Fixation of Tibial Plateau Fractures. Mark E. Nake, MD; James A. Goulet, MD (21 min)

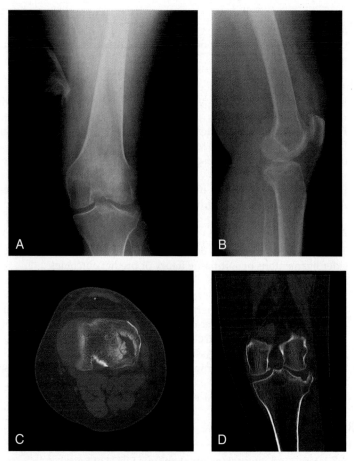

FIGURE 1 AP (**A**) and lateral (**B**) radiographs show a Schatzker type III tibial plateau fracture. Axial (**C**) and coronal (**D**) CT cuts demonstrate a severe articular depression with no associated split in the cortex.

PROCEDURE

Approaches

- Anterolateral approach—For most common fractures (Schatzker types I, II, and III) and fixation of lateral plateau with dual-incision technique in bicondylar fractures
- Lobenhoffer posteromedial approach—For fixation of medial plateau
- Direct posterior approach—Rarely used; for posterior shear–type injuries
- Direct anterior approach—Authors recommend against using

Room Setup/Patient Positioning

- Supine position on radiolucent table for single-incision or dual-incision technique; consider prone position for Lobenhoffer approach
- High-thigh tourniquet
- Radiolucent triangle under knee
- C-arm on contralateral side of table

Special Instruments/Equipment/Implants

- Femoral distractor aids in direct visualization of joint surface and reduction
- 2-mm drill and osteotome for creation of cortical window
- Cannulated reamer from hip compression screw set can also create cortical window
- Bone tamp to reduce depressed fragments
- Autologous iliac crest bone graft, cancellous or cortical allograft, or calcium phosphate cement

Surgical Technique

Anterolateral Approach

- Use standard setup as described previously
- Center incision on Gerdy tubercle in lazy S fashion or using hockey stick shape; make incision midaxial at joint line, sweeping anterior to run 1 to 2 cm lateral to tibial crest
- Proximally, cut iliotibial band in line with its fibers
- Incise fascia over anterior compartment; gently elevate tibialis anterior off metaphysis with Cobb elevator; leave small cuff of fascia attached to tibia to facilitate closure
- Palpate distal joint line; carefully perform submeniscal arthrotomy on anterior aspect of joint only; lateral collateral ligament is at risk
- Place full-thickness stitch through peripheral portion of meniscus to aid retraction and improve joint surface visualization (**Figure 2**)
- May use femoral distractor to further improve articular visualization
- If simple lateral split is present, fracture can be reduced and fixed with precontoured plate, which allows rafting screws under articular surface and closure of submeniscal arthrotomy through its small holes
- In split-depression fractures, open split portion as if opening a book to gain access to compressed fragments
  - ▶ Elevate depressed fragments and backfill with bone graft or bone graft substitute
  - ▶ Close and reduce split; affix with periarticular buttress plate, ensuring that rafting screws are in subchondral bone to support articular surface

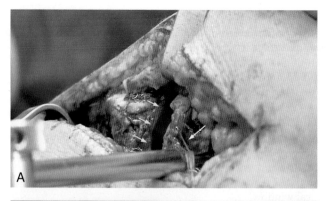

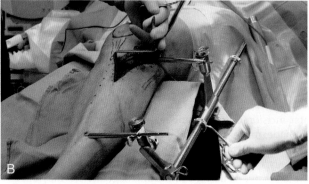

FIGURE 2 Intraoperative photographs show open reduction and internal fixation (ORIF) of a lateral tibial plateau fracture via the anterolateral approach. **A**, Exposure for the ORIF. A submeniscal arthrotomy is made to allow direct evaluation of the joint surface. Care must be taken to not injure the lateral meniscus or lateral collateral ligament. The yellow arrows show the small cuff of the coronary ligament that is left on the tibia for closure. The white arrow highlights stay sutures that are placed for retraction of the meniscus. A headlamp may be required to visualize the joint surface. **B**, A femoral distractor in place on the lateral side of the patient's left knee. The main portion of the distractor remains posterior to the leg so that it does not interfere with access to or imaging of the fracture site.

- Also may use cortical window in depression-type fractures to reduce joint surface
  - Useful when split is nondisplaced or when bookending fragment requires extensive dissection
  - Traditionally, 2-mm drill used to create diamond pattern and osteotome to break cortex; authors place guide pin into depressed fragment, then use cannulated reamer to create cortical window (**Figure 3**)

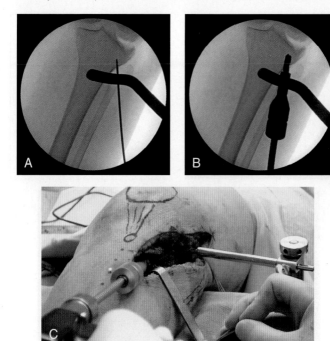

FIGURE 3 Fluoroscopic images show the creation of a cortical window for reduction of the joint surface. **A,** A guide pin is directed at the depressed fragments of the articular surface. **B,** A reamer is used to create a cortical window. **C,** Intraoperative photograph shows the cannulated reamer being directed toward the depression.

- ◗ Use curved bone tamp to reduce depressed joint surface; fill void with autograft, allograft, or cement (**Figure 4**)
- ◗ For both techniques, chosen plate should bypass created window (**Figure 5**)
- • Close arthrotomy, fascia, subcutaneous tissue, skin in layers
- • Authors recommend placing drain

Lobenhoffer Approach

- • Use to access the medial plateau (**Figure 6**)
- • Prone position
- • Incise along border of medial head of gastrocnemius, extending distally 6 to 8 cm from joint line (**Figure 7**)
- • Incise fascia of medial head of gastrocnemius; retract, release, and tag pes anserinus tendons
- • Bluntly dissect to popliteus; release popliteus from fractured fragment in subperiosteal fashion

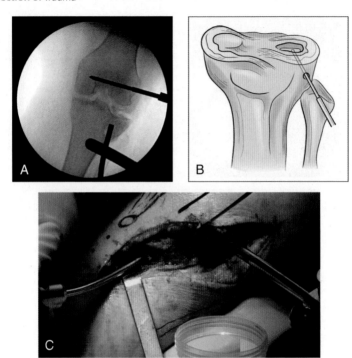

FIGURE 4 Images show the reduction of the area of fracture depression in a Schatzker type III tibial plateau fracture. AP fluoroscopic image (**A**) and illustration (**B**) depict a bone tamp elevating the depressed fragments of the articular surface. **C**, Intraoperative photograph shows allograft cancellous bone being placed through the window to fill the void left in the metaphysis.

- Knee extension, axial traction, anterior-directed force on fragment aid fracture reduction
- Place T-plate in antiglide fashion (**Figure 8**) to stabilize fracture
- Close gastrocnemius, fascia, and skin in layers

COMPLICATIONS
- Uncommon following fixation of low-energy injuries; mostly associated with complex bicondylar fractures
- Most common major complication is infection; careful soft-tissue management, less invasive fixation methods have dramatically reduced incidence
- Malunion, from subsidence at articular surface or loss of anatomic alignment at fracture site
- Deep vein thrombosis rate up to 20% in high-energy injuries
- Secondary arthritis

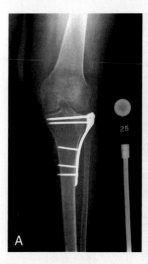
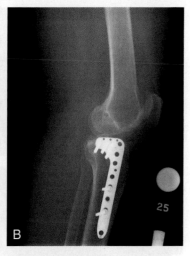

FIGURE 5 Postoperative AP (**A**) and lateral (**B**) radiographs demonstrate open reduction and internal fixation of a Schatzker type III tibial plateau fracture. A periarticular locking plate with a row of rafting screws is used to support the articular reduction. Note that the distal aspect of the plate bypasses the cortical window.

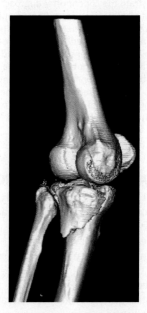

FIGURE 6 Three-dimensional CT reconstruction demonstrates a large posteromedial fragment in a patient with a Schatzker type IV tibial plateau fracture. The apex exits posterolaterally; therefore, a posterior plate will best buttress this fracture.

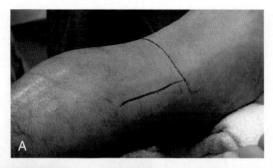

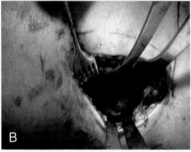

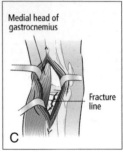

FIGURE 7 Images demonstrate the Lobenhoffer approach for open reduction and internal fixation of a tibial plateau fracture. **A,** Photograph depicts the incision (solid longitudinal line) drawn on the patient's left leg. The patient is prone, and the head is to the right. The incision extends distally over the swollen calf from the joint line; it is 6 to 8 cm in length and runs along the border of the medial head of the gastrocnemius. **B,** Intraoperative photograph shows a posteromedial fragment visualized through the Lobenhoffer approach. The patient's head is to the right, and the foot is to the left. The upper retractors are on the posterior border of the tibia and are retracting the medial head of the gastrocnemius. **C,** Illustration shows the fracture with the anatomy and posteromedial fragment visualized through the Lobenhoffer approach.

POSTOPERATIVE CARE AND REHABILITATION

- Place long leg splint for comfort postoperatively; remove on postoperative day 1 and place unlocked hinged knee brace
- Remove drain on postoperative day 1 or 2
- Toe-touch weight bearing for 12 weeks
- Encourage early gentle range of motion under supervision of physical therapist
- Remove hinged knee brace at week 6
- Initiate low-stress strengthening exercises, aquatic therapy, and use of stationary bike after suture removal
- After Lobenhoffer approach, regaining full extension is main focus of rehabilitation

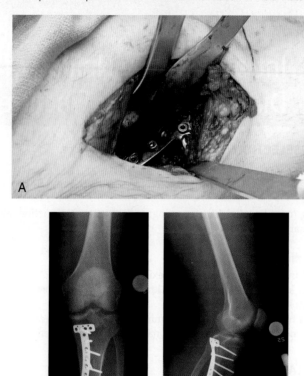

FIGURE 8 Images show open reduction and internal fixation of a Schatzker type IV tibial plateau fracture using a posterior 3.5-mm T-plate to buttress the posteromedial fragment. **A,** Intraoperative photograph shows the T-plate. Four screws are placed distal to the fracture, and two screws are placed across the fracture line in a lag fashion. Postoperative AP (**B**) and lateral (**C**) radiographs show the completed fixation.

PEARLS

- Apply temporary early external fixation for gross instability or severe soft-tissue injury until definitive fixation can be performed.
- MRI evaluation for ligamentous injury in Schatzker type IV fractures before internal hardware is placed can guide surgical treatment.
- Femoral distractor can aid in reduction and visualization of articular surface.
- Can use cannulated reamer to make cortical window in tibial metaphysis to allow reduction of depressed fragments with bone tamp.

77 Intramedullary Nailing of Diaphyseal Tibial Fractures

PATIENT SELECTION

Indications

- Can treat most tibial diaphyseal fractures with intramedullary (IM) nail
- Nailing more beneficial than casting; earlier return to function, alignment maintenance

Contraindications

- Preexisting osseous deformity, preexisting implants
- Relative contraindications—Total knee arthroplasty, morbid obesity (hinders knee flexion)
- In open fractures with gross contamination requiring repeat excisional débridements, delay with staged IM nailing until débridements complete

PREOPERATIVE IMAGING

- AP, lateral radiographs of tibia/fibula, ankle, knee to determine fracture pattern, comminution, bone loss, potential intra-articular extension
- With bone loss, imaging contralateral tibia can help predict symmetric length
- CT helpful if radiographs inconclusive for intra-articular extension or pattern unclear

PROCEDURE

Room Setup/Patient Positioning

- Supine position on radiolucent table with radiolucent bump under hip
- Avoid tourniquet use if possible
- Prepare and drape to midthigh
- C-arm fluoroscopy on contralateral side, monitor at end of bed
- For AP imaging, position C-arm parallel to tibial diaphysis (**Figure 1**)

Based on Jones CB: Intramedullary nailing of diaphyseal tibial fractures, in Colvin AC, Flatow E, eds: Atlas of Essential Orthopaedic Procedures, *ed 2. Rosemont, IL, American Academy of Orthopaedic Surgeons, 2020, pp 622-630.*

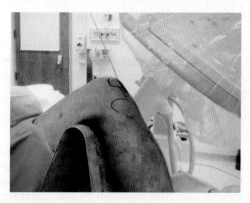

FIGURE 1 Photograph shows fluoroscopic imaging setup for intramedullary nailing of the tibia. For AP imaging, the C-arm is positioned parallel to the tibial diaphysis. (Courtesy of Eben Carroll, MD.)

- Achieve true AP imaging when proximal tibia overlays 50% of fibular head; true lateral imaging occurs when femoral condyles and tibial plateau are collinear
- Position injured leg flexed over radiolucent triangle; should allow knee flexion of 100° to 120°; suspend foot, do not rest on table (**Figure 2**)

Special Instruments/Equipment/Implants

- Complete IM nail set of choice including reamers and ball-tipped guidewire
- Large, medium, small radiolucent triangles for limb positioning
- Multiple small and large retractors
- Multiple large and small Weber bone reduction clamps
- Dental picks

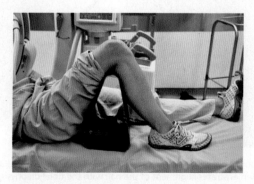

FIGURE 2 Photograph shows incorrect positioning of the foot over the radiolucent triangle. It should be suspended, not impinging or lying on the table. (Courtesy of Eben Carroll, MD, Winston-Salem, NC.)

- Large universal distractor in room, unopened
- Multiple 2.5- and 5.0-mm Schanz pins
- Small-fragment plate and screw set (in room, unopened) for provisional stabilization of open fractures and/or blocking screws
- Additional large drapes to cover fluoroscopy machine during lateral visualization and to cover end of table when knee flexed

Surgical Technique

Approach and Start Site

- With knee in flexion, determine start site fluoroscopically
- Best anatomic start site is along medial aspect of lateral tibial spine on AP view and on apex of anterior tibial slope on lateral view (**Figure 3**)
- To determine start site, place guide pin on skin, confirm position with fluoroscopy (**Figure 4**)
- Medial parapatellar approach
  - ▶ Make 3- to 4-cm incision along medial border of patellar tendon
  - ▶ Reflect paratenon; separate patellar fat pad from posterior aspect of patella; avoid entrapping medial meniscus, coronary ligament
- Lateral parapatellar approach
  - ▶ Useful for proximal third fractures
  - ▶ Make 3- to 4-cm incision along lateral border of patellar tendon
  - ▶ Reflect paratenon; separate patellar fat pad from posterior aspect of patella; avoid entrapping lateral meniscus, coronary ligament
- Patellar tendon–splitting approach
  - ▶ Make 3- to 4-cm incision on middle portion of patellar tendon
  - ▶ Split paratenon; separate patellar fat pad from posterior aspect of patella; avoid entrapping coronary ligament

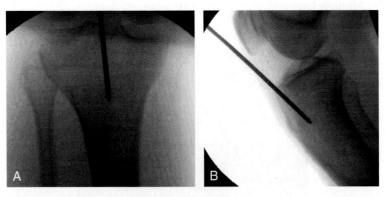

FIGURE 3 Fluoroscopic images show the start site for an intramedullary nail. **A,** AP image demonstrates alignment of the nail with the tibial diaphysis, with a start site just medial to the lateral tibial spine. **B,** Lateral image shows a start site at the apex of the tibial metaphysis and collinear with the tibial diaphysis. (Courtesy of Eben Carroll, MD.)

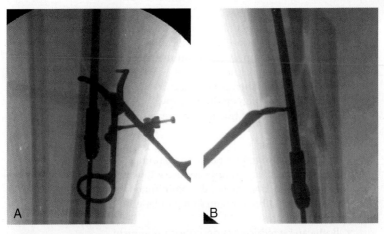

FIGURE 4 AP (**A**) and lateral (**B**) fluoroscopic images demonstrate a percutaneous clamp reducing the fracture and facilitating concentric reaming.

- Percutaneous patellar tendon–splitting approach
  - Make 2-cm incision over distal third of patella
  - Split patellar tendon in proximal-to-distal direction, starting at inferior pole of patella
  - Place guide pin along posterior aspect of patella
  - This approach is author's favorite; avoids cephalad compression/contusion of skin from guide pin, reamers, nail
- Suprapatellar approach
  - With knee flexed in 20° to 30° arc, make 2- to 3-cm incision over rectus
  - Split rectus in line with fibers; insert dilating and instrument cannula
- Medial parapatellar approach with eversion of patella
  - Used in knees with limited flexion from periarticular scarring, patella baja, or knee contracture
  - Make 8- to 10-cm incision over medial half of patella and patellar tendon with knee in extension or slight flexion
  - Incise through medial retinaculum; evert patella laterally
  - Flex knee to desired angle to facilitate pin insertion

Fracture Reduction

- Must reduce fracture before guide pin insertion, reaming, nail insertion
- Can perform fracture reduction many ways
- Transverse fractures
  - Reduce by flexing knee over triangle and applying gentle traction
  - Realign and translate fracture with appropriate distraction
  - "Keying in" of fracture edges ensures reduction, enhances stability
  - Fibular alignment can be used to facilitate fracture rotation

- Oblique or spiral fractures
  - Confirm fracture geometry on preoperative radiographs; use fluoroscopy to determine fracture location and edges
  - Make 5- to 10-mm incisions on medial/lateral and/or anterior/posterior aspects of tibia
  - Spread skin with hemostat; insert Weber clamp through skin; confirm clamp position on fluoroscopy
  - With simultaneous traction and realignment, compress clamp to reduce fracture
- Comminuted fractures
  - Require extensive preoperative planning
  - If fibular fracture is simple, reduce with clamp, plate, or IM device
  - If fibula and tibia are both comminuted, obtain radiographs of contralateral tibia for templating of length
- Segmental fractures
  - Both can be reduced as described previously
  - Can also use open plate fixation to ensure reduction and compression
- Open fractures
  - Require usual excisional débridement and soft-tissue management
  - Can use open wound for clamp positioning, fracture reduction, plate application
  - Plate application can be temporary or permanent
- Associated proximal or distal articular fractures
  - Reduce and stabilize articular/periarticular fractures before nailing
  - Open or percutaneous reduction using Weber clamp
  - Maintain clamp application and/or insert plates or screws to maintain metaphyseal/articular reduction
- Associated ankle and/or syndesmotic fractures
  - Can be reduced, stabilized, and fixed before or after tibial diaphyseal treatment
  - Performing tibial diaphyseal reduction first facilitates syndesmotic treatment by achieving overall length, alignment, rotation
  - Place ankle/syndesmotic implants strategically to avoid impedance of nail insertion
- Delayed or severely shortened fractures
  - Can use closed or open methods, as described previously
  - Can use articulated distraction device attached via 5.0-mm Schanz pins or external fixation
  - Position Schanz pin parallel to tibial plateau and plafond on AP view, posterior to axis of nail insertion on lateral view

Ball-Tipped Guide Rod

- Create opening to IM canal with rigid cannulated reamer over terminally threaded guide pin
- Stop reaming after reamer has entered diaphysis and passed through metaphyseal bone

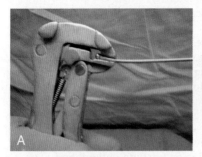
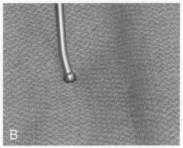

FIGURE 5 Photographs show modification of a ball-tipped guide rod from a straight tip (**A**) to a bent tip (**B**).

- Insert ball-tipped guide rod through medullary opening; balled tip prevents reaming past tip into joint, helps extract any broken cannulated instruments
- Can bend ball-tipped guide rod at tip to facilitate fracture reduction, strategic guide rod positioning (**Figure 5**)

Reaming

- Do not ream until fracture is reduced; doing so prohibits optimal nail insertion, maintenance of reduction
- Push reamer gently through soft tissues without reaming to avoid additional soft-tissue injury or entrapment
- Begin with small-diameter reamer with high rotational speed, slow advancement
- Advance reamer diameter in 1.0- or 0.5-mm increments
- To avoid reamer entrapment or cortical impaction, never stop reamer rotation; instead, vary rotation or advancement speed
- Be wary of fracture fragments pulled into canal and entrapped; if found, place reamer in reverse to dislodge IM fragments; forcefully pulling reamer out can extend or comminute fracture

Nail Insertion

- Base IM nail diameter on surgeon experience, fracture characteristics, final reamer stopping point
- Nail diameter should be 0.5 to 1.0 mm smaller than final reamer diameter
- Determine nail length by comparing length of contralateral leg or by using external rulers
- Do not leave nails prominent proximally; must insert with proper rotation

Compression of Fracture Distraction

- Insert nails down to distal physeal scar; in young dense bone, nail will not pass scar and will distract fracture; in older osteoporotic bone, nail may pass scar easily and enter joint

- When nail is in distal physeal scar, check fracture on AP and lateral fluoroscopy
- If fracture is distracted, requires impaction via backslapping nail, applying longitudinal compression, or repeating nail insertion
- Perform backslapping by placing drill bits or Steinmann pins in distal interlock holes; using final interlocking screws may prestress them, leading to early screw breakage

Proximal Interlocking
- Insert proximal interlocking screws through nail guide drill sleeves
- Use one to three screws, depending on fracture configuration
- Determine trajectory before drilling to avoid penetrating tibial plateau or drilling beyond desired cortex
- Confirm screw length with rollover and rollback AP views or with depth gauge
- Confirm proper nail depth before inserting screws or removing proximal nail guide

Distal Interlocking
- Insert distal interlocking screws freehand or use "perfect circles" technique: keep leg in stable position, translate and rotate C-arm
- Angulation creating elongated hole can create errant drill hole
- After "perfect circle" created, place radiopaque marker on skin to mark incision
- Make vertical incision through skin only; carefully spread soft tissue to avoid damaging underlying neurovasculature
- Insert drill bit, which should be within central portion of radiolucent hole
- Drill cortices; confirm position fluoroscopically

Poller Blocking Screws
- These screws narrow medullary osseous corridors; can use for errant start sites proximally, errant reaming tunnels distally, or with osteoporotic bone to narrow canal width
- Position along concavity of deformity, along lateral aspect of proximal segment to prevent valgus deformity, and along posterior aspect of proximal segment to prevent apex anterior angulation
- Can be placed temporarily or permanently, but should be 3.5 mm or larger
- When reaming with blocking screws, push past site to avoid wear and debris

Interlocking Screw Enhancement
- Some nails allow for proximal nail cap insertion to entrap the most proximal interlocking screw
- Others allow for interlocking screws to thread into nail, providing enhanced stability

Nail Guide Removal
- Remove proximal nail guide only after confirming nail position, interlocking screw insertion, and nail reduction fluoroscopically
- Also confirm no proximal tibial plateau or distal plafond fracture extension or surgeon-induced fractures present fluoroscopically

Incision Closure
- Author recommends 3.0-mm nylon sutures in Allgöwer-Donati fashion rather than mattress or simple interrupted
- Apply full-length elastic skin closure strips without tension across incisions to enhance skin reapproximation, diminish skin tension

Intraoperative Splinting
- Apply splint after sterile bandages, before patient awakens, to reduce pain, equinus ankle deformity
- Flex knee to 90° to relax gastrocnemius; position ankle in neutral (90°) to maintain soft-tissue tension
- Keep splint in place for 2 to 14 days

COMPLICATIONS
- Knee pain most common complication; occurs in up to two-thirds of cases
  - Multifactorial etiology; pain usually resolves with time
  - Focus rehabilitation on improving resultant thigh weakness
- Nonunion second most common complication; occurs in 1% to 50%; more common in open fractures, vascular injury, bone loss, infection, distraction, small nail insertion
- Infection
- Malrotation, malalignment, limb-length discrepancy, leg pain, prominent implants

POSTOPERATIVE CARE AND REHABILITATION
- Remove splint at 2 to 14 days
- Initiate range of motion at home or with physical therapy upon splint removal
- Brace, foot-ankle orthosis, pneumatic boot protects foot when deconditioned patient begins bearing weight
- Start weight bearing based on patient compliance, fracture configuration, stability, surgeon preference
  - Earlier weight bearing for simple transverse middiaphyseal fractures treated with proximal and distal interlocking screws
  - For complex metadiaphyseal and/or comminuted fractures, no weight bearing until callus formation or after delayed bone grafting may be desirable

PEARLS

- A perfect tibial nailing depends on accurate start site, fracture reduction, central reaming; nondistracting nail insertion; and efficient interlocking.
- Only in middiaphyseal fractures with good canal fit of nail can indirect reduction of fracture be accomplished.
- Treatment of tibial diaphyseal fractures early—within 3 to 5 days of injury—facilitates closed methods of alignment, translation, rotational reduction.
- If unable to reduce fracture with single reduction method within 3 to 5 minutes, try another reduction method or revert to minimally open soft-tissue protective method. Do not continue closed methods of reduction that compromise skin or future approaches.

Open Reduction and Internal Fixation of the Tibial Plafond

PATIENT SELECTION
- Articular surface or gross metadiaphyseal malalignment of tibial plafond requires open reduction and internal fixation
- Intrinsic articular surface impaction occurs medially on plafond, from internal rotation/supination, or laterally, from external rotation/pronation from axial load
- Fibular involvement common; Volkmann fragment with or without ligamentous avulsion possible
- Contraindications to surgery include noncompliance with cessation of nicotine use or intravenous drug addictions, venous insufficiency, and systemic disease; evaluate on case-by-case basis

PREOPERATIVE IMAGING
- Plain AP, lateral, and mortise radiographs of ankle (**Figure 1**)
- For tibial plafond fracture, obtain imaging throughout treatment course

PROCEDURE
Room Setup/Patient Positioning
- Use similar surgical setup for index, definitive surgeries
- Supine position on pressure-relieving mattress on radiolucent table
- Place wedge under ipsilateral hip to allow external and internal rotation of ankle
- Index surgery uses more internally rotated position; definitive surgery uses internal and external rotation
- Place ramp pad under ipsilateral limb; allows access for surgery, intraoperative radiographs

Surgical Technique
- Two surgeries are usually necessary
- Index surgery provides gross reduction of ankle through distraction, with talus under tibia, via external fixator
- Obtain CT after external fixation to plan definitive intervention
- Definitive surgery occurs 10 to 21 days after injury

Based on Benirschke SK, Kramer PA: Open reduction and internal fixation of the tibial plafond, in Colvin AC, Flatow E, eds: Atlas of Essential Orthopaedic Procedures, ed 2. Rosemont, IL, American Academy of Orthopaedic Surgeons, 2020, pp 631-638.

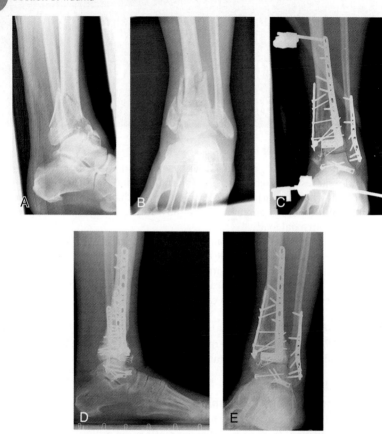

FIGURE 1 Radiographs show initial injury, treatment, and outcome of a tibial plafond injury. Lateral (**A**) and mortise (**B**) radiographs show the injured ankle and foot. **C**, Mortise postoperative radiograph shows a medial buttress plate. The frame was maintained in place for soft-tissue management. Lateral (**D**) and mortise (**E**) radiographs at 1.5-year follow-up.

Index Surgery

- Occurs within hours of presentation
- Early external fixation enables earlier definitive treatment, improved outcomes
- Place Schanz pins carefully to avoid neural and vascular structures
- Address fibular injury first
    - ▸ Must restore correct fibular length, orientation
    - ▸ Fibular reduction more critical with associated tibial plafond injuries; posterior (Volkmann) fragment connected to fibula via posterior tibiofibular ligament

- Unless ligament avulsed, fibular reduction grossly reduces Volkmann fragment; anatomic fibular reduction important for good outcome
- Fibular fixation can wait until trained personnel and the needed equipment are available
- Place external fixator after treating fibula
  - Place basic frame along medial column (**Figure 2, A**); lateral injuries may need bicolumnar frame (**Figure 2, B**)
  - Attach medial column frame to tibia, calcaneus, and medial cuneiform
  - Locate all pins outside anticipated location of incisions
  - Insert calcaneal pin first
    - Terminally threaded, inserted medially for medial column frames; centrally threaded for bicolumnar frames
    - No predrilling required
    - Place in posterior portion of calcaneal tuberosity, posterior to line connecting superior, posterior edges; avoids sural nerve, calcaneal branch of tibial nerve
  - Insert proximal tibial pin
    - Place at proximal middle third junction of tibia through anteromedial surface; avoid saphenous nerve and vein
    - Use 5-mm Schanz half pin
    - Predrilling required
  - Insert third pin through medial, middle, lateral cuneiforms
    - Insert through medial surface of medial cuneiform
    - No predrilling required

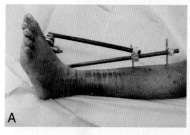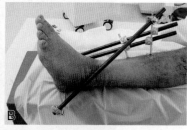

FIGURE 2 Photographs show an external fixation device. **A,** A unicolumnar frame is shown after definitive surgery. The two tibial pins are placed outside the affected area and as far apart as possible. Note the incisional wounds associated with the fibular fixation and the anterolateral approach. **B,** A typical bicolumnar frame is shown. When a bicolumnar external fixation device is needed, the standard arrangement includes two bars to tie the two tibial pins to the medial calcaneus and midfoot (cuneiforms). This arrangement includes the components used in a unicolumnar medial application (**A**), but the calcaneal pin exits the lateral side, and a third bar ties it to the proximal tibial pin (**B**). In the arrangement shown, the midfoot pin through the cuneiforms was not needed to provide adequate stability.

- ❧ Place distal tibial pin last; location determined by tibial fracture; place as distally as possible, while remaining outside fracture area, forthcoming internal fixation
- ❧ Tibial pins require predrilling due to hard cortices
  - – Make small vertical incision; probe down to bone
  - – Insert triple-sleeve drilling attachment; limits soft-tissue injury
  - – Use sharp, 3.2-mm drill to underdrill pilot hole
  - – Copiously irrigate to prevent thermal necrosis
- Complications—Pin-tract infection, early fixator loosening, and failure of fixation
- External fixator slightly distracts ankle joint
  - ❧ Allow 5 mm between talar dome and subchondral fibula
  - ❧ Distraction allows nonimpacted fragments to move; impacted fragments do not; aids preoperative planning
  - ❧ Talus should be centrally located
  - ❧ Ankle in neutral position; do not overstretch tibial, superficial peroneal nerves
- After external fixator placement, assess incisions to ensure skin not under pressure
- After reduction, shorten pins for sterile short leg splint placement
- Obtain CT to aid in definitive surgery planning (**Figure 3**)
- Postoperative care and rehabilitation
  - ❧ Instruct patient to strictly avoid weight bearing and maintain elevation

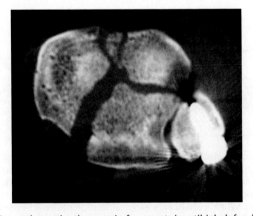

FIGURE 3 CT scan shows the three main fragments in a tibial plafond injury: the posterior or Volkmann fragment that is attached to the fibula via the tibiofibular ligament; the medial fragment, which in this case includes the malleolus; and the anterolateral or Chaput fragment.

- Discontinue splint approximately 10 days after external fixation to assess soft tissues; if swelling resolved, schedule definitive fixation; if swelling remains, reapply splint
- Assess patient compliance based on maintenance of elevation (substantial swelling prompts suspicion); condition of splint, which could indicate weight bearing; harmful habits such as tobacco use
- Perform duplex examination after splint removed
  - Manage deep vein thrombosis (DVT) below popliteus hiatus with perioperative prophylactic anticoagulation, followed by full anticoagulation 48 hours after definitive fixation
  - Manage DVT within 7 cm of popliteus hiatus with prophylactic removable vena cava filter
  - After definitive surgery, remove filter; place patient on therapeutic anticoagulation

Definitive Surgery

- Occurs after swelling has resolved, 10 to 21 days after external fixation
- Surgical approach determined by injury characteristics, fracture pattern
- Anteromedial approach (**Figure 4**)
  - Classic approach to tibial plafond injuries
  - Enables medial impaction to be addressed, visualization of entire plafond, and control of bone fragments
  - Incision begins 1 cm lateral to anterior crest at anticipated proximal edge of plate
  - Extend incision distally to 1 cm distal to medial malleolus tip
  - Retract anterior compartment laterally
  - Lateral plafond difficult to visualize, lateral impaction difficult to reduce with this approach
- Anterolateral approach (**Figure 5**)
  - Used for injuries with substantial lateral disruption
  - Allows optimal access to anterolateral/posterolateral plafond, but medial impaction more difficult to access and manipulate
  - Make incision lateral to anterior crest of tibia, in line with space between fourth and fifth metatarsals, lateral to extensor tendon
  - Retract anterior compartment laterally
  - Cut extensor retinaculum along lateral edge
  - Make separate more proximal incision to place screws through plate (**Figure 2, A**)
- Posteromedial and posterolateral approaches
  - Sometimes useful for highly comminuted posterior injuries
  - Rarely necessary; can lead to complications and limit future salvage options

---

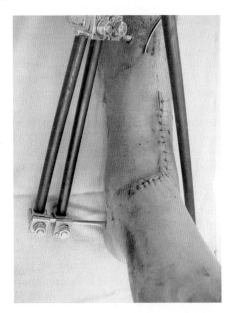

FIGURE 4 Photograph shows the closure of the anteromedial approach. The surgical incision curves gently across the joint from lateral to medial and is closed with Algöwer sutures. Note that part of the bicolumnar external fixation frame is still in place, and the drain exits superiorly.

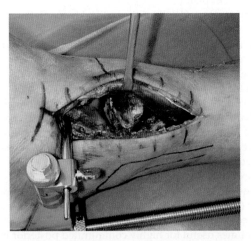

FIGURE 5 Intraoperative photograph shows the anterolateral approach with a Schanz pin in the talar neck, which allows the anterior joint to be distracted.

- After accessing joint, insert Schanz pin into talar neck
  - ▶ Use pin to rotate and distract talus plantarly so anterior edge is open, posterior surface can be visualized (**Figure 5**)
  - ▶ Use Kirschner wires to hold preliminary reductions

Sequence of Reduction

- Addressing fibular anatomy semi-reduces Volkmann fragment unless tibiofibular ligament is avulsed
- In definitive surgery, crucial to first reduce any impaction within Volkmann fragment; inadequately addressed impaction does not provide correct "read" for reducing remaining articular fragments
- Volkmann fragment provides anchor for posteromedial fragment
- Goal is smooth articular surface; any central comminution is brought down to align with Volkmann fragment plus posteromedial plus medial malleolar portion
- Lastly, assemble tubercle of Chaput, which forms anterolateral curve; if fragment is aligned with anteromedial and posterolateral surfaces, reduction is successful
- In summary, reduction proceeds from posterolateral to posteromedial, to anteromedial, to central, and to anterolateral
- Implants are tailored to support particular osseous injury
- Severe comminution requires stiffer implants, such as anteromedial and/or lateral buttress plates
- Kirschner wires provide provisional stabilization
- Screws not integrated into implant rarely used unless medial side requires stability but not buttressing; in such cases, use strut screws

Implants

- Slide plates onto tibia with screws inserted under direct visualization
- With anteromedial incision and plate, visualize through initial incision; with anterolateral approach, make second incision to access upper portion of anterolateral plate; with second incision, move tibialis anterior muscle belly rather than skewering with screws
- Occasionally, anterolateral approach requires medial buttress plate; make small incision anteromedially near distal-most tibia; slide plate proximally along tibia, with screws inserted percutaneously because no muscles are at risk on medial tibial surface
- Remove frame after wound closure; for additional support, maintain frame for three more weeks (**Figure 2, A**)

Closure

- Close ankle joint capsule with 2.0 Vicryl suture (Ethicon) in figure-of-8 pattern
- For anteromedial approach, close tibial periosteal layer with figure-of-8 sutures

---

- For anterolateral approach, suture ankle capsule, extensor retinaculum, superficial tissues
- Close skin with Algöwer sutures (**Figure 4**)
- Place 1/8-in Hemovac drain exiting anteriorly under anterior compartment; leave in for 48 hours
- Apply short leg splint in 5° to 10° of dorsiflexion
- Place continuous indwelling peripheral nerve catheters for pain control for first 48 hours
- Discharge home after drain removal
- Instruct to remain non–weight bearing and elevate foot
- Remove splint 1 to 2 weeks postoperatively; begin active range of motion (ROM) of ankle and subtalar joints and passive ROM of toes
- Apply resting splint in 5° to 10° of dorsiflexion

COMPLICATIONS

- Early complications
  - DVT; consider duplex examination before definitive surgery
  - Delayed wound healing
    - Usually associated with anteromedial approach
    - Can be associated with cellulitis
    - Rare with anterolateral approach (preferred approach)
    - Meticulous intraoperative care of soft tissues important
  - For deep infection, meticulous intraoperative care of soft tissues important
- Late complications
  - Delayed union, nonunion of metadiaphyseal junction
    - Increased risk if insufficiently buttressed
    - If primary implant fails, replace implant, improve buttressing
  - Avascular collapse of articular bone
    - Typically occurs in central plafond, with talus pushing through avascular articular surface
    - With severely comminuted injuries or concern of delayed union, delay weight bearing until radiographic evidence of healing
  - Posttraumatic ankle arthrosis
    - Best avoided with meticulous reconstruction of articular surface
    - Salvage options are limited
  - Nerve complications
    - Result in long-term patient issues
    - Important to preoperatively diagnose sensory deficit caused by initial injury
    - Careful soft-tissue dissection limits intraoperative nerve complications

POSTOPERATIVE CARE AND REHABILITATION

- At 6-week follow-up
  - Radiographs to establish healing
  - Support stocking
  - Continue non–weight bearing, but more aggressive ROM
- At 3-month follow-up
  - Protective sock in normal shoe with insert
  - Progressive weight bearing depends on radiographic evidence of healing
- At 6-month follow-up—Advanced gait training to increase strength and balance
- At 1-year follow-up
  - Most osseous healing is complete (**Figure 1, D** and **E**)
  - Reinforce rehabilitation skills

PEARLS

- External fixation to obtain gross length, alignment, and rotation should occur as soon as possible to protect soft-tissue envelope.
- Place external fixator pins carefully to prevent vascular injury, neural injury, or bone necrosis.
- Fibular length, alignment, and rotation must be anatomically restored; surgical fibular reduction should occur when appropriate personnel and equipment are available.
- Obtain CT images after external fixator placement to help plan for definitive surgical fixation.
- Definitive fixation should involve anatomic reduction of plafond and metadiaphysis.
- Address impaction, particularly of Volkmann fragment, to create anatomic articular surface.

PATIENT SELECTION

- Ankle is most frequently injured weight-bearing joint
- Injury usually results from indirect rotational forces, less commonly due to direct blow; can result in fracture and ligamentous and soft-tissue injury
- Ankle stability depends on bony, ligamentous integrity; injury to both must be recognized, and treated
- Classified based on anatomic site, mechanism of injury
  - Danis-Weber classification based on anatomic site; uses level of lateral malleolar fracture in relation to articular surface
  - Lauge-Hansen classification based on mechanism of injury; predicts position of foot, direction of primary deforming force based on displacement pattern, level, and morphology of fibula fracture
- Individualize treatment decisions based on degree of bony, ligamentous stability, not classification system
- Dislocation or subluxation of talus within ankle mortise is commonly present; even minimal mortise malalignment alters contact pressures, risks arthritis
- Imperative to achieve stable, anatomically reduced mortise by restoring bony and ligamentous structures
- Critical to assess the condition of the soft tissues
  - Marked swelling, fracture blisters, and other skin changes should delay definitive surgery until soft-tissue milieu resolves
  - Can wait up to 3 weeks for definitive management
  - Condition of soft tissues particularly important in elderly and in persons with diabetes
- Most nondisplaced or minimally displaced (<2 mm) monomalleolar fractures, typically medial or lateral, are treated nonsurgically
- Monomalleolar fractures displaced more than 2 mm, bimalleolar and trimalleolar fractures, fracture-dislocations, syndesmotic injuries, and open fractures require surgery

---

Based on Carroll EA, Marquez-Lara A, Medda S, Halvorson JJ: Surgical treatment of ankle fractures, in Colvin AC, Flatow E, eds: Atlas of Essential Orthopaedic Procedures, *ed 2. Rosemont, IL, American Academy of Orthopaedic Surgeons, 2020, pp 639-648.*

- Historically, posterior malleolar fragments greater than 25% of tibial plafond required surgery; recent literature suggests expanding indications for posterior malleolar fixation, including improved fibular reduction, restored syndesmotic integrity

PREOPERATIVE IMAGING

- Ankle injuries require AP, lateral, and mortise radiographs
- Three important radiographic measurements are medial clear space, tibiofibular overlap, and tibiofibular clear space (**Figure 1**)
- Lateral shift of talus at least 2 mm (measured by medial clear space) or fracture displacement greater than 2 mm are surgical indications
- Dynamic stress views can demonstrate talar shift that may be unappreciated on static radiographs (**Figure 2**)
- Syndesmotic injury suggested by tibiofibular clear space >6 mm on AP or mortise radiographs or tibiofibular overlap <6 mm on AP and <1 mm on mortise
- Example of patient with trimalleolar ankle fracture-dislocation (**Figure 3, A** through **C**), who underwent closed reduction under conscious sedation (**Figure 3, C** through **E**) and surgical management 4 days later as soft-tissue milieu allowed

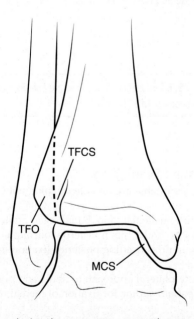

FIGURE 1 Illustration depicts the parameters commonly measured when assessing ankle stability. The medial clear space (MCS) should be 4 mm or less on the AP and mortise views. The tibiofibular overlap (TFO) should be 6 mm or more on the AP view and 1 mm or more on the mortise view. The tibiofibular clear space (TFCS) should be 6 mm or less on AP and mortise views.

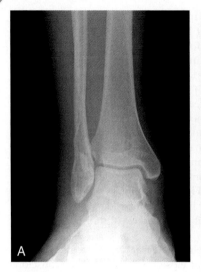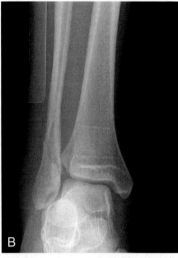

FIGURE 2 AP radiographs show an isolated right distal fibula fracture. **A,** The medial clear space (MCS) appears normal on a static view. **B,** Note the increased MCS, suggestive of widening with gravity stress.

 VIDEO 79.1 Trimalleolar Ankle Fracture Fixation. Eben Carroll, MD; Jason Halvorson, MD (14 min)

PROCEDURE

Room Setup/Patient Positioning

- Surgeon, instrument table are on side of ankle injury, with C-arm on opposite side
- For isolated monomalleolar and bimalleolar ankle injuries, supine position with bump under hip, nonsterile tourniquet
- For trimalleolar injuries needing posterior fixation, lateral position on beanbag
    - Allows posterolateral approach to fibula and posterior malleolus
    - Then, roll patient supine for fixation of medial malleolus

Instruments/Equipment/Implants

- Radiolucent table
- Small-fragment plates and screws
- Fracture-reducing clamps, dental picks, tissue elevators

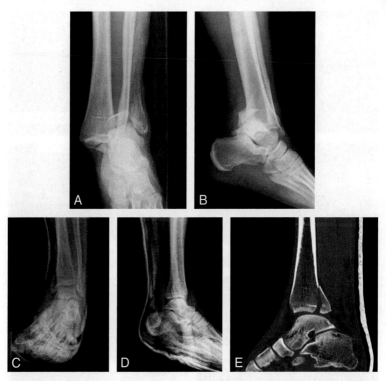

FIGURE 3 AP (**A**) and lateral (**B**) radiographs show a trimalleolar ankle fracture-dislocation in a 76-year-old man. AP (**C**) and lateral (**D**) postreduction radiographs and sagittal reconstruction (**E**) show the posterior malleolar component. Note the now-reduced ankle mortise (**C**) and restoration of the tibiotalar relationship in the lateral plane (**D**). **E,** The size and displacement of the posterior malleolar fracture fragment are evident.

Surgical Technique

- For lateral and posterior malleolar fractures, first position patient laterally to address posterior malleolus and fibula
- Exsanguinate extremity; inflate tourniquet to 250 mm Hg
- Make incision midway between Achilles and posterior border of fibula (**Figure 4, A**)
- Use internervous plane between gastrocnemius-soleus complex and flexor hallucis longus (tibial nerve) and peroneus brevis and longus
- Dissect to deep fascia; avoid short saphenous vein and sural nerve
- Incise deep fascia between peroneus longus and brevis anteriorly and gastrocnemius-soleus complex posteriorly (**Figure 4, B**); retract peroneals anteriorly and gastrocnemius-soleus posteriorly

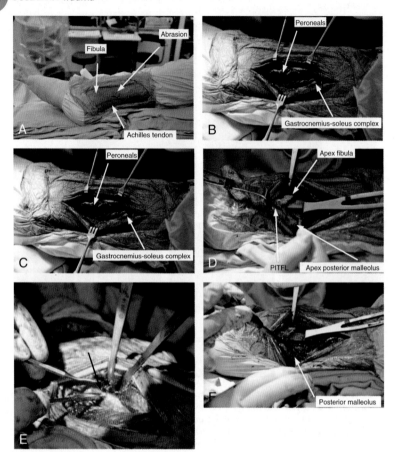

FIGURE 4 Intraoperative photographs show the surgical management of a left posterior malleolar ankle fracture with the patient in the right lateral decubitus position. Distal is to the left. **A,** An incision is made midway between the Achilles complex and the posterior border of the fibula. In this patient, the incision was cheated slightly more posterior secondary to an abrasion in the path of the preferred incision. **B,** The superficial interval is between the peroneal musculature anteriorly and the gastrocnemius-soleus complex posteriorly. **C,** The flexor hallucis longus (FHL) is seen arising from the posterior surface of the fibula. **D,** The apexes of the fibular and posterior malleolar fracture are shown. Note the intact posterior inferior tibiofibular ligament (PITFL). **E,** The fracture apex (arrow; in this figure, the fibula) is reduced with the help of clamps, ball-spike pushers, dental picks, and Kirschner wires (K-wires). **F,** The apex of the posterior malleolar fracture is held provisionally and reduced with a K-wire.

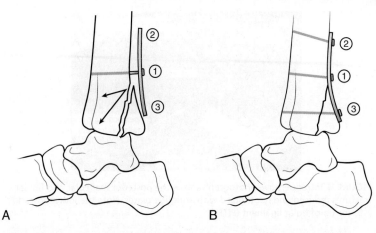

FIGURE 5 Illustration demonstrates reduction and neutralization of a posterior malleolar fracture using an antiglide plating technique. **A**, Screw 1 is inserted first, just proximal to the apex of the fracture line. With tightening of this screw, fracture reduction can be achieved with the distal anterior force vector applied via the plate. **B**, Screw 2 is then placed. Finally, any residual articular gapping is addressed with a lag screw in position 3. In a true antiglide construct, screw 3 may not always be necessary if no articular gapping is present.

- Visualize flexor hallucis longus arising from posterior fibula, detach from its origin, and retract posterior and medial (**Figure 4, C**)
- Take dissection across interosseous membrane to posterior tibia; avoid disrupting posterior syndesmotic ligaments
- Identify apex of fibular and posterior malleolar fractures; clean obstructing soft-tissue debris (**Figure 4, D**); reduction of posterior malleolar fragment aids in reduction and length restoration of fibula and helps gauge fibular rotation
- Reduce fracture and hold provisionally with clamps, ball-spike pushers, dental picks, and Kirschner wires (**Figure 4, E** and **F**)
- Neutralize fracture with antiglide plate; compress with lag screw (**Figure 5**)
- Repeat reduction, fixation for fibula, using one-third tubular small-fragment plates (**Figure 6**)
- In absence of posterior malleolar fracture, address fibula via direct lateral approach, with patient supine
  - ▸ Protect superficial peroneal nerve
  - ▸ Can apply fibular plate posteriorly; more commonly, one-third tubular plate placed directly lateral to neutralize reduced and lagged fibula fracture (**Figure 7**)
  - ▸ Lateral plating may be more prominent
- After posterolateral approach is complete, deflate beanbag; return patient to supine position

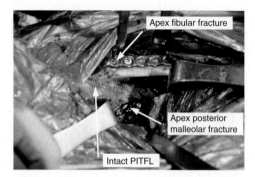

FIGURE 6 Intraoperative photograph shows the posterior malleolar and fibular fractures reduced and neutralized with antiglide plates. Note the intact posterior inferior tibiofibular ligament (PITFL).

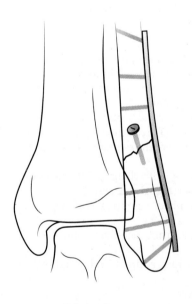

Anterior view

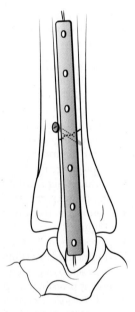

Lateral view

FIGURE 7 Illustration shows a commonly used fixation montage for laterally based fibular fixation. A one-third tubular small fragment plate can be placed directly lateral to neutralize a reduced and lagged fibula fracture. Too much obliquity of the distal screws must be avoided because it increases the risk of problems caused by hardware prominence.

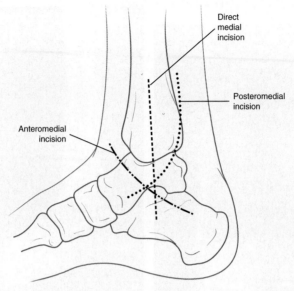

FIGURE 8 Illustration depicts options for incisions to address the medial malleolar fragment.

- External rotation of hip allows access to medial malleolus fracture
- Several options available for medial incision (**Figure 8**); identify and protect long saphenous vein
- Clean fracture of obstructing soft-tissue debris; portions of deltoid ligament or periosteum may be interposed
- If medial malleolar fragment of sufficient size, insert two Kirschner wires to aid in reduction and provide provisional stabilization
- Recommend direct visualization at extra-articular medial fracture line and anteromedial apex of articular surface; do not use fluoroscopy alone
- Perform definitive fixation of medial malleolar fragment with partially threaded 3.5- or 4.0-mm cannulated screws
  - Also can use noncannulated 2.7-, 3.5-, or 4.0-mm screws
  - Achieve compression with partially threaded screws, fully threaded screws with lag technique, or external clamp compression followed by screws
  - Unicortical screws often used, but recent evidence suggests bicortical fixation may be advantageous
- Match screw and fragment size to avoid iatrogenic comminution
- Achieve two points of fixation to prevent rotational displacement (**Figure 9**)
- Scrutinize intraoperative fluoroscopic images and plain radiographs; ensure syndesmotic stability has been restored; syndesmotic injury can occur regardless of level of fibula fracture

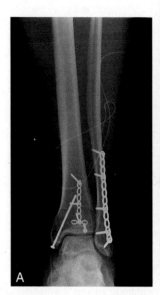 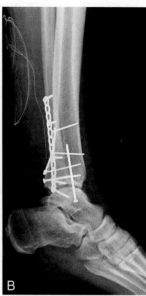

FIGURE 9 Final postoperative radiographs demonstrate reestablishment of mortise congruity and appropriate fixation of the medial and lateral malleoli on the AP view (**A**) and the reduced and neutralized posterior malleolar fracture fragment on the lateral view (**B**).

- If syndesmotic injury, anatomic reduction and fixation is the goal
  - Overreduction is possible and should be avoided
  - May use manual pressure or clamps to reduce syndesmosis
  - Fixation can be 3.5 mm screw(s) or suture button construct
- Copiously irrigate, close wounds in layered fashion with nonabsorbable interrupted sutures, carefully handling soft tissues
- Apply dressings; place well-padded splint with foot in neutral position inversion/eversion and dorsiflexion/plantar flexion

COMPLICATIONS
- Wound problems, infection (4% to 5%)
  - Simple peri-incisional redness and superficial tissue necrosis may be observed or treated with antibiotics
  - Exposed hardware and significant wound breakdown may need plastic surgeon consultation
  - Frank infection needs surgical débridement and culture-directed antibiotic therapy
- Malunion
  - Significantly affects contact pressures in ankle
  - Initial anatomic reduction very important; malunion correction more difficult after index surgery

- Nonunion
  - Uncommon, but can occur with medial malleolus fractures
  - Invagination of soft tissues into fracture may predispose
- Symptomatic hardware
  - Can occur at fibula and medial malleolus due to subcutaneous position
  - Delay hardware removal at least 1 year after surgery
  - Posterolateral fibular plating, less oblique screws, smaller medial malleolar screws may prevent

POSTOPERATIVE CARE AND REHABILITATION

- Maintain splint for 2 weeks
- Some evidence early range of motion is beneficial
- After suture removal, if soft-tissues amenable, place fracture boot; allow gentle range of motion exercises
- Delay weight bearing 6 to 8 weeks
- In patients with diabetes, continue cast immobilization for 8 weeks; delay weight bearing until 12 weeks postoperatively

PEARLS

- Manner of soft-tissue handling has direct implications for postoperative complications, such as wound slough and infection.
- Dynamic radiographs (stress views) required before assuming monomalleolar fibula fracture is stable with intact deltoid ligament.
- Syndesmosis reduction should be achieved under direct visualization and overreduction should be prevented.
- Ankle joint is unforgiving of malreduction; anatomic reduction should be achieved.
- Posterolateral fibular plating, reducing obliquity of distal screws in lateral fibular plate, proper size and location of medial malleolar screws may reduce incidence of symptomatic hardware.
- Progress weight bearing cautiously in patients with diabetes.

Surgical Management of Fractures of the Talus

INTRODUCTION

Anatomy

- Talus consists of the head, neck, body, lateral process, and posterior process (**Figure 1**)
- Flexor hallucis longus (FHL) tendon divides posterior process into medial and lateral tubercle
- Cartilage covers 60% of talus
- No muscles/tendons attach to talus, which plays critical role in midfoot, hindfoot, and ankle motion
- Talus receives blood supply from artery of tarsal canal, deltoid artery, and artery of sinus tarsi; all derive locally from peroneal, anterior tibial, and posterior tibial arteries (**Figure 2**)

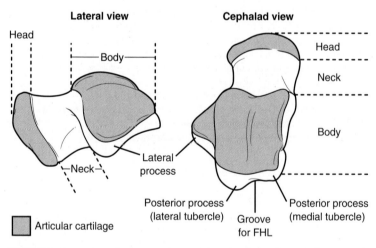

Lateral view

Head

Body

Neck

Lateral process

Cephalad view

Head

Neck

Body

Posterior process (lateral tubercle)

Groove for FHL

Posterior process (medial tubercle)

Articular cartilage

FIGURE 1 Illustrations depict two views of the talus. FHL = flexor hallucis longus

Based on Tabit JM, Webb LX: Surgical management of fractures of the talus, in Colvin AC, Flatow E, eds: Atlas of Essential Orthopaedic Procedures, ed 2. Rosemont, IL, American Academy of Orthopaedic Surgeons, 2020, pp 649-656.

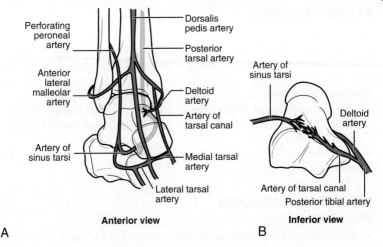

FIGURE 2 Illustrations show anterior (**A**) and inferior (**B**) views of the talus with its blood supply. The blood supply is derived from an anastomotic ring with contributions from the posterior tibial artery by way of its deltoid artery branch and the artery of the tarsal canal. The dorsalis pedis artery and the perforating peroneal artery also contribute, by way of their branches, to the artery of the sinus tarsi and the lateral tarsal artery, respectively. (Adapted from Fortin P, Balazsy J: Talus fractures: Evaluation and treatment. *J Am Acad Orthop Surg* 2001;9[6]:114-127.)

Mechanism of Injury

- Talar neck fractures commonly occur from hyperdorsiflexion force
- Talar neck susceptible to fractures due to its low bone density and small cross-sectional area, as talus strikes denser anterior tibia
- High-energy injuries with significant comminution and displacement; high incidence of associated fractures (64%) and soft-tissue injuries (21% open)

Classification

- Hawkins classification widely used
    - Type I—Nondisplaced
    - Type II—Displaced with subluxation/dislocation of subtalar joint
    - Type III—Displaced with subluxation/dislocation of subtalar and tibiotalar joints
    - Type IV—Displaced with subluxation/dislocation of subtalar, tibiotalar, and talonavicular joints
- Rate of talar body osteonecrosis correlates with Hawkins classification, increasing risk of vascular disruption with extent of displacement
- Hawkins classification confined to talar neck; AO/Orthopaedic Trauma Association classification more broad but rarely used clinically

PATIENT SELECTION

Indications

- Truly nondisplaced fractures can be managed nonsurgically
- Displaced fractures require surgical management (**Figure 3**)

Contraindications

- Preexisting active or indolent bone infection, severe neuropathic foot, uncorrectable vascular impairment with likelihood of wound healing complications
- Isolated nondisplaced lateral or posterior process fractures may be managed nonsurgically

PREOPERATIVE IMAGING

Plain Radiography

- AP, lateral, ankle mortise, and Canale views of ankle and foot
- Lateral view shows talar neck and talonavicular, tibiotalar, talocalcaneal joint incongruencies
- Canale view shows neck in profile; obtain with foot in maximal plantar flexion, 15° internal rotation, with beam angled 75° from horizontal

CT

- Axial CT with sagittal and coronal reformats are recommended
- Aids preoperative planning, characterizing extent of comminution and displacement

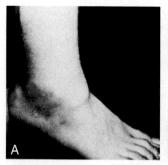 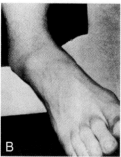 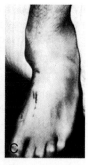

FIGURE 3 Photographs depict deformity associated with the dislocation of the subtalar joint. In this medial subtalar dislocation, the head of the talus is palpable on the dorsum of the foot (**A**), and the heel is displaced medially (**B**). **C**, In this lateral subtalar dislocation, the head of the talus is prominent medially, whereas the rest of the foot is dislocated laterally. (Reproduced with permission from Buckingham WW Jr, LeFlore I: Subtalar dislocation of the foot. *J Trauma* 1973;13[9]:753-765.)

PROCEDURE

Patient Positioning
- Supine position with feet at end of radiolucent table for talar head, neck, and most body fractures
- Place soft bump under buttock of affected extremity
- Place tourniquet on proximal thigh, if desired
- Lateral decubitus position for isolated lateral process fracture
- Prone position for posterior process fractures
- C-arm at opposite side of table

Instruments/Equipment/Implants
- Small, medium Gelpi retractors
- Lamina spreaders
- Headlamp
- Wire driver/drill
- 1.0-, 1.25-, 1.6-, and 2.0-mm Kirschner wires
- Small trocar-tipped terminally threaded Schanz pins
- Small pointed tenaculum (Weber) clamps
- Two dental picks
- Femoral distractor
- Modular foot, minifragment, or small-fragment sets with multiple sizes (1.5-, 2.0-, 2.4-, 2.7-, 3.5-mm) of plates and screws
- Have unopened external fixator set available
- If planning for medial malleolar osteotomy
  - Oscillating saw
  - Small osteotome
  - Partially threaded 4.0-mm screws
- If marginal impaction of articular surface present, may need cancellous allograft and/or juvenile cartilage tissue graft

Surgical Technique

Fractures of Talar Neck and Body
- Approach with medial and lateral incisions to fully assess reduction
- Start medial incision at medial malleolus; extend to navicular tuberosity (**Figure 4, A**)
  - Establish full-thickness flaps; preserve deltoid ligament
  - Incise ankle joint capsule; expose dorsomedial talar neck, anterior part of medial talar body
  - Avoid excessive dissection over dorsum of talus to preserve blood supply
  - Medial malleolar osteotomy facilitates exposure in fractures involving talar body or having posterior body fragments
- Begin lateral incision at anterior border of inferior part of lateral malleolus; continue in line with fourth ray of foot (**Figure 4, B**)
  - Preserve superficial peroneal nerve

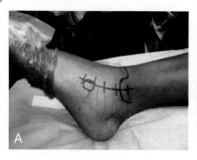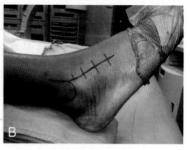

FIGURE 4 Photographs show the medial and lateral incisions for surgical repair of the talus. **A**, The medial incision begins at the medial malleolus and extends to the navicular tuberosity. **B**, The lateral incision begins at the anterior border of the lateral malleolus and is in line with the fourth ray.

- Sharply dissect through extensor retinaculum; develop full-thickness flaps
- Use interval between extensor digitorum longus and extensor brevis
- Excise fat pad of sinus tarsi to visualize lateral talar neck, lateral process, lateral talar head, and lateral talar dome
- Access subtalar joint and lateral process by extending incision proximally
- Address combination talar neck, body fractures in same way (**Figure 5**)

VIDEO 80.1 Talar Neck Fracture and Lateral Process Open Reduction and Internal Fixation. John M. Tabit, DO; Lawrence X. Webb, MD (5 min)

Isolated Displaced Lateral Process Fractures
- Position laterally with affected side up
- Make small, 1- to 2-in incision directed parallel to posterior facet of subtalar joint, just distal to fibula

Displaced Posterior Fractures of Talar Body or Displaced Medial Tubercle Posterior Process Fractures
- Prone position; may require posteromedial approach (**Figure 6, A**)
- Make longitudinal incision in line with and one fingerbreadth medial to Achilles tendon
- May use two-pin distractor, with one pin in calcaneal tuberosity and one in tibia (**Figure 6, B**)
- Protect neurovascular bundle medially
- Elevate and retract FHL
- Sharply incise joint capsule; expose posterior talus

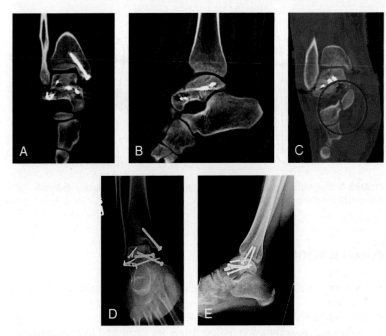

FIGURE 5 CT scans show management of the combination neck and body talar fracture. Postoperative coronal (**A**) and sagittal (**B**) views show good reduction of the talus following a medial malleolar osteotomy. **C**, Coronal view shows satisfactory position of the associated fracture of the sustentaculum (in red circle). AP (**D**) and lateral (**E**) views at 5 months show final reduction. The patient had no swelling or pain. She had resumed weight bearing, reacclimated to shoe wear, and ambulated independently without a limp.

Displaced Fractures of the Lateral Tubercle of the Posterior Process
- Prone position
- Make skin incision parallel to and 1 cm lateral to Achilles tendon (**Figure 7**)
- Dissect medial to sural nerve, in interval between peroneal tendons and FHL
- May use two-pin distractor or external fixator to improve visualization
- After reduction, fix posterior process with minifragment plate and/or screws

Percutaneous Fixation
- Useful when soft tissues preclude formal open reduction and internal fixation and fracture can be accurately reduced by closed or semi-open methods
- Accomplish low-profile fixation through neighboring healthy tissues (**Figure 8**)

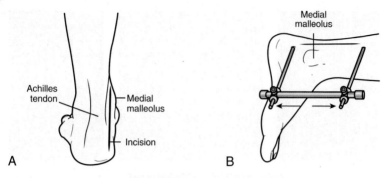

FIGURE 6 Illustrations depict the incision (**A**) and two-pin distraction external fixator (**B**) for the posteromedial approach.

COMPLICATIONS

- Infection
- Osteonecrosis; radiographic incidence 11% to 100% for displaced neck fractures
- Posttraumatic arthritis; incidence 45% to 70%
- Malunion; most common malpositions are varus and hyperextension

POSTOPERATIVE CARE AND REHABILITATION

- Standard closure over medium suction drain
- Consider incisional negative-pressure wound therapy system with continuous suction at −50 mm Hg; has been shown to reduce infection rates

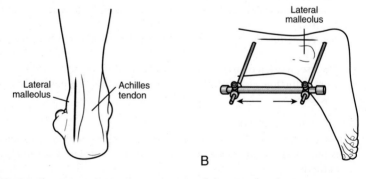

FIGURE 7 Illustrations depict the incision (**A**) and two-pin distraction external fixator (**B**) for a displaced lateral tubercle posterior process fracture.

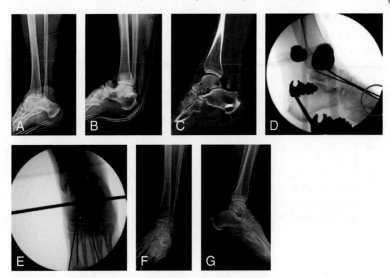

FIGURE 8 Images show open fracture of the talar neck. Significant soft-tissue compromise over the fracture was managed with bridging external fixation and percutaneous pin fixation. **A** and **B**, Orthogonal radiographs show the severely displaced ankle and foot. The talar neck fracture was open, and the wound was débrided. The reduction was stabilized with a bridging external fixation frame and percutaneously applied Schanz pins. **C**, Sagittal CT scan obtained after application of the bridging frame shows excellent position of the neck fracture. Lateral (**D**) and AP/Canale (**E**) fluoroscopic views obtained at "second-look" surgery at 48 hours postoperatively. At this time, the wound was cleaned and the fracture was stabilized by means of three small Schanz pins directed from the normal-appearing area of skin and soft tissue distally on the dorsum (red circle in panel **D**). Postoperative AP (**F**) and lateral (**G**) views of the ankle obtained at 6 months, at which time the patient was fully ambulatory and had no pain, swelling, or limp. A terminal portion of one of the pins had broken off and can be seen in the talar body.

- Apply short leg posterior splint; convert to short leg cast when swelling subsides
- In reliable patients with stable fracture, convert to removable controlled ankle motion boot at 6 weeks, with daily ankle, foot range-of-motion exercises
- No weight bearing for 12 weeks

PEARLS

- High incidence of fractures associated with displaced talar neck fractures; scrutinize CT scans and mortise, lateral ankle, and Canale views for such associated fractures.
- Develop careful preoperative plan; be mindful of blood supply and soft tissues.
- Approach, reduce, and stably fix displaced neck fractures from medial and lateral incisions simultaneously, not sequentially.
- For lateral fixation, can use contoured minifragment plate in axilla of talar neck.
- Remember close relationship of posterior tibial tendon to posterior aspect of medial malleolus when performing medial malleolar osteotomy.
- Negative-pressure wound therapy system protects surgical wound and may help resolve edema that invariably accompanies this injury.

Open Reduction and Internal Fixation of Calcaneal Fractures

PATIENT SELECTION

Indications

- Calcaneus fractures occur from high-energy trauma; result in complex three-dimensional patterns
- Position of foot at impact, extent of force, and bone quality influence fracture pattern, comminution
- Surgical management indicated for displaced intra-articular fractures involving posterior facet

Contraindications

- Use nonsurgical management for patients with nondisplaced intra-articular fractures, severe peripheral vascular disease, type I diabetes, and severe medical comorbidities, and for elderly patients who are minimal ambulators
- Manage fractures with associated severe blistering, edema, or large open wounds later as calcaneal malunion

PREOPERATIVE IMAGING

Plain Radiography

- AP foot, lateral hindfoot, Harris heel view, mortise ankle views
- Calcaneus fractures most easily identified on lateral view of hindfoot (**Figure 1**)
- Loss of height in posterior facet seen with intra-articular fracture
- Decreased Böhler angle, increased crucial angle of Gissane seen in fractures separating posterior facet from sustentaculum and depressed
- Harris heel view shows loss of calcaneal height, increased width, varus angulation of tuberosity fragment

Computed Tomography

- Indicated if plain radiographs reveal intra-articular extension of calcaneal fracture (**Figure 2**)

Based on Clare MP: Open reduction and internal fixation of calcaneal fractures, in Colvin AC, Flatow E, eds: Atlas of Essential Orthopaedic Procedures, ed 2. Rosemont, IL, American Academy of Orthopaedic Surgeons, 2020, pp 657-665.

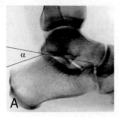 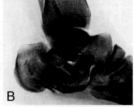 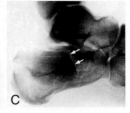

FIGURE 1 Lateral hindfoot radiographs demonstrate radiographic signs used to assess for a calcaneal fracture. **A,** A normal tuber angle of Böhler (angle α) is seen in this uninjured foot. **B,** View of a calcaneal fracture demonstrates a decreased angle of Böhler. Also note the marked loss of calcaneal height with relative horizontalization of the talus. **C,** View of a calcaneal fracture shows impaction of the superolateral fragment, which manifests as a double-density sign (arrows).

- Coronal and sagittal reformats help characterize fracture pattern, displacement, joint depression
- Preoperative planning, review of radiographs, and CT are essential

PATHOANATOMY

- In displaced intra-articular calcaneal fracture, loss of calcaneal height results in shortened, widened heel with varus tuberosity malalignment
- This height loss leads to decreased Böhler angle, ultimate loss of ankle dorsiflexion (**Figure 1**)
- As superolateral fragment is impacted plantarward, lateral wall explodes laterally; may trap peroneal tendons against lateral malleolus, limiting subtalar motion
- Anterior process displaces superiorly, limiting subtalar motion by impinging against lateral process of talus

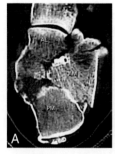 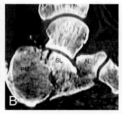 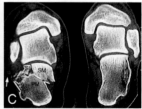

FIGURE 2 Axial (**A**), sagittal (**B**), and semicoronal (**C**) CT images delineate typical calcaneal fracture fragments. In the semicoronal image of the injured side (left image of **C**), note the potential impingement of the expanded lateral wall against the peroneal tendons (arrow). AL = anterolateral, AM = anterior main, PM = posterior main, SL = superolateral, SM = superomedial.

PROCEDURE

Resolution of Soft-Tissue Swelling

- Perform surgery within first 3 weeks after injury, before consolidation but following resolution of soft-tissue swelling
- Initial splint immobilization and limb elevation, later transitioning to compression stocking and fracture boot
- Full resolution of edema demonstrated by wrinkle test

Room Setup/Patient Positioning

- For isolated injuries, lateral decubitus position on beanbag; for bilateral injuries, prone position
- Scissor legs; flex surgical limb at knee, angle toward distal, posterior corner of table
- Adequately pad contralateral limb; create "platform" with blankets, foam for surgical limb (**Figure 3**)

Special Instruments/Equipment/Implants

- Dental picks, freer elevators, sharp and blunt periosteal elevators, Schanz pins, lamina spreaders
- Low-profile, anatomic plates with locking and nonlocking options are available

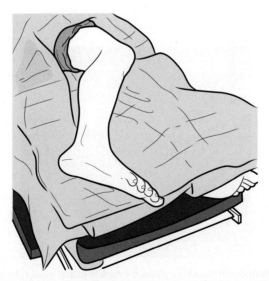

FIGURE 3 Illustration shows intraoperative positioning for the extensile lateral approach for open reduction and internal fixation of a calcaneal fracture. Note the scissor positioning of the surgical and nonsurgical limbs and the operating platform, which facilitate intraoperative fluoroscopy.

- Complete procedure in 120 to 130 minutes of tourniquet time: approach (20 minutes), reduction (60 minutes), stabilization (20 minutes), closure (20 minutes)

Surgical Technique

Incision/Approach

- Soft-tissue complications major source of morbidity; careful incision placement and soft-tissue handling paramount
- For extensile lateral approach, begin incision 2 cm proximal to tip of lateral malleolus, immediately lateral to Achilles tendon; continue vertically at junction of skin of lateral foot and heel pad; extend horizontally to base of fifth metatarsal (**Figure 4**)
- Take dissection straight to bone at calcaneal tuberosity; continue until midpoint of horizontal limb
- Raise full-thickness, subperiosteal flap beginning at apex
- Avoid using retractors until sizable subperiosteal flap is developed
- Sharply release calcaneofibular ligament from lateral calcaneal wall; release peroneal tendons from peroneal tubercle
- Mobilize tendons along distal portion of incision with periosteal elevator to expose anterolateral calcaneus
- Continue deep dissection to sinus tarsi and anterior process region anteriorly, and to superiormost portion of calcaneal tuberosity posteriorly to visualize posterior facet

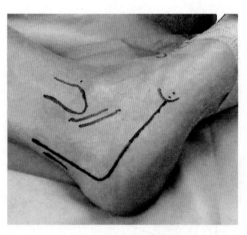

FIGURE 4 Photograph shows the planned extensile lateral incision for open reduction and internal fixation of a calcaneal fracture. The vertical limb, which runs immediately lateral to the Achilles tendon, and thus posterior to the sural nerve and the lateral calcaneal artery, preserves vascular supply to the flap.

- Place 1.6-mm Kirschner wires (K-wires) for retraction of subperiosteal flap: one into fibula, one in talar neck, one in cuboid, one in talar body posteriorly

Mobilization of the Fragments

- Mobilize and débride lateral wall and superolateral articular fragment; preserve on back table in saline
- Assess articular surface for chondral damage (**Figure 5**)
- Introduce blunt periosteal elevator into primary fracture line; lever plantarward to disimpact posterior main fragment from superomedial fragment and restore calcaneal height, length
- Can use 4.5-mm Schanz pin in posteroinferior corner of tuberosity for further manipulation

Reduction of the Articular Surface

- Reintroduce superolateral fragment into wound; place two parallel 1.6-mm K-wires to facilitate reduction
- For two separate fragments, first reduce central articular fragment to superomedial fragment, stabilize with 1.5-mm bioresorbable poly-L-lactide pins; then reduce superolateral fragment, provisionally stabilize with 1.6-mm K-wires

Split Tongue–Type Variant Patterns

- In this pattern, pull of Achilles tendon on tongue fragment may preclude reduction

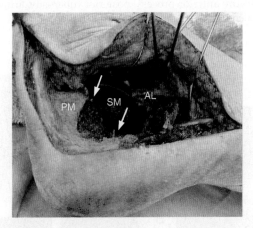

FIGURE 5 Intraoperative view shows excision of the lateral wall fragment and superolateral fragment during open reduction and internal fixation of a calcaneal fracture. Mobilization is through the primary fracture line (white arrows). AL = anterolateral, PM = posterior main, SM = superomedial.

- Use Essex-Lopresti reduction technique; insert 4.5-mm Schanz pin percutaneously into tongue fragment
- Alternate technique is osteotomy of the tongue fragment converting tongue pattern into joint depression pattern

Reduction of the Anterior Process

- Pull anterior process fragments inferiorly; secure provisionally with 1.6-mm K-wires
- May use lamina spreader to facilitate reduction of central fragment
- For transverse fracture line through angle of Gissane, derotate superomedial fragment and stabilize to anterior main fragment
- Verify articular reduction of superolateral, superomedial fragments
- Posterior edge of anterolateral fragment should key into anterior-inferior edge of superolateral fragment, indicating restoration of crucial angle of Gissane
- Lateral wall fragment and body should align with simple valgus manipulation of Schanz pin
- Confirm reduction with lateral, Broden, axial fluoroscopic views (**Figure 6**)

Definitive Fixation

- Secure posterior facet with 2.7- or 3.5-mm cortical lag screws just beneath articular surface, angling toward sustentaculum
- Secure anatomic calcaneal plate with 3.5-mm cortical screws, starting with distalmost screw holes overlying anterior process
- Secure calcaneal tuberosity to plate
- Further secure anterior process, posterior tuberosity, articular surface to plate such that two screws traverse each piece

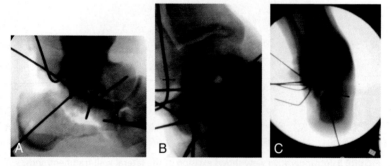

FIGURE 6 Intraoperative lateral (**A**), Broden (**B**), and axial (**C**) fluoroscopic images of a joint depression–type calcaneal fracture pattern demonstrate provisional reduction. Arrows indicate the anatomic alignment of the posterior facet articular surface (**B**) and restoration of calcaneal length (**C**).

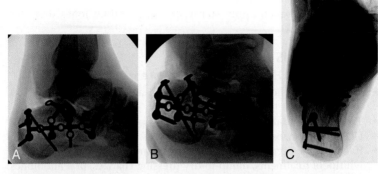

FIGURE 7 Intraoperative lateral (**A**), Broden (**B**), and axial (**C**) fluoroscopic images demonstrate definitive fixation and final reduction of a split tongue–type calcaneal fracture pattern.

- With tongue-type patterns, may place additional screw from superior edge of tuberosity perpendicular to tongue fracture line
- May place additional locking screws beneath posterior facet as rafter screws
- Obtain final lateral, Broden, axial fluoroscopic images (**Figure 7**)

Assessing the Peroneal Tendons

- With K-wire removal, peroneal tendons should reduce into peroneal groove
- Assess stability of peroneal tendons by advancing Freer elevator within tendon sheath to level of lateral malleolus and levering forward
- If superior peroneal retinaculum (SPR) and tendon sheath remain intact, firm end point will be encountered; if elevator easily slides anterior to fibula, SPR repair required

Acute SPR Repair

- Make small (<3-cm) incision along posterolateral edge of lateral malleolus
- Incise peroneal sheath and identify false pouch
- Place two suture anchors along posterolateral rim of lateral malleolus
- Pass sutures in horizontal mattress fashion into detached retinaculum
- With peroneal tendons reduced in groove, tie sutures
- Confirm stability by passively ranging involved limb
- Close tendon sheath with interrupted figure-of-8, No. 2-0 nonabsorbable sutures

Wound Closure

- Close full-thickness flap over deep drain with deep No. 0 absorbable suture, starting at ends and progressing toward apex

- Close skin layer with 3-0 monofilament suture using modified Allgöwer-Donati technique
- Deflate tourniquet, apply sterile dressings, bulky Jones dressing, Weber splint

COMPLICATIONS

Delayed Wound Healing/Wound Dehiscence

- Wound dehiscence most common complication; occurs in up to 25% of cases
- Typically occurs at wound apex; may occur up to 4 weeks postoperatively
- Deep infection, osteomyelitis develop in 1% to 4% of closed fractures
- If dehiscence occurs, discontinue range of motion; manage with serial whirlpool treatments, damp-to-dry dressing changes, oral antibiotics; may use cast immobilization with windowing for dressing changes
- May use negative-pressure wound therapy or "incisional VAC" for recalcitrant wounds

Posttraumatic Subtalar Arthritis

- Despite anatomic reduction, arthritis may develop because of cartilage damage
- May perform implant removal, in situ subtalar arthrodesis

POSTOPERATIVE CARE AND REHABILITATION

- After splint immobilization, use compression stocking, fracture boot at 2 weeks postoperatively; begin early ankle, subtalar range of motion
- Remove sutures after incision fully sealed and dry, at 4 to 5 weeks
- Do not start weight bearing until 10 to 12 weeks
- Gradually transition to regular shoe wear as weight bearing advances
- Emphasize balance, proprioception, eversion strengthening before activity progression

PEARLS

- Must understand pathoanatomy of calcaneal fracture to properly manage injury; learning curve is 100 fractures before reproducible results consistently achieved.
- Soft-tissue management as important as management of bony injury; attention to placement of incision and gentle, meticulous soft-tissue handling paramount.
- Restoring calcaneal morphology—height, length, width, crucial angle of Gissane—as important as reduction of posterior facet articular surface.

- Definitive fixation consists of nonlocking screws placed through anatomic calcaneal plate in box configuration and cortical lag screws stabilizing posterior facet articular fragments. In joint depression patterns, place one or two locking screws beneath articular block for rafter effect to maintain height.
- Before flap closure, assess integrity of SPR. The farther lateral the fracture line in posterior facet extends, the greater likelihood of peroneal tendon dislocation.

Open Reduction and Internal Fixation of Fracture-dislocations of the Tarsometatarsal Joint

PATIENT SELECTION

- Midfoot fracture-dislocations (Lisfranc)
- Injuries to tarsometatarsal (TMT) joint less than 1% of all fractures
- Most common mechanism is axial load to hyper plantarflexed foot
- TMT injuries easily missed; up to 20% missed or misdiagnosed; poor results if treated inappropriately: chronic joint instability, persistent pain, deformity, midfoot arthritis
- Indication for open reduction and internal fixation (ORIF) is TMT injuries with displacement and instability
- Contraindications include active infection, vascular insufficiency
- Consider delaying ORIF for massive midfoot edema; can reduce, provisionally fix with percutaneous pinning or external fixator to prevent skin necrosis, allow soft-tissue recovery (**Figure 1**)
- Plantar ecchymosis can be pathognomonic of high-grade midfoot injury

DIAGNOSTIC IMAGING

- Weight-bearing AP, lateral, oblique views; non–weight-bearing radiographs have 50% misdiagnosis rate (**Figure 2**)
- On AP, assess first, second TMT joints for fracture and diastasis
- On oblique, assess for lateral column alignment
- Fleck sign (small bone avulsion) can indicate unstable injury (**Figure 3**)
- If plain radiographs not diagnostic, consider stress radiographs, CT, MRI
- Stress radiographs performed under anesthesia; can define diastasis at TMT joints
- CT helps identify associated fractures, extent of joint injury
- MRI can identify Lisfranc ligament tear
- Current classification systems focus on mechanisms, patterns of displacement (**Figure 4**)

Based on Philbin TM, Berlet GC: Open reduction and internal fixation of fracture-dislocations of the tarsometatarsal joint, in Colvin AC, Flatow E, eds: Atlas of Essential Orthopaedic Procedures, *ed 2. Rosemont, IL, American Academy of Orthopaedic Surgeons, 2020, pp 666-672.*

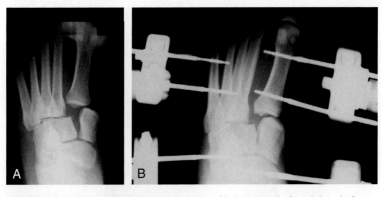

FIGURE 1 AP radiographs show tarsometatarsal joint injury before (**A**) and after (**B**) provisional external fixation.

PROCEDURE

Room Setup/Patient Positioning

- Supine position with bump under ipsilateral hip
- Fluoroscopy on surgical side, opposite surgical table
- Consider preoperative ankle or popliteal block for postoperative pain control

Special Instruments/Equipment/Implants

- Standard small-fragment set with cannulated or solid screws
- Kirschner wires (K-wires), pointed reduction forceps

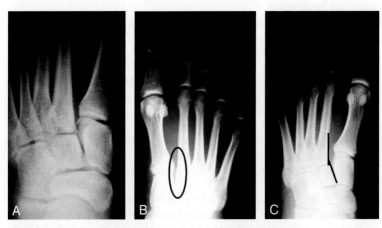

FIGURE 2 Radiographs of a patient with unstable midfoot injury of the left foot. **A**, In non–weight-bearing radiograph of left foot, injury is not apparent. **B**, Unaffected contralateral foot (oval). **C**, Weight-bearing radiograph of left foot demonstrates diastasis (lines).

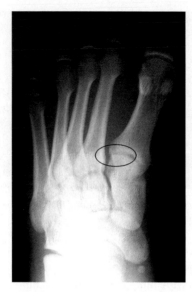

FIGURE 3 AP radiograph of the left foot shows the fleck sign.

- Dental pick
- Anterior cruciate ligament aiming guide
- Long drill bits
- Burr or countersink

Surgical Technique

- Obtain midfoot stress views to determine which joints unstable before incision
- May use dorsomedial and/or dorsolateral incision based on extent of injury
  - ▹ Dorsomedial visualizes first and second TMT, cuneiforms, medial third TMT, and joints proximal in medial column
  - ▹ Dorsolateral occasionally used to expose lateral column, including lateral third TMT, fourth and fifth TMT
  - ▹ Paramount to preserve good soft-tissue bridge between incisions to prevent wound complications
  - ▹ Avoid disrupting dorsalis pedis artery, which is main dorsal flap blood supply
- Make dorsomedial incision directly over first TMT joint (**Figure 5**); deepen between extensor hallucis longus and extensor hallucis brevis tendons
- Protect dorsalis pedis artery and deep peroneal nerve, which are deep to extensor hallucis brevis muscle-tendon junction
- Sharply dissect capsule and periosteum over first and second TMT (and intercuneiform joints, if needed) to expose joints, allow precise reduction

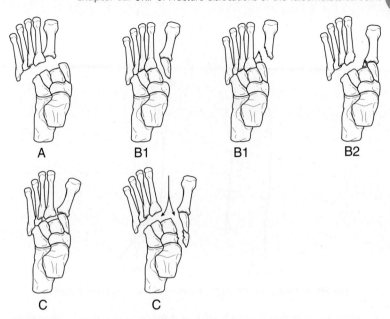

FIGURE 4 Illustrations show the Myerson classification of tarsometatarsal (TMT) fracture. Type A, or total incongruity, is characterized by displacement of all five rays in the lateral or the dorsal-plantar direction. Type B or partial incongruity fractures include B1, indicating medial dislocation of the first ray and B2, with lateral dislocation of the TMT joints. Type C is divergent, with partial or total displacement.

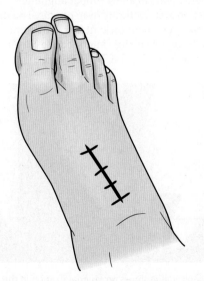

FIGURE 5 Illustration shows the location of the dorsomedial incision.

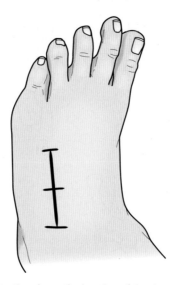

FIGURE 6 Illustration shows the location of the dorsolateral incision.

- Avoid the communicating branch of dorsalis pedis, which dives plantarly between first and second TMT
- Place dorsolateral incision over fourth TMT (**Figure 6**); as incision is deepened, retract extensor digitorum brevis, extensor digitorum communis tendons
- Remove fracture debris to allow proper alignment
- Perform reduction systematically from proximal medial to distal lateral
- Provisionally fix intercuneiform joint first, if fracture unstable (**Figure 7**)
- Use reduction forceps to realign intermediate cuneiform to base of second TMT; provisionally fix first TMT (**Figure 8**)

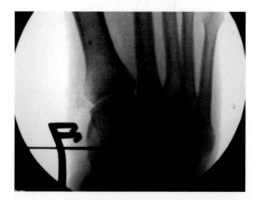

FIGURE 7 Fluoroscopic image shows provisional fixation in the intercuneiform joint.

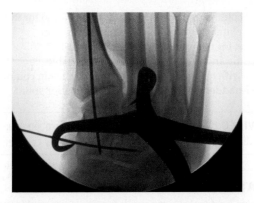

FIGURE 8 Fluoroscopic image shows reduction of the medial cuneiform to the base of the second tarsometatarsal (TMT) joint and provisional fixation in the first TMT joint.

- Important to clinically and radiographically verify anatomic reduction
- Provisionally fix lateral column injury next, if present
- Place first screw medial to lateral across cuneiforms
- Direct first TMT screw distal to proximal across joint
- Countersink to protect dorsal cortex, prevent screw prominence
- Place "home-run" screw from medial cuneiform to base of second TMT (**Figure 9**); use anterior cruciate ligament–type aiming guide to direct screw

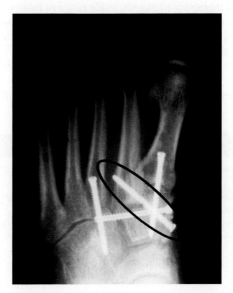

FIGURE 9 AP radiograph shows placement of the "home-run" screw (oval).

- For lateral column injuries, consider screw fixation for third TMT from distal to proximal into middle or lateral cuneiform
- Use K-wires for fixation of fourth and fifth TMT
- Close capsule and periosteum if soft tissue viable
- Close skin with no-touch technique to prevent skin compromise
- Place well-padded dressing, cotton roll, posterior splint

 VIDEO 82.1 Open Reduction and Internal Fixation of an Unstable Midfoot Injury. Terrence M. Philbin, DO; Gregory C. Berlet, MD (1 min)

COMPLICATIONS

- High risk of postoperative wound complications and infection
  - ▶ Prevent with appropriate timing of definitive ORIF
  - ▶ Reduce and provisionally fix significantly displaced fractures until soft tissues ready
- Midfoot arthritis
  - ▶ Manage with NSAIDs, cortisone injections, carbon fiber inserts, rocker-bottom shoe, midfoot fusion
  - ▶ Precise anatomic reduction minimizes need for fusion

POSTOPERATIVE CARE AND REHABILITATION

- No weight bearing for 6 weeks
- At 3 weeks, remove sutures, place controlled ankle motion boot, initiate physical therapy for forefoot, ankle range of motion
- At 6 weeks, remove K-wires, start weight bearing in boot
- At 9 weeks, wean out of boot into custom carbon fiber inserts with supportive shoe wear; progress physical therapy
- At 4 months, remove hardware from high-stress joints, such as first TMT
- NFL athletes return to professional sport median of 11.2 months

PEARLS

- Preoperative planning key for incision location, access of joints, fixation technique.
- Open versus percutaneous reduction recommended for direct visualization of joint reduction.
- Consider bridge plating as alternative to screw fixation through joint.

Open Reduction and Internal Fixation of Proximal Fifth Metatarsal Fractures

PATIENT SELECTION

Indications

- Open reduction and internal fixation (ORIF) indicated for proximal fifth metatarsal fractures in zone II (Jones fractures) or zone III (stress fractures)
- Particularly indicated in setting of delayed union of fracture treated nonsurgically and for acute fracture in athlete

Contraindications

- Skin compromise, active infection on surgical foot, vascular insufficiency, immunocompromised patients, neuropathy, patients with varus heel, and tendency for lateral foot overload
- For varus heel, consider ORIF with concomitant correction of hindfoot malalignment, surgically or with orthoses

PREOPERATIVE IMAGING

- AP, oblique, lateral plain radiographs (**Figure 1**)
- CT, MRI rarely indicated

PROCEDURE

Room Setup/Patient Positioning

- Supine position with bump under ipsilateral hip; foot at edge of table (**Figure 2**)
- May use calf or ankle tourniquet; place distal to fibular head to avoid pressure on common peroneal nerve

Special Instruments/Equipment/Implants

- Fluoroscopy unit
- Cannulated drill system
- Graduated taps

Based on Easley ME, Huh J: Open reduction and internal fixation of proximal fifth metatarsal fractures, in Colvin AC, Flatow E, eds: Atlas of Essential Orthopaedic Procedures, *ed 2. Rosemont, IL, American Academy of Orthopaedic Surgeons, 2020, pp 673-685.*

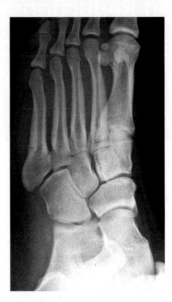

FIGURE 1 Non–weight-bearing oblique radiograph shows the foot of a 22-year-old college athlete with a zone II base-of-the-fifth-metatarsal fracture (Jones fracture). Note that the subtle fracture extends into the articulation between the fourth and fifth metatarsal bases, thus designating this fracture as a zone II injury.

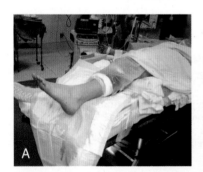
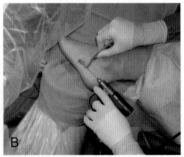

FIGURE 2 Intraoperative photographs show patient positioning for open reduction and internal fixation of a proximal fifth metatarsal fracture. **A**, The patient is positioned on the edge of the operating table with support under the ipsilateral hip and lower leg, allowing satisfactory access to the base of the fifth metatarsal. **B**, The fluoroscopy unit may easily be positioned adjacent to the table so that it can serve as a lateral extension to the operating table, to support the surgical foot during the fluoroscopic portions of the procedure.

- Solid screws
- Dedicated instrument and implant sets

Intramedullary Screw Fixation

- Intramedullary screw fixation is most widely used
- Precontoured hooked plates may be used in cases of comminution, poor bone quality, revision

 VIDEO 83.1 Open Reduction and Internal Fixation of Proximal Fifth Metatarsal Fracture Using Intramedullary Screw. Mark E. Easley, MD (9 min)

Approach

- Make longitudinal incision on lateral foot, 1 cm proximal to base of fifth metatarsal (**Figure 3**); traditional goal is to achieve "high and inside" (superior and medial) starting position for guide pin and screw (**Figure 4**); however, this is coming into question
- Structures at risk include peroneal tendons and sural nerve, which crosses directly at incision site (**Figure 5**); retract sural nerve and peroneus brevis dorsally; retract peroneus longus plantarward

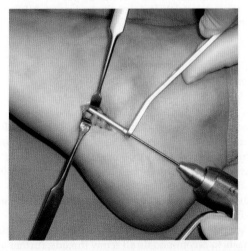

FIGURE 3 Intraoperative photograph shows the surgical approach for open reduction and internal fixation of a proximal fifth metatarsal fracture. An incision is made approximately 1 to 2 cm proximal to the fifth metatarsal base, in line with the fifth metatarsal shaft. The assistant retracts the peroneus brevis tendon and sural nerve dorsally and the peroneus longus tendon plantarward, and the surgeon uses a protective sleeve for guide pin, drill, and tap.

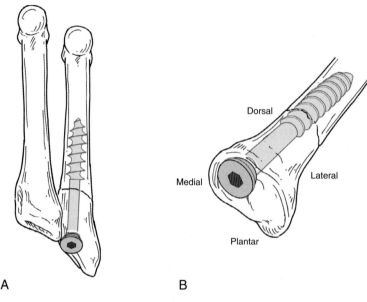

A   B

FIGURE 4 Illustrations demonstrate the "high and inside" starting position for the guide pin and screw for open reduction and internal fixation of a proximal fifth metatarsal fracture. A medial and superior starting position aligns the trajectory of the screw with the metatarsal shaft. **A,** Longitudinal aspect. **B,** End-on view of the proximal fifth metatarsal base.

Guide Pin Positioning and Drilling

- Use drill guide with guide pin, drill, tap to further protect local structures
- Direct guide pin into center of intramedullary canal of fifth metatarsal with optimal high and inside starting position; confirm on AP, lateral, oblique imaging (**Figure 6, A** through **C**)
- Determine ideal starting point before advancing guide pin; difficult to make subtle adjustments after hole is created
- Slowly advance guide pin, confirming trajectory on AP, lateral, oblique imaging (**Figure 6, D** through **F**)
- Advance guide pin, drill, tap, and screw only just beyond fracture/nonunion site to accommodate all screw threads; further advancement can impinge on distal medial cortex of curved metatarsal, creating lateral cortical gap
- After proper positioning, overdrill guide pin with cannulated drill just beyond fracture site
- In nonunion, may remove guide pin and introduce small-diameter drill to drill sclerotic bone at nonunion site and promote healing

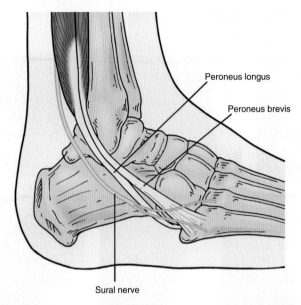

Peroneus longus

Peroneus brevis

Sural nerve

FIGURE 5 Illustration shows the structures at risk in open reduction and internal fixation of a proximal fifth metatarsal fracture. Typically, the peroneus brevis tendon and sural nerve are retracted dorsally, and the peroneus longus tendon is retracted plantarward.

Use of the Tap

- Introduce tap over guide pin
- Tap prepares canal for screw and gauges size of screw affording best purchase in distal fragment
- Tap size that engages distal fragment to point of torqueing it with each turn represents optimal screw size
- No need to advance screw beyond point at which all threads cross fracture/nonunion, so can use relatively large screw diameter
- Remove tap and guide pin from canal

Screws

- Optimal screw diameter is determined by tap diameter that best engages distal fragment
- Optimal screw length is that which allows all threads to cross fracture site
- Screw must not be so long that it contacts distal medial cortex, thus promoting gapping at fracture/nonunion site
- Can determine screw length three ways: by using cannulated depth gauge, measuring difference between two guide pins, or holding screw adjacent to fifth metatarsal base and using fluoroscopy

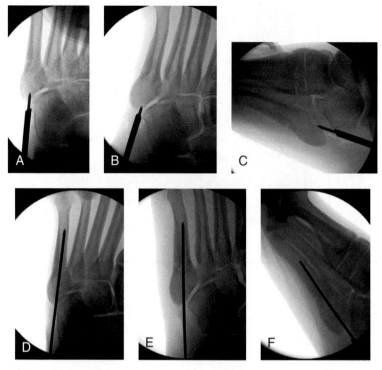

FIGURE 6 Fluoroscopic images show guide pin positioning for open reduction and internal fixation of a proximal fifth metatarsal fracture. AP (**A**), oblique (**B**), and lateral (**C**) views show the starting point for the guide pin/screw. AP (**D**), oblique (**E**), and lateral (**F**) views show the guide pin advanced past the fracture. Note that the guide pin is not advanced the entire length of the metatarsal.

- When ideal screw length, diameter determined, advance screw into prepared canal
- While advancing, resist torque in distal fragment and apply axial force on distal fragment to ensure all threads cross fracture site
- Confirm final position with AP, lateral, oblique fluoroscopic views (**Figure 7**)

Low-Profile Hook Plate Fixation

Approach

- Make longitudinal incision along lateral border of fifth metatarsal starting 1 cm proximal to tuberosity
- Protect peroneal tendons and dorsolateral branch of sural nerve

Reduction

- In fractures requiring reduction, clean fracture edges

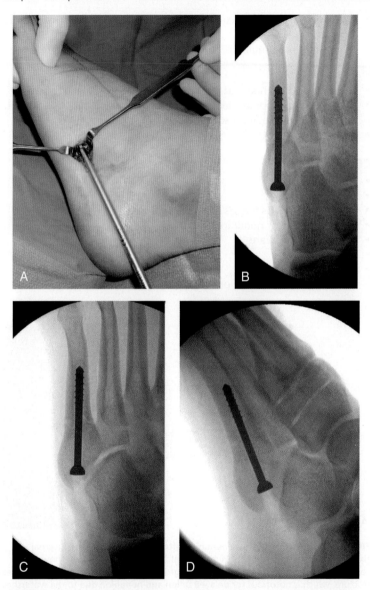

FIGURE 7 Images show screw insertion in open reduction and internal fixation of a proximal fifth metatarsal fracture. **A,** Intraoperative photograph shows the surgeon holding the distal fragment with one hand while placing the screw with the other. This technique allows for axial compression and assessment of how well the screw engages the inner cortex of the distal fragment. Intraoperative AP (**B**), oblique (**C**), and lateral (**D**) fluoroscopic images confirm that the screw is in proper position, the fracture is reduced, and no associated stress fractures are present.

- Use pointed reduction clamp or Kirschner wire to hold provisional fixation
- In nonunion use small drill bit to débride sclerotic bone at site

Plate Application

- Most plates have hooks at proximal end to secure plate to tuberosity
- Determine appropriate length, place against bone and use tamp to engage hooks, use fluoroscopy to check position
- Secure to shaft with screws

COMPLICATIONS

- Infection
- Sural neuralgia
- Injury to peroneus longus or brevis tendons
- Delayed union or nonunion (**Figure 8**)
- Prominent hardware
- Refracture
- Peri-implant fracture
- Delayed wound healing or dehiscence

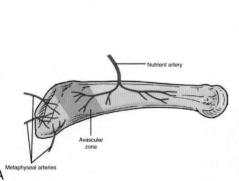
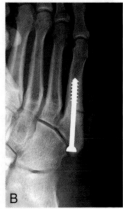

FIGURE 8 Images demonstrate nonunion after open reduction and internal fixation (ORIF) of a proximal fifth metatarsal fracture. **A,** Illustration shows the vascularity of the fifth metatarsal. Zone II (green area) is the location for the Jones fracture, which is notorious for delayed union and nonunion due to the watershed that leaves that segment of the fifth metatarsal with a marginal blood supply. **B,** Oblique radiograph obtained 8 months after ORIF of an acute fifth metatarsal fracture suggests nonunion rather than refracture. This athlete had apparent clinical and radiographic healing 4 months after ORIF but then experienced recurrent symptoms 8 months after surgery, despite 4 months of pain-free participation in sports.

POSTOPERATIVE CARE AND REHABILITATION

- Protected weight bearing in splint, controlled ankle motion (CAM) walker, or cast for 4 to 5 weeks
- Gradually progress weight bearing in CAM walker between weeks 5 and 8
- With radiographic evidence of healing, advance weight bearing in regular shoe
- Restrict athletic activity until fracture site is not tender and radiographs suggest full healing, usually by 10 to 12 weeks
- With evidence of delayed union, restrict weight bearing, continue CAM walker, consider external bone stimulator
- If no radiographic evidence of healing, consider revision surgery with bone grafting, revision ORIF, exchange to larger screw

PEARLS

- Delay in healing of base-of-fifth-metatarsal fractures relatively common; use largest solid screw possible to stabilize fracture.
- Do not extend screw into distal aspect of metatarsal; longer screw can abut against distal medial cortex, creating gap at lateral cortex fracture site, leading to delay in healing or nonunion.
- Procedure involves inserting straight screw into curved bone; insert screw only far enough for threads to cross fracture site; can use relatively large screw diameter, promoting compression at fracture.
- Ideal screw position depends on ideal starting point; insert screw in high and inside (ie, superior and medial) position on proximal end of fifth metatarsal.

Foot and Ankle

6

Section Editor
Michael Pinzur, MD

Ankle Arthroscopy: Diagnostics, Débridement, and Removal of Loose Bodies

PATIENT SELECTION
Indications
- The most common indications for ankle arthroscopy are listed in **Table 1**
- Anterior impingement
  - Common with activities requiring forced dorsiflexion
  - Incidence is up to 45% in football players, 59% in dancers
  - Physical examination reveals pain on anterior joint line, worse with forced dorsiflexion of the ankle
  - Arthroscopy removes anterior osteophytes on the tibia or talus
- Anterolateral soft-tissue impingement
  - Involved structures: Any combination of the superior portion of the anterior inferior tibiofibular ligament (AITFL), the distal portion of the AITFL, along the anterior talofibular ligament (ATFL), lateral gutter near talar dome
  - Physical examination reveals ankle pain worsened by forced dorsiflexion, pain in the lateral gutter

Contraindications
- Infection
- Neuropathy
- Complex regional pain syndrome
- Psychiatric disorder

PREOPERATIVE IMAGING
Radiography
- Lateral ankle view (**Figure 1**) may show anterior osteophytes on tibia, talus with dorsal spur, or signs of dorsal degeneration
- Dorsiflexed lateral ankle view may show impingement

Magnetic Resonance Imaging
- Not indicated in all cases of anterior impingement

Based on Frey C: Ankle arthroscopy: Diagnostics, débridement, and removal of loose bodies, in Colvin AC, Flatow E, eds: Atlas of Essential Orthopaedic Procedures, *ed 2. Rosemont, IL, American Academy of Orthopaedic Surgeons, 2020, pp 687-694.*

TABLE 1 Conditions That Can Be Treated Arthroscopically

Diagnosis/Indications	Percentage of Cases That Can Be Treated Arthroscopically
Ankle arthritis	25
Loose body	90
Synovectomy	90
Acute infection	80
Lateral impingement	95-100
Osteochondral defects	95-100
Anterior osteophytes	90-95
Stabilization	25
Ankle arthrodesis	50
Foreign body	90-100

- Common findings—Cartilage thinning, soft-tissue swelling, osteophyte
- Injury to the AITFL or ATFL is best visualized on short tau inversion recovery and sagittal T1-weighted images (**Figure 2**)
- MRI is 79% accurate and 84% sensitive in diagnosing anterior soft-tissue impingement

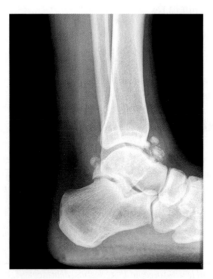

FIGURE 1 A lateral radiograph of the ankle reveals an. anterior tibial spur.

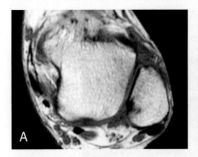 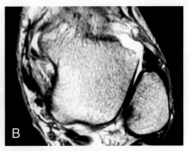

FIGURE 2 Axial T1-weighted (**A**) and fast spin-echo T2-weighted (**B**) MRIs of the ankle of a 39-year-old man with anterolateral ankle impingement. Thickening and scarring of the distal fascicle is evident in these images taken 3 mo after an anterior inferior tibiofibular ligament injury.

Ultrasonography

- Can identify synovial lesions in anterior lateral gutter and ligament injuries
- Can also differentiate soft-tissue impingement from bone impingement
- Will not show osteochondral lesions or stress fractures—may overlook loose bodies

PROCEDURE

Room Setup/Patient Positioning

- Outpatient procedure
- Spinal anesthesia preferred, general acceptable
- Supine position on operating room table
- Well-padded tourniquet on proximal thigh
- Thigh supported with bolster to elevate foot off bed
- Standard preparation and draping
- Distraction through a foot stirrup (**Figure 3**)

Special Instruments/Equipment

- 2.9-mm arthroscope with 30° and 70° options
- 2.9- to 3.5-mm arthroscopic full-radius shaver and acromionizer burr
- Small curets, biters, rasps
- Noninvasive distractor

Surgical Technique

- Outline superficial anatomy—Joint line, greater saphenous vein, superficial peroneal nerve and branches, saphenous nerve, and the dorsalis pedis artery
- Distend joint with saline to start

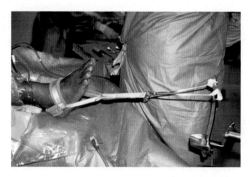

FIGURE 3 Photograph shows the standard setup and patient positioning for ankle arthroscopy.

- Create all portals by small vertical incisions then use mosquito clamp to perform blunt dissection to the level of joint capsule. Use spinal needle as a guide
  - ▶ Place anteromedial portal medial to the tibialis anterior tendon (**Figure 4**)
    - – Placed first
    - – Vertical incision at joint line
    - – Used to visualize medial gutter, anterior joint, deltoid ligament
  - ▶ Place anterolateral portal lateral to the peroneus tertius tendon
    - – Placed second under direct visualization from inside joint
    - – Incision is just distal to the joint line
    - – Used to visualize ATFL, lateral gutter
  - ▶ Place posterolateral portal just lateral to the Achilles tendon (**Figure 5**)
    - – Start just lateral to Achilles tendon, toward medial malleolus
    - – Avoid the lesser saphenous vein, sural nerve, and peroneal tendons, which are at risk
    - – Used to visualize the posterior joint structures; not needed in all scopes
- Approach to the anterior tibial osteophytes
  - ▶ Because of the anterior position of the medial malleolus, it is difficult to visualize fully on medial side
  - ▶ Frequently need a 70° scope to improve visualization (**Figure 6**)
  - ▶ Dorsiflexion and plantar flexion help identify areas of impingement
  - ▶ Remove osteophytes with 4.0-mm burr; use radiofrequency wand or shaver to remove synovium
  - ▶ Acromionizer is useful for removal of exostosis
  - ▶ Before completion of arthroscopy, ensure to inspect for loose bodies

---

 VIDEO 84.1 Subtalar Arthroscopy. Richard D. Ferkel, MD (9 min)

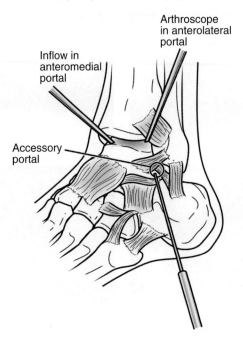

FIGURE 4 Illustration shows the anterolateral and anteromedial portals used for the treatment of anterior ankle impingement. Accessory portals may be helpful.

COMPLICATIONS

- Reported rate is 0.7% to 9%
- Of all complications, 49% are related to nerve injury
- Superficial peroneal nerve most commonly injured

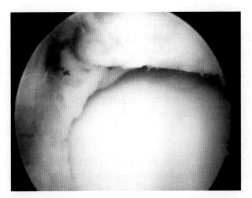

FIGURE 5 Arthroscopic view shows the placement of the posterolateral portal. Care is taken to avoid the sural nerve.

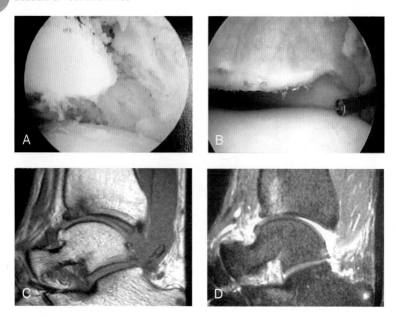

FIGURE 6 Arthroscopic view shows the placement of the posterolateral portal. Care is taken to avoid the sural nerve. Arthroscopic views of a large anterior tibial spur before (**A**) and after (**B**) débridement. Sagittal T1-weighted (**C**) and short tau inversion recovery (**D**) magnetic resonance images show anterior osteophytes of the distal tibia and talus, anterior tibiotalar joint capsular hypertrophy, and subchondral marrow edema within the anterior distal aspect of the tibia.

- Usually a result of direct injury by portal placement
- Other complications—Vascular or tendon injury, chronic regional pain syndrome, infection, deep vein thrombosis, sinus tract formation, skin necrosis, cartilage damage

POSTOPERATIVE CARE AND REHABILITATION
- Weight bearing allowed at 5 days
- Encourage range-of-motion activities and Achilles stretching initially
- Progress to proprioception and strengthening activities
    - Recovery generally 6 weeks; with arthritis, 12 weeks
    - May have swelling for 6 months

OUTCOMES
- For anterior impingement, 92% to 95% good to excellent results
- Results diminish with additional injuries, such as chondral or ligamentous injuries
- Of athletes, 80% return to same level of sports performance
- Most patients continue to lack some dorsiflexion postoperatively

- Better results in patients that are not arthritic
- Grade B evidence for arthroscopy for anterior impingement
- Outcomes same as open surgery, but recovery time is shorter

PEARLS

- Noninvasive distraction is recommended for spur removal to allow better access to the spur and prevent cartilage damage. Do not excessively distract the joint; doing so pulls the synovium and capsule tight against the spur, making visualization and access difficult.
- Dorsiflexion or plantar flexion may be needed to visualize impinging structures.
- Clear excessive synovium using a 3.5- to 4-mm full-radius power shaver. Remove spur with 4-mm power burr. Remove the exostosis with an acromionizer. Smooth the bone surface with 4-mm full-radius shaver or curet. At conclusion, inspect the joint for loose bodies. Posterior portals are not needed for removing anterior spurs on the talus or tibia.
- Arthroscopy is preferred over arthrotomy for removing loose bodies.

Arthroscopic Treatment of Osteochondral Lesions of the Talus

INTRODUCTION

- Definition—An osteochondral lesion of the talus (OLT) is a defect in the articular hyaline cartilage predominantly within the weight-bearing area of the talar dome that has underlying bone involvement
- Etiology—Unclear; history of ankle trauma is implicated in most cases, but some occur without any traumatic events
- Distribution of OLTs
  - Medial, deeper, and likely from impact on tibia: 62%
  - Lateral, thinner, and smaller from shear on fibula: 34%
  - In the central area: 80%
- Symptoms—Ankle pain, instability, swelling, and catching

IMAGING

- Radiographs of the ankle may show some chronic OLT lesions with bony changes and may miss small nondisplaced lesions
  - AP
  - Lateral
  - Mortise weight-bearing
- MRI
  - Sensitive and specific for OLT lesions
  - Localizes lesion and depth
  - Excessive edema can obscure the bony extent of the lesion
- CT is obtained when bone involvement cannot be delineated on MRI (**Figure 1**)

CLASSIFICATION

- The senior author (S.M.R.) has proposed a grading system that combines various modality-specific classification systems (**Figure 2**)
- Stage I OLT lesions involve an isolated cartilage flap without subchondral bone involvement
  - MRI demonstrates bone edema but no fracture

Based on Raikin SM, Mangan JJ: Arthroscopic treatment of osteochondral lesions of the talus, in Colvin AC, Flatow E, eds: Atlas of Essential Orthopaedic Procedures, *ed 2. Rosemont, IL, American Academy of Orthopaedic Surgeons, 2020, pp 695-703.*

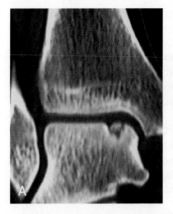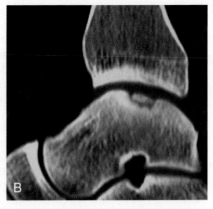

FIGURE 1 Coronal (**A**) and sagittal (**B**) CT scans demonstrate a stage III medial osteochondral lesion of the talus.

- ▶ Radiographs and CT are usually negative
- ▶ Ankle symptoms are mechanical and include painful catching and giving way
- Stage II—Incomplete or completely nondisplaced fracture of underlying bone
  - ▶ MRI and CT show clear signs of fracture
  - ▶ Not visible on radiographs
  - ▶ Stable, may be best managed nonsurgically

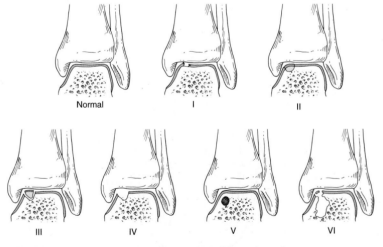

FIGURE 2 Illustrations show the senior author's (S.M.R.'s) grading system for osteochondral lesions of the talus (shown as medial lesions). See text for descriptions.

- Stage III—Unstable and displaced fragment of bone and cartilage
  - Radiographs, MRI, and CT all show lesion
  - Fragments may maintain vascularity and can potentially be reduced and fixed with a bioabsorbable pin, particularly in the acute trauma setting; if avascular, treatment is by arthroscopic reduction, débridement, and microfracture of the lesion base
- Stage IV—Defect with no fragment remaining; frequently has fibrocartilage in the fragment
- Stage V—Subchondral cysts with intact cartilage cap
  - Treat with retrograde drilling and bone grafting
  - Need to confirm healthy cartilage cap
- Stage VI—Large area of chondral damage or cyst with communication to the joint; likely to need some form of osteochondral allograft

TREATMENT OPTIONS/INDICATIONS

- Nonsurgical management for all nondisplaced OLTs
  - No weight bearing with cast immobilization followed by progressive weight bearing and full ambulation by 12 to 16 weeks
  - Success rates with nonsurgical treatment for grades I and II and medial grade III: 45% to 54%
- Acute displaced fragments should be treated surgically in a timely manner
- Before treatment, the surgeon should be familiar with the Raikin classification for localization, based on a 3 × 3 grid of the talar dome (**Figure 3**)

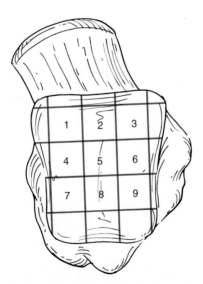

FIGURE 3 Illustration shows the nine-zone localization grid on the talar dome.

- Débridement and bone marrow stimulation via microfracture are standard treatments of lesions less than 15 mm; 88% success in grade III and higher lesions with curettage and/or drilling
- Chondroplasty, retrograde drilling, chondrocyte implantation are also surgical options for larger lesions but have fewer data to support them
- International consensus Group on Cartilage repair of the Ankle advocates repeat bone marrow stimulation in refractory cases, or when patient unwilling to extensive procedure

 VIDEO 85.1 Arthroscopic Treatment of Osteochondral Lesions of the Talus. Steven M. Raikin, MD; Nicholas Slenker, MD (10 min)

PROCEDURE

Setup/Patient Positioning

- General, regional, or local anesthesia
- Supine position with leg in a leg holder and foot of the bed dropped to 90° is preferred for gravity traction
- Tourniquet is set up but used only if needed
- Distraction can be performed by noninvasive stirrup or with tibial/calcaneal pins; no more than 222 N of force for less than 90 minutes to prevent paresthesias of superficial peroneal nerve

Equipment

- 2.7-mm arthroscope with 30° and 70° options
- Small-joint instruments—Small hooked probe, small-joint arthroscopic grasper set, small thin-necked curets, small-joint motorized shaving system, and set of micropicks

Surgical Technique

- Mark out bony and soft-tissue landmarks; avoid superficial peroneal nerve (SPN) and branches
- Distend ankle joint with saline: 20 to 30 mL of saline or lactated Ringer solution using 18- or 20-gauge needle before portal placement at anteromedial ankle joint
- Anteromedial portal made first, 5 mm proximal to medial malleolus and medial to anterior tibialis tendon; great saphenous vein and nerve lie 7 to 9 mm medial to portal and are at risk (**Figure 4**)
- Anterolateral portal is made second, lateral to peroneus tertius tendon at joint line; all branches of the SPN are at risk
- Posterolateral portal is made 1 cm proximal to tip of fibula, just lateral to Achilles tendon; sural nerve and lesser saphenous vein are at risk. Shinning arthroscope light from anteromedial portal to posterolateral aspect of joint will assist with visualization

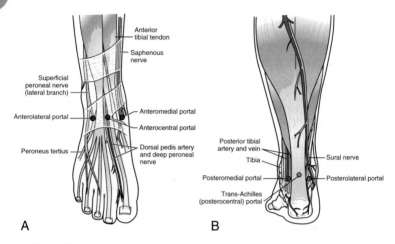

FIGURE 4 Illustrations show portal placement for arthroscopy of the ankle. **A,** Location of the anteromedial, anterolateral, and anterocentral portals. **B,** Location of the posteromedial, trans-Achilles, and posterolateral portals. (Adapted from Stetson WB, Ferkel RD: Ankle arthroscopy: I. Technique and complications. *J Am Acad Orthop Surg* 1996;4:17-23.)

- Make vertical incisions with blunt dissection to the level of the capsule
- Enter joint with blunt probe under traction and joint distension to prevent iatrogenic injury
- Standard diagnostic arthroscopic examination (**Figure 5**)
- Probe lesion borders and débride unstable cartilage and subchondral bone with probe, curets, and shavers (**Figure 6**)
- Move back and forth between portals as necessary to achieve optimal visualization
- Create stable ring of cartilage with stable base of bone

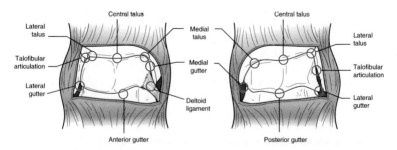

FIGURE 5 Illustration shows the eight-point anterior (left) and seven-point posterior (right) arthroscopic examination. (Adapted from Stetson WB, Ferkel RD: Ankle arthroscopy I: Technique and complications. *J Am Acad Orthop Surg* 1996;4:17-23.)

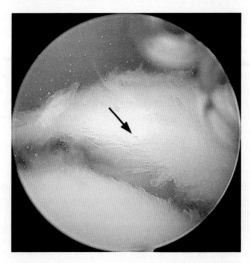

FIGURE 6 Arthroscopic view shows an unstable cartilaginous flap of a medial osteochondral lesion of the talus (arrow) as seen from the lateral portal.

- Mallet the microfracture pick to a depth of 3 to 5 mm to create marrow stimulation; no tourniquet is used during fracture to allow the surgeon to confirm that healthy egress of marrow (fat droplets) and bleeding from the bone has been achieved
- Alternative is to antegrade drill to the lesion using 0.062-in Kirschner wire and arthroscopic targeting guide
- Retrograde drilling can be performed for a stage V lesion with intact cartilage, followed by overdrilling, curetting, and bone grafting (**Figure 6**)

COMPLICATIONS

- Reported complication rate up to 9%, 49% of which are neurologic
- Complications include injury to neurovascular structures, instrument breakage, articular surface damage, neuroma formation, infection, and reflex sympathetic dystrophy
- Injury to the SPN in 56%, to the sural nerve in 22%, and to the saphenous nerve in 18%
- Infection may be related to the type of cannula used and early mobilization

POSTOPERATIVE CARE

- No weight bearing for 6 weeks (especially if microfracture is performed) in a fracture boot; can remove boot for active range-of-motion exercises
- At 6 weeks, transition to full weight bearing in fracture boot

PEARLS

- Portal placement is the most important part of the procedure. Poorly placed incisions limit access to the joint and increase the risk of injury. Identify all topical landmarks before joint distention; these areas could become distorted.
- Distend the joint with a large syringe and 25 to 30 mL of saline before portal placement so the joint can "inflate," easing the entrance of the equipment.
- Débridement of the hypertrophic synovium or adhesed capsule may be needed to maneuver within the joint.
- Invasive or noninvasive distraction devices can enhance access to different areas of the ankle joint, although gravity alone is usually enough. Using additional traction systems can raise the complication rate for this procedure.
- During the two-portal technique, the camera may need to be exchanged between portals to evaluate the joint, before and after addressing the OLT.
- For marrow stimulation techniques that rely on reparative cartilage healing, non–weight bearing with early range of motion postoperatively is vitally important to success.
- Microfracture leads to the formation of fibrocartilage. Limited evidence suggests that the use of bone marrow aspirate concentrate and platelet rich plasma may increase the formation of hyaline cartilage.

PATIENT SELECTION

Indications

- In the United States, 27,000 ankle ligament sprains occur daily
- Most are treated nonsurgically if seen in acute period
- Even chronic injuries should have trial of physical therapy
- Persistent pain, giving way, locking, swelling are reasons for further evaluation
- Osteochondral defects, spurs, and tibiotalar arthritis may develop with persistent instability
- Symptoms of more than 10 years, hyperlaxity, and irreparable ligaments intraoperatively, failed broström procedure may need tendon or fibertape augmentation as opposed to native ligament reconstruction
- Physical examination shows anterior translation with anterior drawer test (**Figure 1**)

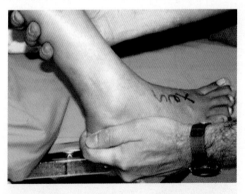

FIGURE 1 Photograph shows the anterior drawer test. The foot is slightly plantar-flexed and internally rotated. The examiner's right hand stabilizes the tibia while the left hand exerts an anterior pull.

Based on Abidi NA: Augmented lateral ankle ligament reconstruction for persistent ankle instability, in Colvin AC, Flatow E, eds: Atlas of Essential Orthopaedic Procedures, *ed 2. Rosemont, IL, American Academy of Orthopaedic Surgeons, 2020, pp 704-714.*

Contraindications

- Arthritis
- Inability to participate in postoperative therapy
- Posterior tibial tendon insufficiency
- Neuropathic/Charcot arthropathy of the foot

PREOPERATIVE IMAGING

- Stress radiographs are no longer recommended
- Weight-bearing radiographs are used to determine articular space and alignment
  - ▶ Varus tibiotalar joint—May need more than just soft-tissue reconstruction, including supramalleolar osteotomy
  - ▶ Varus heel alignment—May need lateralizing calcaneal osteotomy in addition to ligament reconstruction
  - ▶ Plantarflexed first ray—May increase varus moment of hindfoot and require dorsiflexion osteotomy during ligament reconstruction
- MRI can identify injury to anterior talofibular ligament (ATFL) and calcaneofibular ligament (CFL)

PROCEDURE

Room Setup/Patient Positioning

- Semilateral position on beanbag, with affected leg up (**Figure 2**)
- Ensure external rotation of leg to allow placement of a medial arthroscopy portal
- Regional block for saphenous nerve but popliteal block anesthetic overall

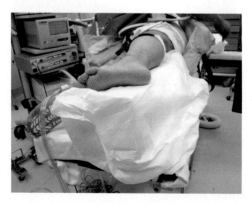

FIGURE 2 Photograph shows setup and patient positioning for lateral ankle ligament reconstruction. The surgical leg is elevated on a foam block. The peroneal nerve of the nonsurgical leg and all bony prominences are shielded from any pressure.

Surgical Technique

 VIDEO 86.1 Augmented Lateral Ankle Ligament Reconstruction.
Nicholas A. Abidi, MD; Brian Martin, PA-C (25 min)

- Ankle arthroscopy—Evaluate ATFL, osteochondral lesions of talus, anterior joint spurs and treat as indicated
- Split peroneus longus autograft augmentation of lateral ankle ligament reconstruction
- Make incision 5 cm proximal to lateral malleolus, distal to the base of fifth metatarsal; avoid injuring sural nerve or peroneal tendons
- Important to visualize ligament attachments to talus and calcaneus
- Sharply detach ATFL; release CFL and lateral joint capsule off fibula leaving proximally retracted periosteal flap
- Identify peroneus longus tendon in peroneal sheath and harvest one-third (4 to 5 mm) of tendon cephalad to superior peroneal retinaculum for approximately 15 cm of graft (**Figure 3**)
- Prepare tendon with a heavy-duty nonabsorbable suture whipstitch at each end (**Figure 4**)
- Calcaneal preparation—Identify insertion of CFL on calcaneus and débride to bleeding bone; place a 4.5-mm bit 20 to 25 mm deep
- Fibula preparation—Place drill bit running from insertion of CFL distally to ATFL insertion anteriorly with 4-mm bit
- Talar preparation—Identify ATFL insertion at distal capsule on talar neck; place 4.5-mm drill bit perpendicular to talar neck and out toward talar head
- Angle talar tunnel plantarward to prevent talar neck fracture or cutout
- Tunnel preparation—After drill holes are placed, use anterior cruciate ligament notch punch to enable fit of tendon and interference screws
- Graft placement
  - Place interference anchor into calcaneus with prepared tendon
  - Pass tendon under the peroneal tendons
  - Pass from distal to anterior through fibula
  - Pass from lateral talus out toward talar head
  - Hold tension on graft with foot in maximum dorsiflexion and eversion when placing final interference screw in talus
- Perform Broström-Karlsson capsular repair with absorbable or nonabsorbable suture to capture the ATFL and CFL to the periosteum of the fibula
- Also perform Gould modification for increased capsular reconstruction
- After skin is closed, place in a bulky Jones dressing and fiberglass splint with foot maximally dorsiflexed while knee is bent

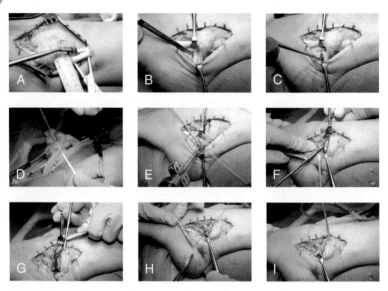

FIGURE 3 Intraoperative photographs demonstrate steps in lateral ankle ligament reconstruction. **A,** A pigtailed tendon stripper is used to harvest a 4-mm-thick section of the peroneus longus tendon above the superior peroneal retinaculum. **B,** The natural origin of the calcaneofibular ligament (CFL) is exposed. **C,** A drill hole is made at the origin of the native CFL. An anterior cruciate ligament notch puncher is used to create a cephalad notch in the drill hole. This notch will create a place to slide the peroneus longus tendon graft alongside the tenodesis interference anchor. **D,** The peroneus longus tendon graft is captured with a No. 2 nonabsorbable suture and the tenodesis interference anchor system. **E,** The first limb of the peroneus longus tendon autograft is placed into the drill hole at the origin of the CFL. The anchor is screwed into the tunnel, providing an interference fit against the whipstitched tendon. **F,** A 4.0-mm cannulated drill bit is drilled over a guide pin in the end of the fibula that travels from the CFL insertion to the anterior talofibular ligament (ATFL) origin. **G,** The two ends of the tunnel in the fibula are connected over a guide pin with a 4.0-mm cannulated drill bit. **H,** A nitinol wire tendon-passing tool is used to pass the peroneus longus tendon graft through the tunnel that was drilled in the fibula. **I,** The peroneus longus graft is passed through the tunnel from the insertion of the CFL to the origin of the ATFL. It is tensioned, and excursion of the tendon is confirmed by examining tensioning at the origin of the CFL.

- Alternative technique: fibertape augmentation of native Broström ligament reconstruction
  - 4 to 6 cm incision made over distal fibula exposing the ATFL and CFL. Detach the ATFL and CFL sharply, develop distal fibular periosteal and prepare bone

    Expose neck of talus and drill with 2.4 mm guide pin. Over drill the pin with a 4.0 cannulated drill bit. Use threaded 4.75 mm tap

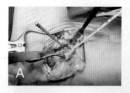
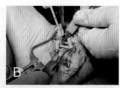
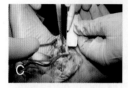
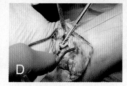
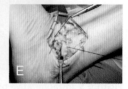

FIGURE 4 Intraoperative photographs demonstrate final steps in lateral ankle ligament reconstruction. **A,** A cannulated guide pin is drilled into the insertion point of the anterior talofibular ligament (ATFL). This will be drilled with a cannulated 4.5-mm drill bit and notched with an anterior cruciate ligament notch puncher. **B,** The peroneus longus tendon autograft is tensioned with the foot held dorsiflexed and externally rotated, and the insertion point at the ATFL is approximated. **C,** The peroneus longus tendon autograft is whipstitched with a nonabsorbable suture 17 mm beyond where the edge of the ATFL insertion point was measured on the tendon. The excess tendon beyond this point is truncated. This 17 mm will represent 15 mm placed within the tunnel and 2 mm as it rounds the edge of the tunnel. **D,** With the foot and ankle dorsiflexed and externally rotated, the peroneus longus tendon autograft is captured with the No. 2 nonabsorbable suture along with the tenodesis anchor system. The tenodesis system is used to place the graft under tension before screwing the interference anchor into place. **E,** The Broström-Karlsson procedure is performed after the tendon transfer by imbricating the periosteal flap that was created at the end of the fibula. This repair also can be augmented with the Gould modification by also imbricating the inferior extensor retinaculum to the edge of the distal periosteal flap.

» One limb of fibertape goes through screw, other outside of the anchor
» Insert PEEK anchor with fibertape in talar neck (**Figure 5**)
» Secure both tails of fibertape into distal fibular with a cannlulated PEEK interference anchor. Hold foot in maximal dorsiflexion (**Figure 6**)
» Imbricate ankle ligaments and capsule with nonabsorbable suture. Secure Inferior extensor retinaculum with Vicryl to the distal periosteal flap
» Follow same postoperative protocols as tendon augmentation

COMPLICATIONS

• Inadequate harvest of peroneus longus graft requiring hamstring or allograft substitute
• Failure of bone anchors from poor bone density

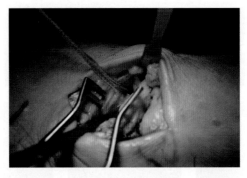

FIGURE 5 Intraoperative photograph shows a 4.75 mm PEEK anchor placed with 2 mm nonabsorbable suture-tape into the hole that was drilled in the talar neck. One limb of the tape is within the anchor while the other limb is in an interference fit between the anchor and the bone tunnel.

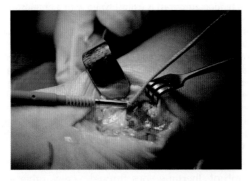

FIGURE 6 Intraoperative photograph shows a 4.75 PEEK Bio-interference anchor with a 19 mm shaft lead and closed peek eyelet tip being used to tension the tails of the 2 mm nonabsorbable suture-tape in the hole in the distal fibula.

POSTOPERATIVE CARE AND REHABILITATION

- Ice and elevate leg for 10 to 14 days with immobilization
- Begin weight bearing at first postoperative visit
- Begin physical therapy at first postoperative visit
- Transition to lace-up ankle brace at 4 weeks, then taper quickly
- By 6 weeks, transition to orthosis to increase subtalar motion
- May begin running in line when at 85% strength
- Cutting and pivoting can begin at 12 weeks

PEARLS

- Exposure to the ligament attachment points on the calcaneus and the talar neck is key. Improper exposure sets up improper biomechanics postoperatively.
- Do not damage the superior peroneal retinaculum during peroneus longus tendon harvesting. Tensioning the graft with the foot held in dorsiflexion and eversion is also important; the graft may stretch with time and should be tightest during surgery.
- When notching the holes, do not make the initial notch too large; it can be made larger but cannot be made smaller.
- It is important to inform patients about the possibility of numbness in the sural nerve distribution postoperatively due to scarring.
- Start rehabilitation early to avoid excessive tightness and scarring after surgery.
- Be careful to decompress the posterior aspect of the ankle when necessary to improve postoperative range of motion and prevent posterior ankle impingement.
- Traditional lateral ankle ligament reconstruction can be augmented reliably with peroneus tendon allograft or autograft with very little morbidity.
- Patients may recover fast with fibertape augmentation when compared to tendon augmentation.

87 Achilles Tendon Rupture Repair

INTRODUCTION

- Achilles tendon rupture is a common sports-related injury in patients in their 40s and 50s
- Examination
  - ▶ Palpable gap in midsubstance of tendon
  - ▶ Thompson test shows no plantar flexion when calf is squeezed
- Recent data show comparable outcomes with surgical and nonsurgical treatment
- Historically, acute surgical repair was normal course of treatment
- Patients who benefit from nonsurgical treatment include those with diabetes, neuropathy, immunocompromised states, peripheral vascular disease, and systemic dermatologic diseases as well as those who are older than 65 years, who smoke, who are sedentary, or who have obesity
- Reduced risk for rerupture is biggest benefit of repair
- Treatment options—Open, limited open, or percutaneous

PROCEDURE

Acute Achilles Tendon Rupture Repair

- Prone position or supine with bump under contralateral hip to access medial heel in figure-of-4 position
- Make incision midline or just medial to midline. Avoids watershed area
- Débride string-like tissue at the ends of the tendons
- For repair, author prefers Krackow stitch with No. 2 nonabsorbable suture (**Figure 1**)
- After repair, gentle range to position of maximum dorsiflexion to determine stability of repair
- Consider a drain for postoperative hematoma control
- Maintain meticulous closure, because wound breakdown is biggest complication
- Immobilize in 5° to 10° equinus

Based on Graves SC, Brown JC: Achilles tendon rupture repair, in Colvin AC, Flatow E, eds: Atlas of Essential Orthopaedic Procedures, *ed 2. Rosemont, IL, American Academy of Orthopaedic Surgeons, 2020, pp 715-720.*

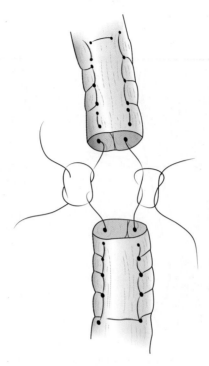

FIGURE 1 Illustration demonstrates tendon reapproximation with a Krackow suture pattern.

Chronic or Neglected Achilles Tendon Rupture

Surgical Planning

- Less well researched, but treatment similar to that of acute rupture
- Examination—Weak active plantar flexion, palpable defect, increased range of dorsiflexion; patient cannot perform single-leg raise
- Consider MRI to determine length of gap
- Reconstruction options
  - ▶ V-Y advancement for gaps of 2 to 3 cm (**Figure 2**)
  - ▶ Fascial turndown for gaps of 3 to 8 cm (**Figure 3**)
  - ▶ Autograft/allograft helps supplement gaps greater than 5 cm
  - ▶ Autograft options—flexor hallucis longus (FHL), fascia lata/iliotibial band, plantaris, hamstring tendons

 VIDEO 87.1 Chronic Achilles Tendon Repair. Stanley C. Graves, MD (8 min)

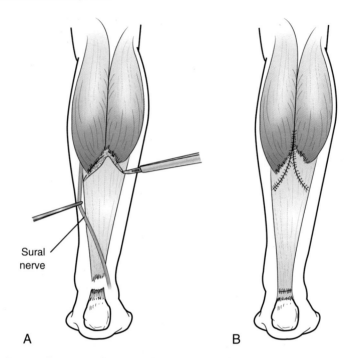

Sural
nerve

A   B

FIGURE 2 Illustrations show V-Y advancement. **A,** After careful dissection proximally to the Achilles aponeurosis and being attentive to the location of the sural nerve, two oblique fascial incisions are made along the inferior border of the muscle. **B,** The Achilles tendon rupture can then be repaired because of the increased extensibility of the gastrocnemius-soleus complex. After the repair has been completed, the fascial incisions are sutured while the foot is held in dorsiflexion, to avoid obtaining a tight Achilles tendon postoperatively.

Surgical Technique Using Flexor Hallucis Longus Autograft

- Supine position with bump under contralateral hip; affected leg in figure-of-4 position
- Make longitudinal incision, 2 mm medial to midline; watch for sural nerve proximally
- Remove unhealthy tendon ends and identify gap
- Identify FHL tendon by opening deep posterior compartment
- Dissect lateral to neurovascular bundle
- Make separate incision in medial arch
  - ⯈ Reflect abductor plantarly
  - ⯈ Divide intermuscular septum
  - ⯈ Identify knot of Henry at intersection of FHL and flexor digitorum longus
- Dissect FHL from the flexor digitorum

- Tenodese distal FHL to flexor digitorum and cut FHL proximally around knot
- Pull FHL tendon into the posterior wound; may require some blind dissection around ankle
- Drill tunnel through calcaneus parallel to tibia
- Pass FHL through tunnel in maximal plantar flexion and sew back onto itself with nonabsorbable suture to set tension; alternatively, can anchor to distal Achilles stump, but author prefers placing tendon through drill hole in calcaneus
- Tension set equal to resting position of contralateral ankle
- Release a 2- to 3-cm rectangle of tendon from underlying muscle of proximal stump to create tissue for reinforcing turndown (**Figure 3**)
- Turn down proximal Achilles stump and suture it to FHL tendon proximally and distally
- Test repair for stability by moving ankle to neutral
- Close wound as for acute repair; maintain meticulous skin closure to prevent wound complications

POSTOPERATIVE CARE AND REHABILITATION

- Postoperative care and rehabilitation are similar for acute and chronic Achilles tendon rupture repair
- Immobilize 1 week postoperatively
- After 1 week, begin active range of motion several times daily; keep in splint at other times

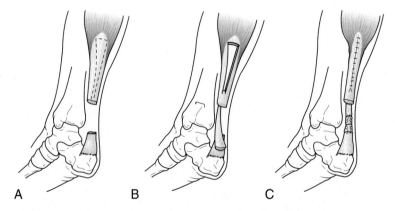

A   B   C

FIGURE 3 Illustrations demonstrate fascial turndown. **A,** The dashed outline shows an incision enabling a repair that matches up the distal component of the tendon uniformly. **B,** The proximal portion of the tendon is reflected anteriorly to minimize palpable thickening where the two tendons overlap. **C,** With the foot held in a neutral position equal to the unaffected side, the rupture site is repaired with the reflected proximal tendon. After the repair has been completed, the harvest site is repaired to produce a stronger tendon overall.

- Allow weight bearing in removable fracture boot when active dorsiflexion reaches 90°, after 3 weeks
- Remove boot at 8 weeks and begin formal physical therapy

COMPLICATIONS

- Most common is skin breakdown, which needs aggressive and early management in conjunction with plastic surgery consultation
- Obese patients with BMI over 30 kg/m² are at increased risk of wound complications
- Rerupture is rare

PEARLS

- Positioning the patient supine allows easier harvesting of the FHL and is not associated with increased infection rates, sural nerve injuries, or rerupture.
- The linear incision along the midline of the leg enables an easily extensible incision, complete visualization of the affected area, and healing, provided the skin is handled with care.
- To achieve a repair that is neither too loose nor too tight, secure the repair with the foot in the same position as the contralateral foot at rest.
- Keep the insertion point of the FHL transfer close to the original insertion of the Achilles tendon to approximate the FHL muscle belly to the Achilles tendon repair and to increase blood supply to promote healing.

PATIENT SELECTION

Indications

- Mainstay of treatment for end-stage ankle arthritis
- Posttraumatic arthritis after ankle and tibial plafond (pilon) fractures
- Rheumatoid arthritis and osteoarthritis
- Failed total ankle arthroplasty
- Chronic ankle instability
- Relative indication—severe ankle deformity (varus, valgus, or equinus)

Contraindications

- Acute or chronic infection
- Osteonecrosis of talar body
- Osteoporosis hinders optimal fixation
- Peripheral neuropathy raises risk of nonunion and infection

PREOPERATIVE IMAGING

- Weight-bearing AP, mortise, and lateral views of ankle
- Evaluate for incongruities, joint malalignment, and signs of arthritis of subtalar joint complex
- CT, MRI as needed to evaluate for bone loss, osteonecrosis, adjacent degeneration
- Nuclear imaging as needed to evaluate for infection

PRINCIPLES OF FUSION

- Rigid fixation, adequate compression, favorable biology are crucial for osseous healing and successful fusion construct
- Special situations
    - External fixator preferred for previous infection, severe osteoporosis
    - Use arthroscopic or mini-open arthrodesis only for minimal deformity
    - Open arthrodesis appropriate for significant deformity
    - Nonunions, osteonecrosis of talus, and Charcot arthropathy need bone grafting, extensive débridement, possible plating

Based on Rubinstein AJ, Mehta SK, Lin SS: Tibiotalar arthrodesis, in Colvin AC, Flatow E, eds: Atlas of Essential Orthopaedic Procedures, *ed 2. Rosemont, IL, American Academy of Orthopaedic Surgeons, 2020, pp 721-730.*

- Position of ankle key to successful outcomes
  - Neutral flexion
  - 5° to 10° of external rotation
  - 5° of valgus
- Optimize patient potential for healing by addressing medical comorbidities and supplementing with orthobiologics as necessary

PROCEDURE
Patient Positioning
- Supine position at edge of table
- Bump under ipsilateral hip
- Tourniquet on upper third of thigh

Special Instruments/Equipment
- Microsagittal saw
- Curets, osteotomes
- 7.3-mm cannulated screws
- 4.0- or 4.5-mm cannulated screws
- Have plating system available

Surgical Technique

VIDEO 88.1 Tibiotalar Arthrodesis. Siddhant K. Mehta, MD; Nicholas A. Abidi, MD; Sheldon S. Lin, MD (6 min)

- Chapter describes open ankle arthrodesis using a two-incision transfibular approach and a transarticular cross-screw fixation technique supplemented with fibular-onlay strut grafting and anterior plating (**Figure 1**)
- Make first incision 10 cm from tip of fibula, distally curving to head down fourth ray
  - Incise superior peroneal retinaculum and reflect tendons back to protect sural nerve

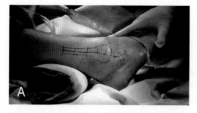
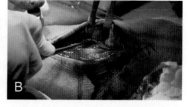

FIGURE 1 Intraoperative photographs show ankle arthrodesis. **A**, The lateral landmarks and planned incision are drawn on the skin. **B**, The periosteum is stripped from the anterior aspect and, minimally, from the posterior aspect to fully expose the distal fibula.

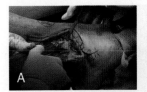 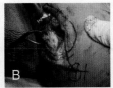 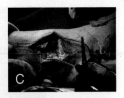

FIGURE 2 Intraoperative photographs show steps in ankle arthrodesis. **A,** A fibular osteotomy is created approximately 4 to 6 cm proximal to the tip of the lateral malleolus. **B,** The distal fibula is split in half in the sagittal plane. The medial fragment will later be morcellized to serve as autologous bone graft, and the lateral fragment will be lagged to the tibia and the talus to provide lateral stability. **C,** The distal fibula is turned down and away from the arthrodesis site to provide adequate exposure to the posteromedial tibia.

- ▶ Maintain full-thickness flaps
- ▶ Strip periosteum anteriorly
- ▶ Carry deep dissection medially subperiosteally to distal tibia and ankle joint, distally to subtalar joint/sinus tarsi (**Figure 2**)
- ▶ Osteotomize fibula 4 to 6 cm proximal to joint, leaving distal posterior ligaments intact to maintain blood supply and act as strut
- ▶ Turn down fibula fragment to expose capsule and joint
- ▶ Clear joint space of any cartilage or debris
- ▶ Sagittal fibula cut is made to resect medial fibular fragment. Use as bone graft
- ▶ Prepare tibiotalar joint
- ▶ (Optional) Perpendicular cut of tibial plafond stopping short of medial malleolus
- ▶ Parallel cut through dome of talus is made resecting 3-5mm of bone
- Make second incision 6 cm proximal to medial malleolus on anteromedial border (**Figure 3**)
  - ▶ Maintain thick flaps on either side
  - ▶ Débride ankle capsule and periosteum
  - ▶ Clear medial ankle of any remaining cartilage
  - ▶ Drill tibial and talar joint surfaces to bleeding bone
- Position joint as described above
- Place guide pins for 7.0- to 7.3-mm cannulated screws (**Figure 4**)
  - ▶ Ensure that the talus is translated posteriorly in ankle mortise
  - ▶ Place first guide pin at base of talar neck directed posteromedially to tibia
  - ▶ Place second guide pin just above posterior facet of talus, anterior to lateral process and directed posteromedially; avoid violating subtalar joint
- Confirm positioning with fluoroscopy; check subtalar joint

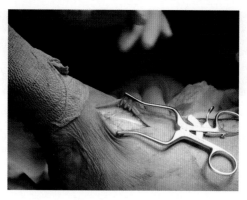

FIGURE 3 Intraoperative photograph shows exposure to the medial aspect of the tibiotalar articulation obtained through a 6-cm anteromedial incision made along the anterior third of the medial malleolus.

- Place 7.3-mm lag screws for compression
- Other screw options (**Figure 5**)
  - ▶ Place first screw from posterolateral tibia directed down center of talus
  - ▶ Place second screw from anterolateral talus directed to medial tibia
  - ▶ Alternatively, place first screw from medial malleolus directed to lateral talus
  - ▶ Place final screw in lateral tibia directed to distal medial talus

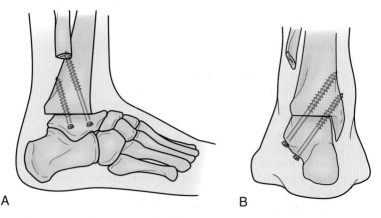

A   B

FIGURE 4 Illustrations of the lateral (**A**) and posterior (**B**) aspects of the foot show the placement of cancellous screws across the arthrodesis site as described by Mann et al.

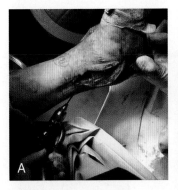 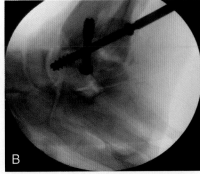

FIGURE 5 Images show the cross-screw fixation technique for ankle arthrodesis. **A,** Intraoperative photograph shows the guide pin for the first cancellous screw being placed from the posterolateral tibia down the center of the talus. **B,** Fluoroscopic image shows the second screw in place, from the anterolateral aspect of the talus directed proximally into the medial cortex of the tibia.

- Use morcellized autologous bone graft to fill in space around mortise; may use bioadjuvants per surgeon discretion
- For fibula fixation, place two 4.0- or 4.5-mm screws—one into the talus and the other across the syndesmosis (**Figure 6**)
- For adjunct plating, place precontoured plates anteriorly after compression screws fixed if necessary. Avoid penetration of subtalar joint
- Close wounds with two-layer technique, taking care to protect adjacent nerves

POSTOPERATIVE CARE AND REHABILITATION
- Place in bulky cast padding padded dressing with plaster splint dressing; maintain for 2 weeks
- Transition to non–weight-bearing cast at follow-up; do not permit weight bearing until radiographic union (8 to 12 weeks)

OUTCOMES
- Procedure results in 60% to 70% loss of sagittal motion and reduced subtalar motion
- Walking speed reduced by 16%
- Overall 83% to 99% union rate

COMPLICATIONS
- Adjacent joint arthritis over time
- Nonunion rate is 10%; risk factors include tobacco use, open fractures, osteonecrosis of talus, neuropathy, infection
- Wound complications
- Neurovascular injury

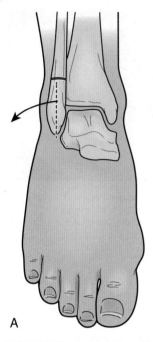 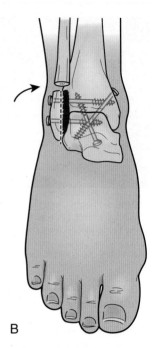

FIGURE 6 Illustrations show ankle arthrodesis. **A,** The fibular osteotomy is achieved while distal fibular soft-tissue attachments are maintained. **B,** After cross-screw fixation, the fibula is lagged to the tibia and the talus in its anatomic position, to serve as a lateral buttress.

PEARLS

- For satisfactory short- and long-term results, it is paramount to achieve correct alignment and to position the ankle in neutral flexion, 5° to 10° of external rotation, and 5° of valgus.

- The amount of rigid fixation used and the technique(s) employed to obtain a successful arthrodesis across the tibiotalar joint are predicated on host factors and bone quality.

- Take care to identify risk factors for impaired osseous healing—advanced age, systemic diseases (eg, diabetes mellitus), smoking, poor nutritional status, chronic use of corticosteroids, and immunosuppressive therapy. In such high-risk patients, bone grafting with or without orthobiologics (eg, local growth factor augmentation with platelet-rich plasma, bone morphogenetic proteins, or recombinant human platelet-derived growth factor) or biophysical bone stimulation with low-intensity pulsed ultrasound, direct current, or pulsed electromagnetic fields may improve clinical outcomes.

89 Total Ankle Replacement

PATIENT SELECTION

Indications

- End-stage degeneration of tibiotalar joint
- Salvage of painful ankle arthrodesis
- Traditionally reserved for patients older than 60 years with low physical demands (expanding with new implants)

Contraindications

- Active infection
- Severe soft-tissue compromise
- Distal neuropathy
- Diminished vascular supply
- Relative contraindications
- Coronal plane deformity > 15°
- Obesity
- Diabetes mellitus
- History of ankle sepsis
- Smoking

PREOPERATIVE IMAGING

- Full-length, orthogonal, weight bearing of tibia and AP/lateral hindfoot views (**Figure 1**)
- Consider maximal dorsiflexion and plantar flexion views as well as lateral obliques
- Consider lateral dorsiflexion and plantar flexion views of hindfoot (**Figure 2**)
- CT—evaluate bone quality, cyst, rotational alignment
- MRI—assess osteonecrosis, ligament damage

Based on Halai MM, Daniels TR: Total ankle replacement, in Colvin AC, Flatow E, eds: Atlas of Essential Orthopaedic Procedures, *ed 2. Rosemont, IL, American Academy of Orthopaedic Surgeons, 2020, pp 731-740.*

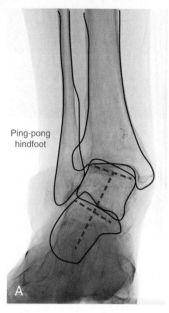
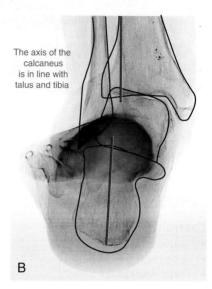

Ping-pong
hindfoot

The axis of the
calcaneus
is in line with
talus and tibia

A

B

FIGURE 1 Artist's illustration of the usefulness of the hindfoot alignment radio-graph. AP ankle radiograph (**A**) and hindfoot alignment radiograph (**B**) in the same patient. Patient with talar valgus and compensatory hindfoot varus (ping-pong hindfoot). This can be best appreciated with a hindfoot alignment view (**B**) where it becomes evident that the calcaneus is not in the same degree of valgus as the talus. The hindfoot alignment view clearly demonstrates that the axis of the calcaneus is parallel to the axis of the tibia. This can create a paradoxical situation where after the ankle joint is packed with a total ankle arthroplasty the remainder of the foot is now behaving as a cavovarus deformity, even though one started with a talar valgus deformity. In these scenarios, the senior author has had to release or perform a posterior tibial to peroneus brevis tendon transfer.

PROCEDURE

Room Setup

- Supine position, bump under affected hip—ensure patella and second toe are pointing to ceiling
- Pad contralateral fibula
- Above-knee tourniquet as proximal as possible
- Mini C-arm lateral to operative extremity

Special Instruments

- Total ankle replacement tray
- Small fragment set
- Cannulated screw set
- Suture anchor system

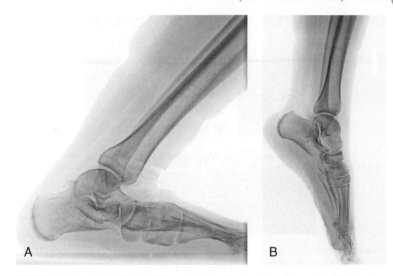

FIGURE 2 Lateral dorsiflexion (**A**) and plantar flexion (**B**) radiographic views of the hindfoot in a patient with pes planus. These can help the surgeon determine correctability of the deformity and are useful for research.

- Small osteotomy
- Laminar spreader

Surgical Technique

- Mark out all anatomical landmarks
- Anterior incision centered over the level of ankle joint, 1 cm lateral to the lateral border of the tibialis anterior (TA) (**Figure 3**)
- Protect the medial branch of superficial peroneal nerve
- Incise the extensor retinaculum in line with skin incision
- Retract the TA and extensor hallucis longus medially; extensor digitorum and neurovascular bundle laterally
- Avoid excessive retraction on skin edges
- Incise ankle joint capsule longitudinally in midline
- Utilize osteotomy to plane off anterior distal tibial plafond
- Medial and lateral ligament release are performed to achieve 25° to 40° of ankle motion (complete with periosteal elevators in medial and lateral gutters)
- Remove large osteophytes off the talar neck

Tibial Preparation

- Tibial jig is centered over the tibial tuberosity proximally; lay cutting block on anterior distal tibial surface (jig must be parallel to joint line and perpendicular to tibial mechanical axis) (**Figure 4**)

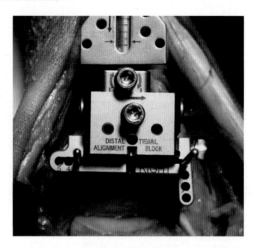

FIGURE 3 Photograph shows anterior ankle joint exposure with the tibial cutting block. The pins in the tibial cutting slot are to prevent transection of the malleoli with the saw.

- Ensure jig is secure and in neutral position
- Utilize mini C-arm and system markers to ensure true AP and lateral radiographs are being taken
- Check rotational alignment; center of tibial cutting block must be in line with second metatarsal

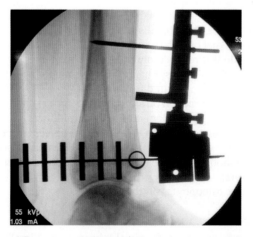

FIGURE 4 Lateral fluoroscopy showing the planned trajectory of the distal tibial saw blade.

- Use saw to make tibial cut; careful when cutting posterior medial aspect of tibia
  - Use weight of saw to make posterior tibial cut
- Remove tibial jig
- Complete vertical limb of medial tibial resection with reciprocating saw or osteotome

Talar Preparation

- Utilize laminar spreaders to place collaterals under full tension (**Figure 5**)
- Place talar cutting guide flush on the talar neck; secure with pins
- Use implant gap sizer; ensure joint will not be too tight
- Check AP and medial/lateral dimensions after cut; choose smaller size if in between two sizes
- Perform anterior and posterior chamfer cuts using specific cutting blocks
  - Check posterior chamfer cut with radiographs as chamfer block tends to sit anteriorly
- Remove talar jig; trial implants
- Check range of motion; ideal to have 25 degrees of plantar flexion/ dorsiflexion
- Wash joint; fill contained cyst with cancellous bone
- Insert final implants, lavage joint, release tourniquet and achieve hemostasis
- Close capsule, retinaculum and buried subcutaneous knots; close skin with staples or monofilament
- Place non–weight bearing below the knee cast and obtain final films

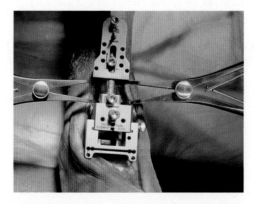

FIGURE 5 Photograph shows superior talus cutting block. Note the use of the laminar spreaders to create the appropriate cut in a tensioned ankle.

POSTOPERATIVE CARE

- Deep vein thrombosis prophylaxis is used for 1 month
- Postoperative radiographs at 2 weeks
- Remove sutures at 2 weeks if incision is healed and place into weight-bearing cast
- Transition patient to weight bearing boot at 6 weeks
- Clinic and imaging evaluations are done again at 3 and 6 months and then annually

COMPLICATIONS

- Persistent unaddressed deformity
- Iatrogenic fracture
- Wound complications (approximately 10%)
- Subsidence of implants
- Periprosthetic infection

PEARLS

- Throughout the entire anterior approach, care is taken not to put excessive traction on the skin edges.
- There are various markers on different systems that allow the surgeon to confirm that they are taking a true AP and lateral radiograph which will make intraoperative comparisons more reliable.
- When making distal tibia cut, it is normal for the posterior lip of the distal tibia to extend more distally compared with the anterior part. Thus it may look as if the cut is taking off slightly more posteriorly than anteriorly, which is normal.
- When a large deformity or the tibial cut has progressed too close to the medial cortex of the tibia, a prophylactic small fragment screw can be placed through the medial malleolus to avoid a fracture.
- Check posterior chamfer with radiographs to avoid cutting the subtalar joint.
- Ancillary procedures to correct deformity, repair ankle ligaments or tendon transfers are required in 60% of patients undergoing TAR.

PATIENT SELECTION

Indications

- Painful osteoarthritis, posttraumatic arthritis, inflammatory arthritis
- Failed nonsurgical management (cortisone injections, medications, inserts, rocker-bottom shoes)
- Primary treatment of comminuted calcaneal fractures

Contraindications

- No absolute contraindications
- Careful patient selection for Charcot arthropathy, smoking, infection, vasculopathy

PREOPERATIVE IMAGING

- AP, lateral, and axial views of hindfoot
- Long weight-bearing axial view of distal tibia (**Figure 1**)
- Brodén views of subtalar joint
- CT definitive imaging modality (weight-bearing CT if available)
- Three-dimensional CT supports better preoperative planning in complex cases
- Consider MRI for subtle symptoms or in cases of osteonecrosis of talus

PROCEDURE

Setup/Patient Positioning

- Supine position, bump under ipsilateral hip
- Can access heel using figure-of-4 position, flexion of the knee so the point of the heel is off the side of the bed, or position that leaves point of heel off foot of bed
- Position C-arm on opposite side of bed
- Large C-arm (opposite side of bed) or small C-arm positioned by surgeon

---

Based on Lee S, Jacobsen SK: Subtalar arthrodesis, in Colvin AC, Flatow E, eds: Atlas of Essential Orthopaedic Procedures, *ed 2. Rosemont, IL, American Academy of Orthopaedic Surgeons, 2020, pp 741-747.*

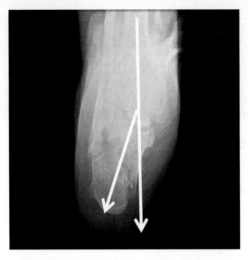

FIGURE 1 Long axial radiograph of the tibia, talus, and calcaneus demonstrates the weight-bearing line falling medial to the calcaneus. The calcaneus is in excessive valgus and thus would require correction if subtalar arthrodesis were performed.

Implants

- 6.5- and 4.0-mm cannulated lag screws
- C-arm
- Tourniquet

Surgical Technique

In Situ Arthrodesis

- Make 4- to 6-cm incision starting distal to fibula tip and overlying anterior process of calcaneus to base of fourth tarsometatarsal joint
- Split or reflect extensor digitorum brevis distally
- Dissect to expose sinus tarsi; resect tissue from sinus tarsi to allow visualization of the talocalcaneal joint
- May release talocalcaneal ligament to increase exposure to middle and anterior facets; may also need to release medial capsule
- Use lamina spreader to open up talocalcaneal space
- Use curets and osteotomes to denude calcaneal and talar joint surfaces to bleeding bone
- Use 2.0-mm drill to make multiple perforations and elevation of thin wedges of bone with osteotome "fish scales"
- Check alignment with real-time fluoroscopy
- Surfaces should ideally have maximal contact; ideal alignment is 7° of valgus; lateral talocalcaneal angle 25° to 40°

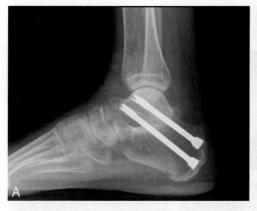 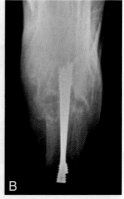

FIGURE 2 A lateral view of the foot (**A**) and axial view of the calcaneus (**B**) showing two screws inserted from the tuberosity into the central body and neck of the talus.

- Perform fixation with two screws (**Figure 2**); countersink both screws to prevent symptomatic hardware
  - ▹ Direct one or two 6.5-8 mm large-fragment screws with short threads from tuberosity of calcaneus to talar body (second screw based on patient's bone quality)
  - ▹ Alternatively, second screw may be place from talar neck to calcaneal tuberosity
  - ▹ Avoid threads across fusion site
    - – Occasionally requires second small incision
    - – Best to assess on axial radiograph

Deformity Correction

- Valgus deformity is most common deformity; from lateral bone loss
- Take care to prepare middle and anterior facets to ensure maximal bony contact
- Release medial subtalar ligaments as needed; medial capsule and talocalcaneal ligament release improves visualization of posterior aspect of joint
- Bone grafts can be added to subtalar joint to maintain lateral talocalcaneal angle greater than 25° (**Figure 3**)
  - ▹ Best applied through posterolateral exposure in lateral decubitus position
  - ▹ Also can help restore bone loss
- Can use structural bone grafts to compensate for bony collapse secondary to calcaneal fracture malunion
- Varus deformity usually correctable with standard bone preparation techniques
- Be sure varus corrected, otherwise forefoot is locked; can cause lateral column overload

---

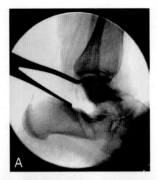

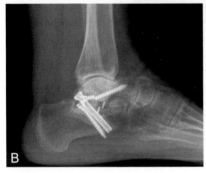
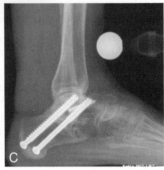

FIGURE 3 **A,** An intraoperative fluoroscopic image shows one method to correct a horizontal talus. The space between the calcaneus and talus is distracted with a lamina spreader. A tricortical bone graft is then placed in the resulting gap. **B,** A preoperative lateral radiograph showing a failed subtalar arthrodesis with loss of lateral talocalcaneal angle and anterior ankle impingement. **C,** Postoperative lateral radiograph showing an interpositional arthrodesis with improved talocalcaneal angle, hindfoot height, and anterior ankle impingement.

COMPLICATIONS

- Nonunion
  - ‣ Rate up to 35% reported at 6 months as seen on CT
  - ‣ May treat with bone stimulators, revision with additional screws, or bone graft
- Malunion
  - ‣ Most commonly varus of calcaneus
  - ‣ Patient notes varus "rolling in" of ankle
  - ‣ Healed varus malunion treated with Dwyer lateral closing wedge osteotomy
  - ‣ Severe malunion may need further osteotomy

POSTOPERATIVE CARE AND REHABILITATION

- No weight bearing for 2 weeks with elevation
- At 2 weeks, apply weight-bearing short leg cast or walker boot
- At 6 weeks, obtain radiograph; walking boot for one additional month then transition to regular shoe wear
- Should see signs of union by 3 months; if healing uncertain on radiograph, move to CT

PEARLS

- Preoperative plan should determine if an in situ arthrodesis is appropriate. Goal is restoration of normal talocalcaneal relationships.
- Correction of deformity usually can be done with capsular release and bone shaping.
- Bone block distraction arthrodesis can correct loss of height as well as calcaneal bone loss.
- Arthroscopic arthrodesis has been described using prone position and two portals.
- Mortise view of ankle will show heel valgus and confirm correct screw placement. Normal valgus will appear as the calcaneus aligned in slight lateral angulation in relation to tibial axis.

91 Arthrodesis of the Tarsometatarsal Joint

INTRODUCTION
- Lisfranc ligament runs from medial cuneiform to base of second metatarsal; strongest part is plantar portion; limits movement
- Tarsometatarsal (TMT) joint movement
  - First joint—5° to 10°
  - Second and third joint—Almost none
  - Fourth and fifth joint—10° to 20°
- Recessed second TMT joint stabilized by plantar ligaments between medial and lateral cuneiforms

PATIENT SELECTION
Indications
- Primary fusion
  - Major ligament disruption with multidirectional instability of Lisfranc joint
  - Comminuted intra-articular fractures at base of first or second metatarsal
  - Crush injuries of midfoot with intra-articular fracture-dislocation
- Secondary fusion
  - Posttraumatic degenerative joint disease (DJD) after Lisfranc injury
  - Idiopathic TMT DJD
  - Rheumatoid arthritis
  - Stable/chronic Charcot neuroarthropathy, other complications of diabetes

CONTRAINDICATIONS
- Skeletal immaturity
- Acute Charcot neuroarthropathy (relative)
- Incomplete ligamentous injuries
- Infection

Based on Coetzee JC, Rippstein P: Arthrodesis of the tarsometatarsal joint, in Colvin AC, Flatow E, eds: Atlas of Essential Orthopaedic Procedures, *ed 2. Rosemont, IL, American Academy of Orthopaedic Surgeons, 2020, pp 748-755.*

PROCEDURE

- Same approach as that for open reduction and internal fixation (ORIF) of Lisfranc injury (**Figure 1**)
- Inflate calf or thigh tourniquet to 250 mm Hg
- Make first incision between first and second metatarsals (**Figure 2**); be careful of dorsalis pedis artery and deep peroneal nerve while dissecting to bone
- Make second incision over fourth metatarsal; incision placement may be aided by fluoroscopic guidance
  - ‣ This should provide access to the lateral cuneiform and cuboid
  - ‣ Err on lateral side of fourth metatarsal on oblique radiograph
  - ‣ Protect lateral branch of superficial peroneal nerve
  - ‣ Incise on lateral side of extensor digitorum longus tendon; divide extensor digitorum brevis muscle belly longitudinally with blunt dissection
- Perform reduction
  - ‣ Evaluate involved joints by direct visualization and forefoot abduction stress fluoroscopy
  - ‣ Débride joints; remove cartilage; expose subchondral bone

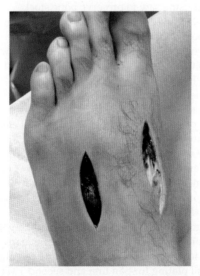

FIGURE 1 Intraoperative photograph shows the surgical approaches for a tarsometatarsal joint fusion in a left foot. The medial incision is between the first and second metatarsals, just lateral to the extensor hallucis tendon. The lateral incision is at least 4 cm farther lateral, overlying the fourth metatarsal.

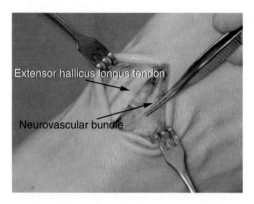

FIGURE 2 Intraoperative photograph of a left foot shows the extensor hallucis longus tendon at the medial side of the incision. The dorsalis pedis artery and the deep peroneal nerve are lateral to the tendon and will be encountered during the exposure. A branch of the superficial peroneal nerve usually runs from lateral to medial across the distal portion of the exposure.

- First TMT joint is about 30 mm deep; expose using laminar spreaders as needed to see plantar aspect and prevent dorsiflexion deformity
  - Avoid using saw to preserve bone stock
  - Stabilize first TMT joint first; build remaining joints in relation to the first TMT
- It is controversial whether acute ligamentous injuries should be fused in situ or treated with open reduction and internal fixation
  - Stabilize first TMT with Kirschner wires
  - Fix medial cuneiform to first metatarsal with 3-, 4-, or 5-mm screws
  - Clamp second metatarsal to first; do not elevate second TMT (**Figure 3**)
  - Place second screw from medial cuneiform to base of second metatarsal
  - Augment with third intercuneiform screw if instability present
  - Compression staples are viable option for fixation if joints are well aligned and reduced
  - Continue to stabilize metatarsals and cuneiforms as needed; do not arthrodese fourth and fifth metatarsals
- Can fuse acute fractures in situ but may need alternate fixation
  - Dorsal plating to span first and second TMT joints (**Figure 4**)
  - Can use combination of plates and free screws
- Chronic DJD or Charcot arthritis (**Figure 5**)
  - Need complete release to mobilize joints
  - Correct abduction and dorsiflexion deformity

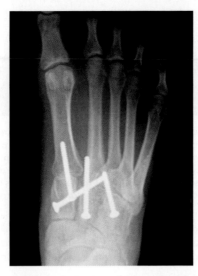

FIGURE 3 AP radiograph shows typical screw placement in reduction of a dislocation of the first through third tarsometatarsal joints. The first ray is immobilized first, followed by the second and then the third.

- Consider plantarmedial incision for removal of osteophyte and adjunct plate fixation
- Occasionally saw is used to make cuts and mobilize bony deformity
- Watch for dorsal and lateral bone loss that may need grafting

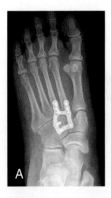
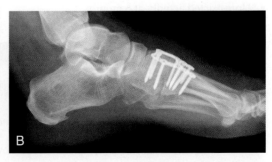

FIGURE 4 AP (**A**) and lateral (**B**) radiographs show plate fixation, which is a better option than screws or staples for significant communication of the metatarsal bases. With the plate construct, the surgeon can maintain length and alignment while immobilizing the joints.

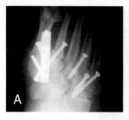
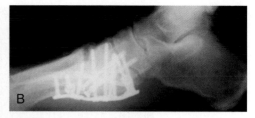

FIGURE 5 Postoperative AP (**A**) and lateral (**B**) radiographs show satisfactory sagittal and coronal plane reduction using a combination of a plantar plate for the medial ray and screws for the lateral rays. A plantar plate can provide excellent strength and stability on the tension side of the joint in severe deformities. This is one of the few cases in which a fusion of the lateral two rays is done to also restore the lateral border after severe collapse due to the Charcot process.

> – Placement of a plantarmedial plate is a good option for stable fixation of first TMT, from which to build construct
> – If deformity minimal, can use just screw construct

COMPLICATIONS
- Nerve and vascular injury
- Skin complications if incisions too close together
- Malunion from malpositioning during exposure

POSTOPERATIVE CARE AND REHABILITATION
- Immobilize in cast or splint
- Keep non–weight bearing in pneumatic walking boot for 6 weeks; encourage ankle range of motion
- Obtain radiographs at 6 weeks to evaluate fusion
- Allow weight bearing in walker boot after 6 weeks
- At 3 months, allow weight bearing without boot
- Unrestricted activity at 6 months

PEARLS

- Protect neurovascular structures.
- Adequate exposure and soft-tissue release are needed for reduction.
- Do not fuse a deformity in situ.
- Use bone graft only as needed, especially if dorsal and lateral defects exist after reduction.
- Must use adequate fixation because of large forces over TMT joints.

Surgical Treatment of Navicular Stress Fractures

PATIENT SELECTION
- Most common in patients who participate in high-impact or explosive athletics (sprinting, jumping) or long-distance running
- Frequently missed; suspect if patient does not respond to treatments for other diagnosis; can be confused with posterior/anterior tibial tendinitis, midfoot sprain, ankle sprain
- Classified as complete versus incomplete, displaced versus nondisplaced
- Nonsurgical care is mainstay for complete nondisplaced and incomplete fractures; minimum of 6 weeks non–weight-bearing (NWB) immobilization
- Noncompliance with NWB, immobilization leads to treatment failure

PREOPERATIVE IMAGING
- Standard weight-bearing AP, oblique, and lateral radiographs of foot; often miss stress fracture, however
- If radiograph negative but clinically suspicious, MRI is next examination (**Figure 1**); MRI may not identify fracture, requiring CT
- If radiograph identifies fracture or sclerosis, CT is next examination (**Figure 2**)
- Bone scans are sensitive but nonspecific for pathology
- Most common fracture is incomplete and in central third of bone traversing from dorsal-medial to plantar-lateral

PROCEDURE
Patient Positioning
- Supine position with bump under ipsilateral hip
- Tourniquet on thigh
- Drape to allow for possible proximal tibial bone harvest

Surgical Technique
- Make dorsal longitudinal incision over navicular (**Figure 3**)
- Protect superficial peroneal nerve branches

Based on Heida K, Walling AK: Surgical treatment of navicular stress fractures, in Colvin AC, Flatow E, eds: Atlas of Essential Orthopaedic Procedures, ed 2. Rosemont, IL, American Academy of Orthopaedic Surgeons, *2020, pp 756-762.*

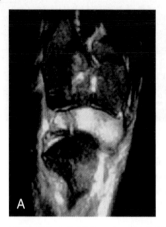
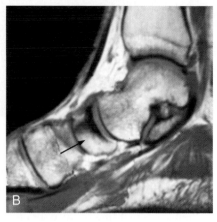

FIGURE 1 Axial (**A**) and sagittal (**B**) magnetic resonance images show a navicular stress fracture (arrow) with associated bone edema and fracture line.

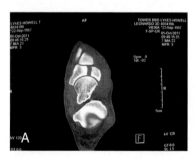
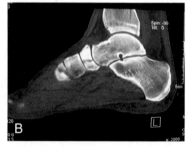

FIGURE 2 Axial (**A**) and sagittal (**B**) CT scan cuts show a complete navicular stress fracture pattern.

- Retract extensor hallucis longus and neurovascular bundle medially to expose talonavicular joint capsule (**Figure 4**)
- Open talonavicular capsule and evaluate talonavicular and navicular cuneiform articular surfaces
- Expose fracture site and débride fibrous tissue
- Place two pins for 4.0-mm partially threaded cannulated screws to affix fracture; place lateral to medial to hold smaller lateral fragment securely (**Figure 5**)
- Alternatively, may use lag by technique for placement of screws and consideration should be given to dorsal plating, as it may provide more points of fixation (**Figure 6**)
- Consider use of solid screws as they are biomechanically superior
- Confirm placement with fluoroscopy
- For large gap or chronic nonunion, consider using bone graft

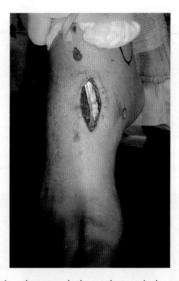

FIGURE 3 Intraoperative photograph shows the surgical approach to the navicular.

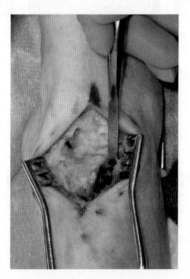

FIGURE 4 Intraoperative photograph shows exposure of the talonavicular joint and identification of the navicular fracture plane.

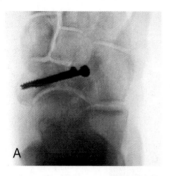 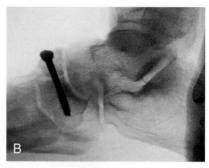

FIGURE 5 AP (**A**) and lateral (**B**) intraoperative fluoroscopic images confirm the placement of two 4.0-mm partially threaded cannulated screws.

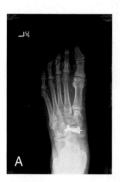 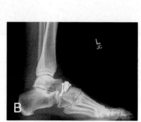 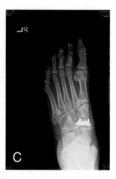

FIGURE 6 AP (**A**), lateral (**B**), and oblique (**C**) postoperative images demonstrating placement of a dorsal plate and screw construct.

COMPLICATIONS

- Delayed union and nonunion most frequent and concerning complications in surgical and nonsurgical management
- Refractures are rare events; some authors consider surgical fixation of all stress fractures to reduce refracture risk upon return to athletics
- Talonavicular arthritis; can treat with arthrodesis

POSTOPERATIVE CARE AND REHABILITATION

- Compliance with NWB and immobilization is critical for successful postoperative care and rehabilitation

For Nondisplaced Fractures

- NWB for 6 weeks in removable boot to allow range of motion once incision is healed
- Progress to weight bearing as tolerated over next 2 to 4 weeks
- If pain persists, repeat CT to assess healing and adjust weight bearing as necessary

For Displaced Fractures

- NWB in cast for 8 to 10 weeks
- Progress to controlled ankle motion walker; slowly wean over 3 weeks
- Physical therapy to manage stiffness
- After pain resolves, can return to preinjury activity and athletics at 4 to 6 months

PEARLS

- Maintain high level of suspicion for navicular stress fracture. For athletes, delay in diagnosis impairs return to play.
- Clear disclosure of treatment expectations to the patient is critical. High-demand athletes will miss the season during treatment; inappropriate return to play will result in failure.
- Lateral to medial direction preferred for placing cannulated 4.0 mm partially threaded screws to affix the fracture.
- The use of locking plates in patient with osteoporotic bone rather than screw fixation does not alter the postoperative NWB protocol.

PATIENT SELECTION

Indications
- Hallux rigidus
- Hallux valgus with arthritis
- Failed surgery of hallux
- Neuromuscular conditions
- Inflammatory disease
- Arthritis
- First metatarsophalangeal joint subluxation, dislocation, or instability

Contraindications
- Infection
- Malignancy
- Tenosynovitis
- Osteochondral defects

Alternative Treatments
- Resection arthroplasty with cheilectomy
- Interposition graft arthroplasty
- Hemiarthroplasty
- Synthetic cartilage implant (unable to address significant deformity with this option)
- Total joint arthroplasty; evidence shows arthrodesis has better long-term results, improved gait mechanics versus total joint arthroplasty

PREOPERATIVE IMAGING
- Weight-bearing radiographs of foot in three planes (**Figure 1**)
- Evaluate proximal aspect of foot; proximal deformity or pathology may affect surgical decisions distally
- Can correct up to a 13° intermetatarsal angle with fusion
- Use intermetatarsal angle, hallux valgus angle, angle of inclination of first metatarsal relative to floor in surgical planning

---

Based on Patel CS, Chou LB: Arthrodesis of the hallux metatarsophalangeal joint, in Colvin AC, Flatow E, eds: Atlas of Essential Orthopaedic Procedures, *ed 2. Rosemont, IL, American Academy of Orthopaedic Surgeons, 2020, pp 763-767.*

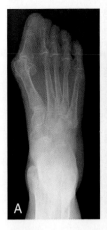
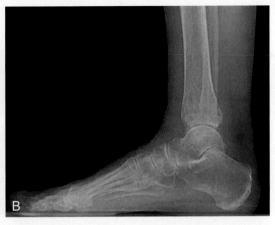

FIGURE 1 Preoperative weight-bearing AP (**A**) and lateral (**B**) radiographs show a right foot. The metatarsophalangeal (MTP) angle is approximately 30°, the intermetatarsal angle is approximately 13°, and the inclination angle of the first metatarsal is approximately 30°. There are signs of first MTP joint arthritis as well: joint space narrowing, sclerosis, osteophytosis, and mild sclerosis. The MTP joint also is subluxated, and the metatarsal head is flattened.

PROCEDURE

Special Equipment and Implants

- Radiolucent table
- Tourniquet
- Mini-fluoroscopy
- Microsagittal saw or Hoke osteotomes
- Low-profile plates

Surgical Technique

- Supine position, generally performed with local or regional anesthesia with sedation
- Place tourniquet
- Make dorsal or medial longitudinal incision over first metatarsophalangeal joint (**Figure 2**)
- Dissect to level of capsule
- Mobilize and retract extensor hallucis longus laterally
- Take care to not injure cutaneous nerves (medial dorsal branch of superficial peroneal)
- Sharply open capsule in line with incision to expose joint
- Sharply elevate capsule and periosteum on both sides of joint
- Remove osteophytes to assess deformity
- Remove cartilage to subchondral bone with saw or Hoke osteotomes
- Can use cup and cone reamers for cartilage removal

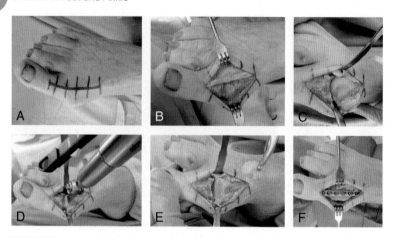

FIGURE 2 Intraoperative photographs demonstrate arthrodesis of the hallux metatarsophalangeal (MTP) joint. **A**, The planned incision for the dorsal approach to the first MTP joint is shown. **B**, The extensor hallucis longus (EHL) tendon is exposed. **C**, The first MTP joint is exposed with hyper–plantar flexion and the EHL tendon retracted laterally. The metatarsal head shows signs of severe arthritis—eburnation, loss of articular cartilage, and flattening of the convex surface. **D**, The first MTP joint is prepared using a flat-cut technique. A microsagittal saw is used to prepare the first metatarsal head. **E**, The first metatarsal head (shown held by a rongeur) is cut and removed from the joint. **F**, The first MTP joint has been prepared and fixed with a lag screw (not seen) and a plate-and-screw construct. Note that the hallux valgus is corrected.

- Position joint in 20° of dorsiflexion, neutral rotation, no more than 15° of valgus; do not overcorrect toe into varus
- Use flat plate to evaluate amount of dorsiflexion of toe; leave few millimeters between plate and pulp of toe (**Figure 3**)
- Leave 3- to 5-mm gap between first and second toe

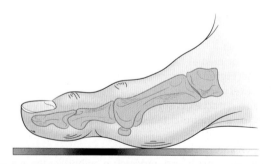

FIGURE 3 Illustration shows use of a flat x-ray plate, which can aid in determining appropriate dorsiflexion. The plate should be parallel to the longitudinal axis of the distal and proximal phalanx on lateral projection when the foot is plantigrade. The toe pad should rest several millimeters off the plate in plantigrade position.

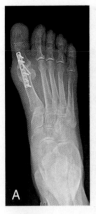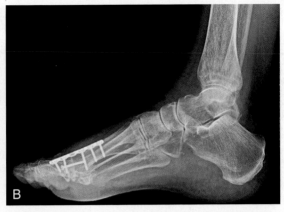

FIGURE 4 Postoperative AP (**A**) and lateral (**B**) radiographs show first metatarsophalangeal (MTP) joint fusion with lag screw and plate construct with corrected MTP angle, intermetatarsal angle (approximately 9°), and dorsiflexion angle (approximately 10°). Note that the pulp of the hallux rests higher than the sole of the foot.

- Hold position with Kirschner wires; verify with fluoroscopy
- Place lag screws distal medially to proximal laterally to gain compression (**Figure 4**)
- Place neutralization plate with bicortical screws for additional fixation
- Alternative options for fixation—two intersecting screws, interfragmentary screws without neutralization plate, plate alone, a single screw, headless screws, compression staples
- Studies suggest no difference between screw versus plate and screw fixation
- Repair capsule over plate; close skin
- Place compression dressing
- Optimize lifestyle (smoking/alcohol cessation), nutrition (vitamin D and calcium)
- Consider bone morphogenetic protein use in high-risk patient groups to decrease nonunion risk

COMPLICATIONS
- Nonunion (consider external bone stimulator and splinting)
- Malunion
- Infection
- Hardware failure or irritation
- Adjacent arthritis

POSTOPERATIVE CARE AND REHABILITATION
- Permit weight bearing with stiff-soled postoperative shoe
- Remove dressing on postoperative day 1 or 2
- Obtain radiographs every 4 to 6 weeks; union seen by 10 to 12 weeks

PEARLS

- Position patient's foot near edge of bed for easy access and maneuvering during the case; bump under the hip can aid with foot positioning.
- Remove osteophytes before joint preparation for better assessment of deformity correction.
- Hyperplantarflex the open joint to improve visualization and access to metatarsal head and proximal phalanx.
- Good fundamental technique is the key to arthrodesis.
- Repairing the capsule and the periosteal layer over the plate minimizes postoperative hardware irritation and toe swelling and improves bone healing. Compression dressing, elevation, and periodic application of ice can also minimize postoperative swelling.

Proximal and Distal First Metatarsal Osteotomies for Hallux Valgus

PATIENT SELECTION

Indications

- Clinically symptomatic moderate to severe hallux valgus deformity with congruent first metatarsophalangeal (MTP) joint (**Figure 1**)
- Uncommon; only 2% to 9% of hallux deformities are congruent
- Radiographic findings—First-second intermetatarsal angle greater than 13°, distal metatarsal articular angle (DMAA) greater than 15° (**Figure 2**)
- Recurrent hallux valgus more common if congruent joint made incongruent
- Triple osteotomies may be indicated for recurrent hallux valgus, hallux valgus interphalangeal deformity, or significant rotational deformity
- Juvenile hallux valgus frequently recurs, likely because of underappreciation of the original deformity

Contraindications

- Cosmetic concerns
- Arthritis of the first MTP joint
- Severe metatarsus adductus
- Spasticity
- Vascular insufficiency
- Infection
- Severe traumatic soft-tissue concerns
- Contracture of first metatarsal phalangeal joint

PREOPERATIVE IMAGING

- Weight-bearing AP, lateral, oblique views of foot centered over tarsometatarsal joint
- Measure hallux valgus angle, first-second intermetatarsal angle, DMAA, first MTP joint congruency

---

Based on Hirose CB, Coughlin MJ: Proximal and distal first metatarsal osteotomies for hallux valgus, in Colvin AC, Flatow E, eds: Atlas of Essential Orthopaedic Procedures, *ed 2. Rosemont, IL, American Academy of Orthopaedic Surgeons, 2020, pp 768-774.*

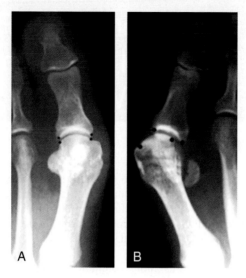

FIGURE 1 AP radiographs show a congruent (**A**) and an incongruent (**B**) first metatarsophalangeal joint.

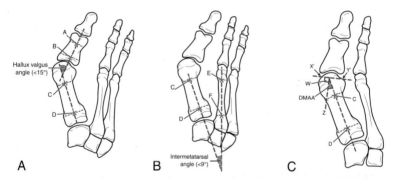

FIGURE 2 Illustrations show measurements that are made on preoperative radiographs to plan surgery for hallux valgus. **A**, Measuring the hallux valgus angle. A normal hallux valgus angle is less than 15°. A line (A) is drawn down the axis of the proximal phalanx and another line (B) is drawn down the axis of the first metatarsal. C and D are reference points midway between the medial and lateral cortex, at a point 1 cm from the end of the bone. **B**, Measuring the first-second intermetatarsal angle. A normal first-second intermetatarsal angle is less than 9°. E and F are reference points midway between the medial and lateral cortex, at a point 1 cm from the end of the bone. **C**, Measuring the distal metatarsal articular angle (DMAA). A normal DMAA is less than 6°. Line C–D delineates the longitudinal axis of the first metatarsal. X′ and Y′ are reference points of the medial and lateral edge of the articular surface. Line W–Z is drawn perpendicular to the line drawn between X′ and Y′. The DMAA is the angle subtended by lines W–Z and C–D.

PROCEDURE

Room Setup/Patient Positioning

- Supine position on standard table
- Bump under ipsilateral hip
- Mini C-arm on surgical side
- Tourniquet

Special Instruments/Equipment/Implants

- Crescentic oscillating saw blade
- Straight oscillating saw blade
- 3.5-mm solid small-fragment screw set
- 0.062-in Kirschner wires (K-wires)
- Proximal first metatarsal plate

Surgical Technique

Distal Metatarsal Osteotomy

- Perform closing osteotomy to correct DMAA (**Figure 3**); goal is to correct to DMAA of less than 6°
- Remove 4- to 6-mm wedge of bone
- Make medial longitudinal incision over first metatarsal head, centered over first MTP joint
- Raise skin flaps; protect dorsal medial cutaneous nerve
- Construct L-shaped capsulotomy: place horizontal limb dorsally, vertical limb proximally
- Expose first MTP joint to inspect cartilage
- Remove medial eminence by excising bone medial to medial edge of diaphysis; smooth bone edges when finished
- Resect medial wedge of bone 1.5 cm proximal to MTP joint and sesamoids
- Close down wedge; hold with K-wires, which run dorsal distal to proximal plantar
- Cut wires and bury under skin

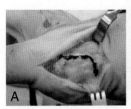 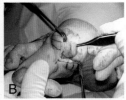 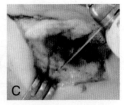

FIGURE 3 Intraoperative photographs demonstrate distal metatarsal osteotomy. **A,** The medial first metatarsophalangeal joint is shown with the capsulotomy outlined. **B,** The medial eminence of the cartilage of the first metatarsal head is resected. **C,** The medial wedge of bone is resected.

VIDEO 94.1 Proximal and Distal First Metatarsal Osteotomy. Christopher B. Hirose, MD; Michael J. Coughlin, MD (6 min)

Proximal Metatarsal Osteotomy

- Make 3-cm incision over dorsal aspect of proximal first metatarsal
- Stay medial to extensor hallucis longus tendon
- Place K-wire into medial cuneiform perpendicular to metatarsal heads; use as reference for position of saw blade for proximal metatarsal cut
- Using crescentic saw blade, start 1 cm distal to tarsometatarsal joint; angle blade halfway between perpendicular to metatarsal and perpendicular to floor (**Figure 4**)
- Keep blade perpendicular to metatarsal heads, parallel to K-wire reference
- Use saw to make cut, osteotome to break medial and lateral cortices
- After cut, swing metatarsal laterally; head is positioned over sesamoids
- Use K-wire to stabilize; place 3.5-mm screw to hold across osteotomy; start screw 1 cm distal to osteotomy site
- In pediatric patient, use multiple K-wires for provisional fixation
- Consider the use dorsal plate for adult population

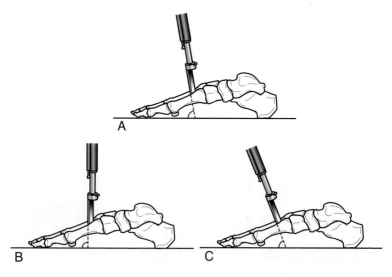

FIGURE 4 Illustration demonstrates proper saw blade orientation for proximal metatarsal osteotomy. The correct orientation (**A**) is neither perpendicular to the plantar surface of the foot (**B**) nor perpendicular to the long axis of the first metatarsal (**C**), but halfway between.

Akin Osteotomy

- Use if, during closure, phalanx still rotates into valgus after two metatarsal osteotomies (**Figure 5**)
- Extend distal incision 2 cm
- Protect extensor hallucis longus and flexor hallucis longus tendons using Hohmann retractors
- Remove 2- to 3-mm wedge of bone from medial aspect of proximal phalanx
- Perform osteotomy at metadiaphyseal junction
- Close down wedge; rotate phalanx as needed
- Pin, using one or two K-wires from distal medial to proximal lateral

Soft-Tissue Release

- Adductor hallucis release occasionally needed if valgus remains, even after three osteotomies
- Adductor release increases incidence of first metatarsal head osteonecrosis to 1.7% to 20%
- Make incision at first web space distal to bifurcation of deep peroneal nerve

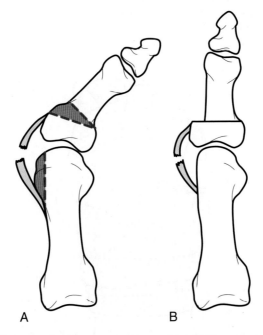

FIGURE 5 Illustration demonstrates an Akin proximal phalanx osteotomy. **A,** Preoperative wedge resection of the proximal phalanx and medial eminence resection of the first metatarsal are shown. **B,** Postoperative reduction of the proximal phalanx is shown.

- Identify conjoint tendon of adductor hallucis
- Use No. 15 blade to identify space between lateral sesamoid, first metatarsal head; amputate metatarsal sesamoid ligament
- Continuing distally, release conjoint tendon off lateral proximal phalanx and lateral sesamoid
- Place stay sutures to anchor adductor tendon stump to lateral first metatarsal head capsule

Closure

- Drill dorsal/plantar hole in distal metaphysis of first MTP
- Using 2-0 Vicryl (Ethicon) on capsule, anchor suture to drill hole
- Hold hallux in neutral position during closure
- Close incisions with interrupted 3-0 monofilament suture
- Dress in forefoot spica gauze-and-tape dressing; wrap in supination (**Figure 6**)
- Apply postoperative shoe; allow weight bearing on heel

COMPLICATIONS

- Nonunion
- Dorsiflexion malunion of proximal osteotomy
- Shortening of first metatarsal by average of 6%
- Metatarsalgia
- Hallux varus

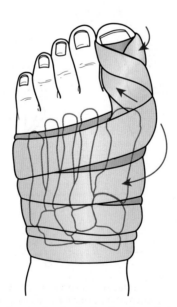

FIGURE 6 Illustration shows a forefoot spica dressing spiraled around the hallux in the direction of supination to counteract a pronated hallux valgus deformity.

- Recurrence
- Physeal arrest in adolescents
- Arthritis of first MTP

POSTOPERATIVE CARE AND REHABILITATION

- Change dressing at 48 hours, continuing to hold toe in neutral position
- Change dressings only every 10 days for 6 to 8 weeks to avoid loss of surgically obtained correction
- Obtain series of three weight-bearing foot radiographs at 7 to 10 days
- Obtain second set of weight-bearing radiographs at week 6; remove pins if healing has occurred
- Begin weight bearing on forefoot at 6 to 8 weeks
- Begin range-of-motion exercises at 8 weeks

PEARLS

- The authors prefer L-shaped capsulotomy over the first MTP joint, with the vertical limb placed proximally. Place a vertically oriented drill hole through the first metatarsal metaphysis and repair the capsule with an absorbable suture through the drill hole. The repair is easily taken down and redone to place the hallux in the proper position if degree of correction unsatisfactory.

- For proximal metatarsal crescentic osteotomy, place the lateral edge of the saw blade so that it will cut through the proximal metatarsal cortex laterally to make a clean and reproducible cut, and then translate the blade through its natural curvature to cut the medial cortex. Complete the osteotomy and open with a 4-mm osteotome.

- For proper reduction of the first-second intermetatarsal angle, place a 4-mm osteotome on the lateral cortex of the proximal portion of the first metatarsal to stabilize it while the distal fragment is shifted laterally. Provisionally pin the osteotomy to check the correction under fluoroscopy and readjust it before final fixation.

Chronic Exertional Compartment Syndrome and Release

PATIENT SELECTION

- Chronic exertional compartment syndrome (CECS) most common in athletes
- Symptoms
    - Pain after certain duration or intensity of exercise
    - Most common bilaterally
    - No inciting event
    - Asymptomatic except during activity
- Pathophysiology
    - Unclear
    - Likely relative ischemia, when muscles cannot expand because of tight fascia during exercise
- Most common in anterior compartment
- Confirm diagnosis by measuring compartment pressures before and after exercising
    - 1-minute postexercise greater than 30 mm Hg
    - 5-minute postexercise greater than 20 mm Hg
    - Postexercise level is greater than preexercise level by 15 mm Hg
- No imaging necessary
- Compartment release contraindicated if pressures do not confirm CECS

PROCEDURE
Anterior and Lateral Compartments

 VIDEO 95.1 Fasciotomy: Two-Incision Technique. Mary Lloyd Ireland, MD (2 min)

- Authors prefer two-incision technique
- Identify anterior intermuscular septum between anterior border of tibia and lateral border of fibula
- Make two 3-cm incisions along intermuscular septum

Based on Wolf BR, Baron J: Chronic exertional compartment syndrome and release, in Colvin AC, Flatow E, eds: Atlas of Essential Orthopaedic Procedures, *ed 2. Rosemont, IL, American Academy of Orthopaedic Surgeons, 2020, pp 775-778*

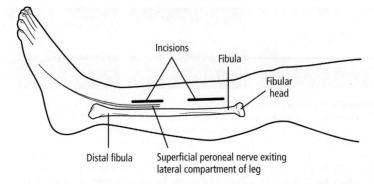

FIGURE 1 Illustration shows skin markings for the two-incision technique for anterior and lateral compartment release.

- Make first incision 10 cm proximal to ankle joint; identify superficial peroneal nerve
- Make second incision 10 cm distal to fibula head (**Figure 1**)
- Incise down to fascia; use blunt dissection to create plane over fascia
- Identify and protect superficial peroneal nerve (**Figure 2**)
- Make 1-cm incision on proximal and distal aspects of anterior and lateral compartments 1 cm anterior and posterior to intermuscular septum, taking care to be continuous with fascial release in distal incision
- The fascia can then be incised and released under the skin bridge

Posterior Compartments
- Authors prefer single-incision technique
- Make 10-cm incision 1 cm posterior to posteromedial border of tibia, at level of gastrocnemius muscle insertion (**Figure 3**)

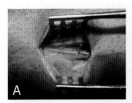
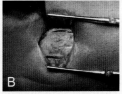
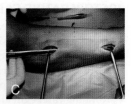

FIGURE 2 Intraoperative photographs show the two-incision technique for anterior and lateral compartment releases. **A,** The superficial peroneal nerve is visualized in the distal lateral incision. **B,** The intermuscular raphe is seen between the fascial incisions. **C,** Fasciotomy is performed using long Metzenbaum scissors in a push-cut fashion. The nerve is visualized directly and protected in the distal incision. (Reproduced with permission from Bederka B, Amendola A: Leg pain and exertional compartment syndromes, in DeLee JC, Drez D, Miller MD, eds: *DeLee and Drez's Orthopaedic Sports Medicine: Principles and Practice,* ed 3. Philadelphia, PA, Saunders Elsevier, 2010, vol. 2, pp 1857-1864.)

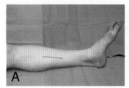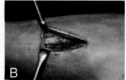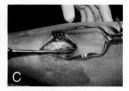

FIGURE 3 Posterior compartment releases. **A,** Photograph shows skin marking for posterior compartment releases. **B,** Intraoperative photograph shows the fascial incision. **C,** Intraoperative photograph shows the muscle fascia being taken directly off the posteromedial border of the tibia. (Reproduced with permission from Bederka B, Amendola A: Leg pain and exertional compartment syndromes, in DeLee JC, Drez D, Miller MD, eds: *DeLee and Drez's Orthopaedic Sports Medicine: Principles and Practice*, ed 3. Philadelphia, PA, Saunders Elsevier, 2010, vol. 2, pp 1857-1864.)

- Identify long saphenous nerve and vein
- Make incision at osseofascial junction of posterior tibia; release the fascia proximally to soleus and distally to posterior tibial tendon along posterior border of tibia
- Make sure release is complete proximally at junction with soleus fascial bridge
- Use Cobb elevator to release posterior tibialis off posterior tibia
- Be sure to stay on bone to protect posterior neurovascular structures
- Release tourniquet prior to wound closure here

COMPLICATIONS
- Hematoma (9%)
- Anterior ankle pain (5%)
- Superficial peroneal nerve injury (2%)
- Recurrence (2%)

POSTOPERATIVE CARE AND REHABILITATION
- Immediate weight bearing as tolerated
- Early active and passive range-of-motion exercises to prevent scarring
- Rest, ice, compression, elevation first 2 days
- Stretching in anterior and posterior compartments three times per day
- Begin physical therapy at 2 weeks
- Running can begin at 5 to 6 weeks postoperatively
- Full return to sports at 3 months

PEARLS

- Most cases of CECS diagnosed with careful and detailed history. Confirm diagnosis with pressure testing in all cases.
- During surgery, take great care to avoid injuring superficial peroneal nerve and saphenous structures.
- Must completely release involved compartments to avoid recurrence or incomplete resolution of symptoms.
- Hemostasis critical to avoid fluid collection complications after surgery.
- Early rehabilitation after surgery recommended for optimal and expedient outcomes.

96 Transtibial Amputation

INTRODUCTION
- Myofascial posterior skin flap initially used to treat peripheral vascular disease
- Mixed data on necessity of tibia/fibula bone bridge
- Ideal tibial bone length 2.5 cm for each 30 cm of height

PATIENT SELECTION
- Ischemic limbs need thorough workup before amputation
  - Ankle-brachial index greater than 0.5
  - Transcutaneous oxygen saturation greater than 20 to 30 mm Hg
  - Albumin level greater than 2.5 g/dL
  - Absolute lymphocyte count greater than 1,500/μL
- Of amputated limbs, 9% to 15% progress to further amputation

Indications
- High-energy trauma, avascular limb, congenital deformity, tumor, infection, chronic pain
- No clear absolute indications with validated outcomes exist for amputation in trauma setting
- Loss of plantar sensation not an indication in the early trauma patient
- Patients with dysvascular limbs considered for amputation have nonreconstructible injuries or are not revascularization candidates
- When considering bone-bridge synostosis, ensure patient can safely endure longer tourniquet times (115 versus 71 minutes) and longer surgical times (179 versus 112 minutes)
- Authors recommend reserving bone-bridge synostosis for young, healthy, active patients
- Those with fibular instability and disruption of interosseous membrane may benefit from bone-bridge synostosis as primary or revision amputation

---

Based on Ficke JR, Stinner DJ: Transtibial amputation, in Colvin AC, Flatow E, eds: Atlas of Essential Orthopaedic Procedures, *ed 2. Rosemont, IL, American Academy of Orthopaedic Surgeons, 2020, pp 779-785.*

Contraindications

- Dysvascular limbs not meeting preoperative assessment criteria
- Consider procedures for optimization of wound healing or higher level amputation

PROCEDURE

Room Setup/Patient Positioning

- Supine position on standard table
- Bump under ipsilateral limb
- Thigh tourniquet

Special Instruments/Equipment/Implants

- Basic major orthopaedic set
- Oscillating saw
- Drill
- Amputation knife optional
- Nonabsorbable suture ligatures for arteries; simple ligatures or vessel clips for veins
- Suction drain
- Small or large fragment set for bone-bridge synostosis or screw fixation
- Appropriate bone-bridge fixation device
- Chisel or osteotome
- C-arm

 VIDEO 96.1 Transtibial Amputation. COL James R. Ficke, MD; MAJ Daniel J. Stinner, MD (5 min)

Surgical Technique

- Perform exsanguination
- Mark tibial tubercle
- Mark skin 1 cm distal to projected tibial cut
- Use hemostat to draw out edges, help minimize dog ears (**Figure 1**)
- Mark posterior skin flap so it is 1.5 times length of transverse cut, to create posterior flap
- Posterior flap should be distal to musculotendinous junction of gastrocnemius
- Incise marked incision through fascia
- Deep medial longitudinal incision should be anterior to long saphenous vein so it is maintained for drainage
- Identify deep, superficial peroneal nerves; pull slight traction and resect sharply
- Identify the anterior tibial artery; tie off and ligate
- If bone bridge planned, follow these steps:

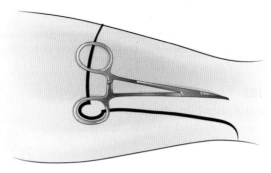

FIGURE 1 Illustration depicts a method of minimizing redundant skin "dog ears."

- ▶ Elevate periosteal flap using single-beveled wide chisel
- ▶ Sharply incise anterior and posterior margins of anteromedial tibial periosteum for 8 to 10 cm distally
- ▶ Raise flap with bevel positioned superficially
- ▶ Small bone fragments are left attached to periosteum (**Figure 2**)
- ▶ Critical to have sufficient periosteum to reach well past lateral edge of fibula
- ▶ Protect flap with moist gauze sponge
- ▶ Isolate remaining tibia using curved periosteal elevator
- ▶ Divide intraosseous membrane and identify and prepare fibula for osteotomy
- Sharply dissect anterior muscle at level of anterior incision or can use electrocautery
- Identify fibula and mark for cut 1 cm proximal to tibia cut
- Transect tibia and fibula using saw; bevel edges with rasp

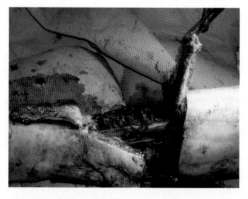

FIGURE 2 Intraoperative photograph shows elevation of the periosteal flap. Multiple small bone fragments can be seen.

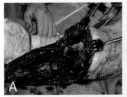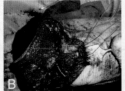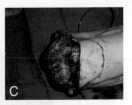

FIGURE 3 Intraoperative photographs show transtibial amputation. **A**, Extended posterior flap with tapered gastrocnemius. Note that the tibial bevel does not encroach on the medullary canal. **B**, Myodesis is achieved with large braided suture to bone. The periosteal flap can be seen underneath, and the submuscular drain is in place. **C**, The completed myodesis is shown. The posterior skin flap overlap is traced before suprafascial skin excision.

- Bevel only anterior cortex of tibia at 45°, without entering canal
- Transect deep posterior compartment muscles at level of tibial cut
- Preserve gastrocnemius fascia
- Once through deep posterior compartment, identify tibial nerve and inject with 1% lidocaine; sharply transect nerve under slight traction at bone cut level; perform same steps for peroneal nerve
- Identify posterior tibial artery and veins; tie off and ligate
- Taper gastrocnemius down to distal posterior flap (**Figure 3**)
- Release tourniquet; attain hemostasis
- Using gastrocnemius, perform fascial myodesis to anterior aspect of tibia
- Perform myodesis via Krackow sutures within aponeurosis; attach to anterior periosteum or via drill holes in anterior tibial cortex and to the anterior compartment fascia
- Myodesis should cross gastrocnemius aponeurosis
- Place small drain into deep space
- Attach borders of gastrocnemius to anterior fascia for deep closure
- When possible, keep anterior closure more proximal and outside of weight-bearing area of tibia
- Close skin with vertical mattress sutures to reduce tension
- Place gauze dressing with plaster splint to keep knee extended

 VIDEO 96.2 Bone Bridging in Transtibial Amputation. Marco A. Guedes de Souza Pinto, MD; Michael S. Pinzur, MD; Lew C. Schon, MD; Douglas G. Smith, MD (13 min)

 VIDEO 96.3 Periosteal Flap Development. COL James R. Ficke, MD; MAJ Daniel J. Stinner, MD (2 min)

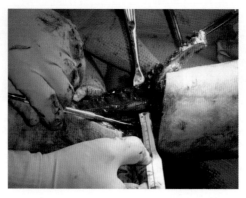

FIGURE 4 Intraoperative photograph shows measurement of the intraosseous distance at the level of tibial transection in preparation for a bone-bridge procedure.

Additional Preparation for Bone-Bridge Procedure

- Do not disrupt tibial periosteum; it is used for sleeve
- When marking out anterior incision, mark vertical line on anterior tibia to protect tibia
- Fibula cut is much longer than traditional level; must add distance between tibia and fibula plus 2 cm for inlay into tibia to usual distal cut (**Figure 4**)
- Make tibia cut in the usual manner
- Make extended distal fibula cut
- Make proximal cut at same level as tibial cut
- Cut a notch in the posterolateral aspect of tibia to completely house fibula
- Notch fibula into tibia and secure using one long 3.5-mm cortical screw running from lateral fibula, through fibula intramedullary canal, into medial cortex of tibia
- Attach tibial periosteal sleeve around transverse fibula fragment and to lateral aspect of fibular periosteum

COMPLICATIONS

- Pain
- Edema
- Knee flexion contractures
- Wound breakdown

POSTOPERATIVE CARE AND REHABILITATION

Phase 1 (Week 1)

- Edema control, bed-to-wheelchair activities, range-of-motion exercises, gait training with walker/crutches, and no prosthesis
- Continue casting to maintain extension

© 2021 American Academy of Orthopaedic Surgeons

- Perioperative antibiotics until drain removal
- Drain removed at 48 hours
- Dressing remains in place for first week
- Rehabilitation goals—Achieve functional mobility/basic ambulation (bed mobility, transfers, ambulation with assistive device, wheelchair use as appropriate), maintain/restore baseline balance and conditioning; appropriate residual limb management/self-care is learned

Phase 2 (Weeks 2 to 10)
- New prosthesis, progressive weight bearing with wheeled walker, walking on uneven surfaces, navigating home environment
- Suture removed at 3 weeks or when wound appears secure (especially in patients with diabetes)
- Begin shrinker use after sutures out
- Continue therapy for mobility and strengthening
- Learn limb care
- Begin wearing prosthesis when skin stable
- Rehabilitation goals—Appropriate exercises performed independently (strengthening, core stability/lumbar stabilization, balance, cardiovascular conditioning); gain sufficient range of motion to allow optimal gait training with use of prosthetic device; achieve independence with mobility and ambulation with appropriate assistive devices; achieve independence with residual limb care

Phase 3 (Weeks 11 and Later)
- Return to active lifestyle
- Advance ambulation
- Independent limb/prosthesis care
- Vocational training
- Rehabilitation goals—Weight-bearing and -shifting activities progressed; rehabilitation exercises performed independently; gait normalized; gait progresses to modified independence or independence with appropriate assistive device; return to high-level/high-impact conditioning, organized and individual sport activity, and vocation-specific training achieved

PEARLS

- Place deep medial longitudinal incision anterior to long saphenous vein to permit venous clearance.
- Clear anterior compartment muscles at or proximal to tibial bone cut to reduce bulk anterolaterally; required for bridge but also eases tension-free skin closure.
- When creating periosteal layer for bone bridge, can use single-bevel chisel to elevate attached bone chips. Place bevel up and use alternating wrist actions to create smaller malleable bone fragments attached to periosteum.

- Vascular ligation requires suture ligature or vascular clip to prevent pulsatile disruption of simple ties—the "rubber band on a newspaper" effect.
- Round the bone ends with rasp to prevent potential sharp corners. A power saw held at angle and pulled across sharp surface is effective power rasp. Make sure anterior bevel does not encroach into medullary canal; can resorb to leave two sharp corners.
- Use braided single-component suture material for myodesis. FiberWire (Arthrex) associated with sterile abscesses.
- When preparing sutures for myodesis, authors make sure material crosses posterior gastrocnemius aponeurosis and is pulled tightly into muscle tissue. Gastrocnemius and associated myodesis can later atrophy and leave suture loose.

CHAPTER

97 Midfoot Amputations

INTRODUCTION
- Most commonly performed midfoot amputation is transmetatarsal, and then Lisfranc and Chopart (**Figure 1**)
- In the United States, 133,235 amputations are performed annually
- 82% related to vascular conditions
- Of lower-extremity amputations, more than 50% are transtibial or transfemoral and 31% are pedal

PATIENT SELECTION
Indications and Contraindications
- Primary indication for midfoot amputation—Extensive soft-tissue compromise of forefoot that does not allow more distal amputation
- Contraindications
  - Inadequate perfusion at level of amputation
  - Infection above level of amputation

PREOPERATIVE EVALUATION
Laboratory and Diagnostic Tests
- Laboratory tests—Complete blood count, absolute lymphocyte count, erythrocyte sedimentation rate, C-reactive protein level, albumin level, protein level
  - White blood cell count greater than 12,000 indicates risk of infection
  - Absolute lymphocyte count greater than 1,500 indicates better healing potential
  - Albumin level greater than 3.0 g/dL, protein level greater than 6.0 g/dL indicate improved wound healing
- Vascular workup
  - Evaluate peripheral pulses
  - Evaluate skin changes, hair growth on foot, capillary refill
  - Ankle-brachial index <0.9 shows impaired profusion; greater than 0.5 shows greater potential for distal stump healing

Based on Van Dyke B, McGann MR, Witt B, Philbin TM: Midfoot amputations, in Colvin AC, Flatow E, eds: Atlas of Essential Orthopaedic Procedures, ed 2. Rosemont, IL, American Academy of Orthopaedic Surgeons, 2020, pp 786-793

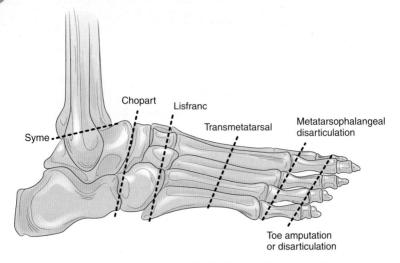

FIGURE 1 Illustration depicts levels of partial foot amputation.

- Arterial Doppler ultrasound—Monophasic waveform shows occlusive disease
- Transcutaneous oxygen pressure less than 30 mm Hg indicates poor healing potential
- Angiography identifies level of disease, possible mechanism for revascularization

Imaging
- Three (preferably weight-bearing) radiographic views of the foot and ankle
- CT to delineate pathologic processes; detect abnormalities missed on plain radiographs; identify tumors, fractures, soft-tissue abscesses
- MRI to evaluate neoplasm or infection (**Figure 2**)
- Nuclear imaging—Indium 111-labeled white blood cell scan specific for osteomyelitis; technetium Tc 99m scan adds accuracy in determining infectious process

PROCEDURE
Room Setup/Patient Positioning
- Supine position, bump under affected hip
- Use Esmarch bandage to exsanguinate foot, ankle
- Use same Esmarch as ankle tourniquet

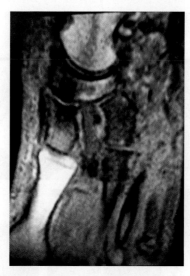

FIGURE 2 T2-weighted magnetic resonance image depicts increased uptake of the first metatarsal bone associated with osteomyelitis.

Surgical Technique

Transmetatarsal Amputation

- Make dorsal medial incision starting at midshaft of first metatarsal over to midshaft level of fifth ray
- Plantar incision is at level of metatarsal heads (**Figure 3**)
- Sharply dissect through peroneal and posterior tibial nerves
- Ligate dorsalis pedis artery and other traversing vasculature
- Place tendons on traction; transect proximally to allow retraction
- Elevate soft tissue off metatarsals distal to proximally
- Connect dorsal, plantar incisions, making "fish mouth" incision
- Use small oscillating saw just proximal to level of dorsal skin incision for metatarsal amputation, aiming dorsal distal to plantar proximal; bevel first and fifth metatarsals toward center of foot to protect soft tissues
- Take care to preserve peroneus brevis
- Debulk plantar flap as needed to allow closure
- Place drain if concerned about infection
- Place absorbable suture to approximate deep fascia; approximate integument using 3-0 nylon horizontal mattress suture or skin staples

Lisfranc Amputation

- Start dorsal incision just dorsomedial aspect of foot, distal to first metatarsocuneiform

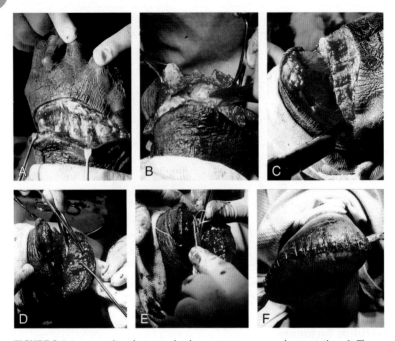

FIGURE 3 Intraoperative photographs show a transmetatarsal amputation. **A**, The dorsal skin incision. **B**, The soft tissues are resected from the plantar surface of the metatarsal bones to maintain a full-thickness myocutaneous flap. **C**, An oscillating saw is used to transect the metatarsal bones at the level of the midshaft in a dorsal distal to plantar proximal direction. **D**, The plantar flap is debulked to allow appropriate closure. **E**, The deep fascia is approximated using absorbable suture. **F**, The completed transmetatarsal amputation, with the skin approximated using skin staples. (Courtesy of Ronald M. Sage, DPM, FACFAS, Department of Orthopaedic Surgery and Rehabilitation, Loyola University Health System, Maywood, IL.)

- Start medial longitudinal incision at medial edge of dorsal incision; continue to just distal to the first metatarsocuneiform to metatarsal neck, curve plantarly
- Start lateral longitudinal incision at lateral edge of dorsal incision; extend to neck of fifth metatarsal, curving plantarly
- The plantar incision connects medial, lateral incisions on plantar surface transversely under metatarsal necks
- Dissect soft tissue as described previously
- Expose tarsometatarsal joints; disarticulate first, third, fourth metatarsals off tarsals sharply
- Must cut second metatarsal at level of cuneiforms because of its recessed position
- Resect fifth metatarsal at level of metaphysis to preserve peroneus brevis attachment
- Smooth off bone edges; perform layered closure as described previously

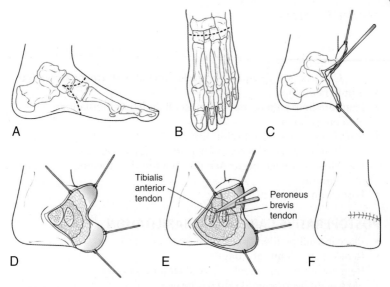

FIGURE 4 Illustrations show Chopart amputation. **A**, Lateral view of incision. **B**, Dorsal view of incision. **C** and **D**, Dorsal and plantar flaps are shown after resection of the distal foot. **E**, Transfer of the tibialis anterior tendon to the talar neck and transfer of the peroneus brevis tendon to the anterior calcaneus are shown. **F**, Appearance of the completed amputation after skin closure.

Chopart Amputation

- Start dorsal incision at dorsomedial aspect of foot, just distal to navicular tuberosity (**Figure 4**); end dorsal incision at midpoint between base of fifth metatarsal and lateral malleolus
- Medial longitudinal incision starts on medial edge of dorsal incision and runs distally to level of midshaft of first metatarsal, curving posteriorly
- Lateral longitudinal incision starts on lateral edge of dorsal incision runs distally to level of midshaft of fifth metatarsal, curving posteriorly
- Plantar incision connects the two longitudinal incisions, running transversely at level of midshaft of metatarsal
- Dissect deep soft tissue as described previously; for Chopart, must preserve anterior tibialis tendon and peroneus brevis tendon
- Visualize talonavicular, calcaneocuboid joints
- Sharply dissect ligaments, tendons to expose joint
- Smooth bony edges of remaining calcaneus; remove exposed articular cartilage
- Reattach anterior tibialis to talus; reattach peroneus brevis to calcaneus
- Close wounds as described previously

COMPLICATIONS

- Infection
  - ▹ May result from inadequate resection of pathologic bone, nonsterile technique
  - ▹ Can lead to subsequent surgeries, including further amputation
- Stump neuromas
- Phantom limb pain occurs in almost all midfoot amputations
- Skin breakdown
- Muscle imbalance/foot deformity; may result in hard-to-fit stump
  - ▹ Equinovarus most common, from Achilles overpull
  - ▹ Most patients need Achilles tendon lengthening to prevent equinus
- Formation of bony exostoses

POSTOPERATIVE CARE AND REHABILITATION

- Place in well-padded splint, with foot in neutral
- Remove any drains at 2 days
- Remove sutures at 3 weeks or until wound is healed
- No weight bearing until skin has healed
- Work on fitting prosthesis after swelling resolves
- Use prosthesis, ankle-foot orthosis (AFO) based on patient function, comfort with ambulation training
- Patients with diabetes require full-length rocker-bottom shoe to keep pressure off foot
- Patients with Lisfranc amputation need longer toe plate, more height to better distribute pressure; patients with Lisfranc amputation also may do well with AFO to protect incision, prevent equinus
- Patients with Chopart amputation generally need full-length shoe and AFO for stability while walking
- Can use Lange partial foot prostheses for more active patients

PEARLS

- ■ Maintain full-thickness myocutaneous skin flaps to avoid wound complications.
- ■ Create long plantar flaps so thick plantar skin can be pulled over distal aspect of stump to prevent wound complications, produce better weight-bearing surface.
- ■ Lisfranc amputation maintain peroneus brevis insertion and function.
- ■ Chopart amputation reinsert the the anterior tibialis to talus and peroneus brevis to calcaneus; prevents equinus deformity.
- ■ To prevent an equinovarus deformity of the stump, an Achilles tendon lengthening procedure is often performed at the time of the midfoot amputation.

Spine

7

Section Editor
Andrew C. Hecht, MD

Anterior Cervical Diskectomy and Fusion

PATIENT SELECTION
- Anterior cervical diskectomy and fusion was first described in the 1950s for treatment of cervical radiculopathy
- Categorize symptoms and examination findings into axial neck pain, radiculopathy, and myelopathy, or a combination of the three

Indications for Treatment of Cervical Radiculopathy
- Failure of a 3-month trial of nonsurgical methods to relieve radicular upper extremity pain with or without neurologic deficit
- Presence of a progressive neurologic deficit
- Neuroradiographic findings must be consistent with signs and symptoms

Indications for Treatment of Cervical Myelopathy
- Progressive myelopathy
- Moderate or severe myelopathy, even if stable and of short duration (<1 year)
- Mild myelopathy that affects activities of daily living
- Emphasize to patient that goal is to prevent neurologic worsening, although most of a patient's neurologic function improves following decompression

Contraindications
- Predominantly dorsal compression of neural elements
- Isolated trauma to posterior elements that is not amenable to anterior approach
- Relative contraindications: soft-tissue destruction or anomalies of the anterior cervical spine (eg, post radiation)

Based on An HS, Cha TD: Anterior cervical diskectomy and fusion, in Colvin AC, Flatow E, eds: Atlas of Essential Orthopaedic Procedures, ed 2. Rosemont, IL, American Academy of Orthopaedic Surgeons, 2020, pp 795-800.

PREOPERATIVE IMAGING

- Plain radiography—AP and lateral; oblique views evaluate narrowing of neuroforamina; flexion-extension views evaluate instability and/or rigidity of sagittal plane deformity
- MRI—Most sensitive for assessing the morphology of the neural elements and compression of spinal cord and/or nerve roots; less effective at detecting foraminal stenosis and demonstrating cortical margins
- CT—Best for evaluating bony morphology (**Figure 1**)
- Myelography—Useful when patient has existing hardware; demonstrates filling defects as a means of assessing neural compression, although cause of contrast blockade cannot be shown

PROCEDURE

Room Setup/Patient Positioning

- Supine position on standard table
- Reverse Trendelenburg position can reduce venous bleeding
- Axial traction with Gardner-Wells tongs (15 to 20 lb); neck slightly extended and positioned in neutral rotation
- Arms adducted and shoulders taped with distal axial traction, which aids in visualizing lower cervical levels

Special Instruments/Equipment/Implants

- Magnification using loupes or microscope
- Lighting to optimize visualization

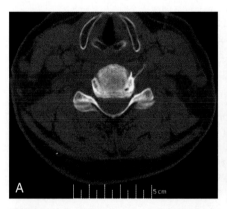 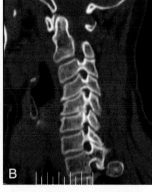

FIGURE 1 CT scans used to evaluate a patient before anterior cervical diskectomy and fusion. **A,** An axial cut through the C5-6 interspace demonstrates foraminal stenosis on the left side from osteophyte formation. **B,** An oblique CT reconstruction demonstrates the specific areas of bony overgrowth into the left C5-6 foramen.

Surgical Technique

- Most commonly employs a transverse incision from midline to middle of the sternocleidomastoid muscle (SCM), which allows exposure of up to three levels
- May use longitudinal incision along anterior border of SCM for exposure of four or more levels (rare)
- Historically, a left-side approach is advocated due to the more consistent course of the recurrent laryngeal nerve (RLN) under the aortic trunk, although a recent review showed no difference in nerve injury from right- or left-side approaches; the right RLN ascends in the neck after passing around subclavian vessels and courses medially and cranially at the C6-7 level, often with the inferior thyroid artery; the left RLN ascends after curving around the aortic arch along the tracheoesophageal groove
- After incision, incise the platysma in line with the incision
- The superior, middle and inferior thyroid arteries extend through the pretracheal fascia from the carotid to the midline
- Superficial layer of the deep cervical fascia is split, followed by the pretracheal fascia, moving the trachea and esophagus medially, while moving the carotid sheath, its contents, and the SCM laterally
- Prevertebral fascia is exposed; a lateral radiograph is taken at this time to determine the level of exposure
- Mobilize longus colli muscles laterally with a Cobb elevator or curet
- Place self-retaining deep retractors laterally; cranial-caudal disk space distraction may be accomplished with the use of Caspar (vertebral) pins at the surgeon's discretion
- Perform diskectomy by incising anulus; remove disk with curets and rongeurs
- Use a high-speed burr to remove anterior osteophytes and create rectangular window to prepare for grafting; preparation continues laterally to uncovertebral joints and posteriorly to the posterior longitudinal ligament
- Remove posterior longitudinal ligament in cases of myelopathy or extruded disk herniation
- Direct decompression of nerve roots can be performed, working from lateral to medial, using a Kerrison rongeur or curets
- Graft choice is at discretion of the surgeon, with many choices available, including autograft, tricortical iliac crest allograft, and polyetheretherketone
- Graft height should be at least 5 and 2 mm greater than the preexisting disk space height; do not distract the disk space more than 4 mm; doing so can result in graft collapse and pseudarthrosis due to overloading of the graft
- Prepare end plates using a high-speed burr to create flat surfaces
- If using tricortical graft, the leading cortical edge faces anteriorly and is set 2 mm posterior to the edge of vertebral bodies

- Choose plate and affix to the anterior surface of the vertebrae with screws that are angled away from the graft; a horizontal screw allows the most resistance to pullout
- Take radiographs to assess plate placement
- Close wound in layers beginning with platysmal approximation and subcutaneous sutures over a suction drain that remains in place for 24 hours

COMPLICATIONS

- Vascular injury
- Esophageal and tracheal injuries
- Vocal cord paralysis (RLN injury)
- Horner syndrome
- Durotomy
- Neural injury
- Infection
- Adjacent segment degeneration
- Graft failure
- Instrumentation failure

POSTOPERATIVE CARE AND REHABILITATION

- Cervical orthosis (soft or hard) depending on surgeon preference
- Monitoring of patients postoperatively for the first 24 hours for airway compromise

PEARLS

- A 45° oblique reconstruction of a preoperative CT scan allows excellent assessment of the neural foramina.
- Reverse Trendelenburg positioning of the bed can reduce venous bleeding.
- Adequate elevation of the longus colli muscles allows proper deep retractor placement, assessment of the midline, and visualization of the uncovertebral joints for foraminal decompression.
- Graft thickness should be 2 mm larger than the preoperative disk space height to allow foraminal distraction.
- Distraction of more than 4 mm can overload the graft, leading to graft collapse or pseudarthrosis.
- A central burr hole in the superior and inferior end plates increases vascularity to the interbody graft while maintaining end-plate structural integrity.
- To assess for esophageal penetration, flush diluted indigo carmine through a nasogastric or orogastric tube at the level of the esophagus to check for extravasation into the surgical field.

Anterior Cervical Corpectomy and Fusion/ Instrumentation

PATIENT SELECTION

Indications

- Most commonly performed for cervical spondylosis, with symptoms of cervical radiculopathy, myelopathy, or both
- Severe or progressive neurologic deficit or pain not responsive to non-surgical management
- Cervical spondylotic myelopathy due to degenerative process with aging, also associated with ossification of posterior longitudinal ligament (OPLL), hypertrophy of ligamentum flavum, or a congenitally narrowed cervical canal; other causes include trauma, instability, tumor, infection, epidural abscess, and kyphotic deformity
- Early surgical management benefits severe or progressive myelopathy with concordant radiographic evidence of cord compression
- Nonprogressive myelopathy with myelopathic symptoms and long-tract signs, Japanese Orthopaedic Association score less than 13 points, radiographic evidence of cord compression
- Nonsurgical management not successful in reversing or permanently preventing progression of myelopathy
- Goals—To decompress spinal cord, prevent further neurologic deterioration, possibly reverse myelopathic symptoms
- Secondary goals—Fusion to stabilize abnormal motion segments, neck pain relief, deformity correction
- Advantages of anterior approach—Can directly decompress structures causing cord compression and nerve root impingement
- Consider corpectomy over multilevel diskectomy in patient with two or three affected levels, developmental stenosis with osseous anterior-posterior canal diameter less than 13 mm, significant fixed cervical kyphosis, posterior osteophytes adjacent to end plate, or free disk fragment migrated posterior to vertebral body, or for significant component of spondylotic neck pain
- Bone graft/interbody spacer needs to fuse two surfaces versus four in two-level anterior cervical diskectomy and fusion

---

Based on Kang DG, Lehman RA Jr, Riew KD: Anterior cervical corpectomy and fusion/ instrumentation, in Colvin AC, Flatow E, eds: Atlas of Essential Orthopaedic Procedures, ed 2. Rosemont, IL, American Academy of Orthopaedic Surgeons, 2020, pp 801-813.

- For three or more levels, perform corpectomy of one level and diskectomies at remaining levels to preserve stability; corpectomy-diskectomy less likely to extrude graft or collapse

CONTRAINDICATIONS

- Tracheoesophageal trauma preventing safe anterior cervical exposure
- Severe osteoporosis
- Consider posterior approach when posterior compression results from buckling of hypertrophic ligamentum flavum or shingling of laminae in patients with hyperlordosis or in the setting of three or more affected levels in patients with no kyphotic deformity or neck pain
- Authors prefer anterior surgery; advantages include lower risk of infection, more direct decompression, less postoperative pain

PREOPERATIVE IMAGING

- AP, lateral, flexion-extension lateral plain radiographic views localize pathology, assess alignment and stability
- MRI evaluates neural structures, soft tissue, vertebral arteries
- CT myelography when MRI cannot be obtained or images difficult to interpret
- Plain CT—For fusion assessment, OPLL or ossification of ligamentum flavum, assessment of diffuse idiopathic skeletal hyperostosis and autofusion of segments, assessment of autofused facets
- Angiography in tumor cases

PROCEDURE

Patient Positioning

- Supine position with arms tucked to sides; bump between scapulae; if iliac crest autograft used, bump underneath hip
- For fibular strut autograft use, place thigh tourniquet with bump underneath ipsilateral hip
- Transcranial motor- and somatosensory-evoked potentials to monitor spinal cord activity
- For severe myelopathy, anesthetic protocol includes awake, fiberoptic, or nasotracheal intubation
- Transient intravenous anesthesia to facilitate motor-evoked potential readings
- Use 3-in silk tape to tape head to table to limit rotation
- Apply Gardner-Wells tongs in corpectomies of three or more levels with initial traction of 15 lb of weight; review evoked potentials before proceeding
- Tape shoulders to bottom of table with 3-in silk tape; avoid overpulling shoulders; traction brachial plexopathy can result

---

Special Instruments/Equipment/Implants

Graft

- Authors prefer freeze-dried allograft fibula or ulna
- Graft should leave 5 to 7 mm of lateral wall
- Determine width of vertebral body preoperatively on axial MRI or CT

Operating Microscope

- Authors use operating microscope; loupe magnification with fiberoptic headlight also may be used
- Microscope advantages over loupes—Magnification easily changed, magnification more powerful than loupe, enhanced lighting and visualization, allows co-surgeon to assist during difficult complication such as dural tear
- Bring microscope into operating field after disk space localized with lateral image, usually from side of assisting surgeon

Approach

- Smith-Robinson anteromedial approach for exposure of middle and lower cervical spine; authors prefer left-side approach but right or left can be used; approach may be dictated by prior anterior cervical exposure
- For revision anterior cervical exposure, preoperative evaluation with direct laryngoscopy needed to identify residual vocal cord paralysis; if present, perform approach on same side as previous surgery; if no paralysis, approach from opposite side

Landmarks for Incision

- Palpate surface landmarks when deciding incision location
- Approximate level of incision by examining preoperative lateral image

Surgical Technique

Superficial Exposure

- For single-level corpectomy, make 3- to 4-cm transverse incision beginning just past midline and extending to medial border of sternocleidomastoid (SCM) muscle
- For multiple-level corpectomy, extend skin incision farther across midline to lateral border of SCM
- Mark skin incision—Draw vertical lines every centimeter to serve as landmarks during closure
- Infiltrate skin as superficially as possible using local anesthetic with epinephrine and 25-gauge needle
- Take localizing radiograph
- Incise skin with No. 10 blade; switch to electrocautery to incise subcutaneous tissue and divide platysma transversely

- Use cautery to develop plane 1 cm cranially and caudally, then finger dissection to create subplatysmal pouches; carefully note location of anterior jugular vein and numerous superficial veins from external jugular system
- Place small Weitlaner self-retaining retractor
- Incise fascia in interval between strap muscles and SCM using cautery followed by Metzenbaum scissors; develop interval with blunt finger dissection; palpate carotid pulse deep to SCM, delineating location of carotid sheath laterally and trachea and esophagus medially; perform blunt dissection through interval posteriorly toward midline to prevertebral fascia and longus colli muscle
- Place appendiceal retractor to aid exposure
- May retract omohyoid muscle medially with trachea or divide to improve exposure; identify it before starting deep dissection
- Keep SCM fascia intact to reduce bleeding, and keep plane of dissection out of carotid sheath; no need to identify recurrent laryngeal nerve

Deep Exposure

- Palpate and visualize anterior vertebral bodies and longus colli
- Divide prevertebral fascia longitudinally with scissors
- Perform exposure of C2 and C3 levels with caution; superior laryngeal and hypoglossal nerves may cross plane of dissection; gently retract them with digastric and stylohyoid muscles
- Inferior thyroid artery/vein encountered at C6, C7 levels; clamp and cauterize or gently retract them to obtain exposure
- Obtain localizing image; if confident about correct level, place 21-gauge spinal needle (bent at two right angles to prevent accidental puncture of cord) into disk space; if doubt exists regarding level, place clamp on edge of longus colli at presumed level to avoid injuring uninvolved disk
- Bring microscope into field; perform rest of procedure under magnification
- Enlarge cranial-caudal extent of the deep dissection
- Mark midline between longus colli in vertebral bodies above and below each disk space with electrocautery; provides landmark for placement of Caspar pins and plate
- Check preoperative magnetic resonance image for presence of anomalous or tortuous vertebral artery
- On localizing radiograph, confirm correct level, correct patient, and correct alignment
- Elevate medial borders of longus colli muscle in full-thickness flaps with bipolar cautery; sympathetic plexus lies superficial to lateral aspect of longus, so avoid lateral dissection (more than 6 to 7 mm) or cauterization on ventral surface of longus; assistant elevates longus with Penfield No. 2 while surgeon cauterizes bleeders with bipolar cautery

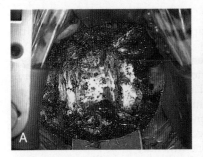
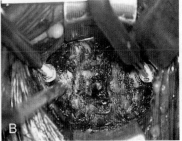

FIGURE 1 Intraoperative photographs show the final steps in deep exposure for anterior cervical corpectomy and fusion. **A**, Adequate visualization includes the vertebral body with the intervertebral disk above and below. **B**, The Caspar pins are placed. Note the 5-mm suction tip used to gauge Caspar pin placement distance from the edge of the disk space.

- Elevate longus colli laterally until costal process of vertebral body and uncovertebral joints exposed
- Place medial-lateral self-retaining retractors under longus colli
- Outline and incise disk space and anterior longitudinal ligament with monopolar cautery (**Figure 1, A**)
- Remove anterior osteophytes with Leksell rongeur and/or burr; irrigate site
- Place Caspar pins (**Figure 1, B**); place cranial pin 8 to 10 mm above superior edge of disk space; place caudal pin 5 mm below caudal edge of disk space; direct pins parallel with disk space
- Make alignment changes by placing bump under shoulders or head or by converging or diverging tips of Caspar pins
- Remove Weitlaner retractor; place Caspar distractor

Disk Removal
- Single-level C6 corpectomy is described here; for multilevel corpectomies, duplicate single-level procedure
- Incise disks above and below vertebral body with No. 15 blade; do not plunge knife deeper than sharp edge of blade (11 mm)
- Remove disk with pituitary; repeat to remove C6-7 disk
- Use largest microcuret that will fit into disk space to scrape disk and cartilaginous end plate off C6 end plate; for concave C5 end plate, turn curet face up and slightly cranially and scrape from bottom up; clean uncinates of disk material
- Repeat for C6-7 disk space
- Relax retractor every 30 to 45 minutes to prevent constant pressure on trachea and esophagus
- To remove posterior disk material, use 2- or 3-mm curet until posterior longitudinal ligament (PLL) exposed
- Remove remaining soft tissue and cartilage with burr

Initial Corpectomy

- Use 2-mm matchstick carbide-tipped burr (side-cutting rather than end-cutting); safer than Kerrison
- Use uncovertebral joints as reference to lateral borders of the vertebral body; lateral vertebral osteophytes can be mistaken for lateral vertebral body, endangering vertebral artery
- Plane off concave C5 end plate into smooth surface by removing ventral overhanging bone; collect bone dust for grafting
- Mark corpectomy width with electrocautery by laying graft on top of vertebral body and removing bone with burr
- Remove cortical bone from superior and inferior end plates and ventral surface of C6 until bleeding cancellous bone exposed
- Use Leksell rongeur to harvest four equal pieces of cancellous bone from body of C6, leaving only posterior cortex and 2 mm of cancellous bone; save removed cancellous bone for grafting
- If bleeding encountered, continue corpectomy without stopping to obtain hemostasis; coagulate bleeding with thrombin-soaked gelfoam or hemostatic liquefied collagen product

---

 VIDEO 99.1 Cervical Corpectomy Part I: Exposure, Diskectomy, and Initial Corpectomy. Daniel G. Kang, MD; Ronald A. Lehman, Jr, MD; K. Daniel Riew, MD (19 min)

Central Decompression

- Perform central decompression at cephalad level (C5-6) using burr; keep burr in one plane without going deeper or shallower while moving it
- Using medial-lateral motion, use burr to thin PLL to 1 mm; at this depth, gradually move cranially and caudally to remove all osteophytes; caudally, remove remaining cortex of C6 until decompression achieved; a 5-mm band of posterior wall usually can be left intact; its removal reduces torsional stability (**Figure 2**)
- Obtain hemostasis with absorbable hemostats or hemostatic matrix and cottonoid patty
- Decompress C6-7 disk space in same manner; if patient has mild OPLL, can be thinned down with same burr; use 1- or 2-mm curet to remove remaining bone; if OPLL is severe, it may involve dura; best to thin area until 1 to 2 mm of bone remains; surrounding bone thinned until ossified dura "floats" ventrally
- Inspect behind PLL for disk herniation fragment with 2-mm curet, and use curet to remove any trapped fragment

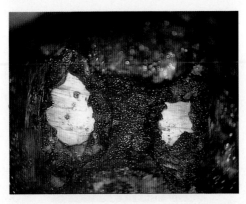

FIGURE 2 Intraoperative photograph shows the surgical area after central decompression for anterior cervical corpectomy and fusion. A burr was used to remove posterior osteophytes, and the posterior longitudinal ligament was thinned to a thickness of approximately 1 mm.

 VIDEO 99.2 Cervical Corpectomy Part II: Central Decompression, Foraminal Decompression, Fusion, and Instrumentation. Daniel G. Kang, MD; Ronald A. Lehman, Jr, MD; K. Daniel Riew, MD (35 min)

Foraminal Decompression and Uncinate Resection

- To protect vertebral artery, clean out contralateral C5-C6 uncinate with 2-mm curet; place Penfield No. 4 lateral to uncinate and tilt side to side to enlarge space; replace with Penfield No. 2; control bleeding with absorbable hemostats and patty; clean out soft tissues in uncinate with pituitary
- Establish lateral border of decompression with burr; to avoid "past pointing," burr in plane parallel with vertebral artery or nerve root in anterior-to-posterior direction, moving laterally until 1 to 2 mm bone remains medial to Penfield No. 2 blade
- To decompress nerve root, start medially where central decompression left off; place burr on PLL and, using medial-lateral burring motion parallel with nerve root, burr off all foraminal osteophytes; remove remaining bone with 1- and 2-mm microcurets; decompression is complete when surgeon can palpate lateral margin of C6 pedicle and no bone overlies root; if severe uncinate hypertrophy is present, resect uncinate by twisting Penfield No. 2 to break off thinned lateral uncinate
- For ipsilateral side, use same technique; hand may obscure visualization, take care to prevent injury to root; less experienced surgeon can move to opposite side of table to finish foraminal decompression (**Figure 3**)

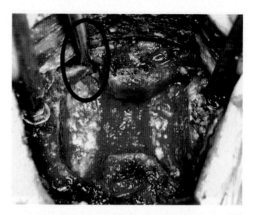

FIGURE 3 Intraoperative photograph shows foraminal decompression and unci-nate resection for anterior cervical corpectomy and fusion. Following a thorough foraminal decompression, all four foramina should be well visualized. A Penfield No. 2 (marked by the oval) points out the extent of the foraminal decompression at C6-7 on the right side.

End-Plate Preparation and Screw Sizing
- Burr off superior end plate of C7 to expose bleeding bone; freshen infe-rior end plate of C5 until bleeding
- Irrigate field copiously
- Place screws into disk level to determine longest screw that can be used; cranial screws (at level when sunk into plate) should just touch dura when placed straight in disk space; start C5 screw close to end plate and angle cranially; choose caudal screw that is 2 mm shy of dura when screw head is held in same depth as when in plate

Graft
- Measure size of bone graft using cervical plates as templates; graft caudal surface is angled to match 15° cranial tilt of C7 superior end plate; cranial surface is straight to minimally lordotic to match end plate of C5
- Fill graft cavity with bone dust, fragments, and demineralized matrix; distract retractor again; place graft into trough under Caspar distrac-tion; tamp into place 2 mm below anterior cortex; release distraction through Caspar pins to load graft
- Burr uncinate area lateral to graft to bleeding bone; shape and wedge chunks of corpectomy bone into gaps (**Figure 4**)

Instrumentation
- Choose shortest plate that spans length of defect; place unicortical fixed-angle screws cranially and variable-angle screws caudally; sup-plement two-level or greater corpectomies with posterior fixation

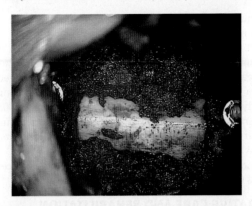

FIGURE 4 Intraoperative photograph shows bone graft in place for anterior cervical corpectomy and fusion. Bone dust and demineralized bone matrix have been used to fill the gaps and cover the graft.

- Remove Caspar pins; fill holes with bone wax
- Angle C5 holes 20° to 30° cranially
- Before securing plate, remove any inadequately removed osteophytes or prominences with high-speed carbide burr so plate can lie flat along anterior aspect of vertebral bodies
- Place plate; thread in C5 screws 90% down
- Use drill guide to drill C7 holes
- Screw in C7 screws; final-tighten C5 screws
- Remove self-retaining retractor
- Verify final plate and screw placement with lateral radiograph

Closure
- Irrigate and inspect for bleeding using appendiceal retractor; place liquefied collagen along medial borders of longus colli, the most common site of postoperative hematoma; coagulate bleeders on esophagus or tracheoesophageal groove with hemostatic agents, not electrocautery
- Place 1/8-in Hemovac drain through separate stab hole so all holes are 2 to 3 cm below hemostatic agents
- Layered closure with figure-of-8 interrupted 3-0 Monocryl suture (Ethicon); approximate subcuticular tissue with interrupted buried 5-0 Monocryl, then apply 0.25-in adhesive skin closure strips and sterile dressings
- Place rigid collar with firm plastic bivalved shell and removable padded liner

COMPLICATIONS
- In immediate postoperative period, perform careful neurologic follow-up; wound hematoma can obstruct breathing and swallowing

- Inflammation and edema from retraction of esophagus; dysphagia is most common complication (24%)
- Recurrent laryngeal nerve injury rates range from 2% to 30%; persistent symptomatic vocal cord paresis ranges from 0.33% to 2.5%
- Esophageal injury from retractor placement, sharp-edged retractors, or trauma by sharp instrument or burr; subsequent risk of infection is potentially life-threatening but incidence is low (0.2% to 0.4%)
- Rate of vertebral artery injury after anterior cervical spine surgery is 0.3%
- Dural tear risk is 3.7%; increased risk in revision anterior surgery or patients with OPLL
- Acute spinal cord injury incidence following anterior cervical spine surgery is 0.2% to 0.9%

POSTOPERATIVE CARE AND REHABILITATION

- If retraction time exceeds 3 hours or intubation difficult, keep patient intubated overnight in intensive care unit; extubate when patient passes cuff leak test
- For severe dysphagia on night of surgery, give 10 mg dexamethasone intravenously, elevate head of bed above 30°
- Continue antibiotic prophylaxis until drain removed, when output less than 20 mL over 8 hours
- Start ambulation morning after surgery; allow progressive walking program 1 to 2 weeks after surgery
- Allow showering 1 day after surgery
- Formal physical therapy usually not necessary; restrict overhead lifting activities until solid fusion obtained
- Cervical collar is worn for 6 weeks; may be removed for few hours daily with minimal neck motion

PEARLS

- Using Gardner-Wells tongs and taping the head to the table in proper orientation decreases rotation of head/spine during surgery, helps prevent asymmetric decompression, and enables proper implant/plate placement.
- Most common reasons for asymmetric corpectomy and injury to vertebral artery are inadequate exposure and failure to maintain midline orientation.
- Creating subplatysmal pouches during superficial exposure facilitates adequate exposure up to six levels through a single transverse incision; transverse incision is cosmetically more pleasing than vertical or oblique incision.
- Improperly placed (ie, off-center) Caspar pins can induce rotatory deformity during decompression and correction.
- Obtain depth of corpectomy by excising all disk material at intervertebral interspace cephalad and caudad to vertebral body being resected.
- A loose bone graft strut generally results from measuring corpectomy site without traction on spine.

100 Posterior Cervical Foraminotomy

INTRODUCTION
- Minimally invasive posterior cervical foraminotomy offers alternative to traditional open techniques with similar outcomes
- Posterior cervical foraminotomy eliminates risk of injuring carotid artery, esophagus, and recurrent laryngeal nerve associated with anterior approach
- Does not require fusion; does not destabilize disk space; easy approach to directly decompress foramen
- Limitation is inability to deal directly with pathology affecting central aspect of canal, compared with anterior approach
- Posterior procedures require more dissection of extensor spine muscle mass, with possible increase in postoperative neck pain
- May modify approach by undercutting spinous process to treat myelopathy; efficacy and safety not demonstrated

PATIENT SELECTION
Indications
- Patients with persistent radiculopathy that correlates with findings on CT, MRI, or myelography
- Failure of nonsurgical management
- Refractory radiculopathy after anterior cervical diskectomy and fusion
- Cervical radiculopathy due to foraminal stenosis, posterolaterally herniated disks, or persistent symptoms after anterior cervical fusion

Contraindications
- Local skin infection
- Cervical myelopathy
- Significant kyphosis
- Mechanical instability of cervical spine
- Spinal cord compression
- Significant disk herniation compressing the nerve root
- Symptomatology not referable to pathology on imaging studies

---

Based on Singh K, Fineberg SJ, Oglesby M, Hoskins JA, Yelavarthi V: Posterior cervical foraminotomy, in Colvin AC, Flatow E, eds: Atlas of Essential Orthopaedic Procedures, *ed 2. Rosemont, IL, American Academy of Orthopaedic Surgeons, 2020, pp 814-817.*

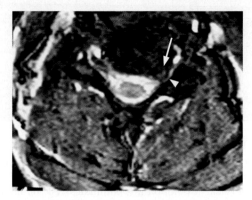

FIGURE 1 T2-weighted axial MRI shows a disk herniation (arrow) in the C5-6 neural foramen compressing the left C5-6 nerve root (arrowhead).

PREOPERATIVE IMAGING

- AP and lateral radiographs to assess cervical alignment
- Dynamic flexion-extension views to identify instability
- MRI to evaluate spinal cord and nerve roots for sites of compression (**Figure 1**)
- If MRI cannot be obtained, CT myelogram is alternative

PROCEDURE

Room Setup/Patient Positioning

- Prone or seated position
- Apply three-pin Mayfield fixation, fixing head to table in prone position
- Place Wilson frame or similar bolsters under torso
- Protect and pad all potential neural compression points
- Extend neck; avoid hyperextension
- Slightly tucking in chin in "military" posture aids in approach
- Reverse Trendelenburg position allows venous drainage, less bleeding
- Position fluoroscopic C-arm under drapes to visualize retractors during procedure
- Tape shoulders down for radiographic visualization of neck
- Flex knees to prevent distal migration of patient

Surgical Technique: Open Posterior Cervical Foraminotomy

Instruments/Equipment

- 1- or 2-mm Kerrison rongeurs
- 2-mm round-tip burr or drill
- Bovie electrocautery
- Self-retaining retractors
- Cobb elevator

Exposure

- Make 2-cm incision slightly lateral (1.5 cm) to midline
- Use electrocautery to carry incision through posterior fascia
- Place self-retaining retractors to spread paraspinal muscles
- Dissect muscle to expose medial half of facet
- Further lateral dissection unnecessary; may destabilize joint

Foraminotomy

- Identify inferior articular process (IAP) of cephalad vertebra
- Remove medial third of IAP and inferior portion of superior lamina with burr
- Visualize superior articular process (SAP) of caudal vertebra
- Use Kerrison rongeur or burr to resect SAP, exposing exiting nerve root
- Create keyhole foraminotomy with nerve root visualized (**Figure 2**)
- Perform decompression until nerve probe is easily placed into neuroforamen

 VIDEO 100.1 Open Cervical Foraminotomy. Kern Singh, MD; Steven J. Fineberg, MD; Matthew Oglesby, BA; Jonathan A. Hoskins, MD; Vamshi Yelavarthi, BA (3 min)

Closure

- Irrigate wound with antibiotics and saline
- Reapproximate fascia; close wound in layers
- Return patient to supine position for extubation

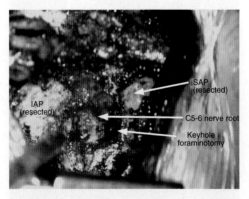

FIGURE 2 Intraoperative photograph demonstrates the nerve root visualized in the keyhole foraminotomy. IAP = inferior articular process, SAP = superior articular process

Surgical Technique: Minimally Invasive Posterior Cervical Foraminotomy

Instruments/Equipment

- Fluoroscopy
- Microscope
- Tubular dilators up to 18 mm
- Tubular retractor system
- Kirschner wires or spinal needle
- Bovie electrocautery
- Kerrison rongeurs
- 2-mm round-tip burr

Exposure

- Use lateral fluoroscopic image to identify level
- Spinal needle or Kirschner wire may help identify level
- Make incision slightly (0.5 cm) lateral to midline
- Use electrocautery to carry incision through fascia
- Under fluoroscopic guidance, place sequential tubular dilators at medial facet joint to spread paraspinal muscles (**Figure 3**)

Foraminotomy

- Expose medial half of facet joint and inferior portion of the superior lamina (**Figure 4, A**)
- Use burr to remove medial one third of IAP of cephalad vertebra (**Figure 4, B**)

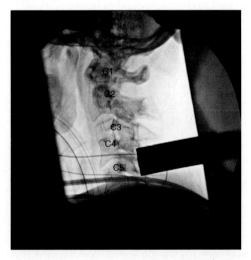

FIGURE 3 Lateral fluoroscopic view shows the final sequential tubular dilator in place.

© 2021 American Academy of Orthopaedic Surgeons

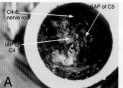 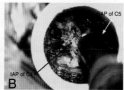 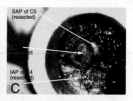

FIGURE 4 Intraoperative photographs demonstrate posterior cervical foraminotomy. **A,** Exposure through the tubular retractor. The medial facet joint and inferior portion of the superior lamina are visualized in the surgical field. **B,** A high-speed burr is used to resect the medial third of the IAP of the cephalad vertebra. **C,** The IAP and SAP have been resected, and the nerve root is visualized. IAP = inferior articular process, SAP = superior articular process

- Use burr or Kerrison rongeur to remove SAP of inferior vertebra
- Visualize nerve root exiting into neuroforamen (**Figure 4, C**)
- Place blunt nerve probe into neuroforamen, ensuring complete decompression achieved

Closure
- Irrigate wound with antibiotics and saline
- Remove retractors, place single stitch in fascia
- Close skin edges with absorbable sutures.
- Return patient to supine position

Controversies
- Minimally invasive posterior cervical foraminotomy demonstrates clinical outcomes comparable to those of open approach
- Critics suggest visualization compromised and not worth benefits of less tissue dissection

COMPLICATIONS
- Infection
- Durotomy
- Postoperative cervical instability
- Persistent radiculopathy due to incomplete decompression

POSTOPERATIVE CARE AND REHABILITATION
- No postoperative immobilization
- Discharge patients home a few hours after surgery
- No restrictions other than routine wound care
- Return to routine activities or work as soon as tolerated

PEARLS

- Minimally invasive techniques reduce tissue trauma and morbidity associated with open approaches.
- Foraminotomy is performed by resecting IAP and inferior lamina of cephalad vertebra, followed by resection of SAP of caudal vertebra.
- Resection of more than 50% of medial facet joint may result in subsequent segmental instability.
- Foraminotomy is complete when blunt nerve probe is easily placed in neuroforamen, ensuring adequate decompression.

Posterior Cervical Laminectomy and Fusion

PATIENT SELECTION
- Cervical degenerative disease is most common acquired disability in patients older than 50 years; radiculopathy, myelopathy, or a combination may be present
- Failure of nonsurgical management indicates surgery
- Surgical approach considerations
  - Alignment of cervical spine
    - Neutral or lordotic—Anterior or posterior approach
    - Kyphotic—Anterior with possible posterior approach
  - Number of levels involved
  - Nature of pathologic process
    - Ventral compression—Anterior approach
    - Intradural tumors—Posterior approach
    - Ossification of posterior longitudinal ligament—Posterior approach
  - Surgeon preference
- Posterior procedure options
  - Laminoplasty with or without foraminotomies
  - Laminectomy and fusion with or without foraminotomies; fusion necessary when performing laminectomy to avoid postlaminectomy cervical kyphosis

PREOPERATIVE IMAGING
- Radiography—Cervical spine standing AP, lateral, flexion, and extension views
- MRI—To assess neural elements and vertebral artery course (**Figure 1**)
- CT—To assess bony anatomy for hardware placement
- CT myelography is indicated if previous instrumentation present

---

Based on Qureshi SA, Hecht AC: Posterior cervical laminectomy and fusion, in Colvin AC, Flatow E, eds: Atlas of Essential Orthopaedic Procedures, *ed 2. Rosemont, IL, American Academy of Orthopaedic Surgeons, 2020, pp 818-824.*

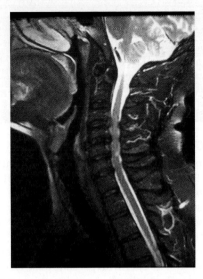

FIGURE 1 Sagittal T2-weighted MRI shows multilevel cervical spinal cord compression.

PROCEDURE

Room Setup

- Intubation
  - ▸ General endotracheal anesthesia
  - ▸ If flexion or extension of neck worsens symptoms, consider awake fiberoptic intubation
- Evoked potential monitoring
  - ▸ Authors use somatosensory-evoked potentials, motor-evoked potentials, and electromyography for all posterior cervical laminectomy and fusion procedures
  - ▸ No evidence for improvement of outcomes but can predict neurologic dysfunction; may help define maneuver or instrumentation placement that irritates nerve roots or impinges on spinal cord
  - ▸ Place bite block

Positioning

- Supine position on Jackson table with flat board
- Place potential monitoring leads; obtain baseline potentials
- Place Gardner-Wells tongs; hang 10 to 20 lb of weight
- Rotisserie turn
  - ▸ Place Jackson four-post frame on top of patient, lock in place, and secure with straps (**Figure 2, A**)
  - ▸ Place facial pillow and disconnect endotracheal tube from circuit

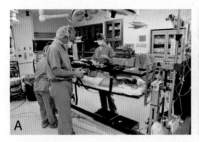 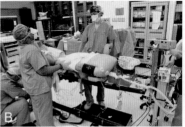

FIGURE 2 Photographs show patient positioning for posterior cervical laminectomy and fusion. **A,** The patient is placed supine on a Jackson table with a flat board. A four-post frame with chest board is placed over the patient, and all pads and pillows are positioned appropriately in preparation for the rotisserie turn. **B,** After the rotisserie turn is completed, the flat board is removed and the patient is now in the prone position on the four-post frame.

- ▹ Rotate 180°, apply rotation lock, and remove flat board (**Figure 2, B**)
- ▹ Recheck potentials, pad bony prominences, and position arms
- • Draping
    - ▹ Fluoroscopy in lateral position, proximal to field; authors prefer three-dimensional fluoroscopy
    - ▹ Shave hair to occipital protuberance, place nonsterile plastic drapes, and apply preparatory solution
    - ▹ Apply iodine-impregnated adhesive drape and sterile fluoroscopy drape
    - ▹ Administer intravenous antibiotics

Instruments
- • Jackson table with flat board and four-post frame
- • Gardner-Wells tongs
- • Insulated electrocautery and bipolar cautery
- • Cerebellar retractors
- • High-speed burr with non–end-cutting drill attachment
- • Angled curets
- • Kerrison and Leksell rongeurs
- • Lateral mass and pedicle screws, rods, and end caps

Surgical Technique
Exposure
- • Use midline skin incision; levels determined by fluoroscopy
- • Maintain meticulous hemostasis
- • Perform subperiosteal dissection of muscle out to lateral masses using electrocautery
- • Release self-retaining retractors periodically to avoid muscle ischemic damage
- • Obtain fluoroscopy to count levels, starting with C2

Laminectomy

- Drill/tap screw tracts before laminectomy
- Make pilot hole with high-speed burr 1 mm medial to midpoint of lateral mass
- Angle drill 30° laterally, 15° cephalad
- Set drill stop at 12 to 14 mm, use ball-tipped probe
- Authors use unicortical screws
- Tap, ball-tipped probe to check integrity of screw tract
- Tap screw tract
- Create troughs (longitudinal) just medial to lateral masses using high-speed burr with non–end-cutting attachment
- Once ligamentum flavum reached, use nerve hook to raise ligamentum and resect it using 2-mm Kerrison rongeurs
- Use Leksell rongeurs to grab spinous processes of most cephalad and caudad segments to provide constant upward pressure
- Tease away adhesions/residual ligamentum as laminae removed en bloc
- Recheck potentials

VIDEO 101.1 Posterior Cervical Laminectomy and Fusion.
Sheeraz A. Qureshi, MD, MBA; Andrew C. Hecht, MD (19 min)

Instrumentation

- Place T1 screws if cervicothoracic junction is to be crossed
  - ▶ Often used if fusion would otherwise include C7 because of high rate of degeneration at cervicothoracic junction
  - ▶ Perform laminoforaminotomy at T1 so medial border of pedicle can be palpated
  - ▶ Use burr to create pilot hole at intersection of midpoint of transverse process and lateral pars
  - ▶ Gearshift turned laterally for 15 mm, then removed; replace with ball-tipped probe aimed medially to confirm tract
- Place lateral mass screws; authors use 3.5-mm–diameter screws with 4.0-mm screws available for rescue
- Confirm placement of screws with fluoroscopy

Fusion and Closure

- Use burr to decorticate facet joints and lateral masses
- Use local bone to achieve biologic arthrodesis; extenders such as demineralized bone matrix or iliac crest graft can be used as needed
- Place rods into screw heads, tighten caps (**Figure 3**)
- Place subfascial drain
- Perform layered closure

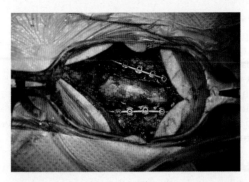

FIGURE 3 Intraoperative photograph shows the decompressed spinal cord following the removal of laminae. Lateral mass instrumentation is in place and interconnected using rods and end caps.

COMPLICATIONS

Vascular
- Vertebral artery injury from lateral mass screw malpositioning
- Very rare; maintain lateral trajectory to minimize risk

Neurologic
- Spinal cord injury
  - Incidence less than 1%
  - Greatest risk during removal of laminae; elevate blood pressure in setting of severe stenosis to prevent ischemia
- Nerve root palsy, most commonly at C5 and usually unilateral
  - Incidence 5% to 10%
  - Possibly from nerve root tethering after posterior migration of spinal cord
  - Prognosis good; usually resolves with observation and physical therapy

Dural Injury
- Incidence 1%
- Repair with suture or patch, seal with fibrin glue
- Use lumbar drain if repair suboptimal

Postlaminectomy Kyphosis
- Laminectomy destabilizes cervical spine; therefore, always combine with fusion procedure
- May place spinal cord at risk
- Treatment—Anterior reconstruction followed by posterior stabilization

Lateral Mass Instrumentation Complications

- Screw impingement on nerve root
- Vertebral artery injury
- Screw loosening
- Screw cut-out
- Rod fracture
- Historically, plate-screw constructs associated with 2% hardware-related radiculopathy; rate with current instrumentation unknown, believed to be low

POSTOPERATIVE CARE AND REHABILITATION

- Place in hard cervical orthosis for 6 weeks
- Restrict overhead activity for 6 weeks
- Remove external sutures/staples after 2 weeks

PEARLS

- Draping fluoroscopy unit into the field saves time and enables accurate placement of instrumentation.
- Subperiosteal dissection and attention to meticulous hemostasis enable perfect visualization of bony anatomy for proper placement of hardware and safe completion of laminectomy.
- Frequent release of self-retaining retractors can prevent ischemic injury to paraspinal musculature.
- Evoked potential monitoring can indicate neurologic injury and helps obviate neurologic issues related to positioning.
- Drilling and tapping lateral mass screw holes before laminectomy minimizes drilling over the exposed neural elements.
- Watertight closure of muscle and fascial layers along with subfascial drains prevent postoperative seroma formation and wound complications.

PATIENT SELECTION

Indications

- Cervical myelopathy due to ossification of posterior longitudinal ligament (OPLL) and multilevel spondylosis involving three or more motion segments (**Figure 1**)
- Spinal cord decompression to salvage failed anterior cervical decompression and fusion (ACDF)
- Recurrent myelopathy due to adjacent segment disease after anterior cervical decompression and fusion
- Myelopathy in patients at increased risk for nonunion (smokers, patients with metabolic bone disease)
- Developmentally narrow spinal canals (midbody AP diameter <12 mm)

Contraindications

- Epidural fibrosis, following infection or prior posterior surgery
- "Hill-shaped" lesions of OPLL occupying 50% to 60% of AP canal diameter
- Axial neck pain as primary clinical symptom
- Morbid obesity and diabetes mellitus (two- to eightfold increase in surgical site infections)
- Lordotic or straight spines have significantly higher functional recovery than kyphotic or sigmoid-shaped curves; lordotic alignment not prerequisite for performing laminoplasty
- Fixed kyphosis (5° to 13°); patients with cervical spines ranging from lordotic to 13° or less of kyphosis are ideal candidates if no cord signal change on T2-weighted MRI; if signal change present, upper limit of kyphosis is 5°

TYPES OF LAMINOPLASTY

- Two main types derive from Hirabayashi "open-door" procedure and Kurokawa "French-door" technique

---

Based on Thakur NA, Freedman BA, Heller JG: Cervical laminoplasty, in Colvin AC, Flatow E, eds: Atlas of Essential Orthopaedic Procedures, ed 2. Rosemont, IL, American Academy of Orthopaedic Surgeons, 2020, pp 825-831.

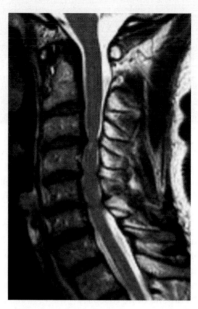

FIGURE 1 T2-weighted sagittal MRI demonstrates multilevel cervical stenosis secondary to spondylosis.

- Techniques differ in how laminae are secured or how exposure is made; initially, hinges were tethered open with suture/wire or propped open with bone grafts/spacers; recent innovations adapted plates and screws to fix in place

PREOPERATIVE IMAGING

- AP, lateral, and flexion-extension radiographic views
- Kyphosis line (K-line) helps determine success of laminoplasty in OPLL; connects midpoints of spinal canal at C2 and C7 on lateral cervical radiograph (**Figure 2**)
- MRI helps determine which levels to include in laminoplasty; helps determine whether C2 dome laminectomy should accompany laminoplasty
- CT affords precise appreciation of bony anatomy including OPLL, ossified ligamentum, foraminal stenosis with osteophyte formation; surgeon can address foraminal stenosis detected on CT with foraminotomy
- CT myelography enhances structural detail; indicated when MRI cannot reveal extent/nature of pathology
- CT determines "occupation ratio" (AP diameter of lesion/AP diameter of canal × 100) for large ventral lesion

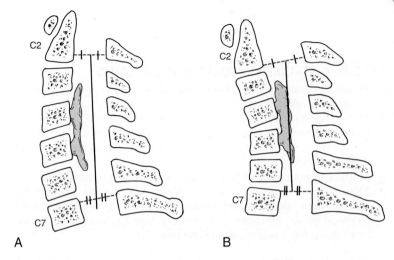

FIGURE 2 Illustrations demonstrate the Kyphosis line (K-line) concept. A positive (+) K-line (**A**) occurs when the compressive pathology ossification of the posterior longitudinal ligament remains ventral to the line. A negative (−) K-line (**B**) is defined by the pathology extending dorsally to or across the line.

PROCEDURE

Room Setup/Patient Positioning

- Prone position
- Assess range of motion (ROM) preoperatively so may position patient in some flexion; reduces overlap or "shingling" of laminae (**Figure 3**)
- Use Mayfield three-pin holder to immobilize cervical spine
- Place longitudinal bolsters on lateral border of chest; takes pressure off central chest/abdomen
- Flex knees, ankles to reduce lower extremity neural tension

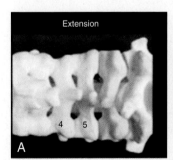
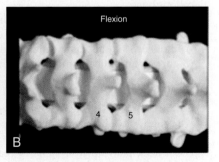

FIGURE 3 Posterior view of cervical spine model shows shingling of laminae in extension (**A**) versus flexion (**B**). (Courtesy of John Rhee, MD, Atlanta, GA.)

- May tape to shift redundant soft tissues when needed.
- Use reverse Trendelenburg position; decreases venous pressure, blood loss

SPECIAL INSTRUMENTS/EQUIPMENT/IMPLANTS

- Monitor somatosensory-evoked potentials (SSEPs) during laminoplasty for myelopathy
- Monitor electromyograms when foraminotomies added to surgery
- Neuromonitoring may identify hypotension or decreases in spinal cord perfusion; early detection enables rapid intervention and neurologic protection
- May use arterial catheter to monitor mean arterial pressure
- Motor-evoked potentials (MEPs) more sensitive to myelopathy changes than somatosensory-evoked potentials; more susceptible to technical issues, however; lack of neuromuscular blockade required by motor-evoked potentials possible safety issue

Surgical Technique

- Authors prefer open-door technique; only two troughs required; more time-efficient than French door; may be harder to control lateral epidural veins, however
- Make hinge and open side troughs at lamina–lateral mass junction; landmarks may be indistinct or obscured; can correlate with preoperative CT
- Create troughs using high-speed burr to depth of approximately 4 mm; too lateral and deep risks damaging vertebral artery; too medial leads to inadequate decompression
- Make open-side trough first; be cautious with burr until visualizing ligamentum flavum at inferior half of lamina; complete remaining cranial opening with burr or with curet and Kerrison rongeur
- Use bipolar cautery to coagulate, divide plexus of veins as lamina is opened
- On hinge side, use burr to remove dorsal cortex and underlying cancellous bone
- Thin inner cortical layer until stiff hinge fashioned; excessive bone removal results in floppy hinge, may displace into canal
- Authors use laminoplasty plate to rigidly fix laminae in open position (**Figure 4**); additional bone grafts with plates not needed

COMPLICATIONS

- Wound infections 3% to 4%; minimize with perioperative antibiotics, watertight fascial closure; can use separate drain for thick subcutaneous layer
- Axial neck pain up to 40% at 10-year follow-up; early active ROM important to reduce pain and stiffness

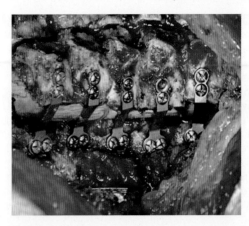

FIGURE 4 Intraoperative photograph shows an open-door laminoplasty from C3-C7, fixed rigidly with segmental plate fixation.

- Kyphosis incidence lower than with laminectomy (0% to 22%); severe kyphosis can lead to poor neurologic recovery, late neurologic deterioration
- Laminar closure reported with various laminoplasty techniques
- Motor root palsies reported at 5% to 12% (C5 most common)
- Weakness of deltoid and biceps muscles; some patients experience sensory dysfunction, radicular symptoms; usual onset 2 to 3 days after surgery but can appear up to 2 months postoperatively; time to recovery is 1 week to 2 years (mean, 21 weeks)

POSTOPERATIVE CARE AND REHABILITATION

- Encourage unrestricted active ROM as soon as tolerated; start isotonic exercises 6 weeks postoperatively
- In interim, encourage daily walking or stationary cycling
- Authors do not recommend brace or collar wear; impedes early active ROM; immobilization risks more axial pain, loss of ROM, possible kyphosis
- Perform clinical assessment with static radiographs at 6 weeks
- Obtain lateral flexion-extension radiographs at 3-month intervals until patient reaches maximal neurologic improvement, expected by 1 year after surgery
- Hinges reliably heal by 6 months; if no instability on dynamic radiographs, patients can engage in any activities, including most sports

PEARLS

- Cervical lordotic alignment is not prerequisite for laminoplasty.
- K-line helps in patient selection; (+) K-line correlates with significantly higher neurologic recovery rate.
- Neuromonitoring can help identify neurologic changes; use electromyography when foraminotomies also performed.
- Preserve as much muscle insertion at C2 as possible; avoid including C7 if does not compromise degree of spinal cord decompression.
- Preserving muscle attachments to C2 and C7 laminae may reduce axial pain and prevent postoperative kyphosis.
- Authors recommend plates to keep lamina open without graft.
- Authors do not use cervical orthosis postoperatively; immediate active ROM without collars prevents postoperative axial pain, stiffness, and kyphosis.

103 Placement of Thoracic Pedicle Screws

PATIENT SELECTION

Indications

- Advantages of thoracic pedicle screw fixation—Achieves stable three-column fixation, improves control of three-dimensional deformities
- Degenerative disorders
- Traumatic injury
- Deformity
- Stabilization of spinal segments
  - After neural decompression for fracture, tumor, infection
  - Facilitate correction of kyphotic or scoliotic deformities

CONTRAINDICATIONS

- Signs or symptoms of infection
- Metal allergies
- Severely deformed, hypoplastic, or absent pedicles
- In trauma setting, medically unstable or underresuscitated patients
- Severe osteoporosis (relative); address inadequate screw purchase with screw augmentation techniques such as polymethyl methacrylate screw augmentation

PREOPERATIVE IMAGING

- AP and lateral radiographs
- CT optional to evaluate pedicle size and anatomy of deformity; assessment of pedicles at rotated levels may be impossible on plain radiographs; if pedicle size appears too small to accept 5-mm screw or plain radiography examination is insufficient, use CT for accurate evaluation
- Pedicles in midthoracic spine have smallest width in patients of all ages; pedicles at apices of concavity of scoliotic curve typically smaller than those on convex side
- Can safely insert screws 80% to 115% of size of outer pedicle diameter through gradual plastic deformation, in a technique known as pediculoplasty, with probe and tap; this deformation is more pronounced in pediatric pedicles

---

Based on Wilson KW, Lehman RA Jr, Lenke LG: Placement of thoracic pedicle screws, in Colvin AC, Flatow E, eds: Atlas of Essential Orthopaedic Procedures, *ed 2. Rosemont, IL, American Academy of Orthopaedic Surgeons, 2020, pp 832-843.*

PROCEDURE
Room Setup/Patient Positioning
- Prone position on radiolucent four-poster frame or OSI table (Orthopaedic Systems) with spine top
- Move patient down toward foot of operating table as much as possible so arm boards can be close to head of table; improves surgeon access while placing screws in proximal thoracic spine
- Place legs in sling to promote systemic venous return
- Consider halo skull traction to facilitate flexing patient's neck and reduce kyphotic angle for easier screw placement
- Use somatosensory-evoked potentials and motor-evoked potentials to monitor spinal cord during screw insertion and correction maneuvers
- Real-time spontaneous electromyography (EMG) monitoring of nerve roots T6 through T12 through the rectus abdominis musculature adds layer of safety; can use triggered EMG to confirm screw placement

Special Instruments/Equipment/Implants
- Fluoroscopic and computer-generated image–guided techniques developed to improve pedicle screw placement accuracy require additional resources; may increase surgery time, blood loss, and infection
- Thoracic gearshift probe
- Flexible ball-tipped pedicle-sounding device
- Variety of screw sizes—4 to 7 mm in diameter; 25 to 55 mm in length
- Monoaxial screw heads allow better manipulation of spine during derotation
- Polyaxial screws aid rod placement after curve correction
- Uniaxial screws combine benefits of monoaxial and multiaxial screw heads

Surgical Technique
Incision and Exposure
- Mark incision from highest planned instrumented vertebra to lowest; make straight vertical line connecting the two points to ensure straight incision after scoliosis correction and confirm with fluoroscopy
- For exposure, incise from spinous process above most cranial vertebra to spinous process of most caudal vertebra to be instrumented
- Anesthesia team paralyzes patient pharmacologically to facilitate exposure of soft tissues; reverse paralysis before instrumentation to avoid interfering with monitoring
- Carry dissection along midline; dissect subperiosteally laterally to tips of transverse processes (**Figure 1**)
- Perform wide facetectomy; use osteotome to remove inferior 3 to 5 mm of inferior facet; scrape exposed cartilage from superior facet

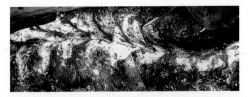

FIGURE 1 Intraoperative photograph shows the posterior elements of the spine exposed to the edge of the transverse processes bilaterally. The inferior facets are removed with a 0.5-in straight osteotome (down to T10) or rongeur (below T10). Articular cartilage is removed from the dorsal side of the superior facet of the inferior vertebra using a small curet. (Reproduced with permission from Kim YJ, Lenke LG, Bridwell KH, Cho YS, Riew KD: Free hand pedicle screw placement in the thoracic spine: Is it safe? *Spine [Phila Pa 1976]* 2004;29[3]:333-342.)

Starting Point and Trajectory

- Most neutrally rotated and most distal instrumented vertebra is good starting level; adjust trajectory of each screw based on screw position of previous level or contralateral pedicle
- Group starting points according to location (**Figure 2**)

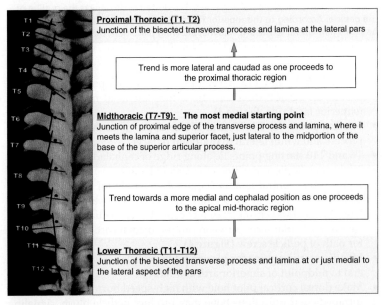

Proximal Thoracic (T1, T2)
Junction of the bisected transverse process and lamina at the lateral pars

Trend is more lateral and caudad as one proceeds to the proximal thoracic region

Midthoracic (T7-T9): **The most medial starting point**
Junction of proximal edge of the transverse process and lamina, where it meets the lamina and superior facet, just lateral to the midportion of the base of the superior articular process.

Trend towards a more medial and cephalad position as one proceeds to the apical mid-thoracic region

Lower Thoracic (T11-T12)
Junction of the bisected transverse process and lamina at or just medial to the lateral aspect of the pars

FIGURE 2 Image shows pedicle screw starting points using a 3.5-mm acorn-tipped burr. The posterior elements are burred to create a posterior cortical breach approximately 5 mm in depth. (Adapted with permission from Kim YJ, Lenke LG, Bridwell KH, Cho YS, Riew KD: Free hand pedicle screw placement in the thoracic spine: Is it safe? *Spine [Phila Pa 1976]* 2004;29[3]:333-342.)

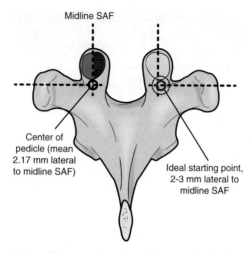

Midline SAF

Center of
pedicle (mean
2.17 mm lateral
to midline SAF)

Ideal starting point,
2-3 mm lateral to
midline SAF

FIGURE 3 Illustration of the posterior view of the vertebra depicts the ideal starting point for a thoracic pedicle screw, determined using the superior facet rule. According to this rule, the screw should not start medial to the midpoint of the superior articular facet (SAF). The medial aspect of the facet is shown in red. In the illustration, the midline of the SAF is marked by the vertical dashed line. The red circle demarcates the ideal starting point. The dotted circle depicts the outline of the pedicle. According to the superior facet rule, the optimal starting point should be 2 to 3 mm lateral to the SAF midline, allowing placement of the screw in the center of the pedicle and avoiding penetration of the canal.

- T1 through T3 and T12 starting points are at midpoint of transverse process in vertical direction and 2 mm lateral to midpoint of facet (superior facet rule, **Figure 3**)
- Starting points for T4, T5, and T11 lie at proximal third of transverse process and 2 mm lateral to midpoint of facet
- T6 and T10 starting points lie along ridge of cephalad aspect of lamina
- T7 through T9 lie at junction of facet and lamina
- Authors use ventral lamina (**Figure 4**) as guide for starting point in pedicle screw placement; because medial cortical wall is thicker than lateral wall, and ventral lamina is consistently medial to midpoint of superior articular facet, surgeon can use medial cortical wall as guide for path of pedicle screw (**Figure 4**)
- Identify starting point for placement of pedicle screws 2 to 3 mm lateral to midpoint of superior articular facet
- Make dorsal cortical pilot hole with high-speed burr
- Intrapedicular cancellous bone may produce pedicle blush, signaling entrance; smaller pedicles may not blush
- Can use anatomic or straight-forward approach to screw trajectory; for anatomic trajectory, pathway follows anatomic axis of pedicle, angled 15° to 22° caudad in sagittal plane; reserve anatomic approach for salvage purposes

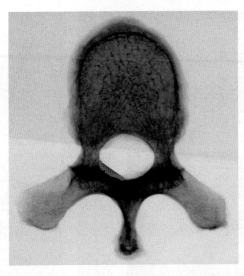

FIGURE 4 Axial fluoroscopic view shows the dissected thoracic vertebra with the ventral lamina outlined in red. As shown here, the ventral lamina forms the roof of the spinal canal and is confluent with the medial pedicle wall.

- Straight-forward approach is recommended for most patients; parallels superior end plate of vertebral body
- Convexity of curve allows reliable and safe placement of pedicle screws with larger pedicle diameter and wider epidural space; concave pedicles often shorter, dysplastic, more sclerotic, and located near spinal cord

Gearshift Probing

- Use thoracic gearshift probe to find cancellous soft spot at entrance of pedicle (**Figure 5**)
- In thoracic spine, direct concavity of gearshift laterally
- Probe pedicle with smooth, consistent movements; sudden shift or advancement signals pedicle wall or vertebral body violation; investigate immediately to avoid complications
- Use nondominant hand to brace gearshift and prevent sudden advancement; anterior and lateral vertebral body cortices most susceptible to penetration by probe
- Point curve of gearshift laterally on entrance to avoid medial wall penetration
- 2-mm tip should "fall" through cancellous inner portion of pedicle, even if quite small
- Carefully sink probe to depth of 15 to 20 mm (beyond medially located spinal canal); be mindful of trajectory and level-specific pedicle anatomy

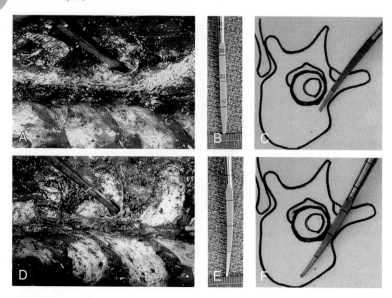

FIGURE 5 Images show gearshift probing for thoracic pedicle screw placement. Initially, the gearshift is directed laterally to a depth of 20 mm, the approximate depth of the pedicle, to diminish the likelihood of medial pedicle perforation. **A,** Intraoperative photograph demonstrates the probe placement with the curve directed laterally. **B,** Standard probes are graduated to gauge the depth of penetration. **C,** Axial diagram shows the curve of the probe directed laterally. Then, the gearshift is removed and redirected medially. The nondominant hand is used to brace the gearshift and prevent sudden advancements. **D,** Intraoperative photograph shows the probe placement with the curve directed medially. **E,** Lateral view of the probe shows the typical curve and graduations. **F,** Axial diagram shows the medially directed curve of the probe. (Reproduced with permission from Kim YJ, Lenke LG, Bridwell KH, Cho YS, Riew KD: Free hand pedicle screw placement in the thoracic spine: Is it safe? *Spine [Phila Pa 1976]* 2004;29[3]:333-342.)

- Remove gearshift; rotate tip 180° to point medially; reenter same tract at base of pedicle and follow it medially, advancing tip of gearshift into body of vertebra; ultimate depth averages 40 to 45 mm in lower thoracic region, 35 to 40 mm in midthoracic region, 30 to 35 mm in proximal thoracic region
- Remove probe; visualize hole to ensure only nonpulsatile blood present, not cerebrospinal fluid; excessive bleeding may signal epidural bleeding from medial wall perforation

Pedicle Sounding

- Use flexible ball-tipped probe to palpate medial, lateral, superior, inferior aspects of pedicle tract and floor to ensure continuity of tract proximal 10 to 15 mm of channel represents isthmus of pedicle; palpate carefully

- Most pedicle wall perforations in isthmus; if perforation identified, remove sounding device, use gearshift probe to redirect tract in more appropriate direction
- Place probe fully into pedicle until abuts bottom of vertebral body; use tonsil hemostat to clamp probe and allow proper measurement of tract length

Tapping, Repalpation, and Screw Placement

- Tap pedicle tract with tap 0.5 to 1 mm smaller in diameter than planned screw diameter
- Undertapping of pedicle provides higher insertion torque than tapping "line to line"
- Evaluate tapped tract with flexible ball-tipped sounding probe
- Insert screw slowly by hand; be mindful of trajectory marked by handle of previously inserted pedicle probe
- Optimize viscoelastic expansion of pedicle walls with slow deliberate insertion of screw; goal is to fit maximum diameter and length of screw without compromising bone integrity

Confirmation of Intraosseous Screws

- Obtain AP and lateral radiographs to assess screw trajectories before proceeding with rods or deformity correction (**Figure 6, A** and **B**); can also use fluoroscopy, which can adjust to true coronal image to assess each screw
- Verify symmetric placement throughout coronal and sagittal planes; sagittal image should show parallel orientation with superior end plate and no penetration of screw tips beyond anterior vertebral body cortex
- Intraoperative plain radiography accurate compared with CT; 1% to 2% of pedicle screws readjusted or removed as result of intraoperative radiographic findings; if length or trajectory of any screw does not correlate with adjacent screws, remove screw so tract integrity can be confirmed with ball-tipped probe
- Can use EMG to validate screw position (**Figure 6, C**); triggered EMG threshold less than 6.0 mA or less than 65% of average of previously stimulated screws signals possible medial pedicle wall breach
- If pedicle wall breached, attempt salvage of that level; lateral wall most common area of breach; if lateral breach suspected, redirect gearshift probe to more medial trajectory
- Base decision to replace or discard screw on repeated pedicle wall palpation, position of screw on radiographs, and assessment of screw purchase; if doubt remains, leave screw out and skip level or substitute laminar hook
- When all screws in position, corrective and bone grafting procedures take place, followed by final instrumentation

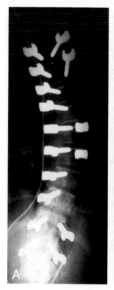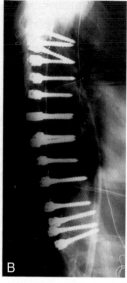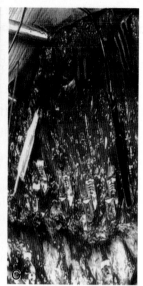

FIGURE 6 Images show confirmation of intraosseous screw placement. AP (**A**) and lateral (**B**) radiographs are obtained after all screws are placed. **C**, Intraoperative photograph depicts the triggered electromyographic testing of the screws. Thoracic screws from T6 to T12 can be monitored with the rectus abdominis muscles. (Adapted with permission from Kim YJ, Lenke LG, Bridwell KH, Cho YS, Riew KD: Free hand pedicle screw placement in the thoracic spine: Is it safe? *Spine [Phila Pa 1976]* 2004;29[3]:333-342.)

Closure

- Irrigate thoroughly
- Reapproximate deep fascia using 1-0 absorbable suture
- Place deep and superficial drains
- Perform deep dermal approximation with buried interrupted 2-0 absorbable suture
- Perform skin approximation with running subcuticular 3-0 absorbable monofilament
- Supplement closure with adhesive strips
- May use liquid topical skin adhesive for moisture barrier; helpful for incisions in patients with poor bowel or bladder control

COMPLICATIONS

- Thoracic pedicle screws have higher risk of neurovascular complications than lumbar screws because of smaller pedicle size
- Most common complication is screw malposition (**Figure 7**)
- Slightly medial (2 mm) or lateral (6 mm) violations have little clinical or anatomic consequence

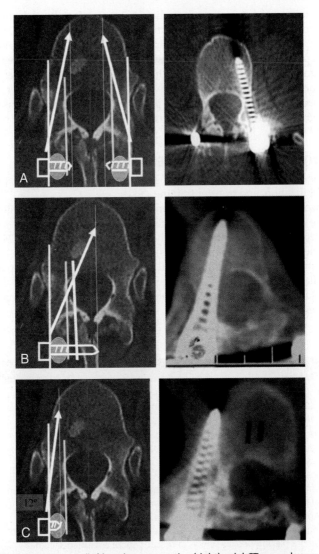

FIGURE 7 Preoperative (left) and postoperative (right) axial CT scans demonstrate thoracic pedicle screw trajectories. The vertical white lines demarcate the boundaries of the pedicle or the lateral and medial cortices. The arrow on the left image corresponds to the final screw trajectory seen on the postoperative image on the right. **A**, The screw axis lies between the outer cortices of the pedicle wall. **B**, A medial breach: the axis of the screw violates the medial cortex. **C**, A lateral breach: the axis of the screw violates the lateral cortex. (Adapted with permission from Lehman RA, Lenke LG, Keeler KA, Kim YJ, Cheh G: Computed tomography evaluation of pedicle screws placed in the pediatric deformed spine over an 8-year period. *Spine [Phila Pa 1976]* 2007;32[24]:2679-2684.)

- Review of pedicle screws in pediatric spinal deformity showed 4.2% malposition rate among 4,570 screws; with postoperative CT, rate of malposition rose to 15.7%; less than 1% required revision surgery for misplaced or loose screws; review did not show major permanent catastrophic neurologic or vascular injury from screw misplacement
- Other studies report intraoperative pedicle fracture (0.50% per screw inserted), dural leaks after screw placement (0.35% per screw inserted)
- Highest reported incidence of screw pullout 0.67%; loosening seen in 0.54%

POSTOPERATIVE CARE AND REHABILITATION

- Standard wound management, pain control, physical therapy for mobilization, and transfer training
- Encourage most deformity patients to get out of bed first postoperative day, depending on hemodynamic status
- Keep drains until output less than 30 mL per 8 hours for 24-hour period (maximum, 48 to 72 hours)
- Restrict diet to clear liquids until return of bowel sounds or passage of flatus
- Obtain weight-bearing AP and lateral radiographs before discharge to assess alignment

PEARLS

- Follow superior facet rule to avoid medial penetration; starting point should be 2 mm lateral to midpoint of superior facet.
- Wide inferior facetectomy improves visualization of superior facet for anatomic landmarks of starting points, allows greater deformity correction, provides local bone graft, and creates greater surface area for fusion.
- To optimize screw diameter, consider pediculoplasty; better fit and fill obtained if cautious during tapping and screw insertion to take advantage of plastic deformation and slow expansion of pedicle.
- Ability to detect presence or absence of pedicle tract violation and location depends on surgeon's level of training; probing pedicle tract before placing pedicle screws in thoracic spine is learned skill that improves with experience.
- Most screw purchase strength variability among pedicle screws explained by regional differences in bone mineral density at bone-screw interface.
- Juxtapedicular technique (in-out-in) and placement of thoracic pedicle screws in costovertebral junction are viable options to obtain fixation.

PATIENT SELECTION

Indications

- Symptomatic lumbar intervertebral disk herniation (IDH) refractory to nonsurgical treatment (oral corticosteroids, NSAIDs, physical therapy, lumbar epidural steroid injection at level of IDH or affected nerve root)
- Patients present with leg pain, or "sciatica," that follows radicular pattern
- Thorough history and physical examination can predict level of IDH before confirmatory imaging studies
- Strongest indication—Progressive loss of motor function (eg, foot-drop) interfering with quality of life
- Most common indication—Intractable pain despite nonsurgical treatment

Contraindications

- No evidence of IDH present on imaging studies
- Pay attention to patients with painless footdrop; differential diagnosis extensive; consider peroneal nerve palsy, tertiary syphilis, diabetic mononeuropathy, fascioscapulohumeral dystrophy, stroke, multiple sclerosis, and amyotrophic lateral sclerosis when paucity of findings present on MRI
- Greater trochanteric pain syndrome commonly causes radiating leg pain; can mimic L5 radiculopathy (pain in gluteus and lateral thigh); not characterized by radiation of pain below proximal calf

PREOPERATIVE IMAGING

- Closed MRI gold standard for identifying suspected herniated nucleus pulposus (HNP)
  - Sagittal T2-weighted sequences (**Figure 1, A**) identify level and degree of foraminal encroachment

Based on Moatz B, Tortolani PJ: Lumbar microdiskectomy, in Colvin AC, Flatow E, eds: Atlas of Essential Orthopaedic Procedures, *ed 2. Rosemont, IL, American Academy of Orthopaedic Surgeons, 2020, pp 844-850.*

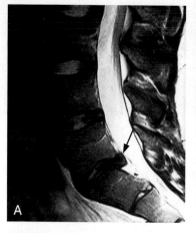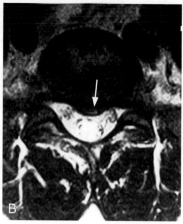

FIGURE 1 T2-weighted MRIs show the spine of a 21-year-old athlete with left S1 radiculopathy. **A**, Sagittal image demonstrates an L5/S1 disk herniation (arrow). **B**, Axial image demonstrates the left paramedian location (arrow).

> ▶ Axial T2-weighted sequences (**Figure 1, B**) determine whether HNP is central, paramedian, subarticular, or far lateral; in far-lateral HNP, axial T1-weighted images may better show HNP because high-signal-intensity fat outside canal contrasts with low-signal-intensity disk material

- Obtain plain radiographs before surgery to evaluate for deformity (scoliosis or spondylolisthesis) or spina bifida occulta (may not show on MRI obtained in supine position)

PROCEDURE

Room Setup/Patient Positioning

- Prone position on Jackson table; pad bony prominences well
- Suspend face and head in padded holder; enables clear visualization of eyes, nose, and endotracheal tube
- Flex knees; pad legs with memory foam pillows
- Bring table into jackknife position; reduces lumbar lordosis and facilitates exposure of disk by increasing interlaminar distance
- Bring C-arm into lateral position; drape out of sterile field after preparing skin

Special Instruments/Equipment/Implants

- C-arm fluoroscope
- Surgical microscope
- Adjustable Jackson table

Surgical Technique for Lumbar Microdiskectomy

 VIDEO 104.1 Lumbar Microdiskectomy. Bradley Moatz, MD; P. Justin Tortolani, MD (30 min)

Preparation
- Identify midline by palpating coccyx and sacrum distally, lumbar spinous processes proximally
- Palpate iliac crest on sides of patient; serves as guide to L4 vertebral level
- Insert spinal needle off midline, directed toward disk of interest; obtain lateral fluoroscopic image to visualize marker, confirming best location for skin incision

Exposure
- Infiltrate with 0.5% bupivacaine with epinephrine; make 3-cm skin incision midline, centered over disk of interest
- Dissect down to level of deep fascia; insert single cerebellar retractor to retract subcutaneous fat and skin
- Make vertical incision in lumbodorsal fascia, just lateral to midline, on side of disk herniation; use Army-Navy retractor alternating in superior and inferior aspect of wound to create fascial incision longer than skin incision, if needed
- Subperiosteally detach lumbodorsal musculature from posterior elements over interspace of interest; for L4-5 disk herniation, expose spinous process and lamina of L4 to level of pars interarticularis proximally and spinous process and lamina of L5 to level of pars interarticularis distally
- Avoid cutting muscle; detach musculotendinous attachments to tip of spinous processes and interspinous ligaments; use laterally directed sweeping motion with 1.5-cm Cobb curet to retract muscles over L4-5 facet joint capsule
- Secure Kocher clamp to inferior edge of cephalad lamina; obtain lateral fluoroscopic image to check that exposed level are correct (**Figure 2**)
- Place Taylor retractor lateral to exposed facet, allowing exposure of deep surgical field, ensuring no muscle creeps into field; can also use tip of Taylor retractor and Penfield 4 as additional check of spinal level on fluoroscopy (**Figure 3**)
- Hold Taylor retractor in position by looping gauze bandage around free end of retractor and surgeon's foot; also may use McCulloch retractor

Decompression
- Bring surgical microscope into field
- Use angled size 2 curet to create plane between ligamentum flavum and lamina of cephalad vertebra

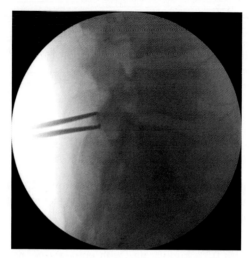

FIGURE 2 Intraoperative lateral fluoroscopic image of the lumbar spine shows a Kocher clamp placed on the inferior lamina of L5, thereby confirming the correct surgical level for L5-S1 microdiskectomy.

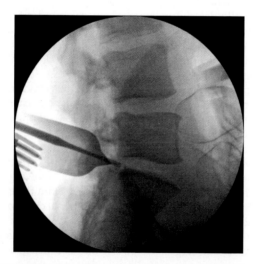

FIGURE 3 Intraoperative lateral fluoroscopic image shows the lumbar spine after the Taylor retractor has been positioned around the lateral aspect of the L5-S1 facet joint. The tip of the Taylor retractor points to the level of the diskectomy. A Penfield 4 is placed along the posterior aspect of the L5-S1 as a final confirmation of the desired surgical level.

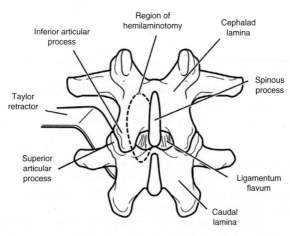

FIGURE 4 Illustration shows the exposure for decompression for lumbar microdiskectomy.

- Use high-speed burr used to thin laminar bone for subsequent hemilaminotomy; laminotomy window extends cephalad from interspace to level of pars interarticularis of superior vertebra and caudad from interspace to superior-most 3 mm of inferior lamina; extend laminotomy laterally to medial edge of facet joint complex (**Figure 4**)
- Ligamentum flavum serves as protective barrier over dura; use 45° Kerrison punch to remove remaining bone and complete laminotomy; can remove ligamentum en bloc by dissecting it free from medial edge of facet; use angled 2-0 microcuret to release adhesions between facet joint capsule and ligamentum
- Resect medial 3 mm of facet with Kerrison punch; perform foraminotomy by angling Kerrison out foramen of traversing nerve root
- Visualize dura; use Penfield 4 to identify lateral edge (shoulder region) of traversing nerve root; mobilize root gently toward midline and hold with nerve root retractor, revealing underlying disk space.
- Control epidural bleeding with bipolar cautery and thrombin-soaked gel foam
- After exposing disk herniation, use No. 15 blade to make incision directly over disk herniation; for smaller herniations without large annular defect, vertical slit incision may be sufficient; authors prefer slit incision; faster healing of anulus and enhanced outcomes
- Suction and micropituitary rongeur may be required for complete removal of fragment; make additional passes into disk space with micropituitary rongeur or angled microcuret to ensure no loose disk fragments are left

Closure

- Absorbable No. 1 Vicryl suture (Ethicon) in deep fascia
- 2-0 Vicryl in subcutaneous tissue
- Close skin with subcuticular suture, staples, or topical skin adhesive

Surgical Technique for Far-Lateral Microdiskectomy

- Far-lateral HNP less common; most direct access via paramedian muscle-splitting approach; after localization with fluoroscopy, make skin incision two fingerbreadths lateral to midline; continue to intermuscular septum between multifidus and longissimus muscles
- Continue subperiosteal dissection to transverse process just cephalad to disk herniation using electrocautery and/or Cobb; use transverse process and associated facet joint as anatomic landmarks
- Confirm correct level with radiography
- Use 4-mm Kerrison rongeur to partially resect lateral margin of superior facet to help expose disk; identify intertransverse ligament and, in medial to lateral direction, partially resect to expose exiting nerve root (**Figure 5**); most common error: not having enough medial exposure
- Identify disk herniation medial to nerve root; may need medial dissection into pars to ensure complete nerve decompression; free fragment found medial and inferior to exiting root

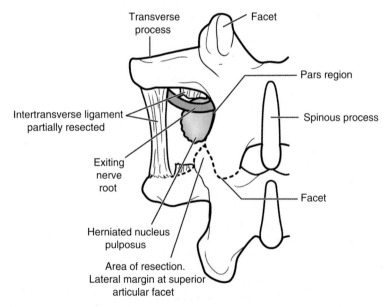

FIGURE 5 Illustration depicts the area of partial facetectomy and intertransverse ligament resection for access to a far-lateral disk herniation.

- Attempt extensive distal dissection only with great care; lumbar vasculature enters lower foramen, and dorsal primary nerve root exits from distal aspects of nerve root
- Remove fragment; flush wound with normal saline to remove loose fragments and dilute chemically irritating mediators of inflammation from nucleus pulposus
- Remove retractors; close wound with absorbable 0 Vicryl suture in fascial layer, 2-0 Vicryl in subcuticular tissue

COMPLICATIONS

- Most feared complication is cauda equina syndrome; occurs from excessive epidural bleeding or with large recurrent disk herniations; use bipolar cautery and gel foam to minimize bleeding at wound closure
- No consensus in literature, but authors do not restart anticoagulation medications until at least 48 hours after surgery; in patients at high risk for bleeding, insert subfascial drain before wound closure
- Nerve root injury, from excessive nerve root retraction during diskectomy; retract nerve root only as far as needed to remove herniation; make largest possible laminotomy window to reduce amount of nerve retraction required
- Close dural tear primarily in watertight fashion with 4-0 Nurolon suture (Ethicon); additional dural sealants or fat graft over dura may reinforce dural closure; if closure of dura required, admit patient and keep flat 24 to 48 hours to reduce hydrostatic pressure on repair site
- Suspect epidural fibrosis in patients with new unremitting radicular pain weeks to months after microdiskectomy; no evidence, but authors place small amount of fat from subcutaneous region over dura and exiting nerve root to reduce risk
- Recurrent radicular pain may occur in recurrent disk herniation after pain-free period; symptoms triggered by activity; knee and hip flexion provide relief; MRI with gadolinium contrast can distinguish recurrent disk herniation from epidural fibrosis
- Surgical site infection very rare with perioperative antibiotics; authors delay surgery in patients with infections of skin, urinary tract, lungs, and teeth, even if under treatment

POSTOPERATIVE CARE AND REHABILITATION

- Discharge patients 3 to 4 hours after lumbar microdiskectomy with oral opiates, stool softeners, and muscle relaxant
- Encourage normal activities of daily living; no waist bending, twisting, upper body lifting more than 10 lb for first 3 weeks
- Provide isometric core and lower extremity exercises, hamstring flexibility routines to perform once per day at home for first 3 weeks; initiate formal outpatient physical therapy program at 3 weeks
- Restrict sports activities for 3 months
- Tailor return to work and driving to patient's circumstances

PEARLS

- Determining correct side and level of IDH to be removed cannot be overemphasized; authors double-check level and side of herniation on MRI before obtaining consent.
- Surgical "time out" is second check; fluoroscopic images obtained with spinal needle pointing to disk and Kocher clamp on cephalad lamina are third and fourth checks.
- Can use tip of Taylor retractor and Penfield 4 as fifth and sixth checks of spinal level with intraoperative fluoroscopy.
- If disk herniation not visualized on exposure, confirm that the surgical level and side are correct before performing diskectomy; retract traversing nerve root laterally (not medially, as described previously), thereby exposing axilla of nerve root; in several cases, IDH has been located in axilla of nerve root.
- For microdiskectomy at L5-S1 level, look for presence of spina bifida occulta on preoperative images to prevent inadvertent surgical plunging into spinal canal and dura during exposure.
- For far-lateral disk procedure, obtain true AP and lateral fluoroscopic views to plan incision.
- Tilting table away from surgeon can improve visualization into foramen and area lateral to pedicle.
- Avoid excessive retraction of dorsal ganglion; can lead to postoperative radiculitis.
- The nerve root usually is displaced superiorly; underlying pedicle blocks any inferior disk migration.

PATIENT SELECTION
- Lumbar stenosis is reduction in size of central, lateral recess, or foraminal lumbar canal
- May present with radiculopathy or neurogenic claudication

Indications
- Unsuccessful nonsurgical treatment of 3 to 6 months—No satisfactory relief, progressive neurologic deficit, impairment of activities of daily living
- Nonsurgical treatment includes weight loss, smoking cessation, physical therapy, injections
- Nonsurgical treatment particularly appropriate for patients with nontraditional symptoms and/or discordant history, imaging, physical examination findings
- Laminectomy indicated after failure of nonsurgical treatment
- Evaluate for spondylolisthesis or instability; both require arthrodesis in addition to decompression

Contraindications
- Contraindication for laminectomy without arthrodesis is severe degenerative disk disease with low back pain
- Elderly patients with multiple comorbidities

PREOPERATIVE IMAGING
- Plain radiographs
  - Weight-bearing AP, lateral
  - Flexion/extension views to assess for instability
- CT—Better assessment of bony anatomy such as ossification of the ligamentum flavum
- MRI—Helps to assess neural elements and soft tissues
- CT/myelography—Helpful if MRI of poor quality, previous surgery with instrumentation, or instrumentation is planned

---

Based on Davis SM, Boden SD: Lumbar laminectomy, in Colvin AC, Flatow E, eds: Atlas of Essential Orthopaedic Procedures, *ed 2. Rosemont, IL, American Academy of Orthopaedic Surgeons, 2020, pp 851-856.*

PROCEDURE

Room Setup/Patient Positioning

- Prone position
- Jackson table or regular table with bolster under anterior superior iliac spine and chest
- Also may position on Wilson frame; creates kyphosis, making decompression easier; may not be beneficial for arthrodesis
- Also may use 90/90 position on Andrews frame
- Abdomen hangs free to decompress epidural venous plexus
- Prepare back in routine fashion
- Perform timeout for all surgical team members
- Localize levels with fluoroscopy

Surgical Technique

- Make midline incision; use monopolar cautery to dissect to level of lumbodorsal fascia
- Dissect fascia to facilitate reapproximation with watertight closure
- Perform subperiosteal dissection to level of lamina
- Expose facet joints carefully to lateral aspect without violating capsule; adequately expose pars interarticularis to avoid excessive thinning, which places it at risk for fracture
- Confirm levels again using metallic marker of surgeon's choice and lateral fluoroscopic image

Three Stages of Decompression

- Central decompression
  - Remove interspinous ligament with Leksell rongeur; remove spinous process or processes overlying disk space to be decompressed using Horsley bone cutter (**Figure 1, A** and **B**)
  - Remove outer cortex of lamina with Leksell (**Figure 1, C**)
  - Separate ligamentum flavum from underside of lamina using curved curets (**Figure 1, D**)
  - Remove inner cortex of lamina with Kerrison rongeurs (**Figure 1, E**)
  - Excise bone rostrally until epidural fat exposed at upper border of ligamentum; exercise extreme caution because ligamentum no longer protects dura mater
  - Remove medial border of facet joint with osteotome or Kerrison
  - Pass Penfield dissector No. 3 between ligamentum and dura to create working space, ensure no adhesions; if adhesions present, use small curet or elevator to separate ligamentum from dura (**Figure 1, F**)
  - Completed central decompression should remove entire lamina and all of ligamentum flavum (**Figure 1, G**)

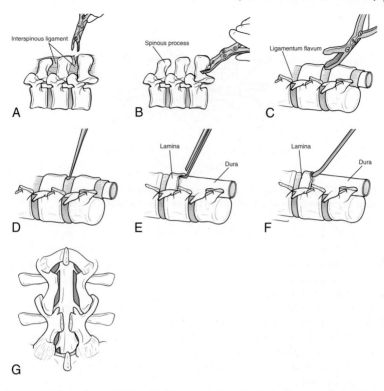

FIGURE 1 Illustrations depict central decompression. **A,** A Leksell rongeur is used to remove the interspinous ligament. **B,** A Horsley bone cutter is used to remove the spinous processes. The interspinous ligament is not present. **C,** A Leksell rongeur is used to remove the lamina overlying the ligamentum flavum. Note that the nose of the rongeur is angled up. **D,** An angled Epstein curet is used to develop a plane between the remaining lamina and the ligamentum flavum to create space for the Kerrison rongeur to work. **E,** A Kerrison rongeur is used to remove the remaining lamina over the dura. **F,** A Penfield dissector is slid between the dura and the undersurface of the lamina to release adhesions. **G,** A complete laminectomy is shown at the superior level; half of the lamina has been removed at the inferior level.

- Lateral recess decompression
  - ▶ Use Woodson elevator to identify space between remaining ligamentum and lateral recess; use elevator to identify areas needing decompression
  - ▶ Place cottonoid patty to protect dura
  - ▶ To prevent catching redundant dura in jaws, use largest Kerrison rongeur possible (**Figure 2**), without compressing neural elements, to decompress

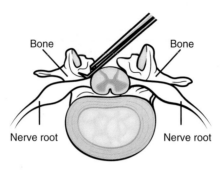

FIGURE 2 Illustration depicts lateral recess decompression. A Kerrison rongeur is used to remove bone and ligamentum flavum from the lateral recess.

- Carry excision to medial border of pedicle, while limiting medial facetectomy to less than 50% of surface area to prevent iatrogenic instability
- Neuroforaminal decompression
    - Use Frazier dural elevator to probe neuroforamina, identify impinging structures (**Figure 3, A**)
    - Use Kerrison to remove osteophytes from superior articular process; rongeur trajectory is in line with that of nerve root (**Figure 3, B**)
    - Use Penfield No. 4 to gently manipulate nerve root and confirm mobility

Closure
- Obtain epidural hemostasis with bipolar cautery
- Obtain intramuscular hemostasis with monopolar cautery

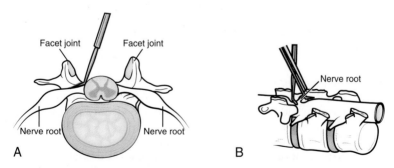

FIGURE 3 Illustrations depict foraminal decompression. **A,** A Frazier dural elevator is used to palpate the foraminal space to assess stenosis. **B,** A Kerrison rongeur is used to remove bone from within the foraminal space. Note that the Kerrison rongeur is angled in the same direction as the nerve root.

- Place Hemovac drain, exiting cephalad
- Close in layers; apply sterile dressing

COMPLICATIONS

- Overall complication rate up to 18.9% in patients older than 85 years having at least three medical comorbidities
- Rate significantly lower in younger patients with no comorbidities
- Postoperative neurologic deficits
- Cerebrospinal fluid leak and fistula
  - Durotomy rate up to 17%
  - Repair any durotomy with nylon suture and/or combination of grafts, patches, fibrin glue
- Facet and/or pars fracture
- Infection
- Most common complications in elderly are postoperative hematoma, renal complications
- Overall mortality rate generally ranges from 1% to 3% depending on age and comorbidities
- Mortality rate 1.4% in patients older than 85 years having at least three comorbidities; in healthier elderly, mortality as low as 0.17%

POSTOPERATIVE CARE AND REHABILITATION

- Postoperative antibiotics for 24 hours
- Patient-controlled anesthesia pump
- Remove drain, catheter as soon as deemed safe by surgeon
- Discontinue patient-controlled anesthesia; transition to oral pain medications
- Physical therapy for gait training and overall mobility
- Bracing at discretion of surgeon
- No bending, lifting, twisting for 6 weeks; coincides with first postoperative visit

PEARLS

- Confirm correct surgical level preoperatively.
- Avoid violation of facet capsule to avoid iatrogenic arthrosis or instability.
- Expose pars interarticularis to safely decompress level of interest.
- Create potential space between bone and ligamentum flavum to allow safe passage of Kerrison rongeur.
- Release adhesions with care to avoid inadvertent durotomy.
- Visualize shoulder of nerve root to ensure adequate decompression of entry zone to the foramen.
- When performing foraminotomy, the Kerrison rongeur should work parallel to trajectory of nerve root.

106 Instrumented Lumbar Fusion

PATIENT SELECTION

- Pedicle screws are anchored in corticocancellous core of vertebral pedicle; strongest point of fixation in spine
- Pedicle screws have biomechanical advantage over hooks, wires, and anterior vertebral body screws
- Enhance arthrodesis rates in lumbar spine
- Important component of transforaminal lumbar interbody fusion, all-posterior correction of idiopathic scoliosis, minimally invasive treatment of fractures, and posterior dynamic stabilization

Indications

- Pedicle screws indicated when lumbar fusion performed
- Spinal conditions treated using instrumented lumbar fusion include stenosis with spondylolisthesis, spinal tumor, fracture, deformity, iatrogenic instability, and recurrent disk herniation

Contraindications

- Absolute contraindications to pedicle screw fixation include pedicle size too small to accept smallest-diameter pedicle screw, congenital absence of pedicle
- Relative contraindications include tumor, other bone lesion unable to support screw, profound osteoporosis

PREOPERATIVE IMAGING

- Plain radiographs to help assess spinal alignment; MRI or CT to assess pedicle dimensions.
- Note rotational deformities, hyperlordosis, and hypolordosis; all affect screw path
- In lumbar spine, visualize starting point for pedicle screw—identified by intersection of line bisecting transverse process horizontally and vertical line along medial aspect of pars interarticularis vertically—on AP view preoperatively

---

Based on Schoenfeld AJ, Bono CM: Instrumented lumbar fusion, in Colvin AC, Flatow E, eds: Atlas of Essential Orthopaedic Procedures, *ed 2. Rosemont, IL, American Academy of Orthopaedic Surgeons, 2020, pp 857-864.*

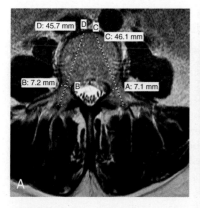 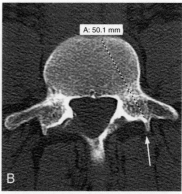

FIGURE 1 Preoperative images used to plan pedicle screw placement. **A**, Axial MRI shows the templating used to determine the appropriate size of pedicle screws. The widths (lines A and B) and lengths (lines C and D) are determined for pedicle screws bilaterally. **B**, Axial CT scan shows how to use the accessory process (arrow) as an anatomic landmark for the screw insertion site.

- Achieve more precise preoperative planning using axial MRI or CT; assess for factors compromising safe screw placement: dysplastic or absent pedicles, aberrant nerve roots, dural ectasia
- Use axial images to measure pedicle diameters, approximate screw lengths at proposed instrumented levels (**Figure 1, A**); determine screw length preoperatively by measuring from posterior aspect of superior articular process to desired depth within vertebral body (**Figure 1, B**); use smallest transverse width of pedicle to determine pedicle screw diameter
- Do not undersize screws; pullout strength of screw depends on interface between cortical bone of pedicle and screw threads; use screws of slightly larger width as "rescue" screws if screw tract compromised
- Careful, slow insertion allows cortical walls to accommodate screws of moderately larger width; no evidence supports using larger-width screws in uncompromised tracts; approximate screw sizes for each level and side transcribed on template paper

PROCEDURE
Room Setup/Patient Positioning
- Proper positioning critical; prone position on well-padded radiolucent table; authors prefer Jackson four-poster frame, with chest pad and supports for iliac crest and thighs
- Abdomen hangs free to reduce intra-abdominal pressure
- Place padding under knees, anterior legs to avoid pressure points
- Shoulders abducted, elbows flexed no more than 90° on well-padded arm boards; bolster anterior shoulder to prevent brachial plexus stretch

- Head positioner keeps neck in neutral position, avoids pressure around eyes, allows access to endotracheal tube
- Secure all wires, lines, catheters to frame of table; allows C-arm to move with less risk of dislodging critical equipment
- Table in center of room, anesthesia station at head; surgeon, assistant on opposite sides of patient
- Position fluoroscopic imaging system where surgeon can see images; have template paper visible
- Before preparing and draping, ensure adequate fluoroscopy can be obtained; adjust table to yield better AP view; use lateral view to mark levels of pedicles to be instrumented to help determine incision size

Special Instruments

- Pedicle screws
- Starter awls, taps, depth gauges
- With screws in place, rod secured to each with "blocker" or set screw; set screws final tightened using manufacturer's torque-limiting driver
- Large 5-mm burr
- Electrophysiologic monitoring, if desired

Surgical Technique

VIDEO 106.1 Lumbar Laminectomy. Howard S. An, MD; Dino Samartzis, BS; Ashok Biyani, MD (4 min)

- Make midline incision for standard posterior approach to lumbar spine (**Figure 2**); can use alternative incisions, such as bilateral paraspinous, if midline structures to be maintained
- Minimize length of skin incision using lateral fluoroscopy to plot incision from spinous process of vertebral level to spinous process of caudal instrumented level
- Strip paraspinal musculature subperiosteally with electrocautery; avoid injuring facet joint capsules
- Dissect lateral to facet capsules; exposure complete once transverse processes, pars interarticularis, laminae, facet joints, spinous processes in zone of fusion are exposed
- Authors prefer to perform decompression at this stage
- Perform pedicle screw insertion with or without live image guidance; at least, obtain plain radiographs after instrumentation placed to check orientation; authors prefer using orthogonal fluoroscopic images during screw insertion
- Identify starting point by identifying junction between horizontal line bisecting transverse process and vertical line running along superior articular process (**Figure 3, A**)

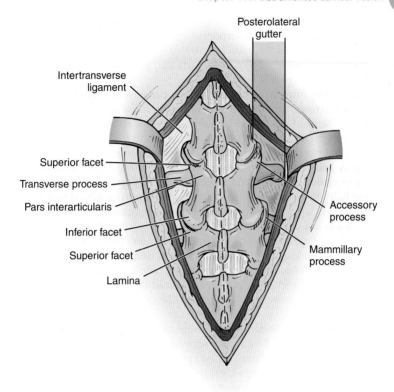

FIGURE 2 Illustration shows the relevant anatomy of the posterior elements of the lumbar spine for lumbar fusion using pedicle screws. The dashed red line indicates the approximate site of the surgical incision.

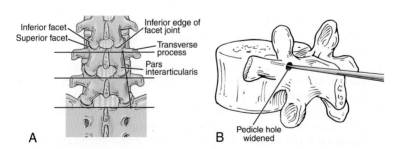

FIGURE 3 Illustrations demonstrate the technique for inserting pedicle screws. **A,** The appropriate starting points (red dots) of pedicle screws within the lumbar spine are shown. **B,** The proper path for cannulating the lumbar pedicle and the tract for screw insertion is shown.

- In some patients, an accessory process may be present (**Figure 2**); can be landmark for screw insertion
- Starting point for S1 pedicle screw is at junction of sacral ala and inferolateral aspect of S1 superior articular process; corresponds to the inferolateral aspect of facet joint
- Facet joints often hypertrophic, which can obscure starting point for pedicle screws; can remove osteophytes to allow localization
- Enter cortex of the bone with rongeur, start awl, or small 3-mm burr; authors prefer burr guided by AP fluoroscopic view; note blush of bleeding from underlying cancellous bone upon entry
- Insert pedicle finder to create screw tract; using lateral fluoroscopy, advance through pedicle into vertebral body (**Figure 3, B**); angle finder medially 10° to 15° until tip reaches posterior portion of vertebral body; once there, apply more aggressive medial angulation; tactile feedback is steady but yielding resistance
- Increasing resistance can indicate abutment with cortical border; sudden "giving-way" suggests penetration of cortical boundary: reposition with image confirmation; advance probe to desired depth, near junction of anterior and middle thirds; bicortical pedicle screw placement not advisable unless screws placed into S1 vertebral body
- Remove pedicle finder, assess screw tract with ball-tipped probe to confirm four intact "walls" (ie, superior, inferior, lateral, medial cortices in pedicle) and "floor" (ie, end point in vertebral body)
- If cortical violation found, create new pedicle tract; may tap screw tract; authors prefer to undertap screw hole
- Screw length judged intraoperatively, screw width determined preoperatively; once screw inserted, confirm position using AP and lateral fluoroscopic views; on perfect AP view, screw tip does not cross midline; on perfect lateral view, screw is confined within bony borders of pedicle
- May use electromyography stimulation to assess thresholds as described previously
- Use flexible rod templates to estimate size; 5.5- or 6.0-mm titanium rods usually used
- Rod should extend beyond margins of cephalad and caudad pedicle screw heads no more than 2 to 3 mm to avoid impinging on facet joints of adjacent nonfused levels
- Fix rod to screw heads by set screws; final tighten using manufacturer's torque-limiting devices, including antitorque sleeve
- Obtain final radiographs to confirm position and alignment of construct; "cross-links," or coupler connections, can enhance biomechanical rigidity of instrumented construct, in setting of osteoporotic bone; not routinely used in short-segment constructs, that is, those spanning three levels or fewer

- Prepare fusion bed and place bone graft; at minimum, transverse processes and facet joints within zone of fusion are decorticated; remove all cartilage from within facet joints in fusion zone; if midline structures present, laminae and spinous processes also decorticated
- Place bone graft along these surfaces
- Irrigate wound; confirm hemostasis; place subfascial drain
- Close wound in layers, with watertight fascial closure; use interrupted sutures to close subcutaneous layers; close skin with running subcuticular absorbable suture, staples, or nylon suture; apply sterile dressing

 VIDEO 106.2 Spinal Fusion. Howard S. An, MD; Dino Samartzis, BS; Ashok Biyani, MD (7 min)

COMPLICATIONS

- Higher risk of complications for instrumented fusion procedures than for stand-alone decompression or uninstrumented fusion
- Overall risk following instrumented fusions is 10% to 20%
- Risk may be higher in cases with deformity, revision surgery, tumor
- Complications include nerve root impingement, fracture of pedicle, dural tear, and injury to great vessels
- Risk of neural compromise greater for screws that breach medial or inferior pedicle wall; inferior pedicle wall breaches in lower lumbar spine at greater risk of nerve root impingement than those at more cephalad levels

POSTOPERATIVE CARE AND REHABILITATION

- Hospital stay extends approximately 3 days after instrumented spinal fusion
- Encourage ambulation on postoperative day 1
- Discontinue catheter when patient can stand or sit at side of bed
- Continue prophylactic postoperative antibiotics for 24 hours
- Keep subfascial drain until output less than 30 mL per shift
- Change surgical dressing on postoperative day 2 unless soiled or saturated
- Obtain standing AP and lateral radiographs once patient has ambulated
- No heavy lifting, twisting at waist, flexion at waist, per surgeon preference; authors recommend avoiding such activities for 12 weeks after fusion
- Clinical and radiographic follow-up at 2 weeks, 3 months, 6 months, and 1 year

PEARLS

- Performing same surgical step at multiple screw insertion sites can be time efficient.
- Failure of pedicle screw driver to maintain medial trajectory following screw insertion may indicate laterally misplaced screw.
- If position of screw is questionable, use C-arm to "rainbow" over pedicle tube so beam is in line with pedicle's trajectory; if pedicle screw placed correctly, image shows screw as a bull's-eye within cortical ring of pedicle; can perform similar maneuver before screw insertion using ball-tipped probe.
- Preparation of fusion bed may be easier if performed before rod or screw insertion.
- Failure to confirm a satisfactory pedicle screw tract with ball-tipped probe increases risk of screw misplacement, damage to adjacent structures.
- Damaging facet joints or facet capsule in regions of spine not included in fusion can raise risk for adjacent segment degeneration.
- Inadequate surgical exposure inhibits successful fusion bed preparation, increases risk of screw misplacement.
- If osteophytes over hypertrophic facet joints are not resected, starting point more difficult to identify, risk of screw misplacement increases.

VIDEO REFERENCE

Video 106.1 An HS, Samartzis D, Biyani A: *Lumbar Spinal Stenosis: Laminoplasty* [video]. Rosemont, IL, American Academy of Orthopaedic Surgeons, 2003.

Transforaminal Lumbar Interbody Fusion

INTRODUCTION
- Transforaminal lumbar interbody fusion (TLIF) first described in 1982
- Enables fusion of spinal segment anteriorly and posteriorly through single posterior procedure; eliminates morbidity, complications of anterior fusion
- Can access disk space through single unilateral posterior approach, preserving contralateral lamina and spinous process, creating larger surface area for posterolateral fusion
- Exposes neural foramen for direct decompression, eliminates need to retract thecal sac, reducing risk of incidental durotomy, neural injury
- Intervertebral disk space ideal for obtaining bony fusion due to compressive forces of anterior column and blood supply provided by prepared end plates
- In lumbar spine, 80% of mechanical load transmitted through vertebral body, 20% through posterior elements; in posterolateral fusion, fusion bed under tensile forces; in interbody fusion, fusion surface under compression
- TLIF combined with posterolateral instrumentation and fusion achieves fusion rates greater than 90% and clinical outcomes comparable to anterior lumbar interbody fusion with posterolateral instrumentation and fusion

PATIENT SELECTION
Indications
- TLIF ideal for treating lumbar spine deformity, degenerative disk disease; interbody fusion restores disk space height and lordosis, indirectly decompressing neural foramen and improving sagittal balance
- Isthmic spondylolisthesis (grades I and II)
- Foraminal intervertebral disk herniations and recurrent disk herniations
- Degenerative disk disease causing mechanical back pain with or without radiculopathy
- Postlaminectomy spondylolisthesis

Based on Tannous OO, Banagan K, Ludwig SC: Transforaminal lumbar interbody fusion, in Colvin AC, Flatow E, eds: Atlas of Essential Orthopaedic Procedures, *ed 2. Rosemont, IL, American Academy of Orthopaedic Surgeons, 2020, pp 865-872.*

- Postlaminectomy kyphosis
- Lumbar coronal or sagittal plane deformities

Contraindications
- Severe osteopenia
- Bleeding disorders
- Relatively contraindicated in active local or systemic infection

PREOPERATIVE IMAGING
- Preoperative AP and lateral radiographs (**Figure 1**)
- CT/MRI

PROCEDURE
Room Setup/Patient Positioning
- Prone position on Jackson table
- Pad bony prominences; free abdomen of compression to relieve intra-abdominal pressure
- Place neuromonitors on lower extremities in lumbar dermatomal distribution
- Anesthesiologist keeps patient in hypotensive state to help reduce blood loss

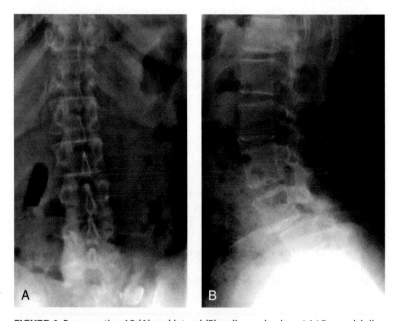

FIGURE 1 Preoperative AP (**A**) and lateral (**B**) radiographs show L4-L5 spondylolisthesis in a 54-year-old woman who presented with reports of worsening back pain and lower extremity radiculopathy.

Special Instruments/Equipment/Implants

- Pedicle screw system
- Structural interbody spacer options: titanium cages, polyetheretherke-tone cages, structural machined allograft, poly-L/D-lactide resorbable spacer
- Bone graft materials
- C-arm
- Neuromonitoring equipment
- Bipolar cautery, straight osteotomes, Kerrison and Leksell rongeurs, straight and curved curets and pituitaries, disk space shavers, disk space dilators, disk space trials, and high-speed burr

Surgical Technique

Open Transforaminal Lumbar Interbody Fusion

- Mark level(s) of interest with fluoroscope; may perform TLIF on side with greatest clinical and/or radiographic abnormality
- Make midline incision; continue dissection in subperiosteal manner, might include transverse process of involved levels
- Place pedicle screws at indicated level(s); create window to access disk space (**Figure 2**)
- Resect inferior articular facet of cephalad vertebra and superior artic-ular facet of caudal vertebra; use straight osteotome to create partial laminotomy in inferior lamina of cephalad vertebra (**Figure 3, A**)

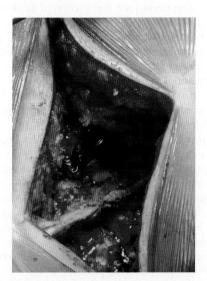

FIGURE 2 Intraoperative photograph shows the transforaminal lumbar interbody fusion window created to access the disk space.

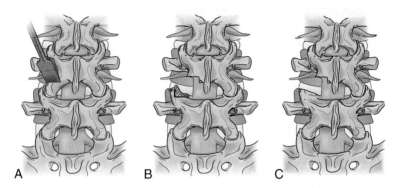

FIGURE 3 Illustrations show a laminotomy during a transforaminal lumbar interbody fusion. **A**, A straight osteotome is used to create a partial laminotomy in the inferior lamina of the cephalad vertebra. **B**, The pars interarticularis of the vertebra above is transected, and the inferior facet is removed. **C**, The superior articular facet of the caudal vertebra is resected, allowing a window of access to the intervertebral disk.

- Transect pars interarticularis; remove inferior facet of vertebra above (**Figure 3, B**); use Kerrison and Leksell rongeurs to resect superior articular facet of caudal vertebra (**Figure 3, C**); save bone for use as graft
- Decompress exiting nerve root; completion of facetectomy allows traversing nerve root to be visualized, freed up
- Apply bipolar cautery to bleeding epidural vessels; place nerve root retractor medially to protect dural sac; achieve exposure of disk space with Penfield dissector
- Create box-cut annulotomy in disk space to begin complete diskectomy; initiate diskectomy with straight pituitary rongeurs, curets (**Figure 4, A**); continue with angled pituitaries, curets (**Figure 4, B**) to access contralateral aspect of disk space
- Use sequential dilators, shavers to open up disk space and facilitate complete diskectomy (**Figure 5**)
- Use lamina spreader to distract at spinous processes; can apply additional distraction force to pedicle screws
- Insert and tamp trial implant anteriorly and medially; confirm fit with tactile feedback and radiographically; remove trial; tamp implant into anterocentral aspect of disk space (**Figure 6**); positioning optimizes load-sharing capacity of implant, helps restore lumbar lordosis
- Place rods; apply compression to compress interbody graft, improve lumbar lordosis
- Perform final tightening; radiographically confirm appropriate implant and graft placement (**Figure 7**)

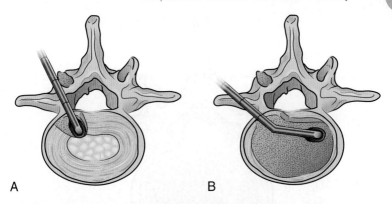

FIGURE 4 Illustrations show a diskectomy during a transforaminal lumbar interbody fusion. The diskectomy is initiated with straight curets (**A**) and is continued with angled curets (**B**) to access the contralateral disk space.

- Decorticate surrounding bone with high-speed burr to form fusion bed; may perform intertransverse process fusion
- Probe foramen and canal to verify no free bone present; irrigate wound; meticulously place bone graft about fusion bed; place wound drains; close wound

Minimally Invasive Transforaminal Lumbar Interbody Fusion

- Steep learning curve
- Under fluoroscopic guidance, make 2- to 5-cm incision 4 to 5 cm lateral to midline, centered over facet joint

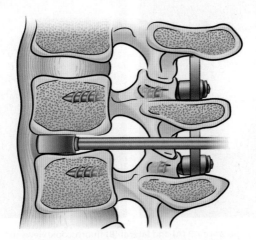

FIGURE 5 Illustration shows insertion of a dilator into the disk space. Sequential dilators are used to distract the disk space and facilitate the performance of a complete diskectomy during a transforaminal lumbar interbody fusion.

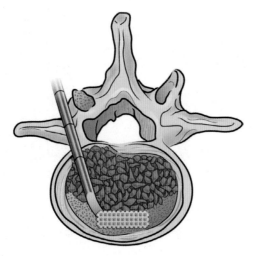

FIGURE 6 Illustration shows placement of the transforaminal lumbar interbody fusion (TLIF) implant. The TLIF implant is tamped into the anterocentral aspect of the disk space. The remainder of the intervertebral space is filled with bone graft.

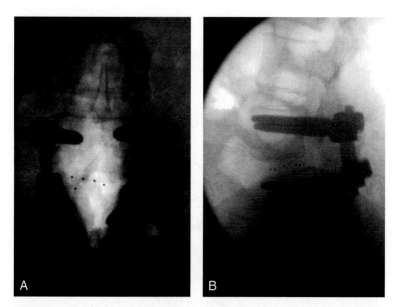

FIGURE 7 Intraoperative AP (**A**) and lateral (**B**) fluoroscopic views show confirmation of screw and interbody placement after implant placement for transforaminal lumbar interbody fusion. The interbody is represented by the dots visible within the disk space.

- Insert guidewire, aiming toward facet with lateral-to-medial vector; control bleeding with electrocautery
- Pass serial dilators over guidewire; insert 22- to 26-mm–diameter tube directly over facet complex
- Use microscope or illuminated tube and loupe combination for remaining steps, which are similar to those of open technique

Minimally Invasive Versus Open Transforaminal Lumbar Interbody Fusion

- Minimally invasive TLIF benefits over open technique include less blood loss, fewer postoperative transfusions, less postoperative back pain, quicker time to ambulation, briefer hospital stay, significantly fewer surgical site infections
- Benefits credited to less extensive, traumatic dissection

COMPLICATIONS

- Infection—Average rate 3.3%
- Incidental durotomy—Average rate 4.8%
- Hematoma—Reported postoperative rate 3% to 4%; revision surgery required
- Postoperative radiculopathy—Average rate 5.3%; defined as new-onset pain or muscle weakness in dermatomal distribution
- Pseudarthrosis—Overall rate 9% for open technique, 5% for minimally invasive method
- Pedicle screw malposition—Rate 1.4% to 2.1%; requires revision surgery for screw removal
- Interbody spacer migration—Rare but serious; related factors include interbody preparation, implant selection, implant placement
- Ileus—Reported incidence 3%; much lower than rate with anterior approach

POSTOPERATIVE CARE AND REHABILITATION

- Immediate postoperative mobilization
- Obtain standing AP, lateral radiographs before discharge
- Consult with physical, occupational therapists for proper ways of bending, lifting, turning
- No restrictions for stair climbing
- No postoperative bracing
- Patients may drive when can react to road, no longer receiving narcotics
- Initiate postoperative outpatient physical therapy at 6 weeks; lift restrictions on activities at 3-month postoperative visit
- Follow patients clinically, radiographically for minimum 1 year or until confirmation of fusion

PEARLS

- Take care to free ligamentum flavum from lamina, especially during revision cases when significant fibrosis present.
- Do not violate pedicles above or below level(s) of interest; use Kerrison rongeur to resect pars interarticularis, high-speed cutting burr to thin down bony elements.
- Protect exiting nerve root in foraminal zone; can damage dorsal root ganglion present in region.
- Achieve complete visualization of exiting, traversing nerve roots before annulotomy.
- Thorough preparation of end plates critical; perform preparation without violating subchondral bone of end plate; can lead to subsidence of implant, nonunion, development of segmental kyphosis.
- Do not violate anterior annulus; can cause anterior migration of cage or bone graft, damage to great vessels.
- Distract cautiously on spinous processes; can cause fractures in osteopenic patients; take similar care when distracting pedicle screws; can cause loosening, loss of fixation.
- Do not insert bone graft into foramen when performing intertransverse process fusion, especially on TLIF side.

Anterior Spinal Column Reconstruction: Anterior, Lateral, and Oblique Approaches to the Spine

ANTERIOR LUMBAR INTERBODY FUSION

INTRODUCTION

- Lumbar levels from L2 to sacrum can be accessed via a single retroperitoneal approach
- Advantages of anterior approach: high fusion rates compared with those of posterolateral intertransverse fusion, especially for L5-S1; better correction of coronal plane deformity; greater graft surface area; and no paraspinal muscle dissection

PATIENT SELECTION

Indications

- Anterior lumbar approach most often performed at L4-L5, L5-S1, with single-level fusion through retroperitoneal approach most commonly
- Most common indication for single-level lower lumbar spine surgery is lumbar disk degeneration with low back pain
- Others include diskitis/osteomyelitis, nonunion after posterior fusion procedure, spinal deformity surgery, recurrent disk herniation, total disk replacement/revision, fractures, tumor surgery
- Failure of nonsurgical treatment
- Alternatives include transabdominal or laparoscopic approaches; both associated with more complications, including prolonged postoperative ileus, bowel injury, retrograde ejaculation

Contraindications

- Revision setting, particularly L4-L5; L5-S1 may be approached from side opposite index approach without significantly increasing vascular injury risk
- Direct lateral approach to levels above L5-S1 may be safer than revision anterior surgery

---

Based on Nimmons SJB, Park AE: Anterior spinal column reconstruction: Anterior, lateral, and oblique approaches to the spine, in Colvin AC, Flatow E, eds: Atlas of Essential Orthopaedic Procedures, *ed 2. Rosemont, IL, American Academy of Orthopaedic Surgeons, 2020, pp 873-889.*

- Before considering revision anterior lumbar exposure, consider direct lateral approach or posterior approach to avoid vascular risks associated with revision anterior retroperitoneal exposure. Morbid obesity is a relative contraindication

DIAGNOSIS

- Diagnosis of degenerative disk disease most commonly encountered at L4-L5, L5-S1; may see multilevel disease
- Presents with long history of low back pain with exacerbations over many years

PREOPERATIVE IMAGING

- Plain radiographs demonstrate height loss on lateral view (**Figure 1**)
- Instability on flexion-extension imaging uncommonly may coexist with degenerative disk
- Be aware of spondylolysis affecting involved motion segment; may affect need for additional fixation
- May see vacuum disk sign on standing, recumbent, flexion-extension radiographs
- MRI changes may include loss of disk space height, loss of signal intensity in nucleus pulposus on T2-weighted image, posterior disk bulge on axial imaging, Modic end-plate changes (**Figure 2**); may see compression of neural elements on axial imaging affecting central canal, subarticular recess, or far lateral zone of neural foramen

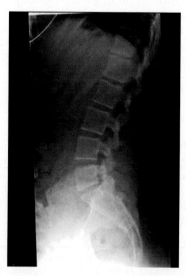

FIGURE 1 Lateral radiograph shows a loss of disk space height at L5-S1.

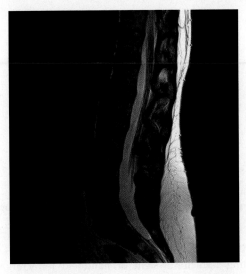

FIGURE 2 Sagittal T2-weighted MRI demonstrates typical changes associated with a symptomatic lumbar degenerative disk.

- Diskography and postdiskography imaging controversial
  - ◗ Introduces variability in technique and interpretation
  - ◗ Inclusion of control level debated, based on theoretical potential for accelerated disk degeneration at control level

PROCEDURE

Room Setup/Patient Positioning

- Use operating table that allows intraoperative fluoroscopic imaging (**Figure 3**)
- Author prefers flat Jackson OSI table (**Figure 4**) or Jackson Axis OSI table (**Figure 5**) (Mizuho OSI); Axis table allows flexion or extension, creating more or less lumbar lordosis (**Figure 6**); may benefit deformity cases or collapsed disk space
- Alternatively, can place inflatable arterial line cuff under lower lumbar spine as bolster to increase lumbar lordosis
- Position patient on operating room table with care to ensure no rotation of pelvis or torso; pad appropriately
- May place arms to side or over chest (**Figures 4** and **5**); arms over chest position allows C-arm to remain in surgical field (lateral position) for imaging without need for multiple drapes; improves sterile technique

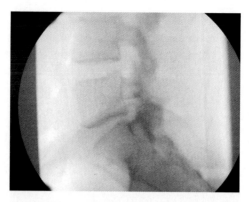

FIGURE 3 True lateral fluoroscopic image demonstrates disk collapse at L5-S1.

Special Instruments

- Self-retaining retractor system or handheld retractors dictated by exposure surgeon
- Handheld vein retractors for managing inferior vena cava and abdominal aorta or iliac vessels (**Figure 7**)
- Variously sized (7 to 15 mm in 1-mm increments) intradiscal distractors to distract disk space open during disk removal
- Sequential dilation of the disk space by alternating disk space distractors from right to left while working the opposite side

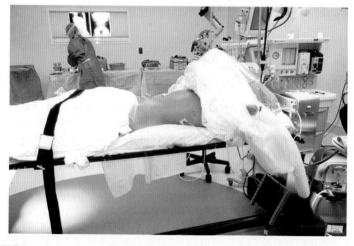

FIGURE 4 Photograph depicts a flat Jackson OSI table. The patient's arms are folded over the chest to allow intraoperative fluoroscopy in the lateral plane.

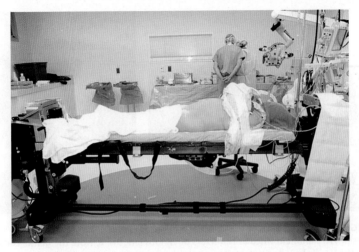

FIGURE 5 A Mizuho OSI Jackson Axis table in the flat position.

Surgical Technique

- Obtain images to confirm no rotation of targeted disk space; also helps localize surgical incision (**Figure 8**); direct access to disk space in plane of disk space is required for insertion of anterior lumbar interbody devices
- May expose anterior spine through relatively small incisions; approach spine through midline vertical fascial incision even if skin is cut transversely

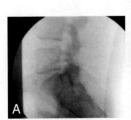
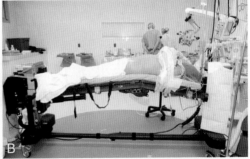

FIGURE 6 Note the increased lordosis at L5-S1 as seen on a lateral fluoroscopic image (**A**) with extension of the operating table using the extension function of the Axis table (**B**).

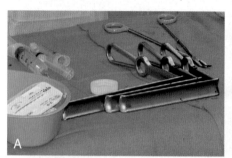
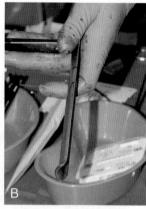

FIGURE 7 Photographs of the instruments used for anterior lumbar interbody fusion. **A**, Handheld vascular retractors of various lengths. **B**, Note the gentle curve at the tip of the vein retractor to assist with retraction and visualization.

- After exposure of disk space, obtain AP and lateral images to confirm surgical level, establish midline of disk space, mark midline on disk space (**Figure 9**) or vertebral body as internal reference for placing implant centrally within disk space
- Many types of interbody devices can reconstruct interspace, achieve solid fusion (**Figure 10**); some have integrated fixation, others can be used alone or with supplemental fixation

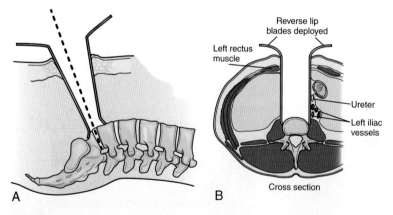

FIGURE 8 Illustration shows localization of the incision. **A**, The view should be parallel to the disk space of the surgical level. The retroperitoneal plane may be approached from either the right or the left side and allows full exposure of the disks while retracting the great vessels. **B**, Illustration shows a left-sided approach. The retractors should not be depressed too firmly, or compression of the neurologic structures within the psoas muscle could result in a neurologic deficit following surgery.

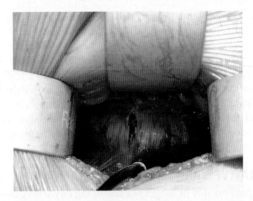

FIGURE 9 Intraoperative photograph shows the marking of the midline of the disk space. This is important for providing a reference point when placing the final implant.

COMPLICATIONS

- Exposure-related complications—Injury to vascular structures, bowel injuries, retrograde ejaculation
- Other complications—Thrombophlebitis, pulmonary embolism, incisional hernia, prolonged ileus
- Management of vascular structures is paramount; invite assistance of general or vascular surgeon familiar with exposure and needed visualization to safely perform diskectomy and reconstruction
- To expose L4-L5 or multiple levels, left-side approach better to ligate iliolumbar vein, usually left-side structure; some suggest right-side retroperitoneal approach acceptable for any level from L2 through sacrum and that retrograde ejaculation less frequent through right-side approach due to avoiding dissection of the left side of the superior hypogastric plexus

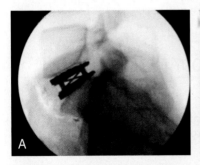
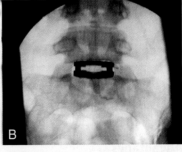

FIGURE 10 Postoperative lateral (**A**) and true AP (**B**) fluoroscopic images show an interbody cage in place. This particular cage is constructed of titanium and comes in four pieces: superior and inferior end-plate devices and two lateral struts. The cage is constructed in situ within the disk space for nontraumatic insertion and expansion of the disk space. Proper imaging is essential to ensure appropriate placement of the reconstructive device.

- Bowel injuries very uncommon with retroperitoneal approach
- Incidence of retrograde ejaculation controversial; literature supports primarily exposure-related incidence; highest frequency in laparoscopic, transperitoneal approaches, least often in retroperitoneal exposures; monopolar electrocautery appears to increase incidence; impact of bone morphogenetic protein–2 (BMP-2) (Infuse, Medtronic) on retrograde ejaculation uncertain
- Deep vein thrombosis, pulmonary embolism are seen with anterior exposure; deep vein thrombosis incidence 3% to 5%; pulmonary embolism less than 1% to 2%

POSTOPERATIVE CARE AND REHABILITATION
- Mobilize patients day of surgery or following day with physical therapy
- External brace at discretion of surgeon
- Remove indwelling catheter when patient mobility allows
- Start clear liquids after bowel sounds return; advance diet to solid foods with return of flatus; usually by day 1 or 2

PEARLS

- Key to safely performing anterior lumbar fusion is management of iliolumbar vasculature; visualization of vascular structures, gentle retraction required to expose disk space for diskectomy and reconstruction.
- Author prefers to alternate disk space distractors from right to left while working on opposite side; allows sequential dilation of disk space while facilitating visualization of side opposite distractor.
- Relax vascular retraction several times during procedure to prevent thrombosis.
- During diskectomy, use temporary disk space distractors to improve visualization, help approximate for trial implants.
- Many different implants and/or bone-graft options may be used with excellent outcomes.

LATERAL LUMBAR INTERBODY FUSION

INTRODUCTION
- Minimally invasive technique that utilizes a lateral incision to access the intervertebral disc via the retroperitoneal space

Advantages
- While lacking long-term literature, several perceived advantages of the lateral lumbar interbody fusion (LLIF) are no direct violation of the spinal ligamentous structures, spinal canal, and neuroforamen, no retraction of nerve roots, less blood loss, and more rapid recovery of function

- Larger interbody cage sizes possible—leading to more graft material, decreased risk of cage subsidence, more cage stability, and a more favorable biomechanical environment for fusion
- Indirect decompression for lateral recess stenosis through restoration of intervertebral height

Disadvantages

- Unfamiliar to many spine surgeons and regional anatomy may be confusing during learning curve
- Postoperative hip flexion pain and weakness is common
- Bowel perforation and ureteral injury are possible during approach
- L5-S1 level is considered inaccessible

PATIENT SELECTION
Indications

- Spinal stenosis, low-grade spondylolisthesis, degenerative scoliosis, disk herniation, degenerative disk disease, discitis that are limited to the L1-L5 levels are indications for an LLIF (**Figure 11**)
- LLIF should be considered for revision surgery to avoid repeat entry through scar that may be adherent to dura and other neural structures

Contraindications

- LLIF is inappropriate to treat pathology of the L5-S1 segment
- Posteriorly locked facets are a relative contraindication to LLIF as the foramen will not readily open in this scenario upon decompression
- Ongoing or prior infection of the retroperitoneal space and severe osteoporosis are other relative contraindications to LLIF
- Oblique lumbar interbody fusion (OLIF) can be performed at the L5-S1 level but should be approached carefully in cases with a low bifurcation of the great vessels

Preoperative Imaging

- Adequate AP and lateral radiographs are critical (**Figure 12**)
- MRI should be evaluated for position of the great vessels, degree of spinal curvature, anatomical relationship between sympathetic plexus, lumbar plexus, and psoas muscle
- Diaphragm should be assessed, specifically if surgery will be on higher lumbar levels

PROCEDURE
Room Setup/Patient Positioning

- Typically, right lateral decubitus position to minimize risk to the inferior vena cava unless right-sided concavity

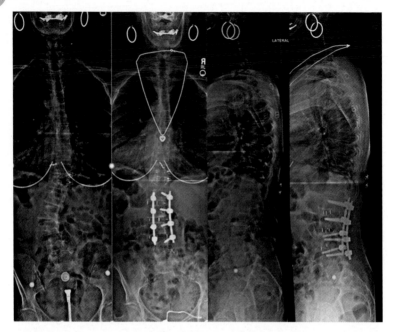

FIGURE 11 Preoperative and postoperative radiographs of a 58-year-old woman with history of juvenile idiopathic scoliosis who presented with right-sided lumbar radiculopathy in L2-L5 distribution. The patient underwent lateral lumbar interbody fusion (LLIF) at L2-L3, L3-L4, and L4-L5, with percutaneous instrumentation posteriorly from L2-L5 and derotation.

- Midpoint of iliac crest at the table break to allow for correction of lumbar deformity with the use of the "table flexion" technique (**Figure 13**)
- Hips and knees flexed to 30° with pressure points padded
- C-arm remains stationary while the orientation of the table is adjusted to obtain true AP/lateral images

Special Instruments
- Handheld electrophysiological monitoring devices used to locate traversing nerve roots

Surgical Technique
- Use multiple parallel transverse incisions for multilevel surgery
- Second posterior incision advocated by some to allow for easier palpation of the retroperitoneal space
- Dissection parallel to the abdominal musculature
- Use large sponge sticks during deep dissection

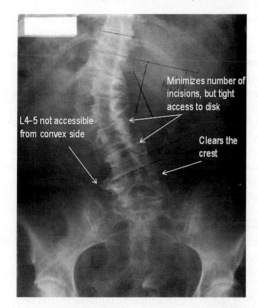

FIGURE 12 Planning of the Lateral lumbar interbody fusion approach using plain radiograph. (Reproduced from Pawar A, Hughes A, Girardi F, Sama A, Lebl D, Cammisa F: Lateral lumbar interbody fusion. *Asian Spine J* 2015;9[6]:978-983.)

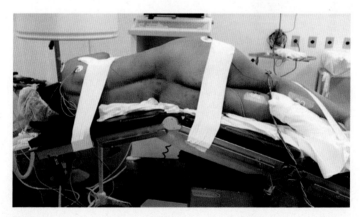

FIGURE 13 Photograph shows lateral positioning of patient, with a break in the table at the level of the greater trochanter. (Reproduced from Pawar A, Hughes A, Girardi F, Sama A, Lebl D, Cammisa F: Lateral lumbar interbody fusion. *Asian Spine J* 2015;9[6]:978-983.)

- Psoas and transverse process should be palpable; the first dilator should be inserted onto the index disk space with the palpating finger acting as a shielding edge
- Confirm index level with fluoroscopy and then advance a Kirschner wire (K-wire) about 3 cm into disk space
- EMG blunt tip probe used to identify the traversing nerve root (should lie posterior)
- Shim deployed to secure retractor posteriorly and blade is inserted anteriorly
- Diskectomy performed with all cartilaginous material removed from the endplates with broad Cobb elevator, avoiding overpenetration to contralateral side
- The appropriate-sized interbody is then inserted

COMPLICATIONS
- The most common complications are transient neurological injury, hip flexion weakness, which are both typically transient
- More serious complications are rare but include vascular injury, visceral injury, and ureter injury
- Subsidence is seen not uncommonly, while vertebral body fracture and infection are relatively rare complications

POSTOPERATIVE CARE AND REHABILITATION
- Postoperative care mimics that of the anterior lumbar interbody fusion from earlier in this chapter

Pediatrics

<big>8</big>

Section Editor
Henry G. Chambers, MD

Closed and Open Reduction of Supracondylar Humerus Fractures

INTRODUCTION

- Supracondylar humerus fractures are among the most common orthopaedic injuries of childhood; annual incidence 60.3 to 71.8 in 100,000 patients
- Peak incidence between age 3 and 10 years; average age 5.5 years for closed injuries
- Most injuries occur from fall onto outstretched, extended, or hyperextended hand
- Nearly 98% are extension type; 2% are flexion type
- Majority treated with cast immobilization alone; however, 24% of fractures require surgical intervention
- Modified Gartland classification system most widely used
    - Type I—Nondisplaced
    - Type II—Moderately displaced with extended distal fragment hinging on intact posterior humeral cortex
    - Type III—Completely displaced
    - Type IV—Loss of periosteal hinge results in multidirectional instability

PATIENT EVALUATION

Physical Examination

- Note neurologic and vascular status, presence or absence of open fracture or compartment syndrome, and condition of skin of antecubital fossa
- Anterior ecchymosis, skin puckering, excessive swelling, skin tenting are red flags for possible evolving neurovascular compromise or compartment syndrome
- Examine adjacent bones; ipsilateral forearm injury increases risk of compartment syndrome or preoperative sensory nerve palsies
- When documenting vascular status, carefully assess pulse and hand perfusion

---

Based on Illingworth KD, Skaggs DL: Closed and open reduction of supracondylar humerus fractures, in Colvin AC, Flatow E, eds: Atlas of Essential Orthopaedic Procedures, *ed 2. Rosemont, IL, American Academy of Orthopaedic Surgeons, 2020, pp 891-902.*

- Recent meta-analysis noted 11% incidence of neurologic injury in patients with displaced supracondylar humerus fractures
  - Anterior interosseous nerve is most frequently affected in extension-type injuries (34% of injuries)
    - Assess the flexion of the thumb interphalangeal joint (FPL function)
  - In flexion-type, 91% of nerve injuries involve ulnar nerve
  - Majority of nerve injuries recovered within six months; however, isolated radial nerve or multiple nerve injuries are associated with longer recovery

PREOPERATIVE IMAGING

- AP and lateral radiographs with evaluation of Baumann angle; decreases in this angle associated with varus angulation
- True lateral required to assess severity of type 2 fractures
- Consider standard orthogonal views of adjacent bones to rule out other injury sites if physical examination is inconclusive

Indications and Contraindications

- Manage type I fractures nonsurgically in long-arm cast bent to no more than 90° in neutral forearm rotation for 3 weeks
- Authors manage type II fractures with closed reduction and percutaneous pinning; benefits outweigh risks
- Types III and IV require surgical management

PROCEDURE

Room Setup/Patient Positioning

- Supine position
- Attach small arm board to table; position patient so elbow can be placed on arm board; in small patients, the head also may need to be placed on table
- Using image intensifier of C-arm as work surface preferred by some, but limits ability to obtain lateral radiograph without moving arm
- Rotate bed 45° away from anesthesiologist; bring C-arm in from foot of bed, parallel to table
- Prepare arm to shoulder
- Place sheet under patient to use as traction device with anesthesiologist helping
- Leave enough room for sterile tourniquet in event open reduction is needed

Surgical Technique

- Reduction maneuver dependent on fracture pattern
- Type 2 fractures treated with gentle elbow flexion (avoid overzealous manipulation resulting in type 4 fracture

---

- Type 3 fractures: begin with axial traction with elbow held in 20° to 30° of flexion with counter-traction applied at axilla by assistant
  - Use pronation (for posteromedially displaced fractures) or supination (for posterolaterally displaced fractures) to help gain further stability; the success of axial rotation is variable (**Figure 3**)
- May address medial and lateral translation by directly manipulating distal fragment Once coronal and axial deformity are corrected, sagittal plane can be addressed
- Direct pressure volarly on tip of olecranon using the surgeon's thumb(s) to level distal fragment anteriorly as arm slowly flexed to approximately 130° (**Figure 1**); the patient's fingers should be able to touch shoulder
- Obtain multiple fluoroscopic views to assess reduction
  - On lateral view, anterior humeral line should cross capitellum
  - On AP view, Baumann angle should be greater than 10°
  - Obtain oblique views to evaluate humeral columns
- Wrap hyperflexed elbow with sterile elastic bandage to maintain fracture reduction so full attention can be paid to pinning
- If adequate reduction cannot be obtained and anterior dimpling is present, consider the so-called milking technique
  - Grasp anterior musculature of arm as proximally as possible while assistant applies countertraction

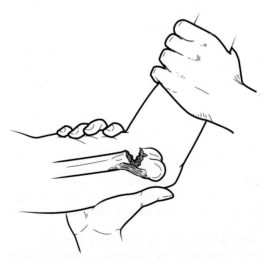

FIGURE 1 Illustration shows fracture reduction for a supracondylar humerus fracture. The reduction maneuver is performed by first applying axial traction to the patient's slightly flexed arm (with countertraction applied in the axilla by an assistant) and then levering the posteriorly displaced distal fragment back into place as the elbow is brought into flexion.

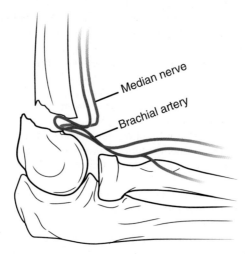

FIGURE 2 Illustration shows inadequate reduction of a supracondylar humerus fracture. The inability to achieve adequate fracture reduction may be associated with interposition of the anterior neurovascular structures within the fracture site.

▶ Apply pressure to anterior musculature in proximal-to-distal direction to guide musculature over spike of proximal fragment; may feel "pop" and see improvement in dimpling

- If adequate closed reduction cannot be obtained and "rubbery" end point to reduction is present, anterior neurovascular structures may be interposed in fracture site; open reduction may be required (**Figure 2**); in most cases, closed reduction will be successful

Fracture Fixation

- For percutaneous pinning, use 0.062-in Kirschner wires; use 2.0-mm Steinmann pins for larger patients
- The first pin should grab adequate fixation of both fragments, so either the lateral or central column pin should be placed; obtain bicortical purchase (**Figure 3**); may advance Kirschner wires across olecranon fossa, in which case four cortices will be purchased; second pin is placed after the first pin has engaged the other cortex and there is a good reduction
- Avoid pins that cross at the fracture site or converge
- Three types of error have been identified in loss of fixation
    ▶ Type A—Failure to engage both fragments with at least two pins
    ▶ Type B—Failure to achieve bicortical purchase with at least two pins
    ▶ Type C—Failure to achieve pin separation of at least 2 mm at fracture site

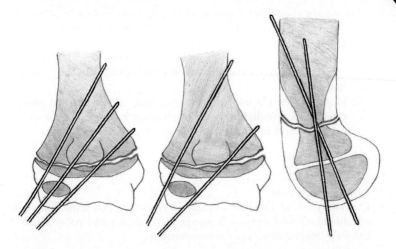

FIGURE 3 Illustration shows pin configuration for fixation of a supracondylar humerus fracture. Two or three pins may be placed in either a parallel or divergent manner, taking care to engage at least two columns of the humerus and to achieve adequate pin spread (>2 mm) at the fracture site. Convergently placed pins should be avoided. (Reproduced with permission from Skaggs DL, Cluck MW, Mostoli A, Hynn JM, Kay RM: Lateral-entry pin fixation in the management of supracondylar fractures in children. *J Bone Joint Surg Am* 2004;86[4]:702-707.)

- Obtain multiple views after two pins are placed to stress the elbow in both sagittal and coronal planes and to make sure the pins are out of the cortex
- If any concern for instability is present, place additional pins
- Final intraoperative fluoroscopic images should include AP (elbow in extension), lateral, and internal/external oblique views

Dressing and Casting
- Bend pins 90°, 1 cm from the skin; cut to a length of 1 to 1.5 cm
- Apply soft felt dressing beneath cut pins
- Authors place strips of 0.5-in–thick sterile foam volarly and dorsally, then dress loosely with cast padding; do not place circumferential dressing deep to foam; this technique obviates the need to split the cast to accommodate swelling
- Apply long-arm cast at 60° to 70° of flexion with arm in neutral position; ensure radial pulse is present in this position

Lateral-Entry Versus Medial-Entry Pins
- Good evidence supports lateral-entry pin constructs only
- Medial-entry pins are associated with iatrogenic ulnar nerve injury at a rate of 4.9%; in study, exposure of entry site did not prevent injury

- Later studies show lateral-entry–only pin fixation omits risk of loss of fracture reduction, diminished range of motion, nerve palsy, cubitus varus, and the need for further surgery
- Some cases (<1%) do require a medial-entry pin, secondary to lateral comminution or a fracture pattern preventing adequate lateral purchase
  - In such cases, place lateral-entry pin first so elbow can be gently extended for medial-entry pin application; helps prevent anterior subluxation of ulnar nerve over medial epicondyle

Special Situations

Flexion-Type Fractures

- Uncommon variant
- One study found 15.4-fold increase in need for open reduction, and additional 6.7-fold increase if preoperative ulnar nerve palsy is present. Reduction is done in relative extension

Type IV Fractures

- They are multidirectionally unstable and require a special reduction maneuver
- Place two lateral-entry pins in distal fragment first; using fluoroscopic images, confirm reduction starting with coronal plane (varus/valgus/rotational)
  - Address sagittal deformity by passive flexion or extension of elbow as well as direct anterior/posterior translation
  - To obtain lateral images, rotate C-arm around table to avoid displacing fracture
- Advance pins across proximal fragment after reduction obtained; add more pins as necessary

Open Reduction

- Indications: open fractures, neurovascular injury warranting exploration, failure to achieve or maintain closed reduction, and/or loss of previously present neurovascular status
- Multiple approaches described; authors prefer anterior approach with sterile tourniquet
  - Make incision in flexion crease starting medial to biceps tendon and moving laterally
  - Avoid neurovascular structures medial to tendon
- For open fracture, clean ends of fracture; during retraction, do not stretch neurovascular structures
- Remove all interposing tissues (brachialis, capsule, periosteum)
- Surgical release of incarcerated nerve results in neurologic recovery by 3 months
- After the impediments to reduction are removed, the fracture is reduced and pinned as a closed fracture

- Up to 20% of displaced supracondylar humerus fractures present with pulseless limb; if vascular status is questioned following closed reduction, approach vessel by extending transverse incision in lazy-S fashion starting proximal and medially and finishing distal and laterally
- Fix fracture in standard fashion

POSTOPERATIVE CARE AND REHABILITATION

- Most children admitted to hospital for routine neurovascular checks
- If no compartment syndrome is present and neurovascular status is stable, child is discharged home
- Must be careful in patients with nerve injuries because compartment syndromes can be missed; these patients require indwelling catheter monitoring
- At 1-week follow-up visit, obtain AP and lateral views and perform neurovascular check; continue cast immobilization
- At third-week visit, obtain radiographs after removing cast. If adequate healing is present pins are removed; allow activities of daily living; restrict aggressive activities
  - If concern for delayed healing (more common in older patients), pins left for additional period not longer than 1 week
- No formal physical therapy; train parents to perform gentle range-of-motion exercises in most cases
- Follow-up visit at 6 to 8 weeks to evaluate range of motion. If no issues, allow return to full activities

PEARLS

- To achieve and maintain adequate reduction
  - Use sterile elastic bandage to hold reduction with elbow hyperflexed while placing pins.
  - Check oblique views to evaluate medial and lateral columns.
  - Most important criteria for assessing reduction are Baumann angle greater than 10° and anterior humeral line intersecting capitellum.
  - Save worst intraoperative fluoroscopic view to be used as comparison later in office.
  - If gap remains at fracture site after reduction or a rubbery feel is present, neurovascular structures may be interposed; proceed with open reduction.
- To avoid technical errors in pin placement
  - Engage medial and lateral columns just proximal to fracture with lateral pins
  - Achieve bicortical fixation with each pin.
  - Maximize pin spread at fracture site.

- Ensure bony purchase in distal fragment; do not start too posteriorly or too near lateral edge.
- Avoid pins crossing at fracture site; they function as one pin.
- Recognize persistent instability or inadequate fixation by performing stress views of fracture in AP and lateral planes.
- Protect neurovascular structures by extending elbow during medial-entry pin placement.
- Pay attention to soft tissues and neurovascular status of arm
  - Avoid tight circumferential dressings.
  - Use sterile foam to accommodate swelling in cast.
  - Avoid elbow flexion greater than 70° in postoperative cast.
  - Recheck radial pulse after fracture reduction.

110

Reduction and Fixation of Lateral Condyle Fractures of the Distal Humerus

PATIENT SELECTION

- These fractures typically occur after falling onto outstretched hand or from a height
- Jakob classification describes these fractures (**Figure 1**)
- Treatment is based on extent of displacement, not location of fracture
- Reserve nonsurgical management for nondisplaced or minimally displaced fractures (<2 mm)
- Surgery is recommended for displaced (>2 mm) or rotated fractures
  - ▶ Closed reduction with percutaneous pinning may be indicated for minimally displaced fractures
  - ▶ Open reduction and internal fixation is warranted for significantly displaced (>4 mm) or unstable fragments

PREOPERATIVE IMAGING

- AP, lateral, and internal oblique views of elbow
- Oblique view helps visualize true displacement
- Often larger than visualized on plain films due to cartilaginous component
- Hinging is difficult to assess on plain radiographs; MRI or magnetic resonance arthrography can help
- Most treatment decisions are made from plain radiographs; advanced imaging rarely used because of cost and required patient sedation

PROCEDURE

Special Instruments/Equipment/Implants

- Fluoroscopic unit
- Sterile tourniquet
- Small right-angle retractors for open reduction
- Kirschner wires (0.062-in); a small cannulated screw/washer can be used for older children with a bony fragment

---

Based on Patel NM, Flynn JM: Reduction and fixation of lateral condyle fractures of the distal humerus, in Colvin AC, Flatow E, eds: Atlas of Essential Orthopaedic Procedures, *ed 2. Rosemont, IL, American Academy of Orthopaedic Surgeons, 2020, pp 903-908.*

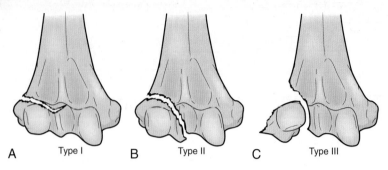

FIGURE 1 Illustrations show the Jakob classification of lateral condyle fractures. **A,** Type I: displaced less than 2 mm with no violation of the articular surface. **B,** Type II: displaced 2 mm or more with no violation of the articular surface. **C,** Type III: displaced 2 mm or more with disruption of the articular surface.

Surgical Technique

Closed Reduction and Percutaneous Pinning

- Evaluate fracture stability under dynamic fluoroscopy
- Closed reduction performed with direct manual manipulation. Ensured with arthrography
- After successful closed reduction, place two divergent Kirschner wires from distal-lateral to proximal-medial (**Figure 2**)
- Bend pins to 90° and cut outside the skin
- Place petrolatum gauze infused with 3% bismuth tribromophenate at base of pins to protect skin-pin interface
- Immobilize elbow in cast or splint at 80° of flexion

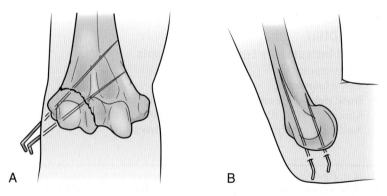

FIGURE 2 Illustrations of the anterior (**A**) and lateral (**B**) aspects of the elbow demonstrate optimal pin placement for a lateral condyle fracture.

Open Reduction and Internal Fixation

- Make lateral Kocher-type incision with 2 to 3 cm of the incision above the elbow joint
  - ▷ Posterior approach preferred by some, but limited long-term data
- Place incision slightly anterior for improved visualization
- As incision is carried through subcutaneous tissues, the plane into joint becomes apparent; fracture trauma has done most of dissection
- Evacuate hematoma to enhance visualization
- Keep dissection anterior and avoid stripping posterior tissues; blood supply enters distal fragment posteriorly
- When fracture fragment can be seen all the way medially, exposure is complete
- Use long right-angle retractor to elevate capsule and anterior structures
- Place first pin percutaneously through posterior flap and drill into fragment, penetrating just enough to verify a central position
- Reduce fragment; advance pin through medial cortex
- After fracture is reduced, visualize joint surface to evaluate reduction
- After fluoroscopy has confirmed reduction, place second pin in divergent fashion; one or both pins may go through olecranon fossa
- Reassess under fluoroscopy; include stress views; add additional pins until stable
- When feasible, suture periosteal flap to reduce risk of bone spur formation
- Bend pins to 90° and cut outside the skin
  - ▷ Some surgeons bury pins; this causes skin irritation and requires additional surgery to remove
- Place petrolatum gauze infused with 3% bismuth tribromophenate at base of pins to protect skin-pin interface
- Immobilize elbow in cast or splint at 80° of flexion
- Bend pins to 90° and cut outside the skin
- Place petrolatum gauze infused with 3% bismuth tribromophenate at base of pins to protect skin-pin interface
- Immobilize elbow in cast or splint at 80° of flexion
- Screw fixation gaining popularity for older patients with large metaphyseal fragment,
  - ▷ Proponents advocate improved construct stability allows for earlier postoperative elbow motion, lowering risk of loss of reduction, nonunion and stiffness
  - ▷ Typically two screws for rotational stability, should not traverse olecranon fossa

COMPLICATIONS

- Osteonecrosis, from original injury or excessive intraoperative tissue stripping posteriorly
- Delayed union and nonunion; may require casting up to 12 weeks or further surgery
- Pin-tract infection, growth arrest, tardy ulnar nerve palsy

POSTOPERATIVE CARE AND REHABILITATION

- Place long arm cast in operating room; may bivalve to accommodate swelling
- First follow-up is at 4 weeks; take radiographs with cast off and pins left in; can remove pins if callus is present; pins should be removed at 4 weeks, but new cast may need to be applied
- At least 6 weeks of immobilization followed by gentle range of motion exercises
- Physical therapy rarely needed; consider if range of motion fails to improve after 4 weeks out of cast

PEARLS

- Avoid posterior dissection.
- Divergent, bicortical pins enhance fracture stability. May need more pins if stressing fracture results in displacement.
- In older patients, one of more compression screws may provide increase construct stability allowed for earlier postoperative elbow motion.
- Close periosteum to avoid bone spur formation.
- Avoid open reduction of patients who present three or more weeks after injury; amount of periosteal stripping can result in significant complications.

Intramedullary Fixation of Radial and Ulnar Shaft Fractures in Skeletally Immature Patients

PATIENT SELECTION

- Only ~10% of pediatric forearm fractures require surgical fixation due to remodeling potential of growing bone. Plates and screws are not commonly used in skeletally immature patients although this is the mainstay of treatment in adults
- Stiffness in children is rare, so postoperative immobilization is not a concern
- Intramedullary (IM) fixation
  - ◗ Minimally invasive, safe method to manage fractures not amenable to closed treatment with a cast
  - ◗ Minimizes soft-tissue disruption and scarring; easy implant removal
- Complication rate between 14 and 21%, increasing with age of patient
  - ◗ No difference in complication rate between IM and plate/screw fixation methods

Indications

- IM fixation can stabilize and maintain reduction in high-energy, open fractures or those that cannot be acceptably reduced closed
- IM fixation manages fractures requiring fasciotomies; can obviate the need for a cast, which can increase compartment pressures
- Patient with multiple fractures requiring the use of the arm
- Acceptable displacement varies by age and location within forearm (**Table 1**)
  - ◗ Remodeling is more likely in younger patients and in fractures close to distal physes
  - ◗ Rotational malalignment is unlikely to remodel
- When assessing malalignment, if the true angle of maximal displacement is not orthogonal to radiographs, magnitude of deformity may be underestimated

---

Based on Pring ME, Gottschalk HP, Chambers HG: Intramedullary fixation of radial and ulnar shaft fractures in skeletally immature patients, in Colvin AC, Flatow E, eds: Atlas of Essential Orthopaedic Procedures, *ed 2. Rosemont, IL, American Academy of Orthopaedic Surgeons, 2020, pp 909-917.*

TABLE 1 General Guidelines for Acceptable Values in Both-Bone Forearm Fractures

Age	Acceptable Angulation	Acceptable Translation	Acceptable Rotation
Younger than 9 yr	<15°	Bayonet	≤45°
9 yr or older with >2 yr of growth remaining	≤10° for proximal fractures, ≤15° for distal fractures	100%	≤30°

Data from Noonan KJ, Price CT: Forearm and distal radius fractures in children. *J Am Acad Orthop Surg* 1998;6(3):146-156.

Contraindications

- In children younger than 5 years, IM fixation is rarely indicated, given potential for remodeling
- IM fixation may not be rigid enough for skeletally mature patients
- Intra-articular fractures, gross contamination, significant comminution, and extensive soft-tissue loss may benefit from external fixation

PREOPERATIVE IMAGING

- AP and lateral radiographs of forearm
- Dedicated views of elbow and wrist to evaluate proximal and distal radioulnar joints
- Galeazzi or Monteggia fractures can be missed on inadequate radiographs

PROCEDURE

Room Setup/Patient Positioning

- Organize room to enable appropriate imaging and visualization of the images (**Figure 1**)
- Position arm on a radiolucent arm board perpendicular to the operating table

Special Instruments/Equipment/Implants

- Various titanium or stainless steel IM implants are available; titanium is more flexible than steel. Implant choice is based on fracture pattern and stability
- Kirschner wires can be used in younger children
- No matter the implant type, measure width of IM canal at narrowest point and choose implant that provides 40% to 80% fill of canal

VIDEO 111.1 Distal Forearm Fractures: Both-Bone Forearm Fracture Intramedullary Nailing: Step 1. Kelly D Charmichael, MD; Chris English, MD (25 min)

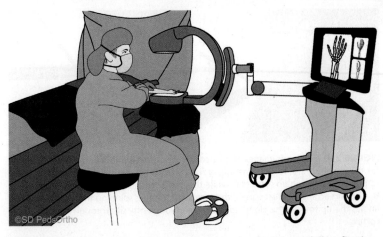

FIGURE 1 Illustration shows the operating room setup for intramedullary fixation of a forearm fracture.

Surgical Technique

- Controversy exists regarding which bone to fix first; authors recommend starting with the more difficult bone first, usually the radius
- Ulna is more subcutaneous, therefore easier to manipulate and easier to fix after the radius is fixed

Fixing the Radius

- Implant should be precontoured to recreate the radial bow
- Lay implant on forearm with tip curved toward bicipital tuberosity
- Mark end of bone and fracture which will be the point of maximal bow
- Use contouring tool to create a gentle curve from tip to where implant will exit bone
- S-shaped bend helps with later rotation once fracture site is crossed
- Ideal entry point is 1.5 cm proximal to distal radial physis
- Make a 1.5-cm incision on dorsal-lateral side of distal radius
- Avoid injuring dorsal sensory branch of radial nerve
- Enter interval between first and second compartments or second and third compartments; tip of implant should not rest under a tendon; rupture can occur
- Bluntly dissect down to bone; use drill or awl to enter bone; entry point should be at proximal end of incision to allow easy passage of implant
  - Enter at an angle so IM implant can be passed proximally without impinging on the medial cortex (**Figure 2**)
  - Make sure to go through only one cortex
- Advance implant to fracture site with gentle oscillating motion
- Reduce radial fracture

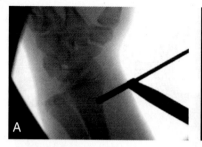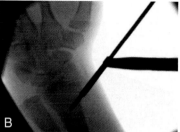

FIGURE 2 Fluoroscopic images of a forearm with a both-bone fracture show drilling for the nail entry site for intramedullary fixation of the radius. **A,** A drill guide is used to prevent wrapping up soft tissue while the drill is started perpendicular to the bone. **B,** After breaching the first cortex, the surgeon continues spinning the drill bit and angles the tip toward the elbow to create an oblong entry site through only one cortex.

- Sometimes manual traction is sufficient; if not, use implant as a lever to manipulate distal fragment to proximal fragment.
- Gently advance end of implant out of distal fragment; use tip to "catch" canal of proximal fragment to aid in reduction
- Multiple false passes have been linked to compartment syndrome.
- After three unsuccessful attempts, make a small incision (either volar "Henry" or dorsal "Thompson" approach) at fracture site to aid in open reduction
- Consider fasciotomies if multiple false passes are made
- Once IM implant is passed across the fracture, advance it to the bicipital tuberosity and rotate it to restore the radial bow
- Cut implant with enough length to make later retrieval possible without making implant unnecessarily prominent

Fixing the Ulna
- Ulnar implant does not require precontouring unless Kirschner wires are used and tip catches far cortex instead pf passing down the canal
- Three options for approach: tip of olecranon, lateral aspect of olecranon, or distal ulna
  - Lateral aspect of olecranon is the most common with fewest complications
  - Tip of olecranon provides straightest trajectory down canal; however, tip of nail is often symptomatic
  - Distal ulnar entry site is more useful for proximal fractures; however, more it is a difficult trajectory and puts dorsal sensory branch of ulnar nerve at risk

- For the lateral/proximal approach, make a small incision lateral and distal to tip of olecranon
- Incise directly down to the bone
- Advance drill or awl from starting point halfway between joint and posterior cortex; angle to avoid far cortex
- Advance implant to fracture site; use similar reduction techniques as in radius. If fracture cannot be reduced, make a small incision at fracture site to aid in reduction
- Advance implant to distal physis and cut close to its entry point
- Occasionally the ulnar medullary canal is so small that the curved tip will not pass down the canal. One can turn the intramedullary device around and pass the blunt end into the distal canal

Closure and Casting
- Close skin with absorbable suture
- Confirm correct rotational alignment before casting
  - Radial styloid should be 180° from biceps tuberosity on an AP radiograph with forearm supinated
  - Assess pronation and supination
  - Ensure radiocapitellar and distal radial ulnar joints are reduced
- Splint or cast forearm
  - In younger children, casting is preferred; risk of stiffness is minimal and cast protects child from reinjury
  - Implants are not designed for rigid stability; micromotion occurs and postoperative immobilization helps prevent discomfort
  - If using a cast, univalve or bivalve, and monitor post-op as there is a known risk of compartment syndrome following IM fixation of both-bone forearm fractures

COMPLICATIONS
- Wound infections, osteomyelitis, hardware migration, refracture after implant removal, tendon rupture, nerve injury, decreased range of motion, and muscle entrapment have been reported
- Risk of compartment syndrome rises with multiple false passages; follow "three-pass rule": make small incision to aid in reduction after three false passes and consider fasciotomy

POSTOPERATIVE CARE AND REHABILITATION
- After 3 to 4 weeks, enough healing has occurred to remove immobilization and start gentle motion
- In skeletally immature children, we remove implants 6 to 12 months after surgery.
  - Use original incisions to remove implants
  - Can use vice-grip pliers or large needle driver to remove IM nails
- If bone is removed to help extract retained implants, postoperative casting is prudent; otherwise, warn family about fracture risk

---

PEARLS

- Dedicated views of the wrist and the elbow should be obtained to ensure that the proximal radioulnar joint and the distal radioulnar joint are intact.
- Use an implant that is 40%-80% of the canal diameter.
- Contour the radial implant; to recreate the radial bow.
- Implant should have a gradual curve with the apex at the fracture site.
- Curving IM implant too aggressively can bind it in canal, preventing advancement.
- Follow "three-pass rule."

VIDEO REFERENCE

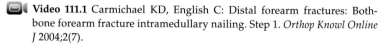 **Video 111.1** Carmichael KD, English C: Distal forearm fractures: Both-bone forearm fracture intramedullary nailing. Step 1. *Orthop Knowl Online J* 2004;2(7).

PATIENT SELECTION

- Diagnosis of septic arthritis can be difficult; must be considered for any child with atraumatic history who refuses to bear weight
- Delay in diagnosis can be catastrophic
- Treatment options include simple joint aspiration under ultrasonography guidance, formal anterior arthrotomy, and arthroscopic lavage and decompression
- Most commonly affects children younger than 4 years
- History of progressive reluctance to use or bear weight on affected leg; malaise and fever
- May be remote history of trauma, often noncontributory
- Neonates lack fever or higher inflammatory markers; pseudoparalysis or irritability of limb should arouse suspicion
- With effusion, child flexes, abducts, and externally rotates hip to reduce intracapsular pressure
- Rotation is poorly tolerated
- Palpation of effusion usually not possible

PREOPERATIVE IMAGING/TESTING

- AP pelvic radiograph helps rule out other pathology; greater than 2 mm of side-to-side difference from medial femoral head to medial acetabulum is diagnostic of effusion
- Ultrasonography helps diagnose effusion; presents chance to obtain diagnostic aspiration
- Blood work includes erythrocyte sedimentation rate, C-reactive protein, complete blood count with differential, blood culture, antistreptolysin O titer, and, where geographically indicated, Lyme titer
- Differentiating between septic arthritis and transient synovitis of hip can be done using four independent, multivariate predictors: fever (temperature >39.5°C), not bearing weight on affected limb, erythrocyte sedimentation rate greater than 40 mm/hr, serum white blood cell (WBC) count greater than 12,000 cells/mm^3

Based on Shore B, Kocher MS: Incision and drainage of the septic hip, in Colvin AC, Flatow E, eds: Atlas of Essential Orthopaedic Procedures, *ed 2. Rosemont, IL, American Academy of Orthopaedic Surgeons, 2020, pp 918-922.*

- Elevated C-reactive protein level (>20 mg/L) was later added as fifth independent predictor of septic arthritis
- Aspirate from hip that yields synovial WBC count greater than 50,000 cells/mm^3 is diagnostic of septic hip
- Aspirate with less than 25,000 cells/mm^3 may reflect an inflammatory process, such as transient synovitis
- WBC value between 25,000 and 50,000 cells/mm^3 requires clinical examination, inflammatory markers, and aspiration results
- Authors' institution performs MRI of hip in unclear cases to differentiate septic arthritis and osteomyelitis
- Base ultimate decision for surgical incision and drainage on clinical judgment

PROCEDURE

Room Setup/Patient Positioning

- Supine position with small bump under affected side to elevate 25°
- Prepare and drape entire extremity free

Special Instruments/Equipment/Implants

- If diagnosis still uncertain, use long 18- or 20-gauge spinal needle to aspirate hip; use fluoroscopy to confirm location
- Use drain or Penrose catheter to decompress

Surgical Technique

Hip Aspiration

- Preferred approach is medial with patient in a "frog-leg" position
- Place 18- or 20-gauge needle inferior to adductor longus and advance toward ipsilateral nipple at 45° angle relative to floor
- Inject small amount of radiopaque dye mixed 1:1 with sterile saline to confirm needle placement within joint

Incision and Drainage

- Make standard anterior skin incision within crease created by flexing hip to 90°, 1 to 2 cm below crest of anterior superior iliac spine
- Center incision over anterior inferior iliac spine (**Figure 1, A**)
- Perform sharp dissection through skin and fat
- First internervous interval reached is between sartorius and tensor fasciae latae muscles
  - Lateral femoral cutaneous nerve (LFCN) crosses this interval; identify and retract throughout case (**Figure 1, B**)
  - The LFCN usually runs along sartorius, then crosses field to lie with tensor fasciae latae, 4.5 cm distal to anterior superior iliac spine
  - The lateral femoral circumflex vessels can run at base of incision; coagulate if necessary without fear of causing osteonecrosis

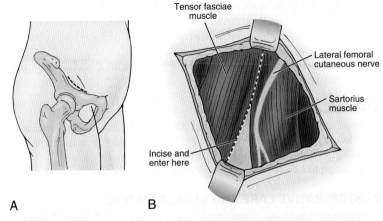

FIGURE 1 Illustrations show the skin incision and superficial dissection for drainage of a septic hip. **A,** The incision is centered over the anterior inferior iliac spine in line with a skin crease of the anterior hip. **B,** The superficial interval between the tensor fasciae latae and sartorius muscles is shown. The surgeon should try to keep the lateral femoral cutaneous nerve medially with the sartorius if possible when accessing the deeper interval.

- Deep within interval, identify direct head of rectus femoris tendon; it may be covered by fatty fibrous tissue (this tissue is present in some children even without infection)
- Elevate and retract direct head medially via blunt dissection; this step reveals the iliopsoas tendon and capsule
  - Local swelling and edema can make identification of these structures difficult
  - Use Cobb elevator or peanut retractor to sweep soft tissues off capsule
  - If needed, can release reflected head of rectus tendon to aid visualization
- Digital palpation of femoral head while rotating can show correct location of joint
- After confirming correct location, remove 1- to 2-cm window of capsule anteriorly
  - Obtain cultures, Gram stain, and cell count from fluid within joint
  - Perform copious irrigation until all purulent material removed
- Authors do not routinely drill proximal femoral metaphysis unless suspicion for osteomyelitis exists (controversial, may depend on whether a preoperative MRI was performed)

- Check hip for stability; in children younger than 18 months instability from septic arthritis and from the arthrotomy can develop; if instability is identified, place hip spica cast for 3 weeks; in younger children, a Pavlik harness can be utilized
- Place drain; close only superficial tissues with absorbable suture
- Remove drain at 48 hours

COMPLICATIONS

- Most complications are associated with delay in diagnosis, resulting in osteonecrosis, destruction of femoral head, capital growth arrest, and subsequent limb-length discrepancy
- Damage to LFCN resulting in painful neuroma is rare

POSTOPERATIVE CARE AND REHABILITATION

- Initiate intravenous antibiotics; base duration on Boston Children's Hospital guidelines
  - If patient improves after 72 hours of intravenous antibiotics and is negative for methicillin-resistant *Staphylococcus aureus* (MRSA), transition patient to oral antibiotics for 21 days, with weekly follow-up
  - If inflammatory markers remain elevated and patient does not improve clinically after 48 hours, repeat irrigation and débridement
- Encourage physical therapy in early postoperative period
- Keep patient non–weight-bearing for 6 weeks

PEARLS

- Timely diagnosis and treatment is critical. Aspirate hip when in doubt.
- Better to err on side of surgical drainage when presented with confusing clinical picture; complications of delay in treatment are catastrophic.
- Carry out close clinical follow-up in immediate postoperative period. Failure to improve should prompt evaluation for MRSA or other etiology; collaborate with infectious disease services; MRI is excellent adjuvant modality to investigate for conditions associated with MRSA bone and joint infections.

Percutaneous In Situ Fixation of Slipped Capital Femoral Epiphysis

INTRODUCTION

- Slipped capital femoral epiphysis (SCFE)—Adolescent hip disorder involving slip of posterior and inferior proximal femoral epiphysis relative to metaphysis
- Most (>95%) are stable; very good prognosis for stable SCFE
- Unstable SCFE has osteonecrosis (ON) rates up to 50%
- Presentation can vary
  - History can include intermittent limp; thigh, knee, or groin pain; loss of internal and spontaneous external rotation; reduced abduction and flexion; shortening of lower extremity; limb-length discrepancy
  - Hip pain may or may not be present

PATIENT SELECTION

- All patients with a stable SCFE and open physes
- Treatment goals
  - Prevent slip progression
  - Avoid osteonecrosis and chondrolysis
  - Maintain adequate hip function
- Standard treatment for stable SCFE includes internal fixation that crosses the physis (in situ) with single screw
  - Single or double screw for unstable; controversial
  - Some authors recommend acute osteotomy correction; controversial
- Secondary osteotomies can be performed after complete physeal closure occurs
- Patients with endocrinopathies, those taking growth hormone supplementation, and the very young (open triradiate physes) warrant prophylactic pinning of contralateral femur

PREOPERATIVE IMAGING

- Stable SCFE
  - AP and lateral pelvis (frog-lateral or cross-table) radiographs
  - Carefully check other side; bilateral cases approach 20%

Based on Loder RT: Percutaneous in situ fixation of slipped capital femoral epiphysis, in Colvin AC, Flatow E, eds: Atlas of Essential Orthopaedic Procedures, *ed 2. Rosemont, IL, American Academy of Orthopaedic Surgeons, 2020, pp 923-929.*

- Unstable SCFE—AP and cross-table lateral only
- Measure slip magnitude using epiphyseal-shaft angle on lateral radiograph
  - ▶ Draw line between anterior and posterior tips of epiphysis; draw another line perpendicular to first line
  - ▶ Draw line along shaft of femur
  - ▶ Epiphyseal-shaft angle lies at intersection of perpendicular line and femoral shaft line; measure for both hips
  - ▶ Magnitude of slip displacement is angle of affected hip minus angle of contralateral hip; for bilateral slips, use 10° to 12° as unaffected hip angle
  - ▶ Classify slips as mild (<30°), moderate (30° to 50°), or severe (>50°)

PROCEDURE

- Treat SCFE with single cannulated screw in situ; use stainless steel screw (titanium has higher complication rate: breakage and difficulty removing)
- For stable SCFE, place screw in center of femoral head epiphysis on both the AP and lateral radiograph

Room Setup/Patient Positioning

- Can use fracture table or radiolucent flat table; author prefers fracture table
- Supine position on fracture table; place C-arm to allow easy movement during case
- When positioning patient, do not aggressively manipulate leg; can lead to osteonecrosis.
- Place cannulated screw guide pin on skin overlying center of epiphysis and perpendicular to physis on AP and lateral views
  - ▶ Draw lines on skin to record guide pin projection for AP and lateral views
  - ▶ Pin enters skin at intersection of lines (**Figure 1**)

Surgical Technique

- Use small incision to introduce guide pin through skin; incise through fascia latae to prevent tethering of guide pin
- Introduce guide pin through anterolateral cortex; confirm correct entry point and angulation on two orthogonal images (**Figure 2**)
- Advance pin into epiphysis after correct placement is confirmed
  - ▶ Advanced pin should lie at least 5 mm from subchondral bone
  - ▶ Avoid superior pin placement to prevent osteonecrosis

VIDEO 113.1 Single Screw Fixation for Slipped Capital Femoral Epiphysis. David D. Aronsson, MD (5 min)

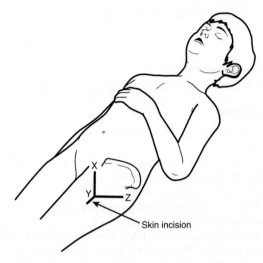

FIGURE 1 Illustration shows the skin lines drawn to record the position of the guide pin; the incision is made at the intersection of the skin lines. X = anterior line, Y = lateral line, Z = skin incision. (Adapted from Loder RT, Aronsson DD, Dobbs MB, Weinstein SL: Slipped capital femoral epiphysis. *Instr Course Lect* 2001;50:555-570.)

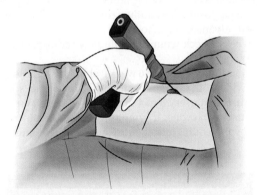

FIGURE 2 Illustration shows the guide pin for the cannulated screw being inserted after a small incision is made at the intersection of the skin marking lines. Note that the guide pin follows the trajectory of both skin marking lines.

- Measure for appropriate screw length
- Place screw after drilling and/or tapping as needed
  - Screw should be at least 6.5 mm in diameter
  - Carefully monitor pin to avoid breakage, acetabular or abdominal penetration, and withdrawal

- Use one of the following techniques to confirm that screw threads do not penetrate subchondral bone
  - Intraoperative live fluoroscopy
  - Approach-withdraw
  - Intraoperative arthrography
- Close incision after confirming screw position and depth

COMPLICATIONS

- Joint penetration; can result in chondrolysis
- Pin breakage
  - If pin breaks, attempt retrieval if pin is at or near anterolateral cortex, otherwise try another path
  - To avoid, use careful technique
    - Drill along same trajectory as guide pin
    - Avoid levering/angling pin
    - Ensure quick release chuck does not notch pin (**Figure 3**)
- Stress risers can form after multiple passes of pin; can result in fracture
- Ensure that starting point of pin is above the lesser trochanter to prevent later fracture

POSTOPERATIVE CARE AND REHABILITATION

- Obtain permanent radiographs in operating room or recovery room
- Allow toe-touch weight bearing immediately if radiographs demonstrate adequate positioning; author continues for 4 to 6 weeks; many children self-advance long before
- At 1 to 2 weeks, check wound, obtain new radiographs to ensure no loss of fixation
- Next postoperative visit at 4 to 6 weeks; obtain new radiographs; allow normal activities, but no running, jumping, or contact sports
- Require return visit every 3 to 4 months until skeletal maturity; counsel patient to return sooner if symptoms appear in either hip
- Screw removal is controversial; most surgeons do not recommend

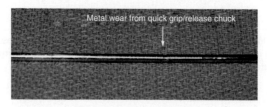

FIGURE 3 Photograph shows the notching of a guide pin from a cannulated screw set caused by an automatic grip/release chuck.

PEARLS

- Must obtain good AP and lateral fluoroscopic images before prepping and draping.
- Avoid levering on the guide pin during insertion through the fascia latae and onto the bone. Levering will frequently bend the pin, which can result in inadvertent cutting of the pin when drilling over it.
- One pass of guidewire is ideal. More passes create stress risers in the bone and increase the risk of postoperative fracture.
- The surgeon must be able to visualize the tip of the screw in multiple planes before closure.

114 Fixation of Pediatric Femur Fractures

PATIENT SELECTION
- Surgical stabilization is treatment of choice for children older than 5 years
  - Faster return to school
  - Lower overall costs than casting and traction
- Several fixation options available; choice depends on patient age, size, fracture location and pattern, surgeon preference
- Chapter describes techniques of submuscular plating, elastic intramedullary nailing, and lateral trochanteric-entry nailing

SUBMUSCULAR PLATING
- Plate osteosynthesis is proven method of stabilizing pediatric fractures
- Submuscular plating technique has similar advantages as plate osteosynthesis and minimizes soft-tissue disturbance

Indications
- Submuscular plating recommended for patients aged 5 years to skeletal maturity with comminuted or long oblique length-unstable femur fractures
- Also can be used in proximal or distal-third fractures, assuming at least two screws can be placed in proximal or distal fragments

Preoperative Imaging
- AP, lateral views of femur; include ipsilateral knee and femoral neck
- Evaluate for other injuries, especially to ipsilateral hip and knee

Procedure
Room Setup/Patient Positioning
- Supine position on fracture table
  - Small (~3%) risk of nerve palsy incidence, minimize time in traction as much as feasibly possible
- Obtain provisional reduction via boot traction; evaluate length and angulation with special attention toward rotation

---

Based on Sink EL, Peck J: Fixation of pediatric femur fractures, in Colvin AC, Flatow E, eds: Atlas of Essential Orthopaedic Procedures, *ed 2. Rosemont, IL, American Academy of Orthopaedic Surgeons, 2020, pp 930-941.*

- Place contralateral leg in extension and abduction or in well-leg holder to obtain true lateral image; perfect lateral is imperative if percutaneous techniques will be used
- Can use standard radiolucent table if appropriate assistance is available

Special Instruments/Equipment/Implants

- Author prefers long, narrow 4.5-mm plate; readily available, easy to contour, fits most femurs
- Other options are available; choose per surgeon preference
  - Can use 3.5-mm plate system for smaller children
  - Custom pediatric implants with bowed plates are available
  - Can use standard or locking systems
    - Reserve locking plates for patients with poor bone quality or very proximal or distal fractures
    - Nonlocking screws help reduce fracture; if choosing locking plate system, use hybrid approach
    - Self-tapping screws facilitate percutaneous insertion
- Plate length usually has 10 to 16 holes; need three holes for fixation proximally and three distally
- Precontour plate to match lateral femoral cortex using hand or table benders
  - Account for greater trochanteric and distal metaphyseal flares; to maximize rigidity, plate should run length of femur
  - Final position of femur will match bend, so the bending should be done carefully

Surgical Technique

- Make 3- to 5-cm incision proximal to the physis along lateral thigh
- After incising the iliotibial fascia, identify the vastus lateralis
- Carefully elevate vastus lateralis to expose periosteum
- Insert plate in this interval (above the periosteum); carefully advance proximally, maintaining contact with femur (**Figure 1**)
- Plate may be difficult to pass past fracture site; surgeon may need to pull plate back and redirect; use fluoroscopy judiciously and adjust as necessary
- After plate rests in intended position, obtain AP and lateral images before placing screws
- Fix plate provisionally in desired position with 2-mm Kirschner wires placed in most proximal and distal screw holes
- Apply principles of external fixation pin placement for submuscular bridge plating
  - Place one screw close to proximal and distal limits of fracture; place rest of screws at ends of plate
  - Use three screws proximal and three screws distal to fracture; can use two screws in locking plate or in very proximal fractures when two screws obtain significant purchase

---

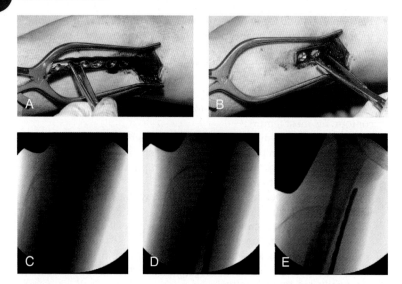

FIGURE 1 Intraoperative photographs (**A** and **B**) and fluoroscopic images (**C** through **E**) show tunneling of the plate through the plane between the vastus lateralis and the periosteum of the lateral femur.

- Place first screw in fragment farthest from plate; this screw acts as reduction screw (**Figure 2**)
  - ▶ Use "perfect circles" technique; drill both cortices
  - ▶ Measure screw length by laying depth gauge or screw on top of femur; use fluoroscopy to estimate
  - ▶ Tie 0 absorbable suture around screw head to prevent losing screw in soft tissues
  - ▶ As screw enters femur, fragment will reduce to plate
- Place remaining screws; close incisions; place soft dressing

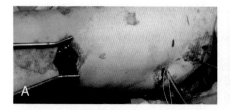

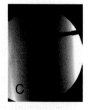

FIGURE 2 Intraoperative photograph (**A**) and fluoroscopic images (**B** and **C**) demonstrate the reduction of the femur to the precontoured plate with percutaneous screw placement in a pediatric femur fracture. (Panel A is reproduced with permission from Sink EL, Hedequist D, Morgan SJ, Hresko T: Results and technique of unstable pediatric femoral fractures treated with submuscular bridge plating. *J Pediatr Orthop* 2006;26[2]:177-181.)

Complications

- One reported case of plate failure was with a titanium 3.5-mm plate; none with stainless steel and 4.5-mm plates
- One reported case of refracture following plate removal attributed to premature plate removal
- Minimize malunion, especially in rotation, by careful preoperative evaluation and comparison of ipsilateral and contralateral limbs

Postoperative Care and Rehabilitation

- Use knee immobilizer for comfort during immediate postoperative period
- Encourage early range of motion; prohibit full weight bearing until bridging callus is seen, usually at 6 to 10 weeks
- Plate removal recommended after 6 months as failure to remove can result in valgus deformity, leg length discrepancy, stress shielding, and medial thigh screw tip prominence
  - ‣ If removal is delayed, tissue and bone ingrowth may complicate or prevent percutaneous removal
  - ‣ After removing screws, slide Cobb elevator, sharp end away from bone, beneath plate to free it
  - ‣ Patients may bear full weight; no sports for 6 weeks

PEARLS

- Submuscular bridge plating is best for comminuted or long oblique pediatric femur fractures.
- For rigid stabilization, plate should span from greater trochanter apophysis to distal femoral metaphysis.
- Precontour 4.5-mm stainless steel plate to accommodate bend of proximal and distal metaphyses. Place plate on anterior aspect of thigh before insertion. Use fluoroscopy to shadow lateral cortex and confirm contour.
- Place first nonlocking screw at margin of fracture where femur is farthest from plate. After screw engages far cortex, femur will reduce to plate.
- Obtain as much screw spread as possible with remaining screws for stability.

ELASTIC INTRAMEDULLARY NAILING

Patient Selection

- Best for transverse or stable fracture patterns in children aged 5 to 11 years
- Location of fracture should be within middle 60% of femur
- Restrict use of implants to patients weighing less than 50 kg; complications are common in heavier patients

Procedure

Room Setup/Patient Positioning
- Setup identical to that for submuscular plating
- Access to medial and lateral sides of knee is imperative

Special Instruments/Equipment/Implants
- Titanium and steel implants are readily available
  - Stainless steel (Ender) nails benefit from increased stability as well as decreased rate of malunion and cost
- Standard method of implantation is retrograde, using two C-shaped nails; antegrade implantation requires one C-shaped nail and one S-shaped nail
- Implants should obtain 80% fill of medullary canal; if canal width measures 10 mm, two 4-mm nails will fill 8 mm, or 80%
- Some titanium nails come in standard length and need to be cut to appropriate length, while stainless steel nails come in preset lengths
  - Lateral nail should extend to level of greater trochanter, medial nail to base of femoral neck

Surgical Technique
- Most common insertion points are at medial and lateral flares of distal metaphysis
- Mark physis; make incision roughly from superior pole of patella to two fingerbreadths above superior pole of patella using the same approach as described in submuscular plating section
- Use similar approach medially, noting insertion should be anterior to ridge of bone present on medial flare. It is usually beneath the vastus medialis muscle. Confirm entry point position on fluoroscopy; create entry point using either 4.5-mm drill bit or an awl (**Figure 3**); angled drill position facilitates implant insertion
- Contour implants before implantation to maximize contact at fracture site; if asymmetry of bend exists or if two different nail sizes are selected, unwanted angulation can occur at fracture site
- Insert nails up to fracture site; then advance nails across, one at a time
  - Order of nail insertion is at surgeon's discretion; author prefers lateral first
  - Rotate first nail until optimal reduction achieved, then advance the other nail
  - Do not intertwine implants while rotating
  - Do not advance rod too far past fracture site until second rod has passed fracture site; doing so will make passing of second rod difficult or impossible
  - Use fluoroscopy to confirm adequacy of reduction and to check for distraction

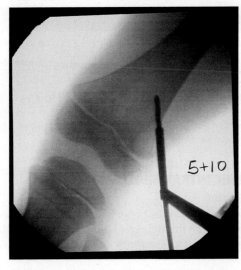

FIGURE 3 Fluoroscopic image shows the insertion point for a flexible intramedullary nail.

▶ Rarely, third or fourth nail is needed for stability; place before either of previous two is fully advanced; the third nail can lead to angulation if different diameter used
   – When using stainless steel Enders nails, cortical screws can be placed through eyelets for additional construct stability
▶ Cut nails and advance to final positions
   – Final advancement performed using bone tamp
   – View lateral image of femoral neck to ensure nail does not exit the posterior metaphysis or femoral neck
▶ Nails should not be more than 1 to 2 cm proud; should rest along flare
▶ Apply knee immobilizer for comfort; very rarely, use hip spica cast to enhance stability

Complications

• Nail prominence; to prevent, cut nails so they rest just proximal to physis
• Pain
• Malunion is reduced by adhering to the age/weight restrictions
• Fracture site shortening seen in more unstable fracture patterns and patients older than 11 years
• Stainless steel Enders nails may reduce risk of shortening when compared to titanium nails. Avoid complications by using largest diameter nail possible, using similarly sized nails with a bend opposite to each other, cutting nails short, using nails in stable fractures in middle 60% of femur

PEARLS

- Use in stable fractures in middle 60% of femur in patients age 5 to 11 years.
- Insert nail through oblique hole at upper portion of metaphyseal flare to facilitate proper nail positioning.
- Advance both nails to fracture site before crossing fracture.
- Advance nail requiring less manipulation to cross fracture first and rotate to align fracture anatomically. Then pass second rod before advancing both rods to upper femur.

TROCHANTERIC INTRAMEDULLARY FIXATION

Patient Selection

- Rigid intramedullary implants can be appropriate for adolescents
- Lateral entry points through greater trochanter theoretically reduce risks associated with piriformis entry nails (osteonecrosis, coxa valga)
- Author uses lateral trochanteric-entry nails in children older than 11 years who have femur large enough to accept implant

Procedure

Surgical Technique

- Can position on fracture table or radiolucent table
- Details of entry point vary among manufacturers, but all use entry point lateral to tip of greater trochanteric apophysis
- After performing reduction, most important part of case is ensuring that the guidewire and opening reamer are lateral to tip of greater trochanter and angle of entry pin is correct
  - If entry angle is too shallow, nail can be difficult to pass
  - Aim at, or just inferior to, lesser trochanter
- Remaining steps vary among manufacturers; consult respective guides
- Proximal and distal fixation is recommended
- If fixation within neck is required, remember and account for increased anteversion in pediatric femurs
- Can start postoperative weight bearing immediately, at least partially; progress to full weight bearing within 6 weeks

Complications

- Increased OR time as well as higher estimated blood loss than flexible nails
- Nonunion extremely rare in this age group; minimize by making sure fracture site is not distracted
- Implant irritation
- Uncommonly, coxa valga secondary to proximal femoral growth disturbance and osteonecrosis of femoral head

PEARLS

- Suitable for children 12 years and older with either stable or unstable fracture weighing greater than 50 kg.
- Guidewire placement is critical.
- Start lateral to tip of greater trochanter and aim for center of femur at level of lesser trochanter.

INTRODUCTION

- Nondisplaced fractures can be treated with long leg cast in 10° to 15° knee flexion
- Minimally displaced fracture may be reduced closed and then casted
- If there is displacement, there may be entrapment of one of the menisci or intermeniscal ligament; may also have meniscal tear
- High potential of arthrofibrosis after surgery

PATIENT SELECTION

Indications

- Tibial spine fractures displaced 3 mm or more
- Fracture that cannot be reduced in extension
- Suggestion of extension of fracture into the weight-bearing articular cartilage

Contraindications

- Nondisplaced fractures or fractures able to be closed reduced and casted
- Lateral view on plain radiographs most helpful
- Can identify meniscal entrapment on MRI
- CT or MRI can demonstrate comminution or extension to weight-bearing surface not easily seen on plain radiographs

PROCEDURE

Treatment Selection

- Surgical treatment with three No. 2 sutures is stronger than single 4-mm screw; sutures minimize risk of impingement
- Screw fixation best suited for large fragments

Nonsurgical Treatment

- May manipulate mildly displaced fractures, especially those hinged posteriorly, to acceptable position of less than 3 mm
- Aspiration, 10 mL lidocaine injection can aid reduction
- Perform reduction by putting ankle on bolster and knee in extension

---

Based on Wall E, Lewis K: Surgical reduction and fixation of tibial spine fractures in children, in Colvin AC, Flatow E, eds: Atlas of Essential Orthopaedic Procedures, *ed 2. Rosemont, IL, American Academy of Orthopaedic Surgeons, 2020, pp 942-949.*

- Confirm with lateral radiograph
- Place cast in near full extension (10° to 15°)

Room Setup/Patient Positioning

- Position knee to allow lateral intraoperative imaging
- Suture fixation requires about 20° knee flexion; screw fixation requires 60° to 90° flexion
- Paint roller can be placed at end of table to flex knee to 60°
  - Bump under ipsilateral hip prevents knee from falling outwards

Special Instruments/Equipment/Implants

- For suture fixation
  - No. 2 reinforced braided nonabsorbable suture
  - 45° or 90° suture passer
  - Anterior cruciate ligament (ACL) tibial drill guide, guide pin
  - Microfracture awl/pick
  - Arthroscopic curette
  - Suture lasso
  - 3.5-mm drill guide
  - 30°, 70° arthroscopes
  - Arthroscopy camera and shaver
- For screw fixation
  - 4.0- or 4.5-mm cannulated screw and washer
  - Curette
  - Arthroscopy shaver
  - Microfracture awl/pick
  - Kirschner wire set
  - Nonabsorbable suture to tag washer

Surgical Technique

For Suture Fixation and Screw Fixation

- Inflate tourniquet
- Perform arthroscopic irrigation; can use outflow portal to clear hemarthrosis
- Clot shaved and curetted from fracture site
- Identify anterior horn of medial meniscus, transverse intermeniscal ligament; ensure ligament not entrapped
- Explore medial and lateral compartment for meniscal tear, fracture extension
- Elevate anterior tibial spine fragment to continue clot and crater débridement
- For adequate reduction, visualization of fragment needed to ensure postoperative impingement does not occur; can be accomplished by pulling in anterior, medial, distal direction (**Figure 1**)
- If medial meniscus entrapped, pull it forward; confirm reduction with lateral view

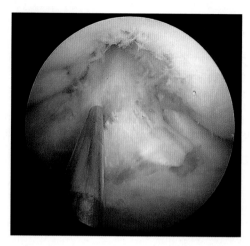

FIGURE 1 Arthroscopic view of a knee with a displaced Meyers and McKeever type III tibial spine fracture shows the notch and the medial compartment. An arthroscopic probe is seen reducing the fracture fragment inferiorly and medially into the crater.

For Suture Fixation Only

- Using ACL tibial guide, place first guide pin medial to patellar tendon; aim to exit at anterolateral rim of crater (**Figure 2**); second pin enters ~10 mm more medially, exits at anteromedial rim; process creates two all-epiphyseal tunnels (**Figure 3, A** and **B**)

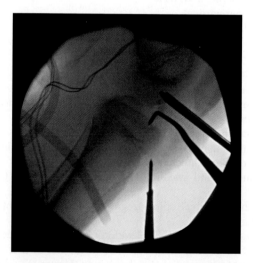

FIGURE 2 Intraoperative fluoroscopic image shows a tibial tunnel anterior cruciate ligament guide used to place a guidewire into the anterior rim of the fracture crater without passing through the growth plate (all-epiphyseal).

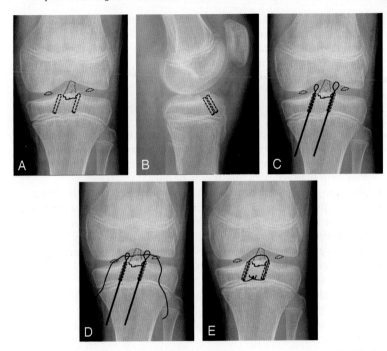

FIGURE 3 AP (**A**) and lateral (**B**) radiographs show two epiphyseal tunnels drilled percutaneously with an anterior cruciate ligament (ACL) guide and a guide pin anteromedial and anterolateral to the fracture. Tunnels are placed only in the epiphysis, with both tunnels medial to the patellar tendon. **B,** Lateral view shows the same two epiphyseal bone tunnels from a different angle. **C,** Suture lassos are placed up through the tibial tunnels using a drill guide so the tunnel is not lost in the soft tissue during the guide pin–to–suture lasso exchange. **D,** Reinforced suture is placed with a 90° suture passer through both suture lassos and the ACL at its insertion into the tibial fracture fragment. **E,** Sutures are tied securely over a bone bridge in the epiphysis.

- Create 10-mm-long horizontal skin incision connecting pins; do not disturb physis
- Use drill guide over guide pin to mark pin site; advance suture lasso into joint; repeat on other pin (**Figure 3, C**)
- Using suture passer, pass No. 2 suture through first lasso; penetrate ACL distally where it attaches to fragment, then pass through other lasso **Figure 3, D**); repeat with second suture
  - First suture placed transversely through the center of the ACL insertion onto the fracture fragment
  - Second suture placed in front of the first, about 5 mm behind the anterior edge of the fracture fragment
- Withdraw lassos

- With knee in about 30° flexion, reduce fracture with microfracture pick; tie sutures (**Figure 3, E**)
- Range knee; test stability; ideally, fragment stability should allow immediate range of motion (ROM)

For Screw Fixation Only

- Make accessory portal medial to equator of patella with knee flexed 60° to 90°
- Place guide pin through accessory portal; take care to not damage femoral condyle; reduce fracture with microfracture awl; place guide pin 5 mm posterior to anteromedial rim of fragment; second Kirschner wire may help hold fixation; drill fragment only
- Measure guide pin to determine the screw length (typically 22 mm)
- If bone purchase weak, use larger screw or consider crossing physis; take care to not penetrate posterior cortex with guide pin or drill; check by rotating leg 30° in both directions under fluoroscopy (**Figure 4**); confirm proper screw placement with arthroscopy, fluoroscopy
- Check screw head to ensure no impingement; small notchplasty may be necessary
- Tie nonabsorbable suture with 2-cm tail to washer to aid in future implant removal
- Screw placed across physis should be removed at about 8 weeks to prevent growth arrest

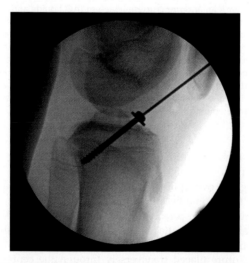

FIGURE 4 Postoperative fluoroscopic image shows anatomic reduction of the fracture with secure fixation to the posterior metaphyseal cortex. Notice that the guide pin starts just medial to the patella at its equator. Caution must be exercised to avoid overpenetrating the posterior metaphyseal cortex with the guide pin or the screw, which could cause serious neurovascular injury.

Open Surgical Fixation

- May need open fixation if fracture fails to reduce with arthroscopic treatment
- Medial parapatellar often is best approach because this is area of maximal displacement
- Headlight strongly recommended
- Fracture fragment often much deeper than expected; can improve visualization with partial fat pad excision
- Care must be taken to avoid injury to medial meniscus during incision into capsule
- Fixation technique similar to arthroscopic method

COMPLICATIONS

- Knee stiffness secondary to arthrofibrosis rare, perilous
  - Consider manipulation under anesthesia and/or arthroscopic lysis of adhesions if less motion less than 10° to 90° at 3 to 4 weeks
- Loss of full extension and joint laxity can be asymptomatic complications of surgical management

POSTOPERATIVE CARE AND REHABILITATION

- Fixation (of either type) must be secure enough to enable early ROM
- Start physical therapy on postoperative day 3
  - Toe-touch weight bearing
  - Do not restrict active or passive ROM
  - Wean immobilizer by 1 week
  - Full weight bearing gradually achieved over 6 weeks

PEARLS

- Place drill guide before exchanging ACL tibial guide pin for suture lasso to mark hole.
- For screw fixation, use second wire to hold reduction.
- Make sure wire, drill, screw do not damage condyle on insertion.
- Do not penetrate posterior cortex.
- In 50% of cases, screw fixation across physis is required to achieve adequate fixation.
- Place tag suture around washer to aid later retrieval.
- Patients who do not regain ROM of 5° to 90° 3 to 4 weeks after surgery need gentle manipulation under anesthesia.
- For resistance to motion, perform arthroscopic lysis of adhesions before manipulation.
- Adhesions may need removal from articular surface with shaver to reduce fracture risk during manipulation.
- Initiate epidural catheter, continuous passive motion, aggressive physical therapy to maintain ROM.

Treatment of Clubfoot Using the Ponseti Method

PATIENT SELECTION

Indications

- Ponseti method appropriate for all clubfoot types
- Children older than 2 years, those having had surgery for clubfoot may undergo Ponseti treatment to minimize extent of surgery, prevent further surgery

Contraindications

- No absolute contraindications
- Premature infants, infants with jaundice or poor feeding/growth, those with unstable cardiorespiratory status may benefit from delay in treatment until condition improves

Evaluation

- Clubfoot has four components: cavus, forefoot adductus, hindfoot varus, equinus
- Thorough examination required to rule out underlying conditions
- Radiographs not required before casting of idiopathic clubfoot
- Later, forced dorsiflexion images can help determine whether Achilles tenotomy required at end of casting
- Prenatal ultrasonography can identify clubfoot as early as 12 weeks; false-positive rate 20%
- Of infants with prenatally diagnosed clubfeet, more than 50% have associated anomalies

PROCEDURE

Room Setup/Patient Positioning

- Perform casting with patient supine; position parents at head to comfort child
- Older child may sit in parent's lap or at edge of table for lower-leg portion of casting, then recline for long-leg cast
- Two practitioners required; one holds, other wraps
- Same supine positioning for Achilles tenotomy

Based on Nemeth BA, Noonan KJ: Treatment of clubfoot using the Ponseti method, in Colvin AC, Flatow E, eds: Atlas of Essential Orthopaedic Procedures, *ed 2. Rosemont, IL, American Academy of Orthopaedic Surgeons, 2020, pp 950-956.*

Special Instruments/Equipment/Implants

- Plaster casting preferable to fiberglass
- In larger patient, may use fiberglass to reinforce plaster
- For tenotomy, may use standard No. 11 or No. 15 blade; authors prefer 5,100 or 6,900 eye blade

Surgical Technique

 VIDEO 116.1 Treatment of Congenital Clubfoot. Ignacio V. Ponseti, MD (24 min)

Serial Casting

- First, stretch foot
- Use one hand to abduct: right hand for right foot and vice versa
  - Place index finger along medial aspect of foot
  - Use third, fourth, fifth fingers to support plantar aspect
  - Place contralateral index finger behind lateral malleolus; place thumb over lateral head of talus
  - Do not place pressure over lateral calcaneus; will prevent correction
- First cast corrects cavus
- Elevate first ray; keep first ray elevated during subsequent castings to align metatarsals, prevent recurrence of cavus
- After stretching foot, apply cast in position of maximum stretch, without overstretching
- Start at toes by wrapping two to three layers of cast padding up calf while other practitioner holds toes
- Apply plaster in two to three layers into short-leg cast
- Mold cast around malleoli, posteriorly above calcaneus with gentle pressure around lateral talar head; avoid causing pressure sores from persistent pressure
- Extend cast up leg into long-leg cast with knee flexed at 90°
  - In stronger children, may reinforce cast with anterior splint
  - For complex clubfeet, flex cast up to 120° to prevent slippage
- Trim cast; leave toe plate to stretch toe flexors
- Change casts weekly; four to six casts usually required before tenotomy
- After achieving 70° abduction relative to sagittal plane and less than 15° of dorsiflexion, perform tenotomy to correct equinus deformity
- After tenotomy, place final cast with foot in maximal dorsiflexion and abduction; check that 15° of dorsiflexion is present without midfoot breach on lateral radiograph

Complex Clubfoot

- Atypical clubfoot may be identified during treatment
- Foot may become swollen, red, irritated, difficult to cast (**Figure 1**)

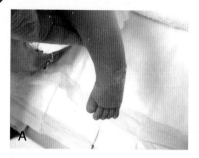
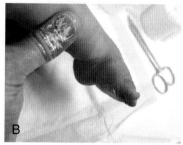

FIGURE 1 Clinical photographs show complex clubfoot. After two casts, retraction of the great toe (**A**) and pronounced cavus deformity (**B**) are evident.

- Great toe may start to retract; cavus will remain pronounced
- Complex clubfoot requires changing standard Ponseti technique; abducting foot to 70° causes midfoot breakdown
- Instead, stretch plantar and posterior contractures
  - ▶ Place both thumbs under metatarsal heads, dorsiflexing foot against counterpressure applied dorsally against talar neck using index fingers; use middle fingers to mold behind malleoli, above calcaneus (**Figure 2**); apply posterior splint down to foot to provide more support
  - ▶ Perform percutaneous tenotomy after abducting foot to 40°

Teratologic Clubfoot
- Use standard casting technique
- Change to complex clubfoot technique if great toe retracts or cavus is accentuated

Percutaneous Achilles Tenotomy
- Perform tenotomy after achieving appropriate abduction—60° to 70° for standard clubfoot, 40° to 60° for teratologic, 40° for complex
- Tenotomy indicated if foot does not dorsiflex enough

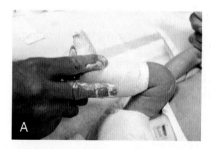
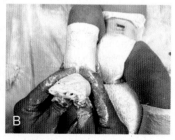

FIGURE 2 Clinical photographs show modified Ponseti casting technique for a complex clubfoot as seen medially (**A**) and anteriorly (**B**).

- If performed under local, use topical anesthetic cream, injection, or both
- Perform sterile preparation
- Assistant holds knee flexed 90° with foot in dorsiflexion
- Insert blade 1 to 1.5 cm proximal to calcaneus
  - Insert blade through skin medially, parallel to tendon; turn blade 90° when tip passes lateral border of tendon; cut tendon
  - Alternatively, insert blade at 45° angle to skin with blade pointing posteriorly; lift handle anteriorly when blade deep enough; use contralateral finger or thumb to push tendon through blade
- Take great care to avoid posterior tibial artery; may be only artery present in clubfoot; do not buttonhole skin
- Apply pressure; wash away any sterilizing solution to prevent irritation
- Extend standard short-leg cast to long-leg cast; make sure posterior trim line does not impinge the popliteal fossa

COMPLICATIONS

- Vasospasm occurs following dorsiflexion after tenotomy; pallor may be striking (**Figure 3**) but resolves within minutes; if not, remove and reapply cast with less dorsiflexion
- Evaluate excessive bleeding (>2 cm) seen on cast
- Pseudoaneurysm has been reported
- Pressure sores from cast
- Patients with myelomeningocele at high risk of sores due to stiff feet, insensitive skin
- Tibial fractures reported in patients with myelomeningocele

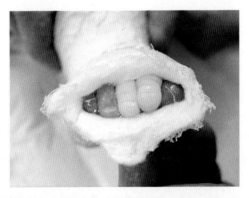

FIGURE 3 Clinical photograph shows an infant's foot following release of dorsiflexion during casting after percutaneous Achilles tenotomy for clubfoot. Pallor of the second and third toes is seen; the first, fourth, and fifth toes demonstrate return of blood flow. Perfusion of the second and third toes returned within seconds.

POSTOPERATIVE CARE AND REHABILITATION

- After percutaneous tenotomy, leave final cast in place for 3 weeks
- Then place foot in foot abduction orthosis
  - Amount of abduction should parallel final abduction achieved in cast
  - In unilateral cases, place unaffected foot in 30° abduction
- Child wears brace full time for 3 months; nighttime, naptime wear continues until age 4 years
  - Recurrence occurs in 80% of cases of noncompliance
  - Compliance improves with close telephone and clinic follow-ups
  - Intolerance of brace can occur if fit is poor or correction incomplete
- Repeat tenotomy may be indicated if less than 15° dorsiflexion (<5° in complex/teratologic feet) present after repeat casting; should perform in operating room
- For persistent recurrence, limited soft-tissue surgery—Achilles tendon lengthening with posterior release—may be required
- Perform transfer of tibialis anterior to lateral cuneiform for dynamic supination/persistent varus after lateral cuneiform is ossified

PEARLS

- Avoid pronation during correction.
- Manipulate foot before casting to assess deformity, progress of correction.
- Recognize features of complex clubfoot; understand how to correct it.
- Educate caregivers on compliance and appropriate brace use.

PATIENT SELECTION

- Patients present with myriad symptoms: foot pain, foot deformity, recent or prior foot or ankle injuries
- Suspect tarsal coalition in teenager with multiple ankle sprains
- Careful history, physical examination help identify coalitions
- Stiff flatfoot is hallmark of tarsal coalition; can be dramatic when unilateral (**Figure 1, A**)
- Calcaneonavicular coalitions
  - ◗ Restricted subtalar motion
  - ◗ Palpable bony ridge in sinus tarsi
  - ◗ Restricted plantar flexion (**Figure 1, B**)
- Talocalcaneal coalitions
  - ◗ Restricted subtalar motion
  - ◗ Tender bony prominence around sustentaculum tali
- Author asserts nonsurgical management has no long-term benefit; recommends excision for all young patients; temporary cast relief outweighed by altered biomechanics, long-term effects, including adjacent joint degeneration

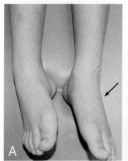 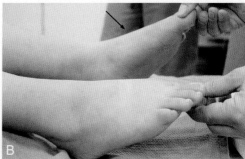

FIGURE 1 Clinical photographs show a patient with a unilateral calcaneonavicular coalition. In the supine position, the affected foot (arrows) fails to form an arch (**A**) and has diminished plantar flexion (**B**).

Based on Mubarak SJ: Treatment of tarsal coalitions, in Colvin AC, Flatow E, eds: Atlas of Essential Orthopaedic Procedures, *ed 2. Rosemont, IL, American Academy of Orthopaedic Surgeons, 2020, pp 957-964.*

PREOPERATIVE IMAGING

- Coalition types have classic radiologic signs: anteater sign for calcaneonavicular coalitions (**Figure 2, A**), C-sign for talocalcaneal coalitions (**Figure 2, B**)
- CT of both feet preferred for all preoperative cases; CT with three-dimensional reconstructions even more helpful
- MRI can identify fibrous coalitions

PROCEDURE

Room Setup/Patient Positioning

- Position foot near end of table so team can be seated
- Place sterile tourniquet; perform Esmarch exsanguination

Special Instruments/Equipment/Implants

- C-arm
- Kerrison rongeurs (3 or 4 mm)
- Osteotomes
- High-speed burr (3 or 4 mm)

Surgical Technique

Calcaneonavicular Coalition Resection

- Make oblique modified Ollier incision along Langer lines directly overlying coalition
- Identify extensor digitorum brevis (EDB); carefully reflect its insertion, avoiding superficial peroneal nerve

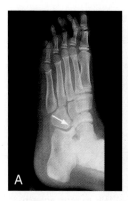 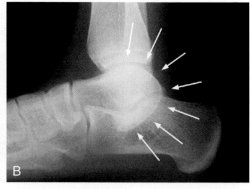

FIGURE 2 Radiographs demonstrate typical findings of a tarsal coalition. **A,** Internal rotation oblique view demonstrates the calcaneonavicular coalition (arrow). **B,** Lateral view shows the C-sign, which indicates a talocalcaneal coalition. This sign is present when the posterior margin of the talus appears to be continuous with the sustentaculum tali (arrows). The C-sign also can be seen in flexible flatfoot.

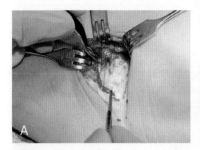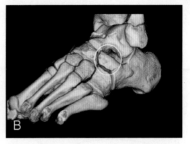

FIGURE 3 Images demonstrate the exposure for calcaneonavicular coalition resection. **A,** Intraoperative photograph shows the extensor digitorum brevis elevated off the coalition by proximal release at its origin. The coalition is visible directly beneath the elevated muscle. **B,** Three-dimensional CT scan is used to ensure that the intended plane of dissection is the correct one.

- Coalition is visible beneath EDB
- Plane of resection is guided by preoperative three-dimensional CT (**Figure 3**)
- Identify synchondrosis by elevating bone with curette at junction between calcaneus and navicular; protect calcaneocuboid and talonavicular joints with retractors
- Use 1-cm osteotome first, followed by 0.5-cm osteotome to resect the coalition; take care to not damage prominent cuboid or talar head
- After excising coalition, use Kerrison rongeurs to complete resection until achieving 1-cm × 1-cm gap
- Check internal oblique C-arm images to confirm completion
  - Also assess subtalar range of motion (ROM), which should have improved but still may be abnormal
- Insert harvested fat graft (see below for description) to fill gap
- Suture EDB back down with 0 absorbable to enable normal contouring of foot postoperatively
- Close fat graft site; close skin of foot; place foot in split short-leg cast to allow for swelling

Talocalcaneal Coalition Resection
- Make incision 1.5 to 2 cm distal to medial malleolus; should be long enough to expose entire subtalar joint
- Coagulate crossing branches of saphenous vein
- Identify tendons of tarsal tunnels in their sheaths
  - Retract tibialis posterior dorsally
  - Retract flexor digitorum longus and flexor hallucis longus plantarly
  - Incise deep sheath to expose coalition
- Good exposure should enable visualization of coalition borders from proximal to distal

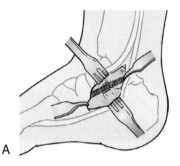
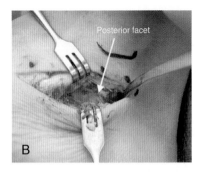

FIGURE 4 Images demonstrate resection of talonavicular coalition. Illustration (**A**) and intraoperative photograph (**B**) show the completed resection. Resection is not complete until the posterior facet is visualized and motion can be seen to occur within the subtalar joint.

- Use preoperative CT scan to guide plane of resection if synchondrosis not readily visible; easy to get lost if plane of coalition not understood
- Use combination of osteotomes, followed by rongeurs and high-speed burrs to resect the coalition; author prefers to start with osteotomes
- Perform resection until cartilage is visualized anteriorly and, especially, posteriorly (**Figure 4**)
  - Some coalitions can be very large
  - If small hook is left posteriorly, it will still restrict ROM
- Carefully use Freer elevator to release subtalar adhesions and help improve ROM
- After ROM is significantly improved and posterior facet is visualized, resection is complete
- Consider intraoperative CT to verify complete removal of coalition
- Harvest and insert fat graft
- Close deep sheath with No. 1 absorbable suture
- Close skin; apply short-leg cast and split it to allow for postoperative swelling

Fat Graft Harvest
- After resection of coalition, obtain fat graft
- Author prefers to use fat from ipsilateral gluteal crease; leaves cosmetic scar and always contains enough fat, even in thin patients
- Required size is 3 cm × 1 cm × 1 cm for calcaneonavicular coalitions, slightly smaller for talocalcaneal coalitions
- Make 4-cm incision; take through dermis only
- Elevate dermis off fat 1 cm around wound; do not buttonhole skin
- Use Allis clamp to gain traction and resect 3-cm-long × 1-cm-wide × 1-cm-deep piece of fat; place fat in saline-soaked sponge

- When ready for closure, close deep portion with 0 absorbable suture; use 3-0 absorbable sutures to approximate skin and running 3-0 absorbable subcuticular suture; author also uses 0 absorbable retention sutures to prevent dehiscence

COMPLICATIONS
- Early wound dehiscence at buttock wound if retention sutures not used
- Wound infections extremely rare
- Continued pain, stiffness, deformity possible long-term complications
- Follow-up CT may help rule out recurrence if pain persists

POSTOPERATIVE CARE AND REHABILITATION
- Author's preference is to admit all patients overnight for observation (optional)
- Encourage immediate weight bearing as tolerated in univalved cast
- Follow up at 1 week for cast closure, at 2 to 3 weeks for cast removal
- After cast removal, encourage patient to use foot and ankle; counsel that foot may not feel normal for up to 6 months
- At 6 weeks, clear patient for activities as tolerated; some patients may require physical therapy
- See patient at 3 months, 6 months, 1 year, and 2 years postoperatively; obtain radiographs at 1 year

PEARLS

- Understanding resection subtypes will help avoid pitfalls.
- In type I calcaneonavicular coalitions, do not excise the prominent, but normal, cuboid.
- In types II and V talocalcaneal coalitions, resect the posterior component.
- In type IV talocalcaneal coalitions, no physis is evident. Begin with small rongeurs and use fluoroscopy to aid in resection.
- Severe pes planus will not improve after resection and may require future surgery; counsel families about this fact preoperatively.
- Author recommends correction if lateral ankle or foot pain or deformity persists for 6 to 12 months. About 20% of calcaneonavicular coalitions need further surgery.

INTRODUCTION

- Cerebral palsy (CP) is an abnormality of motor function resulting from insult to the brain during early development
- Brain injury is considered static; musculoskeletal manifestations are progressive
- Delay surgery until the patient is at least 6 years old; spasticity management is important adjunct
- For multiple deformities, single-event multilevel surgery is recommended to prevent decompensation from unbalanced correction
- Gross Motor Function Classification System (GMFCS) categorizes patients with CP based on function (**Figure 1**)
- Functional Mobility Scale (FMS) rates ambulatory function at 5, 50, 500 m
- Classification is important because surgery goals vary depending on whether the patient is ambulatory (GMFCS I through III) or nonambulatory (GMFCS IV and V)

Ambulatory Patients

- Surgeon must understand gait abnormalities to identify correct treatment and procedure
  - May be assessed via observational or instrumented gait analysis
- Common abnormal gait patterns include scissoring gait, crouch gait, jump gait, stiff-knee gait, recurvatum gait
- At the foot and ankle, patterns include pure equinus, equinovarus, pes planovalgus
- Rotational abnormalities also may be present and need to be addressed; children with CP often cannot compensate for lever-arm dysfunction
- Surgical options for ambulatory CP patients are listed in **Table 1**; before selecting one or more options, the surgeon must consider:
  - Gait abnormality
  - Soft-tissue, bony rotational issues causing dysfunction

Based on Pandya NK, Chambers HG: Lower extremity surgery in children with cerebral palsy, in Colvin AC, Flatow E, eds: Atlas of Essential Orthopaedic Procedures, ed 2. Rosemont, IL, American Academy of Orthopaedic Surgeons, 2020, pp 965-982.

GMFCS E & R between 6ᵗʰ and 12ᵗʰ birthday: Descriptors and illustrations

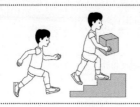

GMFCS Level I

Children walk at home, school, outdoors and in the community. They can climb stairs without the use of a railing. Children perform gross motor skills such as running and jumping, but speed, balance and coordination are limited.

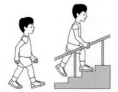

GMFCS Level II

Children walk in most settings and climb stairs holding onto a railing. They may experience difficulty walking long distances and balancing on uneven terrain, inclines, in crowded areas or confined spaces. Children may walk with physical assistance, a hand-held mobility device or used wheeled mobility over long distances. Children have only minimal ability to perform gross motor skills such as running and jumping.

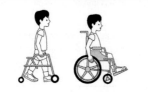

GMFCS Level III

Children walk using a hand-held mobility device in most indoor settings. They may climb stairs holding onto a railing with supervision or assistance. Children use wheeled mobility when traveling long distances and may self-propel for shorter distances.

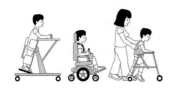

GMFCS Level IV

Children use methods of mobility that require physical assistance or powered mobility in most settings. They may walk for short distances at home with physical assistance or use powered mobility or a body support walker when positioned. At school, outdoors and in the community children are transported in a manual wheelchair or use powered mobility.

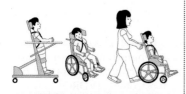

GMFCS Level V

Children are transported in a manual wheelchair in all settings. Children are limited in their ability to maintain antigravity head and trunk postures and control leg and arm movements.

GMFCS descriptors: Palisano et al. (1997) Dev Med Child Neurol 39:214-23
CanChild: www.canchild.ca

Illustrations Version 2 © Bill Reid, Kate Willoughby, Adrienne Harvey and Kerr Graham,
The Royal Children's Hospital Melbourne   ERC151050

FIGURE 1 Illustration of the Gross Motor Function Classification System (GMFCS) for cerebral palsy. Levels I through III (ambulatory). Levels IV and V (nonambulatory). E & R = expanded and revised. (© Kerr Graham, Bill Reid, and Adrienne Harvey, The Royal Children's Hospital, Melbourne, Australia. Data from Palisano R, Rosenbaum P, Walter S, Russell D, Wood E, Galuppi B: Development and reliability of a system to classify gross motor function in children with cerebral palsy. *Dev Med Child Neurol* 1997;39[4]:214-223 and data from CanChild Centre for Childhood Disability Research Institute for Applied Health Sciences, Ontario, Canada.)

TABLE 1 Typical Abnormalities and Potential Surgical Options in Ambulatory Patients With Cerebral Palsy

Abnormality	Potential Surgical Treatments
Hip adduction contracture	Adductor tenotomy
Hip flexion contracture	Psoas release at pelvic brim
Knee flexion contracture	Distal hamstring lengthening
	Distal femoral extension osteotomy with patellar tendon advancement
Knee recurvatum	Ankle plantar flexor lengthening
Stiff-knee gait	Rectus femoris transfer
Equinus contracture	Ankle plantar flexor lengthening
Equinovarus deformity of the foot	Posterior tibialis lengthening, split posterior tibial tendon transfer, split anterior tibialis transfer, ankle plantar flexor lengthening
Pes planovalgus deformity	Peroneus brevis lengthening, calcaneal lengthening osteotomy (±cuneiform osteotomy), calcaneal sliding osteotomy (±cuboid and cuneiform osteotomy), subtalar arthrodesis, triple arthrodesis

- Appropriate procedure to correct gait based on contractures/imbalances
- Rotational components, which should be treated more aggressively in patients with CP than in typically developing children

Nonambulatory Patients

- Hip subluxations, dislocations can cause sitting issues and can exacerbate scoliosis
- Address this problem with combination of procedures, including proximal adductor, hamstring, psoas lengthenings; open reduction with capsulorrhaphy of hip (>50% subluxation); pericapsular pelvic osteotomy; femoral varus derotational osteotomy (VDRO)
- Manage knee flexion contractures with hamstring lengthenings
- Manage foot, ankle issues with surgeries similar to those used for ambulatory patients

SOFT-TISSUE LENGTHENING PROCEDURES
Adductor Lengthening
Indications

- Scissoring gait
- Spastic hip subluxation/dislocation

Preoperative Imaging

- Usually not required in isolation
- When part of hip reconstruction, obtain AP, frog-leg lateral views of pelvis, bilateral hips; possibly CT with three-dimensional reconstructions

Surgical Technique

- Supine position
- Make transverse incision one fingerbreadth distal to groin crease
- Incise fascia overlying adductor longus tendon in line with its fibers
- Isolate adductor longus with right-angle clamp and cut as proximally as possible with electrocautery
- Transect gracilis muscle similarly if limited abduction present with hip in extension
- If still further abduction required, transect adductor brevis until 45° of abduction is achieved; identify and preserve the anterior branch of obturator nerve lying across this muscle
- Close wound in layers

Complications

- Hematoma formation
- Inadvertent transection of obturator nerve branches

Postoperative Care and Rehabilitation

- Place in Petrie casts with abduction bar for 4 weeks
- Abduction brace may be worn instead; maintained at night for 6 months

PEARLS

- Do not extend the incision beyond the lateral border of the adductor longus tendon to avoid the femoral neurovascular bundle.

Distal Hamstring Lengthening

Indications

- Crouch gait, jump gait, knee flexion contractures
- Patient should have popliteal angle greater than 40° and posterior pelvic tilt;
  - Risk of worsening gait if performed in patients with anterior pelvic tilt

Surgical Technique

- Prone position if performed as isolated procedure, with single midline incision
- Supine position when performed with other surgeries via two-incision technique (medial and lateral)
  - ▶ Start incisions slightly anterior to hamstring tendons, 1 to 2 cm proximal to knee joint and extend proximally 5 to 7 cm
- Medial Hamstrings
  - ▶ Dissection taken posterior to sartorius muscle to open fascia overlying gracilis
  - ▶ Section tendon of gracilis over muscle belly with electrocautery or knife
  - ▶ Identify semitendinosus tendon; section through fascia overlying muscle or perform Z-lengthening if more length needed
  - ▶ Semimembranosus muscle is deep, broad; can section its fascia once or twice as needed
  - ▶ Avoid injuring sciatic nerve by excessively stretching knee into extension
- Lateral Hamstrings
  - ▶ Rarely indicated
  - ▶ Approach anterior to biceps to protect peroneal nerve
  - ▶ Transect tendon overlying biceps muscle belly

Complications

- Sciatic nerve stretch or transection
- Sciatic nerve palsy

Postoperative Care and Rehabilitation

- Place in knee immobilizer for 4 weeks, and then begin stretching program
- Carefully monitor sciatic nerve postoperatively

Lengthening of the Gastrocnemius-Soleus

Indications

- Equinus contracture, jump gait, recurvatum gait
- In the vast majority of children with diplegia, only the gastrocnemius is lengthened; in hemiplegia, both muscles are lengthened
- Discourage Z-lengthenings of the Achilles tendon; risk of overlengthening, weakens muscles

Surgical Technique

- Supine position
- Make incision medially in middle third of calf
- Identify sural nerve, lesser saphenous vein; isolate and protect them

- Open fascia and lengthen tendon overlying muscles from medial to lateral under direct visualization, taking care to preserve muscle underneath
- Perform gentle dorsiflexion after completing transection

Complications
- Rupture of Achilles tendon
- Sural nerve injury
- Overlengthening

Postoperative Care and Rehabilitation
- Short-leg walking cast with foot in neutral for 4 to 6 weeks
- Transition to ankle-foot orthosis (AFO)

PEARLS
- Do not overlengthen.
- The incision can be made medially or laterally, depending on the need to lengthen other tendons, such as the tibialis posterior and peroneus brevis, respectively.

Peroneus Brevis Lengthening
- Indicated for pes planovalgus
- Can perform with gastrocnemius-soleus lengthening through single lateral incision
- Obtain weight-bearing foot radiographs as part of larger procedure

Surgical Technique
- Supine position
- Make posterolateral incision over distal third of fibula, approaching posteriorly to protect superficial peroneal nerve
- Open sheath; identify peroneus longus tendon lateral to peroneus brevis tendon, which has muscle belly at this level
- Protect peroneus longus; transect peroneus brevis tendon over belly, with distraction provided by inverting foot

Complications and Postoperative Care and Rehabilitation
- Primary complication is superficial nerve injury
- Rarely performed in isolation; postoperative care depends on larger procedure

Pearl
- Can be performed concomitantly with gastrocnemius-soleus lengthening through lateral incision.

Posterior Tibial Tendon Lengthening

Indication and Surgical Technique

- Indicated for equinovarus
- Supine position with bump under hip
- Make 3-cm incision medially at the junction of the middle and distal thirds of the leg
- Identify posterior border of tibia; enter deep posterior compartment
- Flexor digitorum longus (FDL) is encountered first, medial to the posterior tibialis tendon, when entering the compartment; do not confuse with posterior tibialis tendon; retract the FDL posteriorly
- Section tendon overlying posterior tibialis

Complications and Postoperative Care and Rehabilitation

- Complications include inadvertent lengthening of the FDL, injury to the posterior tibial vessels and tibial nerve
- Rarely performed in isolation; postoperative care depends on larger procedure

Pearl

- Be sure to properly identify FDL and PT tendons as they are in close proximity.
- Can be performed concomitantly with gastrocnemius-soleus lengthening through medial incision.

Psoas Release at the Pelvic Brim

Indications

- Hip flexion contracture
- Spastic hip subluxation/dislocation

Preoperative Imaging

- Not required in isolation
- When part of procedure for spastic hip subluxation/dislocation, obtain AP, frog-leg lateral views of pelvis, bilateral hips, and possibly CT with three-dimensional reconstructions

Surgical Technique

- Supine position
- Palpate and mark femoral artery
- Make oblique incision parallel and inferior to anterior hip flexion crease
- Dissect down to iliac fascia, which is divided lateral to femoral vessels
- Identify femoral nerve and retract medially with Penrose drain
- Identify iliopsoas muscle; roll medial border laterally against pelvis, with hip in flexion and external rotation, to help visualize psoas tendon

- Transect the psoas tendon without transecting any iliacus fibers
- Important to stay inferior to inguinal ligament

Complications and Postoperative Care and Rehabilitation
- Hematoma
- Femoral nerve injury
- Rarely performed in isolation; postoperative care depends on larger procedure

Pearl
- Essential to retract inguinal ligament proximally and palpate rim of pelvis to ensure release at appropriate level.

SOFT-TISSUE TRANSFER PROCEDURES
Rectus Femoris Transfer to the Hamstrings
Indication
- Primary indication is stiff-knee gait in swing phase

Surgical Technique
- Supine position
- Incise from proximal pole of patella 10 cm proximally
- Incise fascia overlying quadriceps; isolate rectus femoris and release distally
  - ▷ Avoid penetration into knee joint
- Make second incision medially down to hamstrings
- Suture semitendinosus to semimembranosus at musculotendinous junction; transect semitendinosus tendon distally
- Create tunnel in adipose tissue from rectus to hamstrings
- Suture free end of semitendinosus to rectus femoris tendon using Pulvertaft technique

Complications
- Primary complication is inadequate excursion of the rectus femoris and continued stiff-knee gait

Postoperative Care and Rehabilitation
- Place in knee immobilizer for 3 weeks; immediate weight bearing and range of motion

Pearl
- Can also use gracilis and fascia lata as anchor points for transfer.

Split Posterior Tibial Tendon Transfer
Indications
- Dynamic equinovarus, particularly hindfoot varus
- Preoperative gait analysis can help exclude tibialis anterior as deforming force

Surgical Technique
- Supine position
- Use four incisions
  - First, approach the tibialis posterior tendon medially from navicular to medial malleolus; free inferior half of tendon
  - Make second, 5-cm incision at junction of distal and middle thirds of tibia medially; open fascia and pass the tibialis posterior tendon proximally, splitting tendon up to musculotendinous junction with either scissors or suture tape
  - Make a third incision behind lateral malleolus extending from tip of malleolus to point 5 to 7 cm proximal and enter lateral compartment; open sheaths of peroneal tendons; tendon passer should pass from medial wound against posterior tibia, then out laterally anterior to peroneal tendons; close medial wounds at this point
  - Make fourth incision overlying peroneus brevis tendon at base of fifth metatarsal; pass posterior tibial tendon into sheath of peroneus brevis tendon and suture into peroneus brevis tendon with foot held in neutral position. Close lateral wounds in standard fashion

Complications
- Complications are neurovascular damage and transection of split tendon

Postoperative Care and Rehabilitation
- Short leg weight-bearing cast for 4 to 6 weeks, followed by AFO

Pearl
- Preoperative gait analysis is helpful to ensure tibialis anterior is not deforming force.

BONE PROCEDURES
Combined Procedure for Spastic Hip Subluxation/Dislocation
Indications
- Indicated for spastic hip subluxation/dislocation
- Includes adductor tenotomy, psoas lengthening, proximal hamstring tenotomy, acetabuloplasty, VDRO of femur, hip open reduction and capsulorrhaphy

Preoperative Imaging
- AP, frog-leg lateral radiographs of pelvis
- Three-dimensional CT optional

Implants
- Pediatric blade plate
- Pediatric proximal femoral locking compression plate

Surgical Technique

- Supine position, bump under ipsilateral thorax
- Make first incision in perineum to lengthen adductors as described previously
- Make second incision 1 cm lateral to iliac crest, extending anterior to anterior superior iliac spine; perform standard Smith Petersen approach
- Split iliac apophysis medially and laterally down to sciatic notch and anterior inferior iliac spine, respectively
- Cut the reflected indirect head and direct heads of rectus femoris distally
- Open capsule in T-shaped manner
- Resect ligamentum teres; remove all blocks to reduction; can lengthen psoas through this approach
- Make third incision for VDRO, using standard lateral approach to femur
- After subperiosteal exposure, introduce Kirschner wire (K-wire) to mark neck anteversion; place second wire to allow selected fixation to create 110° neck-shaft angle
- Advance chisel up to calcar
- Place rotational K-wires to aid in planning for derotation
- Make three cuts in femur
  - One parallel to chisel
  - One perpendicular to shaft
  - One to bevel lateral edge of proximal fragment to seat blade
- Remove chisel; carefully seat blade; hold plate to distal segment with clamp
- Place screws in compression mode; this step can be delayed until the pelvic osteotomy has been performed
- Place at least five nonabsorbable capsulorrhaphy sutures
- Perform acetabuloplasty, starting with straight osteotome, to create opening in outer table in curvilinear fashion from anterior inferior iliac spine to sciatic notch (**Figure 2**)
- Use Kerrison rongeur to complete corner cuts
- Complete osteotomy with curved osteotome that approaches triradiate cartilage
- Hold osteotomy open 1.0 to 1.5 cm with laminar spreader; in pelvis, can use graft from femur or iliac crest (the femoral graft is more robust)
- No fixation is needed to hold wedge in place
- Reduce hip; tie sutures of capsulorrhaphy with hip in internal rotation, abduction
- Repair apophysis with heavy absorbable suture

Complications

- Sciatic nerve injury
- Osteonecrosis

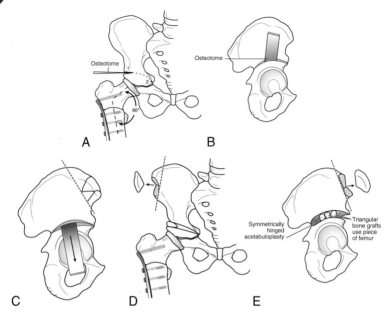

FIGURE 2 Illustrations demonstrate the surgical technique for a bending acetabuloplasty. Anterior (**A**) and lateral (**B**) views show the intended path of the acetabuloplasty. A straight No. 1 and curved No. 2 osteotome are used to perform the acetabuloplasty and correction of the coxa valga with a varus derotational osteotomy. **C**, Lateral view shows a curved osteotome directed toward the triradiate cartilage to perform the bending acetabuloplasty. Anterior (**D**) and lateral (**E**) views show the bicortical graft taken from the iliac crest and used to hold open the acetabuloplasty.

- Iatrogenic fracture
- Loss of hip reduction

Postoperative Care and Rehabilitation
- Some choose not to cast
- Authors place a one and one-half hip spica cast for 2 to 3 weeks, for pain relief

PEARLS

- Visualize the sciatic notch posteriorly for safe osteotomy.
- Keep the reduced hip in abducted, internally rotated position during closure, casting.

Proximal Femoral Rotational Osteotomy

Indications
- Increased femoral anteversion
- Lever-arm syndrome

Preoperative Imaging
- AP, frog-leg lateral radiographs of pelvis, bilateral hips
- CT rotational profile optional

Implants
- Pediatric blade plate
- Pediatric proximal femoral locking compression plate

Surgical Technique
- Prone or supine position
- Make straight lateral incision over lateral aspect of the proximal thigh from just below tip of the greater trochanter and extending distally 6 cm. Full subperiosteal exposure is required; introduce K-wire to mark neck anteversion; place second wire to aid planning for derotation and achieve 10° to 20° anteversion postoperatively
- For blade plate, use procedure described previously
- For locking compression plate, use 6-hole plate
- Drill, measure proximal holes; perform transverse osteotomy; derotate limb
- Apply plate; place screws
- Check rotation
- Perform standard wound closure

Complications
- Malunion/nonunion
- Overcorrection
- Angular deformity

Postoperative Care and Rehabilitation
- Place one and one-half hip spica cast for 4 to 6 weeks
- If bone quality allows, cast not required, per some authors

Pearl
- Expose femur subperiosteally to fully assess rotation

Tibial Derotation Osteotomy

Indications
- Tibial torsion
- Lever-arm syndrome

Preoperative Imaging

- AP and lateral radiographs of the knee, tibia, and ankle
- Three-dimensional CT with rotational profile optional

Implants

- 6-hole 3.5-mm compression plate
- K-wires

Surgical Technique

- Supine position
- If more than 20° to 30° of correction required, consider fibular osteotomy, which is performed 3 to 4 cm proximal to ankle; protect superficial peroneal nerve
- Approach tibia medial to tibialis anterior tendon, which is reflected off tibia
- Expose tibia in subperiosteal fashion
- Place two K-wires, one proximal and one distal to osteotomy; they should diverge by intended degree of derotation (**Figure 3, A**)
- If using a compression plate, drill and measure three proximal holes; perform osteotomy, followed by final placement of the plate and screws
- Can use crossed K-wires in young children with good bone (**Figure 3, B**)
- Monitor closely for compartment syndrome

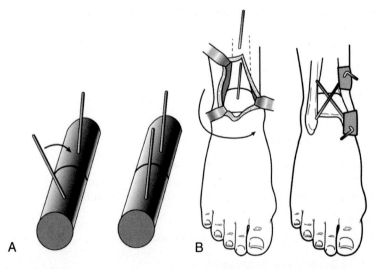

FIGURE 3 Illustrations show the use of Kirschner wires (K-wires) in distal tibial/fibular derotational osteotomy. **A,** Rotational K-wires are placed in the tibial segments. **B,** The crossed K-wires are placed across the osteotomy site for fixation in younger patients.

Complications

- Nonunion/malunion
- Compartment syndrome
- Overcorrection or undercorrection
- Varus or valgus
- Hardware irritation

Postoperative Care and Rehabilitation

- Use short leg, non–weight-bearing cast for 4 weeks; pull pins, if present
- Weight-bearing cast for 4 more weeks

Pearl

- Important to monitor for compartment syndrome postoperatively.

Distal Femoral Extension Osteotomy With Patellar Tendon Advancement

Indications and Preoperative Imaging

- Knee flexion contracture
- Crouch gait
- AP, lateral knee radiographs

Implants

- 90° pediatric blade plate or distal femoral locking plate
- 3.5- or 4.5-mm screws

Surgical Technique

- Supine position, bump under hip
- Incision over lateral aspect of distal femur, posterior to vastus lateralis and proximal to joint and physis (if open)
- Expose femur in subperiosteal fashion
- Place K-wire just proximal to physis; if blade plate used, place chisel proximal to the physis; angle of chisel should be perpendicular to tibia shaft to correct deformity.
- Remove shortening anterior wedge
- Remove chisel; fix blade plate to proximal fragment
- Make second incision over tibial tubercle and patella
- Isolate patellar tendon from retinacula
- Free the tendon from its insertion distally by elevating it off the tubercle
- Incise periosteum distal to tubercle in T-shaped fashion
- Advance patellar tendon and patella until inferior pole of patella is at level ofBlumensaat's line (**Figure 4**) and attach to periosteum
- If patient is skeletally mature, can use bone block instead
- Use tension band to back up fixation

Complications

- Nonunion/malunion
- Anterior knee pain

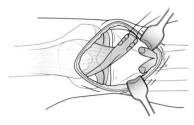

FIGURE 4 Illustration demonstrates placement of medial and lateral Krackow sutures in the patellar tendon for advancement in the technique of distal femoral extension osteotomy.

- Tendon rupture
- Sciatic nerve palsy
- Extensor mechanism disruption
- Compartment syndrome
- Symptomatic hardware

Postoperative Care and Rehabilitation
- Knee range of motion brace in 10° to 20° of flexion for 2 weeks
- Advance motion gradually over 4 to 6 weeks until osteotomy heals

PEARLS
- In skeletally immature patient, can imbricate and suture patellar tendon to itself using nonabsorbable suture.
- Keep knee slightly flexed until swelling has resolved to protect sciatic nerve.

Calcaneal Lengthening Osteotomy
Indication
- Pes planovalgus foot

Preoperative Imaging
- Standing AP, lateral, oblique, Harris radiographs of feet
- Three-dimensional CT optional

Surgical Technique
- Supine position, with bump under hip
- Approach lateral border of calcaneus proximal to level of calcaneocuboid joint
- Protect sural nerve; lengthen peroneus brevis tendon
- Make medial incision to approach talonavicular capsule; remove an ellipse from capsule

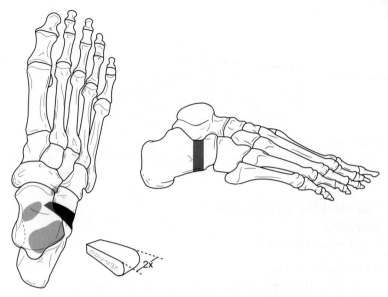

FIGURE 5 Illustration demonstrates the intended path of the osteotomy for calcaneal lengthening, exiting between the anterior and middle facets.

- At lateral incision, subperiosteally expose calcaneus 2 to 2.5 cm proximal to calcaneocuboid joint, which is pinned in reduced position
- Make osteotomy in oblique plane between anterior and middle facets (**Figure 5**)
- Place trapezoid wedge into osteotomy; may fix with K-wire
- At medial incision, imbricate talonavicular capsule with heavy nonabsorbable suture
- Perform plantar closing wedge osteotomy of medial cuneiform to plantarflex medial column

Complications
- Malunion/nonunion
- Iatrogenic lengthening of peroneus longus

Postoperative Care and Rehabilitation
- Short leg non–weight-bearing cast for 4 weeks; pull pins at 4 weeks
- Follow with weight-bearing cast for 4 more weeks; AFO may then be used

PEARLS
- Fixation of calcaneal osteotomy is optional because of inherent stability.
- Protect areas plantar and dorsal to calcaneus during osteotomy.

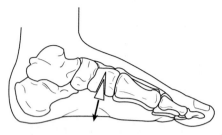

FIGURE 6 Illustration demonstrates correction of residual forefoot supination with a plantar-based closing-wedge osteotomy of the medial cuneiform at the end of the calcaneal sliding osteotomy procedure.

Calcaneal Sliding Osteotomy

Indication
- Pes planovalgus foot

Preoperative Imaging
- Standing AP, lateral, oblique, and Harris radiographs of feet
- Three-dimensional CT optional

Surgical Technique
- Supine position; bump under hip
- Approach lateral border of calcaneus proximal to level of cuboid–fifth metatarsal joint
- Protect sural nerve; lengthen peroneus brevis
- Retract peroneal tendons; expose calcaneus from Achilles insertion to calcaneocuboid joint
- Subperiosteally dissect osteotomy plane, which is parallel to posterior facet and perpendicular to calcaneus in lateral-to-medial direction
- Begin osteotomy with saw; finish with osteotome
- Slide calcaneus 1 cm medially; fix with two K-wires
- Continue incision distally to expose lateral border of cuboid; perform vertical osteotomy centrally
- Make medial incision to identify medial cuneiform
- Perform plantar closing wedge osteotomy (**Figure 6**)
- Place wedge in cuboid as opening-wedge osteotomy
- Place K-wires across the lateral and medial columns

Complications
- Lateral wound necrosis
- Nonunion/malunion

Postoperative Care and Rehabilitation
- Short leg non–weight-bearing cast for 4 weeks; pull pins at 4 weeks
- Follow with weight-bearing cast for 4 more weeks; may then use AFO

PEARLS

- Meticulous lateral wound closure is required to prevent wound complications. Use interrupted horizontal mattress absorbable sutures instead of subcuticular sutures.
- Use an osteotome to complete calcaneus cut to prevent neurovascular damage.
- A gastrocnemius-soleus recession and/or peroneus brevis lengthening may be necessary.

Index

Note: Page numbers followed by "f" indicate figures, "t" indicates tables and "b" indicates boxes.

U

Ulnar collateral ligament (UCL)
    reconstruction
  complications, 68
  contraindications, 64
  indications, 63–64
  patient positioning/special equip-
    ment, 65
  patient selection, 63–64
  pearls, 69b
  postoperative care and rehabilitation,
    68
  preoperative planning, 64
  surgical technique, 65–68, 66f–67f

W

Wide awake hand surgery
  complications, 388
  contraindications, 386
  patient selection and indications,
    386
  pearls, 389b
  postoperative care and rehabilita-
    tion, 388
  room setup/patient positioning,
    386
  special instruments/equipment/
    implants, 387
  surgical technique, 387–388